THE WOMEN'S HEALTH BOOK

A Complete Guide to Health & Wellbeing for Women of All Ages

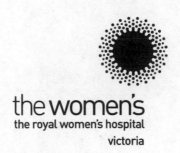

the women's
the royal women's hospital
victoria

WILLIAM HEINEMANN: AUSTRALIA

A William Heinemann book
Published by Random House Australia Pty Ltd
Level 3, 100 Pacific Highway, North Sydney NSW 2060
www.randomhouse.com.au

First published by William Heinemann in 2014

Diagrams and drawings on pp. 75, 87, 105, 106, 110, 132, 143, 218, 233, 247,
263, 400, 415, 630 © Beth Croce; on pp. 293, 296, 303, 305, 306, 601, 606, 607,
609, 610, 641, 642 © Bill Reid; on pp. 7, 227 © Carmel Reilly

Addresses for companies within the Random House Group can be found at
www.randomhouse.com.au/offices.

National Library of Australia
Cataloguing-in-Publication Entry

The women's health book/The Royal Women's Hospital

ISBN 978 1 74275 724 7 (paperback)

Women – Health and hygiene
Women – Psychology
Women – Diseases

Other Authors/Contributors:
Royal Women's Hospital (Melbourne, VIC)

613.04244

Cover illustration by Getty Images
Cover design by Christabella Designs
Internal design by Midland Typesetters, Australia
Typeset in 11/14 pt Minion by Midland Typesetters, Australia
Printed in Australia by Griffin Press, an accredited ISO AS/NZS 14001:2004
Environmental Management System printer

Random House Australia uses papers that are natural, renewable and recyclable
products and made from wood grown in sustainable forests. The logging
and manufacturing processes are expected to conform to the environmental
regulations of the country of origin.

Contents

MIDLIFE

LATER YEARS

Preface

The Women's Health Book has been written to help improve the health and wellbeing of all the women in our lives: us, our partners, our mothers, our daughters, our sisters, our aunties and our friends. Information is power. Good health information can give *you* the personal power to take control of your health and your life.

In the absence of any complete Australian women's health guide, Victoria's Royal Women's Hospital has brought together its experts to craft a comprehensive women's health resource that can be utilised at any stage of a woman's life.

Enjoying your fundamental right to good health and wellbeing is dependent on understanding the factors that impact your health. So throughout the pages of this book you will read about general health and wellbeing; sexual and reproductive health; pregnancy and childbirth; the role of both gender and sex in health; mental health; violence against women, and many other social issues that impact our health.

It has long been recognised that we need health information specifically for women; historically, that information has been anchored in the reproductive phase of a woman's life, as well as cancers peculiar to women. Yet women's health is so much more than this. Over many years, the health system has been designed and developed around general health issues, and thus there has been an unconscious bias against women and how general disease manifests differently in women. This has left us with a healthcare system researched and designed for men and then applied to women.

The good news is there is now greater understanding of this structural inequity as well as international evidence that applying a gender lens to health care improves healthcare programs for women *and* men. Sex and gender do matter. In a civilised society, equity is not a vision, it is a responsibility.

I hope that the knowledge and insight you gain from this book will encourage you to advocate for the health and wellbeing of *all* women, and to understand the need for a health system developed for both women and men, which focuses not only on the biological issues but also the social issues that impact on health. This will drive the changes necessary to ensure the health and wellbeing for future generations of women.

Dale Fisher
Chief Executive, Royal Women's Hospital,
Melbourne, 2004–2013

Introduction

Leslie Reti

In a digital, socially connected world flooded with information, why another resource on women's health? Well, we at the Royal Women's Hospital believe there is a need to distil some crystal-clear drops from that flood. We understand from our daily clinical experience that women want authoritative, plain-language information on their health issues in an easily accessible form. This book is written to provide a comprehensive single source of reference.

We see hundreds of women every year, many of whom are overwhelmed by the health system; their health issue; pregnancy and impending parenthood; having to negotiate their own health needs and those of their family; and by the enormous amount of information (and misinformation) they have to trawl through to make well-informed decisions. The Royal Women's Hospital in Melbourne, fondly and generally known as the Women's, is well placed to provide that information.

The Women's, the largest health facility in Australia specialising in women's health, provides approximately 220,000 occasions of care to women each year. On these occasions we offer health advice, sometimes in small packets and at other times in larger amounts during complex consultations. This body of experience is broad and we hope to share much of it with you in the following pages.

We agree with the World Health Organization's concept of health as a state of complete physical, mental and social wellbeing – not merely the absence of disease. In this book we start with the social determinants of health, and discuss many different manifestations of physical and mental health in the subsequent chapters. These are well-women-centred and evidence-based and they draw on the depth of experience at the Women's.

The book is divided into life stages. (Some matters, such as sexuality, depression and nutrition, are covered at each of these stages, because the specific issues vary throughout life.) It is not intended as a reference for in-depth discussion of any particular aspect of a woman's health, so resources are provided at the end of the book for readers who want further information. Rather, it is a guide to women's health that informs readers when health events or concerns arise in their life. We expect women will use this book to dip into periodically, as they need to find out about an issue or a concern, although many will read it from cover to cover.

We hope you find it helpful, accessible and informative, and that it provides a lifelong guide to maintaining your health and wellbeing, and the wellbeing of those in your care.

The Editorial Group who guided the production of the book so expertly comprised:

Associate Professor Leslie Reti (Chair)
Dr Jan Davies
Ms Dale Fisher
Professor Suzanne Garland
Professor Martha Hickey
Ms Maureen Johnson
Professor Fiona Judd
Ms Tanya Maloney
Dr Jennifer Marino
Associate Professor John McBain
Miss Orla McNally
Dr Ines Rio
Dr Sarah White

1

Why women's health matters

Dale Fisher

It sounds obvious, but women are different from men. Women and men experience life differently, both when they are healthy and when they are unwell. What might come as a surprise to you, though, is to learn that nearly all health research, health information and healthcare treatments approach women and men as if they were exactly the same.

Think about this for a moment. Health care doesn't take into account that women have menstrual periods and a uterus while men do not; that women have dominantly oestrogen but men have dominantly testosterone; or even that men have a prostate and women do not. It is blindingly obvious that different anatomies, different hormones and different genetics must impact health differently … and yet health care treats women and men as if they were exactly the same.

As you'll read in this chapter, the health differences between women and men – and among different groups of women – are caused by both biological and social factors. If we don't have health care that takes into account these factors, we won't achieve the best health and wellbeing for women (or men).

Medical research provides us with the information we need to prevent, diagnose and treat health problems, but less than one-third of participants in medical research and drug trials are women. This means that most medical research has been done on men and then *applied* to women.

This continues to happen even though we know that women often have different symptoms and experience different outcomes of health problems from men, and that women respond differently to many medicines. As a result, many diagnoses, treatments and even prevention strategies aren't as appropriate for women as for men. Women are often treated when there is little evidence supporting that treatment in women. In fact, some medicines that have been shown to be safe for men may be potentially dangerous for women.

Research needs to include both women and men, and the results for women and men need to be analysed separately. This is the only way we will begin to answer questions such as why the rate of lung cancer in women is rising while the rate in men is falling, and why women who have heart attacks are more likely than men to die from them.

So let's start by outlining the differences between women and men:

- **Women are biologically different from men – *this is the sex difference.*** This means that women's anatomy, physiology, hormones and genetics are different. Because of these differences, some health conditions are more likely to affect women (such as osteoporosis, arthritis, migraines and depression), some health conditions affect women differently from men (such as schizophrenia and lung cancer), and women respond differently from men to some medicines (such as those used for anaesthesia, epilepsy and depression). Women's biology also means that some health issues, such as endometriosis, pregnancy, menopause and gynaecological cancers, only affect them.

- **Women are positioned differently in society from men – *this is the gender difference.*** This means women are more likely than men to have a lower income, less secure employment, to be carers, and to be exposed to domestic violence. These differences have a profound impact on women's health. For example, women are more likely than men to experience depression and anxiety, and this affects their relationships and ability to function at work and in the community.

- **There are *demographic differences* between women that affect health.** Some women, such as those living in rural areas, Aboriginal and Torres Strait Islander women, and women with disabilities, are at much higher risk of poor health.

- **A woman's *life stage* also has a direct impact on her health.** Women's health changes at each life stage, and having access to the right information and services at the right time helps them to make the best choices for their health.

All these factors need to be considered together to help women access better health care and experience better health.

Reading health information (such as this book) written specifically for women by health professionals who *specialise* in women's health is a good place to start. This book will also point you in the direction of health services that take into account the wide range of factors that affect women's health. This is called taking a gendered approach to health, an approach that results in better health for you as an individual, and that flows on to your family and the wider community. A gendered approach to health is a win-win-win.

The rest of this chapter will take a closer look at the ways sex, gender, demographics and life stage affect women's health. And, most importantly, it will help you ask questions, start a conversation and find more information and services that can lead to better health at any stage of your life.

Sex versus gender

Many people use the terms 'sex' and 'gender' interchangeably, but the terms mean quite different things, as we have described here. 'Sex' refers to the biological differences between women and men, whereas 'gender' refers to the social differences between women and men. Both sex and gender influence women's health.

The sex difference

Biology, anatomy and genetics at every level influence nearly everything about the way women's and men's bodies work. This influences the health problems women are more likely to experience, how women experience them, and how women respond to treatment.

For example, we know that women tend to develop schizophrenia at a later age, have different symptoms from men, and tend to have a less severe version of the illness. These differences may be due, at least in part, to a protective effect the hormone oestrogen has against schizophrenia.

Another example of sex affecting a health problem is the incidence of migraine, which is three times more common in women than in men. Hormones are also one of the main influences here. When preventing and treating migraine in women, taking each woman's life stage – for example, adolescence, pregnancy or menopause – and hormonal state into account will give the best chance of treatment success.

These are just two examples of how sex affects health. For a long time, the basic differences between women and men have been ignored in medical research, but this is slowly beginning to change. More research is starting to focus on women's experiences of health, resulting in better treatments for such conditions as schizophrenia. But we still have a very long way to go. This is partly because the differences between women and men are complex: they involve much more than biological difference. Social or gender differences between women and men have a huge impact on women's health and these also need to be taken into account when research studies are designed and analysed and when new treatments are developed.

The gender difference

Women have different economic, social, political and cultural positions and opportunities than men. This is called the gender difference. These gender differences interact with sex differences to impact women's health and wellbeing, often by affecting the health services women are able to access and the outcomes of treatment.

One of the key differences is that women are more likely than men to be financially disadvantaged. This is because women generally have less access to education than men, have lower incomes than men, live in poorer housing, and have less secure employment and less super-annuation. Women are also more likely than men to spend time out of the paid workforce while caring for children and/or elderly parents. These factors can also lead to social isolation.

According to the 2010 Australian National Women's Health Policy, women who are socially or financially disadvantaged are more likely to have poor health, and have a high chance of having children with poor health. The reasons for this are many and complex. We know that the most disadvantaged women have the highest exposure to risk factors that can damage their health. They also have more barriers that prevent them from taking up healthy behaviours. A 2008 report from the Australian Institute of Health and Welfare found that these women are more likely to be overweight, to smoke, to experience family violence, to have fewer social networks, to be less physically active and to eat less fruit and vege-tables. All these factors increase a woman's chance of developing many health problems, including type 2 diabetes, heart disease, certain cancers, respiratory diseases and mental health problems.

The Australian Bureau of Statistics reported in 2007 that anxiety and depression are almost twice as common in women than in men, and for women the Institute of Health and Welfare lists these as the leading causes of healthy years of life lost due to disability. Anxiety and depression affect women at all stages of life and affect their ability to function in jobs and in the wider community. These illnesses also have a significant impact on women's relationships.

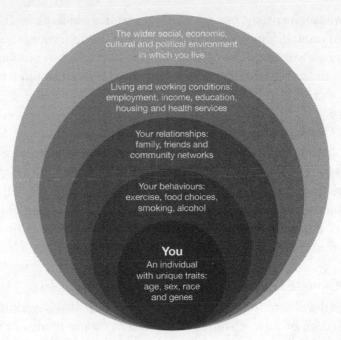

The wider social, economic, cultural and political environment in which you live

Living and working conditions: employment, income, education, housing and health services

Your relationships: family, friends and community networks

Your behaviours: exercise, food choices, smoking, alcohol

You
An individual with unique traits: age, sex, race and genes

Influences on health

A range of gender factors contributes to higher rates of anxiety and depression in women. These include higher levels of financial disadvantage, lower levels of education, lower rates of working outside the home, the higher burden of being a carer, and higher exposure to discrimination, harassment, and family or intimate partner violence (which used to be called domestic violence).

More research is being undertaken to better understand the sex and gender effects on women's mental health. Prevention and treatment programs that take a woman-centred approach and take into account her social, cultural and economic situation will help to ensure the best outcomes for women's mental health.

Many people are shocked to learn how common violence against women is in Australia: nearly one in five adult women is subject to intimate partner violence. A 2004 Australian study found that intimate partner violence is responsible for more ill health, disability and premature death in women under the age of 45 than any of the other well-known risk factors, including high blood pressure, obesity and smoking. Women who have been exposed to violence have a greater risk of developing many health problems, including depression, anxiety, eating disorders and substance abuse. Intimate partner violence also impacts on women's reproductive health, with an increased risk of sexually transmitted infections, abnormal Pap tests, unplanned pregnancies, pregnancy complications, abortions and miscarriage.

Violence against women is a complex problem, but we do know that cultural, social and economic factors all play a part. One main underlying factor is the unequal access to power and money between women and men, which has been noted by the World Health Organization. Intimate partner violence is so common and has such an overwhelming effect on women's health, but it's rarely discussed or given much publicity. There is emerging recognition that violence against women is more than just a law enforcement issue: just like high blood pressure, smoking and obesity, violence is a major women's health issue. You can read more about family violence and where to get help in chapter 30.

Demographic differences between women

As well as the differences between women and men, demographic differences between groups of women affect health. Some groups of women experience greater inequalities that increase their exposure to health risks, affect their attitudes to health and reduce their ability to access health information and services. These groups include women living in rural and remote areas, Aboriginal and Torres Strait Islander women, women with disabilities, women from non-English-speaking backgrounds, and lesbian, bisexual and transgender women. Understanding the needs of these women using a social model of health, which takes into account social and environmental factors that affect health as well as sex and gender factors, allows us to continually improve the health information and services we develop.

Let's look at some key examples of how demographic differences affect particular groups of women.

- **Women living in rural and remote areas** are more likely to be socially and financially disadvantaged and have less access to general practitioners (GPs), specialist health care, family planning services and counselling services. Where healthcare services are available, many women worry about accessing them confidentially because 'everyone knows everyone' in a country town.

- **Aboriginal and Torres Strait Islander women** have lower levels of education, lower incomes, higher rates of unemployment and a higher risk of exposure to violence than other Australian women. As a result of these and other factors, Aboriginal and Torres Strait Islander women have poorer physical and mental health than other Australian women.

- **Women from non-English-speaking backgrounds** often have difficulty accessing health information in their own language or in accessing information or services that take their cultural needs into account.

- **Women with a disability** are more likely to have lower incomes and have more difficulties with transport and accessing services. They also have less daily contact with friends and family and are more likely to experience intimate partner violence. According to 2003 figures from the Australian Bureau of Statistics, one in five Australian women is living with a disability that causes many challenges in her everyday life.

- **Lesbian, bisexual and transgender women** experience greater levels of discrimination and violence, which impact on their health and result in higher rates of depression and isolation. The fear of insensitive treatment or discrimination can be a major barrier for these women in accessing health care.

A social model of health

A social model of health provides a framework or a big picture way of thinking about health. When we think about health in this way, it becomes clear that better health results from considering the social and environmental factors that affect health *as well as* the biological and medical factors. This means that you have the best opportunity for good health when you are treated as an individual who is a member of a family and a member of a wider community, which in turn dictates the political, social and economic environment you live in.

To do this, we need continued investment in women's health. We need to focus on the social and economic factors that influence women's health and start making positive changes to the environments in which women live, work and socialise, so that women from all backgrounds have access to tools that can improve their health. Women are the centre of families and communities, and research shows that looking after women's health results in healthier families and a healthier community.

An important first step in addressing the health needs of women in these different groups is developing health information and services that are sensitive to their needs and are easier for them to access. See the Resources section at the end of this book for information and services that focus on the needs of all women as well as different groups of women.

Different needs at different life stages

Women's health needs change throughout their lives and it is very important for them to have access to the right information and services at the right time to achieve the best health. Women have many important transition points in their lives. The social, emotional, economic and hormonal changes women experience at these transition points can make them especially vulnerable to health problems. Having access to the information and services you need at each of these stages can give you better control of your preventative health care and health-management decisions and can help prevent health risk factors from 'adding up' throughout your life.

Young women can be under pressure to be successful at school and university, to be popular, to conform to stereotypes and to look attractive. All of this can increase the chance of risky behaviours such as drinking too much alcohol and having unprotected sex, and can lead to an unhealthy body image and eating disorders. The Australian Bureau of Statistics reported in 2007 that nearly one in three young women has a mental health disorder.

When women begin to think about having a family, they face a whole new set of health issues. Because these days women are older when they have children, they may not find it as easy to get pregnant as they hoped. Women who are pregnant or who have recently become mothers have a high risk of depression, and balancing parenting and work responsibilities can affect women's health in many ways.

In midlife women often experience more life events and changes than at any other time. This is a time of physical transition, when menopause may cause a range of physical symptoms, depression and anxiety, as well as an increased risk of other health problems such as osteoporosis and heart disease. At the same time, adult children may be leaving home and new opportunities for work and leisure may open up. Many women in this life stage, however, take on the role of caring for an elderly parent, which creates another range of emotional and physical challenges.

Women are making up a larger proportion of the old and very old population groups in Australia. Older women have specific health needs that are often influenced by outliving their partners, being less economically secure than men, and having much higher rates of age-related health problems such as dementia, arthritis and osteoporosis than men of the same age. Older women are often invisible in Australian society, and yet this is a time when, with the right support and a positive outlook, they may have many opportunities to enjoy life in ways there wasn't time for when they were younger. This is also the time to enjoy the wisdom that only comes with many years of life experience!

Because your experience of life and health is influenced so heavily by different life stages, we have divided this book into sections that relate to women's four major life stages. The information in each section will help you navigate each life stage, making the most of the opportunities and reducing any health risks you face.

Transition points in women's lives

Have a look at this list and think about how many of these transition points you have already experienced:

- starting school
- adolescence
- entering the workforce
- living with a partner
- pregnancy and childbirth
- being a new mum
- returning to the workforce

- menopause
- children leaving home
- leaving the paid workforce
- caring for ageing parents or a partner
- death of a partner
- older age

Did you experience new health challenges and stresses at these times? What advice would you give a younger woman about finding health information and services and looking after herself well at these stages? How do you think you can prepare for the transition points you will experience in the future?

What does all this mean for you?

Just by reading this book, you are on the right path to enjoying better health. *The Women's Health Book* has been developed in *partnership* with women and health professionals.

The first thing we did when we were developing this book was talk to women about what they wanted to see in a women's health book. Women told us that it was important for this book to help them understand more about their bodies and what it means to be healthy. They told us they wanted a book that acknowledges that while we are all women, we are also different groups of women.

We are younger women, midlife women, older women, mothers, carers, independent women and women with disabilities. We are single, married, lesbian, divorced and widowed women. We are Aboriginal and Torres Strait Islander women, we are Australians descended from migrants and refugees, from Africa, Asia and Europe. We are professional women and women on low incomes. We are women living with cancer, women managing menopause symptoms and women with mental health problems. Often, we are women dealing with any number of life and health issues at the one time.

What unites all women is their need to be respected, to be treated with dignity, and to have access to health information and services that make a clear connection between their health and the lives they lead every day.

When we were writing this book, we considered the needs of women from different backgrounds to ensure that all women will find information and stories in it to which they can relate personally.

You will also find that this book covers many topics you may not find in other health books but that many women told us are important, such as unplanned pregnancy, drugs and alcohol, violence at home, being a carer and the positive side of getting older.

All the information in this book is written by health professionals who specialise in women's health. Working with women every day, they understand the issues that affect women, how health problems affect women differently from men, and how social factors – such as employment, income and relationships – affect women's health. They also understand the difficulties many women face in finding the information and care they need. *The Women's Health Book* is designed to give you the information you need to participate as an equal partner in your health care. Armed with the real facts, you will be able to ask more questions and make better choices to help improve your health and even prevent future problems.

Here are some more practical ideas to head you in the right direction towards better health:

- **Look for women-centred health services and support groups in the community.** There are many services and groups for women with specific health needs, and these can help you to feel connected, to make new friends and learn ways to live well.

- **Start a conversation with your mum, daughter, sister or girlfriend.** Did they know that women experience many health conditions differently from men? What have their experiences been in dealing with the health system?

- **Talk about your own health and life experiences (good and bad) as openly as you can.** When you start talking to a trusted friend or healthcare professional about difficult subjects – such as having an abusive partner, or starting to rely on tranquillisers too much, or the tough conditions at work – you help other women open up and start talking too. Talking to someone is often the point when we realise things really aren't right and we need some extra help to get things back on track.

- **Ask your healthcare professionals more questions.** Ask if there is a clinic with a woman-centred approach to your health problem. Ask if the symptoms or treatment of your health problem might be different in women from men. You might not always get a clear answer, but asking questions is a good way to get everyone thinking about these issues.

- **Look at the 'big picture' of your health.** As well as seeing a health professional and taking your medicine, think about your lifestyle choices and how your work and family situation influence your health. How can you start changing some of these factors so you can feel healthier? Perhaps you can ask some friends to start walking with you a couple of times a week. If the changes are more difficult ones, like finding a job with better conditions and less stress, ask for the support you need to make these changes.

- **Celebrate being a woman.** Although women have higher rates of certain health problems, women are also better than men at surrounding themselves with good friends and using social networks to stay connected. Make an effort to see friends, talk about important issues and have fun together. It's all good for your health.

- **Remember that taking care of your health** is the most important step in creating a healthy, happy family and a thriving community. The best opportunities for good health come from a *combination* of individual choices – such as being more active, eating more fresh vegies and going easy on alcohol – and through improving the wider social and economic factors that affect your health. Most importantly, it means putting your own health first.

2
Staying healthy

Alison Bean-Hodges, Christina Bryant, Orla McNally, Ines Rio

Most of what we do to stay well and healthy has little to do with seeing doctors or interacting with the healthcare system.

Most of it is about keeping our bodies in the best shape we can by staying within a normal weight range; staying active; eating well; sleeping well; preventing injury, sexually transmitted infections and unplanned pregnancy; ensuring adequate sun protection; undertaking dental hygiene; and not using substances that are detrimental for us. It's also about keeping our minds healthy by having good relationships, keeping our brains active, contributing to society and feeling valued.

In this chapter we outline some of the things you can do to make and keep yourself healthy, and how you can interact with your GP and the healthcare system to best achieve this.

Physical wellbeing

Smoking

We all know that smoking has many harmful effects on many parts of the body. Some of these harmful effects include many types of cancers, lung disease (such as chronic obstructive airway disease and asthma), cardio-vascular disease (such as heart attack and stroke), osteoporosis, decreased fertility and poorer pregnancy outcomes, tooth loss and premature ageing of skin. Tobacco use is the leading cause of preventable death in Australia and was responsible for the deaths of more than 14,000 Australians in the 2004–05 financial year. One in two lifetime smokers is predicted to die from a disease caused by their smoking. Smoking is also increasingly known to have harmful effects on those exposed to smoke (secondary or passive smoking), including a developing baby, infants and children.

Australia has made great gains in decreasing its smoking rates. In 1945, 72 per cent of men and 26 per cent of women smoked; in 1976, it was

43 per cent of men and 33 per cent of women; in 1995, 29 per cent of men and 23 per cent of women; and in 2011, 18 per cent of men and 15 per cent of women. This change has seen a marked reduction in the community of health problems such as lung cancer.

The good news is that if you do smoke, quitting smoking is doable and it's never too late to achieve health benefits. Many harmful effects of smoking begin to decline as soon as a person stops smoking. Some aspects of health return rapidly, and after a long period of cessation some disease risks return to the same level as in people who have never smoked (while others do not).

Although most people find quitting difficult, and it often takes a number of tries, there are more ex-smokers in Australia than there are smokers. So if you smoke, phone a helpline to have a chat and see your doctor.

See chapter 11 for more on smoking.

Alcohol and drugs

Alcohol is the most widely used drug in Australia and it affects people in different ways depending on their gender, age, body weight, other medicine and drugs they may use, their health and the way their body metabolises alcohol. Therefore, *there is no amount of alcohol that can be said to be safe for everyone.*

Drinking alcohol to excess can cause heart, liver and brain damage and high blood pressure, and increases the risk of obesity, diabetes and many cancers. Women who drink alcohol to excess are generally at a greater risk of developing many of these alcohol-related diseases, including some cancers, than men who drink alcohol.

It is estimated that between 1996 and 2005, more than 32,000 Australians aged over 15 died from alcohol-related injury and disease. These health risks from alcohol accumulate over a lifetime – this means that the more you drink over a longer time period, the greater the risk.

The more immediate (acute) effects of alcohol on brain function, reasoning and the body also increase the risk of injury and violence through sexual assault, rape, unplanned pregnancy, sexually transmitted infections, road trauma, violence, falls and accidental death.

Responsible drinking is about balancing your enjoyment of alcohol with the potential risks and harm that may arise from drinking. Australian guidelines recommend that:

- for healthy women and men, drinking no more than two standard drinks on any day reduces the risk of harm from alcohol-related disease or injury over a lifetime, and drinking no more than four standard drinks on a single occasion reduces the risk of alcohol-related injury on that occasion
- for children and young people under the age of 18, *not* drinking alcohol is the safest option; children under the age of 15 are at the greatest risk of harm from drinking and for this age group, not drinking alcohol is especially important
- for young people aged 15–17, the safest option is to delay the initiation of drinking alcohol for as long as possible
- for women who are pregnant, planning a pregnancy or breastfeeding, *not* drinking alcohol is the safest option

It is important to note that a standard drink contains 10 grams of pure alcohol, but that drink serving sizes in Australia are not standard and there is often more than one standard drink in a glass. The label on an alcoholic drink container tells you the number of standard drinks in that container.

There are also myriad illicit drugs, some of which have been used for many centuries, while others are more recent and evolving 'designer drugs'. All can cause harmful effects. Although largely unstudied and unknown, they are likely to cause both long-term and short-term harm. So don't make the mistake of thinking that because the harms may not be widely known for the drug you choose to use or are considering using, there is little or no harm – many people made that mistake in the 1950s about tobacco use. These drugs may also be associated with harm in other ways, such as what they are mixed with, how they are administered (e.g. via injection), the activities and groups associated with their obtainment or use, and the effects on communities and people involved in the growing, manufacturing, transport and distribution of these drugs.

See chapter 11 for more on alcohol and drugs.

Your teeth and mouth

There is a lot you can do to keep your teeth and mouth healthy – and a healthy mouth means less tooth loss and pain, better smelling breath and a better looking and feeling mouth.

To keep your mouth healthy you should:

- use fluorides (see below)

- have a healthy diet
- maintain good oral hygiene
- not smoke
- protect your mouth against trauma

Use fluorides
Fluoride is a normal part of the human body and is involved in the mineralisation (hardening) of both teeth and bones.

Fluoride intake from most foods is low, but about two-thirds of Australians drink fluoridated water, which is well recognised by public health groups and scientific bodies around the world as an important, safe and effective way of decreasing tooth disease.

If you live in an area where the water is not fluoridated and there is insufficient natural fluoride (less than 0.3 milligrams per litre), talk to your dentist about taking fluoride supplements.

Have a healthy diet
Diet is linked to tooth problems in three different ways:

- Diets high in sugar increase the risk of tooth decay, as bacteria in plaques on the teeth take up the sugar in the food we eat to produce acids. These acids lead to the loss of tooth enamel and subsequently to holes in the teeth (dental cavities). Sugars that are refined, taken frequently or combined with food acids are particularly bad. A person's individual susceptibility is also important.

- Acidic substances in food and drink can directly cause the loss of tooth enamel. Foods and drinks that cause this include soft drinks, sports drinks, fruit and fruit juices, wine, pickles and chewable vitamin tablets.

- While severe malnutrition is extremely rare in Australia, it can be associated with damage to the structure of teeth and their supporting tissues.

Maintain good oral hygiene
A regular daily oral hygiene routine, preferably from the time you get your first teeth, is very important in keeping your mouth healthy. It reduces not only the plaques on teeth and the bacteria in them that cause acid build-up and the resulting loss of tooth enamel, but also the overall numbers of harmful bacteria and other substances that can cause problems for the

gums and teeth. It also increases tooth-surface resistance and the ability of the mouth to repair itself.

As an adult, it is recommended that you:

- brush your teeth at least twice daily with fluoride toothpaste
- floss your teeth daily
- have regular check-ups with a dentist or dental hygienist

Don't smoke

As we saw above, smoking is bad for many parts of the body. It also is bad for the mouth, as it increases the risk of cancers of the mouth, tooth loss, gum problems and staining of teeth. We know, however, that stopping smoking usually allows the mouth to return to a relatively healthy state over a fairly short time period. So if you do smoke, please see your GP to discuss how they can help you quit.

Protect your mouth against trauma

Damage to teeth is often complex, expensive and difficult to repair. While oral injuries can occur at any time, certain sports, leisure activities and workplaces can pose particular risks. So think about what you do and how you can decrease the risk of mouth injuries, such as using a mouthguard when playing a contact sport.

Your skin

Good skin care and healthy lifestyle choices can help prevent various skin problems and delay the natural ageing process.

Protect yourself from the sun

One of the most important ways to take care of your skin is to protect it from the sun. A lifetime of sun exposure can cause wrinkles, age spots and other skin problems – as well as increase the risk of skin cancer.

For sun protection, remember the Cancer Council's slogan 'Slip, slop, slap, seek and slide':

- *Slip* on some sun-protective clothing that covers as much skin as possible.
- *Slop* on broad-spectrum, water-resistant sunscreen of at least SPF30+. Put it on 20 minutes before you go outdoors and every two hours afterwards. Never use sunscreen to extend the time you spend in the sun.

- *Slap* on a hat – broadbrim or legionnaire-style – to protect your face, head, neck and ears.
- *Seek* shade. Avoid the sun when the sun's rays are strongest.
- *Slide* on some sunglasses – make sure they meet Australian standards.

Don't smoke

Smoking makes your skin look older and contributes to wrinkles. It narrows the tiny blood vessels in the outermost layers of skin, which decreases blood flow and thus the amount of oxygen and nutrients reaching the skin. Smoking also damages the collagen and elastin fibres that give your skin its strength and elasticity. In addition, the repetitive facial expressions you make when smoking – such as pursing your lips and squinting your eyes to keep out smoke – can contribute to wrinkles.

If you smoke, ask your GP for tips or treatments to help you.

Treat your skin gently

Daily cleansing can take a toll on your skin. Be gentle to your skin by doing the following:

- Limit bath time. Hot water and long showers or baths remove oils from your skin. Keep your bath or shower time to a minimum, and use warm rather than hot water.
- Avoid strong soaps. Use a mild, non-drying soap and avoid scrubbing or repeated skin washing.
- Moisturise dry skin. If your skin is dry, use a moisturiser that fits your skin type. It doesn't need to be expensive. On sun-exposed areas, consider a moisturiser that contains a sunscreen of at least SPF30+.
- Eat a healthy diet. Because your skin is a reflection of what is going on inside your body, you should eat a healthy, balanced diet and keep well hydrated. Eat plenty of fruits, vegetables, whole grains and lean proteins. The association between diet, acne and healthy skin isn't clear, but some research suggests that diets high in sugar, refined carbohydrates, other foods with a high glycaemic index (GI; i.e. that raise your blood sugar level quickly after eating) and milk may be related to worsening acne, and a diet rich in vitamin C and low in refined sugars, carbohydrates, other high-GI foods and unhealthy fats might promote younger-looking skin. There is no evidence from research that chocolate, nuts, salt or greasy foods cause acne. Foods that contain chocolate and salt do, however, often have other high-GI ingredients.

- Maintain a healthy body weight. Constantly gaining and losing weight is bad for your skin. When the skin frequently expands and contracts it eventually loses its elasticity, which causes lines and wrinkles.

Manage stress
It is possible that stress may make your skin more sensitive and trigger acne breakouts and other skin problems. To encourage healthy skin, and a healthy mind, take steps to manage your stress in a positive way.

Get enough sleep
During sleep, the time when most cellular repair and turnover occurs, collagen production in the skin seems to be accelerated. Collagen firms the skin and increases skin hydration. Conversely, lack of restful sleep suppresses the immune system, which can lead to skin-related problems such as rashes.

The ideal amount of uninterrupted sleep ranges from seven to nine hours.

Exercise regularly
Increasing blood circulation through exercise increases the amounts of oxygen and vital nutrients reaching your skin.

Drink alcohol only in moderation
Alcohol causes blood vessels to dilate, especially the small ones near the skin's surface, causing flushing and redness. After some time this can result in permanent facial redness. It also dehydrates the skin.

Don't pick or squeeze your pimples
Picking pimples can force bacteria deeper into the skin, causing greater inflammation, and can lead to scars and pigmentation.

Well women's check

To maximise your health, it is crucial to have a GP you can talk to and you feel listens to you. Your GP gets to know you and your circumstances over time, and you get to know that they are providing good care and advice, working in your best interests and advocating for you in our complex healthcare system.

If you don't have a GP, try asking your friends, family, colleagues or a health professional for recommendations. It's important to find a GP you can relate to and who relates to you, so keep trying until you do.

It's also important to have your own Medicare card so you can access health care without others knowing if you choose to. Make sure you have one, and if you have a teenage daughter, help arrange one for her.

All women, even healthy women, need to have regular check-ups, which can detect problems early and enable early interventions to decrease the likelihood of ill health. Most of these will be done by your GP, but they may send you to a nurse or another health professional for others. Sometimes, as is the case with BreastScreen Australia, you can also access these checks directly and ask for the results to be sent to you as well as to your GP.

What you need to do in consultation with your GP to keep well depends on your circumstances, including your age, weight, personal and family history, genetic predispositions, hobbies, occupation, medicine use, smoking, and alcohol and drug intake, as well as your own preferences. For example:

- If you smoke, your GP can provide very effective counselling and medicine to help you quit.
- If you developed diabetes when you were pregnant or are at high risk of developing diabetes, your GP will order regular blood glucose tests.
- If you have had heart disease such as angina or a heart attack, your GP will prescribe medicine to decrease the likelihood of it recurring, will regularly test your blood pressure, lipids and glucose, and will give you advice about physical activity and your weight.
- If you have broken a bone easily or have other risk factors for osteoporosis, your doctor will organise a test for your bone density.
- If you have a family history of haemochromatosis (where your body accumulates too much iron), your GP will suggest blood tests to see if you inherited the gene.
- If you are planning a pregnancy, your GP will give you special dietary and supplementation advice (e.g. take folate and iodine), organise tests and arrange vaccination as required – such as for chickenpox, rubella (German measles), influenza (flu) and pertussis (whooping cough).
- If you are at increased risk of glaucoma, your GP may refer you for an eye check, including an eye pressure test.
- If you are a childcare or healthcare professional, your GP may recommend additional immunisation.
- If you are at higher risk of depression or other psychosocial problems, your GP may ask you some questions about these things to ensure your mental health is the best it can be.

So tell your GP about your own history, your family history, and your health and life circumstances so that they can advise you on the best preventative measures to keep you as healthy and well as you can be.

The rest of this chapter outlines the *general* recommendations for vaccinations, checks and tests for all Australian women (but not children). Remember, depending on your individual circumstances, you may require more frequent tests, different starting times for tests or different vaccinations, checks and tests.

Vaccination

Vaccination is the administration of a vaccine to stimulate your immune system so you develop protection against a bacterium or virus that causes an infectious disease. A vaccine contains an inactivated (non-infective), attenuated (with reduced infectivity) or parts of the bacteria or virus that causes the infectious disease. In this way, your body's immune system develops fighters (antibodies) that are used if you then come into contact with the real infectious disease, thus helping you fight or prevent the bacteria or virus from taking hold, to help you avoid getting the disease.

Vaccination is one of the most effective ways of preventing infectious diseases, and widespread immunity due to vaccination is largely responsible for the worldwide eradication of smallpox, the eradication of polio from much of the world, and the fact that measles and tetanus are now rare in Australia.

The following vaccinations are recommended in adolescents or adults. Recommended schedules alter in different states and change with time, so ask your GP what you should have.

Human papillomavirus (HPV) vaccination

Human papillomavirus (HPV) is a highly contagious virus. There are more than 100 types of the virus, including those responsible for common warts, plantar (foot) warts and genital warts.

More than 40 HPV types are sexually transmitted and affect the genital areas. Most people become infected soon after becoming sexually active, with around 80 per cent of people infected with at least one genital type of HPV at some stage in their life. Because it is so common, doctors often call it the 'common cold of sexually transmitted infections'.

These infections generally have no symptoms; you don't usually get warts, and as a rule your body just gets rid of the infection with time.

However, infection can cause genital warts, cervical cancer (and its precursors) and some other cancers of the genital tract.

As there are often no symptoms and the time taken for any symptoms to declare themselves if you do get them varies, it is unlikely you would know when you were infected or by whom. Also, just because an infected partner has no symptoms doesn't guarantee you will show no symptoms if you are infected. There is no screening test to check for overall 'HPV status'.

There are currently 15 types of HPV designated as 'high risk' for the development of cervical cancer; those called types 16 and 18 cause around 70 per cent of all cervical cancers.

The progression from HPV infection to cervical cancer is well understood and takes a number of years. While a HPV infection may result in low-grade (minor) changes to the cervix (the opening of the uterus) and may resolve itself, some high-risk HPV infections go on to cause high-grade (serious) changes that over many years can develop into cervical cancer. A Pap test is a smear of cells from the cervix taken by a doctor or nurse using a speculum that is inserted into the vagina. A speculum is a metal or plastic device the doctor or nurse inserts gently into the vagina and opens up so they can get a better look at the cervix and the vagina. The cervix is gently scraped with a disposable implement so that some cells can be collected. These cells are then smeared on a microscope slide so they can be viewed in a laboratory. The test aims to identify the precursors to cervical cancer so they can be removed before a cancer has time to develop.

HPV vaccination immunises girls (and boys) at the age of 10–15, before they become sexually active, against the high-risk type 16 and 18 HPVs. HPV vaccines are made by producing virus-like proteins in the laboratory. They do not contain DNA from the virus, so they are not infectious and do not have any cancer-causing potential.

It is extremely important for all women to have regular Pap tests, even if they have been vaccinated against HPV. This is because the vaccination does not stop all cervical cancers; it only covers two or four of the many HPVs that can cause infection.

HPV vaccination

Vaccination is recommended at the age of 10–15 and involves three doses of HPV vaccine over six months.

Hepatitis B vaccination

Hepatitis B is one of several different viruses that can cause liver infections and damage. It can be found in the body fluids of infected people and spreads through contact with bodily fluids such as blood, saliva, semen and vaginal fluid. It can therefore be spread from an infected person through sexual contact; sharing of saliva and open-wound contact (e.g. household contacts and childcare); sharing drug-injecting equipment, toothbrushes or razors; needle-stick injury; mother-to-baby contact (usually during child-birth); and blood transfusions (not usually in Australia).

All babies born in Australia since May 2000 should have received hepatitis B vaccination as part of their routine childhood vaccinations.

Vaccination is also recommended for adults at higher risk of contracting hepatitis B, namely:

- those with household, close or sexual contact with people who have hepatitis B
- migrants from areas with high rates of hepatitis B
- Aboriginal and Torres Strait Islander people
- those on kidney dialysis
- those who are HIV-positive or otherwise have impaired immunity
- those with chronic liver disease or hepatitis C
- those who inject drugs
- recipients of certain blood products, such as plasma, red blood cells or platelets
- residents and staff of facilities for people with intellectual disabilities
- prison inmates
- sex industry workers
- those who come into contact with bodily fluid as part of their work, such as police, healthcare workers, childcare workers, funeral workers, tattooists and body piercers
- those travelling to areas with high rates of hepatitis B

Hepatitis B vaccination

Vaccination at the age of 10–13 is recommended for those who did not receive a primary course of hepatitis B vaccine as a child. In some states this is recommended for all children. High-risk adults should also be vaccinated.

Varicella (chickenpox) vaccination

Varicella (chickenpox) is a highly contagious infection caused by the varicella zoster virus. The disease is spread by direct contact with people who are infected. A blood test can indicate if you have immunity against varicella.

In healthy children it is usually a mild disease that lasts a short time. However, it is often more serious in adults and may cause serious and even fatal complications in people of any age. Varicella virus can also reactivate many years after the initial infection and cause shingles (herpes zoster). If a non-immune woman gets varicella when she is pregnant, it is usually much more severe and can also cause congenital abnormalities in her baby.

Varicella vaccine is a live attenuated vaccine, which means it is from the virus that causes chickenpox, but it has been altered so it is less infective and does not cause disease. As it is a live vaccine, however, it should not be given to anyone with impaired immunity or pregnant women. Varicella vaccination is a routine childhood vaccination (starting in late 2005 for 18-month-old children). In non-immune people from the age of 14, two doses of varicella vaccine at least four weeks apart are required to achieve immunity.

It is also recommended that the following adults be vaccinated if they are not immune, as they are at higher risk of complications or passing on varicella:

- women planning for pregnancy
- healthcare workers
- those who have household contact with people with impaired immunity

---

Varicella vaccination

Varicella vaccination is recommended at the age of 10–13 if there is no history of chickenpox or vaccination. A booster dose of varicella vaccine can be given at this time even for those who received childhood vaccination. High-risk adults should also be vaccinated.

Diphtheria, tetanus and pertussis (whooping cough) vaccination

Combined diphtheria, tetanus and pertussis immunisation has been given as a routine childhood vaccination since the 1950s.

Diphtheria is an illness caused by a bacterium spread in droplets (from coughing or sneezing) or direct contact with contaminated wounds and materials. Toxins (poisonous substances) are produced by the bacteria, which affect breathing, the nervous system and the heart. Diphtheria is fatal in 7 per cent of people who contract it.

Tetanus is caused by a bacterium from the environment (usually soil or manure) getting into deep open wounds, where it can enter the bloodstream. You do not catch tetanus from other people. Tetanus is often fatal, as the toxin made by the bacteria attacks the nervous system, causing severe muscle spasms, including in the neck and jaw muscles (lockjaw), convulsions, breathing problems and heart problems.

Pertussis (whooping cough) is caused by a highly infectious bacterium spread through droplets in the air. It is most serious in babies under the age of 12 months, as the mother's antibodies do not provide reliable protection. Babies are at greatest risk of infection until they have had at least two doses of the vaccine (the earliest at four months old). Most babies who contract pertussis get it from their parents or close carers.

Symptoms include coughing and 'whooping' (the sound made when trying to draw in breath after a bout of coughing), which can continue for months. Complications include pneumonia and hypoxic encephalopathy (lack of oxygen to the brain), leading to brain damage and possibly death.

Diphtheria, tetanus and pertussis vaccination

It is recommended that a booster dose of diphtheria, tetanus and pertussis be given at:

- the age of 10–17
- the age of 50 unless you have had a booster in the previous 10 years

To protect babies against pertussis, a booster dose is also recommended for women who are planning pregnancy, unless they have had a booster dose in the last five years (if this is missed it can be given late in pregnancy or just after the baby is born); fathers and other close carers before the birth of a baby; and healthcare and childcare workers every 10 years.

Influenza vaccination

Influenza (flu) is caused by two types of virus in humans (influenza A and B), which have many strains or subtypes. It is spread easily through infected droplets in the air from coughing or sneezing or from contact with the droplets on surfaces. Complications from flu (such as pneumonia) cause many thousands of deaths in Australia every year.

Influenza viruses change very easily, so every year different strains cause the majority of flu. The components of the annual influenza vaccine therefore change every year, depending on what is believed will be the major strains likely to cause disease that year (based, for example, on the northern hemisphere flu season and circulating strains).

This means that people at risk need the influenza vaccine every year. The vaccine is not a live vaccine, but is made from either parts of or inactivated (dead) virus and is currently made in hens' eggs. People with severe egg allergy should therefore not receive the vaccine, and should discuss this with their doctor.

People at increased risk of complications from flu include:

- anyone aged 65 and older
- Aboriginal and Torres Strait Islander people aged 15 and older
- people over the age of six months with conditions predisposing them to severe influenza (such as heart, lung, kidney and neurological disease, diabetes, Down syndrome or being immune-compromised). Only some brands can be given to children.
- those with significant obesity
- pregnant women
- homeless people
- residents of aged-care and long-term residential facilities

People who may potentially transmit influenza to those at risk should also be immunised, including healthcare workers, staff at nursing homes and family members of people who are at high risk.

Influenza vaccination

Vaccination for influenza is very effective in preventing influenza and its complications, including death, and is recommended every year if you are at increased risk, may infect those at high risk or wish to decrease your likelihood of illness from influenza.

Pneumococcal vaccination

Pneumococcal vaccination gives protection against invasive pneumococcal disease (IPD), which is caused by a bacterium that is commonly carried in the respiratory tract without any problems. IPD can cause pneumonia, blood infection, meningitis and death.

The vaccine is made of parts of the bacterium and is not live; it has been given as a routine childhood vaccination to all Australian children born since 2003.

People at increased risk of IPD include:

- anyone aged 65 and older
- Aboriginal and Torres Strait Islander people aged 50 and older
- smokers
- those with a range of underlying medical conditions
- those without a functional spleen

Pneumococcal vaccination

It is recommended anyone aged 65 and over, and Aboriginal and Torres Strait Islander people aged 50 and over, be vaccinated against pneumococcal disease. People at higher risk may require vaccination earlier. One to two booster doses are needed, depending on the risk group you fall into.

Checks and tests

This section deals with tests and checks to find important and treatable health problems for which there are proven benefits in early identification and treatment. Identifying them may also have implications for advice and tests recommended for your relatives, so do consider letting them know.

It is important to understand that all the following tests and schedules are for healthy people without problems or symptoms.

If you are in a higher risk group, the tests your GP orders may well be different, so do let them know if you have had problems in the past or if you have a family history of a problem.

Keep your GP informed

If you have or develop any problems or symptoms, you need to tell your GP about it as different tests may well be needed. Even if you just had a test that came back fine and you then develop a problem, you need to go back and tell your GP.

Recommended checks and tests for healthy women

Check for	What the test involves	Age to start (years)	How often	Some higher risk groups
Breast cancer	Mammogram	50	Every two years	Personal or family history of breast cancer Carrying a gene for breast cancer Family history of cancers Early menopause Long-term hormone replacement therapy (HRT) Your mother had the drug diethylstilboestrol (DES) when she was pregnant with you
Cervical cancer	Pap test (smear of cervix)	18–20 or one to two years after first sexual encounter (whichever is later)	Every two years	History of cervical cancer Previous abnormal Pap tests Your mother took diethylstilboestrol (DES) when she was pregnant with you Being immune-compromised, e.g. you have had a transplant of some type or chemotherapy for another condition
Bowel cancer	Test of stools (faeces)	50	Every two years	Personal history of bowel cancer or polyps Family history of bowel cancer or polyps Chronic bowel problem such as ulcerative colitis or Crohn's disease
Ovarian cancer	Not routine – be aware of problems and tell your GP			Family history of ovarian cancer Carrying a gene for breast cancer
Skin cancer	Not routine – be aware of problems and tell your GP			Personal history of melanoma or many atypical or dysplastic naevi (strange-looking freckles) Family history of melanoma

Check for	What the test involves	Age to start (years)	How often	Some higher risk groups
Chlamydia	Urine sample or cervical swab	From first sexual encounter until 29	Every year ideally, or with Pap test every two years	Within six months of a new sexual partner (irrespective of age)
High blood pressure	Blood pressure check	18	Every two years until 50, then every year	Being an Aboriginal or Torres Strait Islander Cardiovascular disease (CVD) Diabetes Kidney disease High cholesterol Being overweight Family history of early CVD Excessive alcohol intake
High lipids	Fasting blood test for cholesterol and triglycerides	45	Every five years	Being an Aboriginal or Torres Strait Islander Cardiovascular disease (CVD) Higher risk of CVD (such as high cholesterol, high blood pressure, diabetes, kidney disease, being overweight, family history of early CVD) Family history of high lipids
Diabetes	Questionnaire	40	Every three years	Aboriginal or Torres Strait Islander, Pacific Island, Indian subcontinent or Chinese cultural background The questionnaire places you in a higher risk category Diabetes when you were pregnant (gestational diabetes) Cardiovascular disease (CVD) Family history of diabetes Polycystic ovarian syndrome Taking antipsychotic medicines Abnormal blood glucose in the past, but not diabetes

Check for	What the test involves	Age to start (years)	How often	Some higher risk groups
Kidney disease	Blood pressure check, urine check and sometimes a blood test	From 35 if at increased risk	Every one to two years	Being an Aboriginal or Torres Strait Islander Diabetes High blood pressure Obesity Family history of kidney disease Long-term smoking
Osteoporosis (thin bones)	Assessment of risk factors for osteoporosis	45 for women (50 for men)	Every year	A low-impact fracture or vertebral fracture Family history of osteoporosis Certain health conditions (including some thyroid and other hormone problems, rheumatoid arthritis, coeliac disease, kidney and liver problems and multiple myeloma) Taking some medicines (e.g. long-term steroid use, some breast cancer medicines) History of early menopause, anorexia nervosa or another reason period stopped for more than six consecutive months under the age of 45 (excluding pregnancy or hysterectomy) Smoking High alcohol intake Vitamin D deficiency Being significantly underweight Low levels of physical activity Recurrent falls
Teeth and mouth problems	Examination of mouth (by a dentist or dental hygienist)	From childhood	Every year	Being an Aboriginal or Torres Strait Islander Being a recent refugee Having reduced saliva (e.g. as a result of head and neck radiation or some medicines) Poor diet Smoking Exposure to excessive amounts of sunlight (lip cancer)

Check for	What the test involves	Age to start (years)	How often	Some higher risk groups
Falls	Questions	65	Every year	Poor vision Health problems affecting balance, strength, coordination, walking, joints and blood pressure Some medicines Alcohol or other substances that result in confusion, sedation, light-headedness or poor coordination
Eye problems	Eye check	65	Every year	Family history of glaucoma or macular degeneration Diabetes Being very near-sighted (short-sighted) African descent if you are over the age of 40 Long-term steroid use Poorly controlled high blood pressure
Hearing problems	Whispered voice test or questions about hearing	65	Every year	Exposure to regular loud sounds over the years (occupational or recreational) Some medicines (some chemotherapy, long-term gentamicin, and some antimalarials)
Urinary incontinence (see chapter 39)	Not routine – be aware of problems and tell your GP			Being pregnant or having given birth Being overweight Certain medical conditions (respiratory problems, diabetes, stroke, heart problems, recent surgery, neurological problems) Being older and frail Living in residential care

Check for	What the test involves	Age to start (years)	How often	Some higher risk groups
Dementia	Not routine – be aware of problems and tell your GP			Increasing age Family history of Alzheimer's disease Higher risk of cardiovascular disease (CVD) History of significant head trauma Down syndrome
Depression	Not routine – be aware of problems and tell your GP			Personal or family history of depression Other psychiatric problems Alcohol or drug abuse Family violence or child abuse
Intimate partner violence (IPV) (domestic violence; see chapters 29 and 30)	Not routine – be aware of problems and tell your GP			Being pregnant Being young Having a partner with alcohol or substance-abuse problems, or who were abused or witnessed IPV or have problems dealing with anger

Breast cancer screening

Breast check

If you are healthy, we don't recommend examining your breasts each month. Instead of doing a single check each month, it is better to be 'breast aware'; in other words, know what your breasts normally feel and look like at different times of the month, so that you can notice any important changes right away.

If you are still having monthly periods, you may notice changes in your breasts during your monthly cycle. Women who are using hormonal medications such as the Pill or hormone replacement therapy (HRT) may also notice some changes in their breast texture.

The cessation of your periods with menopause is another time you may notice changes in your breasts, and of course there will be substantial changes if you are pregnant or breastfeeding.

It is a good idea to have your breasts examined by your doctor or nurse when you attend for your Pap test or other checks. Some abnormal breast symptoms indicate you should seek prompt medical advice. These symptoms include breast thickenings or lumps, discharge from your nipples or inversion of your nipples, and changes to breast skin colour or texture.

Breast cancer is a major health issue for women: it is the second most common cause of cancer-related death in Australian women. In 2007, 2680 Australian women died from breast cancer. The lifetime risk of women developing breast cancer before the age of 75 is one in 11. Screening with a mammogram can substantially reduce deaths from breast cancer and is recommended every two years between the ages of 50 and 69.

Cervical cancer screening

Cervical cancer screening should start between the ages of 18 and 20. In Australia it is recommended that every woman have a Pap test every two years until the age of 70, from the age of 18 if she has ever been sexually active, or one to two years after her first sexual encounter, whichever is later. Guidance on screening is currently under review in light of the success of the cervical cancer vaccine now being given to Australian schoolchildren. It's best to double-check with your GP about the right screening schedule for you as it might depend on your age, previous Pap test results and whether you have had the cervical cancer vaccine or not.

Colorectal cancer screening

Bowel cancer is common: one in 12 Australians is diagnosed with bowel cancer by the time they reach the age of 85. If caught in time, 90 per cent of bowel cancer can be cured.

In a colorectal cancer screen – called a faecal occult blood test (FOBT) – a faeces (stool) sample is checked to see if it contains any blood that is not visible to the naked eye. FOBT screening is only for people who do not have any symptoms of bowel cancer. If you have symptoms your doctor may order different tests.

Symptoms of bowel cancer include:

- recent, persistent change in bowel habits or feeling that the bowel does not empty completely
- blood in the stool (either bright red or very dark)
- bloating, fullness or cramps
- stools that are narrower than usual
- a lump or mass in the abdomen
- weight loss for no known reason
- persistent abdominal pain or frequent gas pains

There are different types of tests. With some tests you collect your stools and put them in a container; with some you smear a bit of your stool on a slide. You usually have to take a few samples over a few days. It is very important that you follow the instructions for these tests carefully, including any dietary restrictions and the number of stools taken.

FOBT is a screening test for colon and rectal cancers (types of cancer of the bowel). It won't diagnose them, but will indicate if further testing

---

Screening for colorectal cancer

It is recommended that all Australians have an FOBT every two years from the age of 50.

If you are at higher risk – for example, you have a blood relative who had colorectal cancer, you come from a family where bowel cancers or polyps are hereditary, you have had bowel polyps or you have a chronic bowel problem such as ulcerative colitis or Crohn's disease – you may need earlier and different testing. Talk to your GP about it.

is needed. For those who have a positive FOBT, the likelihood of having a cancer is about 30–50 per cent.

If your FOBT is positive, your GP will arrange for your rectum and colon to be investigated, usually by colonoscopy.

Ovarian cancer screening

Despite numerous international studies, no recognisable 'pre-cancer' stage to ovarian cancer has yet been identified that would allow screening and reduce death rates. There is also no current consensus of screening in women at high risk of ovarian cancer, such as those who have a BRCA gene mutation.

See chapter 35 for more information on ovarian cancer.

Skin cancer screening

Australia has one of the highest rates of skin cancer in the world. At least two in three Australians will be diagnosed with skin cancer by the age of 70, more than 1000 Australians are treated for skin cancer every day and more than 1830 Australians die from skin cancer each year.

The good news is that skin cancer is one of the most preventable forms of cancer in Australia. More than 95 per cent of skin cancers can be successfully treated if found early.

Sun exposure is the cause of most skin cancers in Australia, but other factors can increase the risk of skin cancer, such as:

- a family history of melanoma
- a fair complexion
- past history of skin cancer
- many atypical or dysplastic naevi (funny-looking freckles)

See chapter 5 for more on skin.

Testing for skin cancer is not routine. You should be alert for any new or changing skin lesion or spot by looking for changes every three months, especially if you are over the age of 40.

If you have had a melanoma in the past, or have many atypical or dysplastic naevi, you should consider seeing your doctor at least every year to be examined and assessed.

Sexual health check for well women

Once you start having sexual experiences with partners, awareness of your sexual health is important, regardless of your age. Good sexual health care is best provided where the communication between you and your doctor or nurse is open, comfortable and professional. In some instances, you may feel unable to discuss these issues with your regular GP. Fortunately, there are sexual healthcare services staffed by doctors and nurses who specialise in this area.

During a sexual health consultation your doctor or nurse will ask you about any problems you are experiencing (such as genital itching, pain, lumps or abnormal discharge or bleeding) and about your partner(s) and sexual history, health and practices. In this way they can determine your risk of having a variety of sexually transmitted infections and therefore what swabs need to be taken during the consultation and what blood tests (if any) should be considered.

This is likely to be followed by an examination of your genital area and a vaginal examination undertaken with a speculum, when swabs will be taken for the detection of sexually transmitted infections (STIs). If your Pap test is due, this might also be performed. Depending on your risks, the doctor/nurse may also discuss having blood tests for syphilis, hepatitis B, hepatitis C and human immunodeficiency virus (HIV).

For well women who are not experiencing any abnormal symptoms, simple tests for two common infections are recommended for maintaining sexual health. Both chlamydia and *Mycoplasma genitalium* are bacterial infections you may not be aware you have contracted, but which can be easily detected with either a urine test or a swab from the cervix. Both infections are usually treated with a very short course of antibiotic tablets for you and your sexual partner(s).

Many women will have heard about chlamydia, the most common STI in Australia, but you may not yet have heard of *Mycoplasma genitalium*, which has only recently been recognised as an STI. You may find therefore that testing for *Mycoplasma genitalium* is not yet readily available at your local GP.

Because younger women tend to change their sexual partners more often, if you are aged less than 29 we recommend that you have chlamydia and *Mycoplasma genitalium* tests. We also recommend these tests, regardless of your age, when you change your sexual partner. If your Pap test is due, this can be performed at the same time. Of course, if you are experiencing any symptoms such as an unusual vaginal discharge, pain with passing urine or with sex, or bleeding between your periods or after sex, it is important to see your doctor or nurse for a complete sexual health check.

Good communication with your sexual partner is the best protection for your sexual health. This may involve agreeing with your partner to use condoms or dental dams until both of you have been tested and also disclosing if either of you have additional sexual partners outside your relationship. See chapter 8 for more information on STIs.

In addition to your local GP, a wide range of services provide sexual health testing (see the Resources section at the end of this book).

Blood pressure check

Blood pressure is the pressure that blood exerts on the walls of the arteries as it is pumped by the heart around the body. It is written as one number above another – for example, 120/80 mmHg. The higher pressure (systolic) is the pressure when the left side of the heart is contracting and the lower pressure (diastolic) is the pressure when the left side relaxes between contractions. Hypertension (high blood pressure) is indicated by a systolic pressure of 140 mmHg or more and/or a diastolic pressure of 90 mmHg or more.

As blood pressure normally changes throughout the day, your doctor needs to have taken several high blood pressure readings on separate occasions before they will diagnose you with hypertension.

It is estimated that around 3.7 million Australians aged over 25 have hypertension. It is important to identify and treat hypertension because it is a major risk factor for cardiovascular disease (CVD) such as stroke, coronary heart disease (heart attacks and angina) and heart failure; kidney failure; and some eye problems.

The higher the blood pressure, the higher the risk of problems. A more sensitive assessment of your risk of CVD is the 'absolute' risk, which takes into account not only the presence and degree of hypertension but also other risk factors for CVD, such as age, gender, smoking status, obesity, cholesterol, kidney problems, diabetes and physical inactivity.

If you are diagnosed with hypertension, your doctor will usually do a number of tests, including tests:

- to see if there is a reason you developed hypertension, such as kidney problems. In most cases there is no identifiable cause and it is called *essential* or *primary* hypertension. This often runs in families, but other contributors include excessive alcohol intake, obesity and lack of physical activity.

- to check for other risk factors for CVD, such as high cholesterol or diabetes
- to see if the high blood pressure has caused your heart muscle to thicken (by an ECG) or to see if the vessels in your eyes have been affected (by referring you for an eye check)

There is very good evidence that reducing blood pressure decreases the risk of CVD. Your doctor will talk to you about managing any contributing factors for your hypertension and other risk factors for CVD. The decision whether to prescribe anti-hypertensive medicine is influenced by the level of the high blood pressure and an assessment of other risk factors for CVD.

See chapter 32 for more on hypertension and CVD.

Blood pressure checks

All adults should have their blood pressure assessed every two years between the ages of 18 and 50 and every year over the age of 50. If you are at higher risk of CVD or high blood pressure, your GP should check your blood pressure more often. This includes if you are an Aboriginal or Torres Strait Islander, have diabetes, kidney disease or high cholesterol, are overweight, have been assessed as having an increased risk of CVD, or have a family history of early CVD.

Blood lipid (cholesterol and triglycerides) check

Cholesterol is a fatty substance (lipid) made naturally by your liver, which performs many different functions in the body. Some people make a lot of cholesterol, and this often runs in families.

In addition, we get cholesterol from some foods, especially foods high in saturated fats, such as animal fats, and trans fats.

Your total blood cholesterol level includes two types of blood cholesterol:

- low-density lipoprotein (LDL), also known as 'bad' cholesterol because it can add to the build-up of plaque in arteries and increase the risk of CVD

- high-density lipoprotein (HDL), also known as 'good' cholesterol because it helps protect against CVD

Most of the total cholesterol in blood is made up of LDL (or 'bad') cholesterol, with only a small part made up of HDL cholesterol. It is best to aim for a low LDL cholesterol level and a high HDL cholesterol level.

Triglycerides, another fat normally found in the body, are used by the body to store unused calories. You may have high triglycerides if your diet is high in sugars and other high-carbohydrate foods or high in alcohol, if you have poorly controlled diabetes, kidney or liver problems, or if you have a family history of high triglycerides.

High total and LDL cholesterol and/or high triglycerides are common and are risk factors for CVD, as they contribute to the atherosclerotic plaques that cause CVD.

See chapter 32 for more on lipids.

Blood lipid checks

- All adults should have their lipids checked every five years from the age of 45.

- If you are an Aboriginal or Torres Strait Islander this should start at the age of 35.

- If you are at increased risk of CVD or high lipids, your lipids should be checked more often by your GP.

Diabetes check

Diabetes is a chronic (long-term) disease in which the pancreas doesn't produce enough insulin and/or there is a problem with how the body's cells respond to the insulin the pancreas does produce. This means that when a person with diabetes eats glucose, which is in many foods, it can't be adequately taken up into their cells and converted into energy, and instead stays in the blood. This is why blood glucose levels are higher in people with diabetes.

Type 2 diabetes mellitus (usually just called type 2 diabetes) is the most common type of diabetes, affecting 85–95 per cent of all people with diabetes and around 8 per cent of Australians aged 25 or older. While it usually affects older adults, younger people, even children, are now getting type 2 diabetes. Its incidence is increasing rapidly, and is estimated to almost double by 2030. This increase is linked to lifestyle factors (see below).

In type 2 diabetes, the pancreas makes some insulin but it is not produced in the amount the body needs, or the body's cells don't respond properly to the insulin produced – most people with diabetes have both of these problems.

There is no single cause of type 2 diabetes; it results from a combination of lifestyle factors and genetics. The risk of type 2 diabetes increases:

- if you have a family history of diabetes
- with age – it is most common after the age of 40, although the age of onset can be earlier
- if you are overweight, especially with the classic 'apple shape' body where extra weight is carried around the waist; most, but not all, people with type 2 diabetes are overweight
- with insufficient physical activity
- with poor diet
- if you are from a certain cultural background, such as Aboriginal or Torres Strait Islander, Pacific Island, Indian subcontinent or Chinese
- if you had a baby whose birth weight was more than 4.5 kilograms or you had diabetes when you were pregnant (gestational diabetes)
- if you have a condition known as polycystic ovarian syndrome (see chapters 6 and 24)
- if you take antipsychotic medicine
- if you had abnormal blood glucose in the past, but not diabetes (called glucose intolerance)

It is estimated that a healthy lifestyle would prevent more than half of type 2 diabetes cases, and would enable the rest to be better managed and have fewer complications. A healthy lifestyle includes:

- maintaining a healthy weight
- engaging in regular physical activity
- making healthy food choices
- managing blood pressure
- managing cholesterol levels
- not smoking

Many people do not have any symptoms at all when they develop type 2 diabetes, while others experience problems such as tiredness, lack of energy, blurred vision, headaches, dizziness, leg cramps, slower healing of sores or more frequent infections. These symptoms may be subtle and easily dismissed as a part of 'getting older'. Unfortunately, often by the time type 2 diabetes is diagnosed, complications may already be present. Regular check-ups are therefore needed to diagnose type 2 diabetes early, so it can be well managed and complications can be minimised.

See chapter 32 for more on diabetes.

Tests for diabetes

All adults over the age of 40 and all Aboriginal or Torres Strait Islanders over the age of 18 should be assessed by their doctor every three years for their risk of type 2 diabetes (possibly using the questionnaire 'The Australian Type 2 Diabetes Risk Assessment Tool', or AUSDRISK). If this shows you are at higher risk, you will need to have a blood test.

If you or your GP already know you are at higher risk, you don't have to answer a questionnaire, but should go straight to a blood sugar test every three years. This includes if you have CVD; had gestational diabetes; have polycystic ovarian syndrome; or are taking antipsychotic medicines.

If you have had abnormal blood glucose in the past, but not diabetes (impaired glucose tolerance or impaired fasting glucose), you need a blood sugar check every year.

Kidney disease check

The kidneys are essential organs with several functions, including maintaining the body's salt and water balance and acid–base balance, and regulating blood pressure. They also filter the blood, and remove wastes such as urea, excreting them via our urine.

Chronic kidney disease can lead to kidney failure, as well as high blood pressure and all its consequences; it is also a risk factor for CVD.

End-stage kidney disease is a serious health problem that requires dialysis (or similar) or kidney transplantation for survival. More than 2000 Australians start dialysis every year, and the rates are rising, largely because the rates of diabetes are rising. Besides chronic kidney diseases causing hypertension (high blood pressure) and being a risk factor for

CVD, both hypertension and CVD are risk factors for chronic kidney disease, as they compromise the blood flow through and functioning of the kidneys.

Risk factors for chronic kidney disease include the risk factors for CVD, such as being an Aboriginal or Torres Strait Islander, diabetes, hypertension, smoking, obesity, physical inactivity and poor diet. A family history of kidney disease is also a risk factor.

Early detection and treatment for chronic kidney disease can halt or reduce the progression of kidney problems to end-stage kidney disease. Routine checking usually consists of a blood pressure check, a urine check and sometimes a blood test.

The urine test is to see if there is too much protein in the urine, which is one indication of kidney problems. The appearance of protein in the urine may be the first sign of an otherwise silent kidney problem. If a test indicates too much protein in your urine, your doctor is likely to repeat the test to see if it persists.

If you are at higher risk, your doctor may also order a blood test so your kidney function (glomerular filtration rate, or GFR) can be estimated.

Tests for kidney disease

All adults who are at increased risk of kidney disease, including those with hypertension (high blood pressure), obesity, a family history of kidney disease or of Aboriginal or Torres Strait Islander descent, should have a kidney health check consisting of a urine check and blood pressure check and sometimes a blood test every one or two years from the age of 35.

If you have diabetes these checks need to start when your diabetes is diagnosed and you should have them every year.

Osteoporosis

Osteoporosis is a condition in which the bones become fragile and brittle, leading to a higher risk of fractures (breaks or cracks) than in normal bone.

Osteoporosis occurs when bones lose minerals, such as calcium, more quickly than they can be replaced, leading to a loss of bone thickness (bone mass or density). In this case, even a minor bump or accident can break a bone. These are known as minimal trauma fractures. One in two women and one in three men over the age of 60 in Australia will have such a fracture during their lifetime.

Osteoporosis checks

Every woman from the age of 45 should see her GP every year to have her risk factors for osteoporosis assessed and get advice on prevention.

If you are older than 45 and have had a low-impact fracture or vertebral fracture, or have other risk factors, you should discuss with your doctor if you should have a test to check your bone density.

As you cannot see or feel your bones getting thinner, the only way to establish your bone density is by having a bone density test (sometimes called a bone mass measurement). There are a number of different ways bone density can be measured, but it is usually performed using a special form of X-ray scanning, called dual-energy X-ray absorptiometry (DEXA).

Women are at a greater risk of developing osteoporosis than men. This is mainly due to the rapid decline in oestrogen levels after menopause. Oestrogen is an important hormone for maintaining healthy bones, so when oestrogen levels decrease after menopause, bones lose calcium (and other minerals) at a much faster rate.

Other risk factors for developing osteoporosis or osteoporotic fractures include:

- a low-impact fracture or vertebral fracture in the past
- a family history of osteoporosis and fractures
- certain conditions including rheumatoid arthritis, overactive thyroid (hyperthyroidism) or parathyroid glands, coeliac disease and other chronic gut conditions, liver and kidney disease and multiple myeloma
- some medicines, such as long-term use of steroids and some breast cancer medicines
- early menopause
- a history of anorexia nervosa or another reason for periods stopping for six consecutive months (excluding pregnancy, menopause or hysterectomy) under the age of 45
- smoking
- high alcohol consumption
- lack of calcium in the diet and/or vitamin D deficiency
- an inactive lifestyle over many years

- being significantly underweight
- recurrent falls

See chapter 32 for more on osteoporosis.

Depression screening

Depression is common, occurring in around 1 million Australian adults and 100,000 young people. On average, one in six people will experience depression in their lifetime: one in five women and one in eight men.

There is very effective treatment for depression, but left untreated the consequences can be dire. Testing for depression is not routine, but if you have any symptoms or are concerned you are at risk, please talk to your GP about it.

See chapters 10, 22, 40 and 44 for more on depression.

Intimate partner violence

See chapters 29 and 30 for more on intimate partner violence and violence against women.

Urinary incontinence

See chapter 39 for more on urinary incontinence.

Falls risk screening

Falls in the elderly are common: about 30 per cent of Australians over the age of 65 fall every year and 10 per cent of these falls lead to injury. In people over the age of 65, falls are the biggest single reason for admission to hospital and presentations to the emergency department. The most commonly injured areas requiring hospitalisation are the hip and thigh. Along with cognitive impairment and incontinence, falls are one of the major factors in precipitating admission to residential aged-care facilities. Preventing falls and minimising their harmful effects is therefore critical.

Falls can be caused by many things, and often the cause is a combination of many of these factors. An increase in falling as people get older is associated with:

- decreased muscle tone, strength and fitness as a result of physical inactivity
- problems with balance and walking due to arthritis, stroke or Parkinson's disease

- poor vision
- cardiovascular problems resulting in light-headedness or loss of consciousness
- cognitive problems such as dementia
- medicine for other conditions that result in sedation, light-headedness or poor coordination
- excessive intake of alcohol or other substances resulting in confusion, sedation, light-headedness or poor coordination
- incontinence (and thus the need to get to the toilet very quickly)
- extrinsic factors such as poor lighting, stairs, uneven floor surfaces, poorly fitting footwear and lack of equipment or aids

Falls often require a number of health professionals to help with assessment and management, including treating and aiding recovery from any injuries sustained during the fall, and preventing any future falls.

Assessment of falls risk

All Australians over the age of 65 should see their GP every year so their risk of falls can be assessed. If you have had a fall or are at higher risk, you should have any underlying factors identified and remedied if possible, and undertake a physical activity program.

Vision and hearing impairment

Vision and hearing can rapidly deteriorate with increased age, causing a decrease in enjoyment and involvement in life and contributing to other problems such as falls and injuries, road accidents, problems with taking medicine and difficulty communicating.

Visual problems can be due to a number of conditions, including cataracts, glaucoma, macular degeneration, diabetic retinopathy and retinal detachment.

Besides advancing age, risk factors for eye and visual problems include:

- a family history of glaucoma (increased pressure in the eye) or macular degeneration
- diabetes
- long-term steroid use

- being very near-sighted (short-sighted)
- poorly controlled high blood pressure
- a history of eye trauma
- migraine
- African descent if you are over the age of 40

Eye and hearing checks

All Australians from the age of 65 should see their GP or optometrist every year to have their eyesight checked with an eye chart.

If you are at higher risk for visual problems, you should start having your eyes checked at an earlier age and see an ophthalmologist or optometrist for a more thorough examination of your eyes. If you have a family history of glaucoma, examinations should start five to 10 years earlier than the age of onset of glaucoma in your affected relative. If you have diabetes, these checks need to start when your diabetes is diagnosed.

All Australians from the age of 65 should have their hearing screened every year by their GP (the GP whispers out of your field of vision and at 50 centimetres away, rubs their fingers together at 5 centimetres away or asks about your hearing).

Dementia screening

Dementia describes a collection of problems affecting the brain that results in a progressive decline in a person's functioning. It usually affects a number of areas of brain functioning, such as memory, attention, language, problem-solving skills, thinking and behaviour. It affects a person's ability to perform everyday tasks enough to interfere with their normal social or working life. Symptoms normally need to be present for at least six months for dementia to be diagnosed.

Higher thinking functions are affected first, and the early signs of dementia are usually vague, non-specific and often not very obvious. Some common symptoms may include:

- memory loss
- confusion
- disorientation

- personality change
- loss of interest and apathy
- loss of ability to perform everyday tasks

These symptoms are often easily dismissed or put down to depression, anxiety or normal ageing. In fact, depression or anxiety often coexists with dementia, affecting about 30–50 per cent of people with dementia. Most people who develop dementia are over the age of 65, but it is not a normal part of ageing; not all older people get dementia and some people in their 40s and 50s can develop dementia.

Dementia is not caused by one disease; many different diseases may cause it, and it may in fact be multifactorial (caused by more than one disease). Some more common causes of dementia include Alzheimer's disease, vascular dementia/multi-infarct dementia (from lots of small strokes), alcohol-related dementia and Parkinson's disease.

The risk of dementia is increased with:

- a family history of Alzheimer's disease
- a history of repeated head trauma
- Down syndrome
- a history of excessive alcohol intake
- poorly controlled CVD
- poorly controlled diabetes

An increasing number of management options are available for people with dementia. It is important to have it diagnosed early so that its cause or causes can be determined and its progression can be minimised.

> ### Dementia testing
> Testing for dementia is not routine, but if you notice any problems in you or a family member, do go and speak to your GP about it.

Maintaining mental and emotional wellbeing

Mental and emotional health problems such as depression and anxiety are common, but developing and maintaining mental and emotional wellbeing will decrease your risk of developing such problems, and may help you manage them better if they do develop. In that way you can decrease the effects of anxiety or depression on yourself or your family. Being emotionally and mentally healthy doesn't mean never going through bad times or experiencing emotional or relationship problems. We all go through disappointments, loss and change, and some people have to face great hardships. And while most of these are normal parts of life, they still do cause sadness, anxiety and stress. However, just like feeling bad is not the same as feeling good, being mentally and emotionally healthy is much more than being free of depression, anxiety or other mental and emotional health problems. Rather, it allows you to participate fully in life through productive, meaningful activities and strong relationships, and helps you cope when faced with life's challenges and stresses.

People who are emotionally and mentally healthy have the tools to cope better and are more resilient in the face of difficulties. People cope in a variety of ways, including by maintaining a more balanced outlook, balancing stress and emotions better, having the ability to remain focused, being flexible and creative in bad times as well as good, having an ability to recognise their emotions and express them in constructive ways, and learning and moving on with life. This helps them bounce back from adversity, trauma and stress, and avoid getting stuck in depression, anxiety and other negative mood states.

Your mental and emotional health has been, and will continue to be, shaped by your experiences and upbringing. Early childhood experiences are especially significant. Genetic and biological factors also play a role. Whatever factors have shaped your mental and emotional health, it's never too late to make changes to improve it.

There are many things you can do to help you achieve mental and emotional health. But just as it requires thought and effort to build and maintain physical health, so it is with mental and emotional health. The activities you engage in and the daily choices you make affect the way you feel physically and emotionally. Everyone is different; not all things will be equally beneficial to all people. The important thing is to find a mindset, strategies and activities that work for you.

Here are some ideas for maintaining your mental and emotional wellbeing.

Stay healthy and active

Our physical health affects our mind much more than we realise, so to have good mental and emotional health, it's important to take care of your body. Many people find that if they improve their physical health, they experience greater mental and emotional wellbeing.

Be physically active

Regular physical activity raises the levels of chemicals in the brain that appear to improve mood and reduce depression and anxiety, such as endorphins, adrenaline, serotonin and dopamine. They may even enhance creativity and imagination. Some studies have shown that physical exercise in a social context (such as walking with a friend or in a group) is particularly beneficial, and that physical activity is good for the brain as well as the rest of the body.

Some people find activities that focus on breathing, relaxation and meditation, such as yoga and Pilates, especially helpful for combating stress, anxiety and sleeplessness.

Eat well

The food we eat provides both the energy and nutrition our brain needs to function, so the more you practise good nutrition, the better for your brain.

Get enough sleep

Sleep recharges the brain and body and enables the brain to process the day's events. Most people need seven to nine hours of sleep each night in order to function optimally.

Limit alcohol and avoid cigarettes and other drugs

These are substances that may unnaturally make you feel good in the short term, but have long-term negative consequences for mood and emotional health.

Get outside every day

This exposes you to fresh air and a dose of sunlight, which lifts your mood and connects you to nature. Studies show that simply walking through a garden can lower blood pressure and reduce stress, so if you really take the time to notice your surroundings you can add psychological value to your physical exercise.

Maintain positive, strong, supportive relationships

We are social creatures with an emotional need for relationships and positive connections to others. We're not meant to survive, let alone thrive, in isolation. We need others to share our experiences and thoughts, to support us through tough times and to share good times. Others can also give us alternative perspectives we can learn from and help us see situations with more balance.

Develop, invest in and maintain good relationships and friendships. Develop networks of people around you who make you feel good, who you feel listen to you, whom you can trust, talk to, turn to, respect and value, and who support and value you.

Keep your brain healthy

Keep your brain active

Keep your brain fit by exercising it – challenge it by stretching it and learning something new, whether through stimulating conversation, crosswords, or learning a language, a new skill or a musical instrument.

Stimulate your senses

Our senses need to be kept alive, too. Appeal to the five senses: sight, sound, touch, smell and taste. Listen to music that lifts your mood, place flowers where you will see and smell them, massage your hands and feet, or sip a warm drink.

Engage in meaningful, creative work

Do things that challenge your creativity, make you feel productive and have a positive impact on others, whether or not you get paid for them. Being useful to others and being valued for what you do can help build self-esteem.

Strive for balance

Try to maintain a balance between your daily responsibilities, looking after yourself and doing the things you enjoy. Balance the time, effort and energy you put into yourself, your study and work, and your family, friends, community, hobbies and other activities. Balance gives you better perspective, makes you and your life more interesting, and gives you the skills and connections you need to be better prepared to deal with challenges if and when they arise.

Learn to appreciate the moment

Life is short and we so often get caught up in the whirlwind that we forget to live in the present moment. Practise enjoying the moment you are in and the things you are doing.

Learn to reflect

Make time for contemplation and appreciation. Meditate, pray, enjoy the sunset or something you find beautiful, incorporate a relaxation technique into your daily routine or simply take a moment to pay attention to what is good, positive and beautiful as you go about your day.

Think about what you read, and find out how you can use the information in your life. Look into yourself and into your mind, and try to find out what it is that makes you feel conscious, alive and happy.

Work towards goals

Having something to work towards is good for everybody. What that something is depends on you and your life. The achievement of milestones towards goals and the self-discipline required naturally leads to a sense of hopefulness and a greater ability to overcome despair, helplessness and other negative thoughts.

Learn and maintain good ways of dealing with difficulties

Be positive

Be optimistic. Try to recognise and be grateful for whatever it is that brings happiness and fulfilment to your life. Think positively and develop the happiness habit, by choosing a predisposition towards happiness. Open the door for the positive and don't let the negative dwell. Happiness comes from within. Don't let the outside world decide your happiness for you.

Learn from life's lessons

Learn from difficult situations, accept they have happened, face their reality, take responsibility for your part in them, learn and move on with life. We have all made mistakes and poor decisions in our lives, but we have all made good ones, too. So learn and leave regrets behind, because regretting cannot change the mistakes we've made.

Limit unhealthy mental habits like worrying and regret

Try to avoid becoming absorbed by repetitive mental habits such as worry, regret and negative thoughts about yourself and the world. They waste time, drain your energy, trigger feelings of anxiety, fear and depression and don't lead to positive outcomes. Consider whether what you are worrying about really matters, and if it does, try to generate a solution to the problem. If you find that you are worrying about something that might never happen, try to let it go, or even distract yourself with a physical or social activity.

Learn to release anger and let go of grudges

Anger can be constructive as long as it is expressed acceptably. We sometimes need it to give us the momentum to deal with injustices, make changes in our lives or deal with issues. So work constructively through anger via positive actions towards better outcomes. Holding on to anger or resentment builds emotional toxicity, which ultimately affects your overall health.

Manage your stress levels and learn to relax

Stress takes a heavy toll on mental and emotional health, so it's important to keep it under control. While not all stressors can be avoided, stress management strategies and learning to relax can help you bring things back into balance.

The strategies that work for you will be individual to you, but make them positive ones and have a number of methods to fall back on. You may want to take some yoga classes, learn to meditate or incorporate a relaxation technique into your routine. You may want to exercise, listen to or play music, garden or paint, cook or play with your children.

Besides having fun and not taking yourself too seriously, it's a good idea to integrate relaxation strategies into your routine for those times when life gets somewhat overwhelming.

When to seek professional help for emotional problems

If you've made consistent efforts to improve your mental and emotional health and you still don't feel good, then it's time to see your GP.

Feelings and behaviours that indicate you should see a doctor include:

- difficulty sleeping
- feeling down, hopeless or helpless most of the time
- concentration problems that interfere with your work or home life
- using nicotine, food, alcohol or drugs to cope with difficult emotions
- negative, destructive or self-destructive thoughts or fears that you can't control
- thoughts of death or suicide

Keeping our physical, mental and emotional health as good as we can is one of the most important aspects of our lives. Not all of it is in our control: there are things in our lives we have, or have had, little or no control over. Health issues will come our way that we need to manage as best we can, with many of us currently dealing with or being faced with chronic and serious health conditions in ourselves or our loved ones. Remember our tips to:

- live as healthy a lifestyle as you can: physically, mentally and emotionally
- develop a strong partnership with a GP and healthcare team
- undertake the recommended screening tests and preventative health interventions for you
- understand the health issues you have or may be at particular risk of and how they can be best prevented, identified and managed
- seek early quality information and help
- develop constructive ways of dealing with problems and adversity

These positive choices, decisions and paths will all assist in decreasing the likelihood of chronic and serious conditions, minimising their effects and improving their management.

3

Getting the most out of your health consultation

Leslie Reti

In our busy lives we often arrive at a medical consultation not quite prepared, with perhaps one question or concern in our minds. Some of us might find the experience a little intimidating, confronting or anxiety-provoking. Women sometimes leave a consultation unsatisfied or later think of a question they should have asked. There are also some points you may not have thought to ask about. The time allocated is necessarily limited, so it is useful to plan your consultation at home to maximise its effectiveness. The following is a useful guide.

Planning a health consultation

Make a list of the issues you want to discuss and prioritise them. Ensure that the 'must ask' topics are covered, but don't allow your list to get so long that you don't have enough time to air some important issues towards the bottom. To develop your list it can be helpful to do some research. Familiarity with your concern will often uncover additional questions you may want to ask.

Do some research

One of the purposes of this book is exactly that: to provide some sound background knowledge on your particular topic. The internet can also be a good source, but it has its limitations. The reliability of consumer-oriented health sites is variable, so use a few checks. Look at who runs the website and what its purpose is. If it is run by a reliable health organisation, a medical school or a government agency, it is likely to be reliable. Sources that contain .edu, .org or .gov are more likely to be accurate, and sources that end in .au are more likely to be relevant. Be wary if its purpose is to promote a product or raise money rather than simply inform. You should also check how current the information is. Health information especially needs to be regularly updated as medical knowledge improves. Most websites will have a currency date at the bottom of each page. Finally, you should be cautious of websites that make claims that are too good to be true or claim results better than everyone else's.

Describe what is wrong

When visiting your doctor, describe your symptoms chronologically and in detail, including any aggravating factors. For instance, you might say something like: 'My pain is worse when …'

Don't be afraid to discuss sensitive topics. If you feel inhibited, start by saying there is something you are concerned about but you have difficulty explaining. A skilled doctor will often help you approach such topics with sensitivity and privacy. If you still don't feel comfortable, it may be worth seeking another doctor. There are also specialist clinics in large hospitals and in the community that deal with such things as psychological, sexual and private social issues. Your local doctor or community health nurse can refer you to these.

Take someone with you

If privacy is not an issue for you, some people find bringing a friend or a relative to the consultation helpful if they have difficulty remembering what they want to say or need extra support. This is becoming an increasingly common practice and you should feel comfortable about it. A friend can prompt you to ask questions you may have forgotten or remind you after the consultation of things you were told.

Ask all your questions

Don't leave something out because you're worried about taking up too much time. Having prioritised your questions, you're likely to get through the important ones, but if some remain say so, and either ask for extra time or a further appointment. Ask what contact is appropriate after the consultation. Most doctors accept telephone calls if you remember an outstanding issue after your consultation has finished, although this is often not practical following consultations in large hospital clinics. After the appointment the doctor may not have immediate access to your records and they can't discuss problems with you without reference to these.

Know your medications

Bring a list of all the prescribed drugs you are taking, as well as non-prescription medicines and herbal medicines. (Sometimes when you've been on a medicine for years, you get so used to it you may forget to mention it.) This is important because anything new that is prescribed for you may interact with what you're already taking, and sometimes doctors find out about existing medical conditions you have forgotten to mention from the drugs you're on. It's important to remember that even if some remedies are termed 'natural', that does not necessarily mean they are free from side effects, and they may still interact with prescribed medicines. For instance, chamomile can interact with anticoagulants, and St John's wort should not be taken with antidepressants such as fluoxetine (Prozac).

If you are a smoker, make sure you mention this. It's also important to tell your doctor about any recreational drugs you might be using. The frequency and amount of alcohol you drink is also clinically important. Don't forget, this is all confidential.

Ask for an interpreter if you need one

Women who have difficulty with English should ensure the availability of an interpreter. A professional interpreter organised by one's doctor or sourced privately is far preferable to a relative. An interpreter, especially one who specialises in health matters, can not only translate technical medical terminology into lay language that is easily understood but can also accurately communicate concerns and symptoms to the doctor.

Make sure you understand

A lot of women find it useful to takes notes during a consultation. After being offered advice, be sure to ask if there are any risks or side effects. It is important to understand the likelihood of these risks: are they common or rare? It is not only the common ones that are important. Potential serious side effects are also important even if they are not common. Also ask what the likely course of events is if you leave things alone without treatment and what other management options are available. Just because you have a condition doesn't mean it needs treatment; for instance, most people with fibroids or mild prolapse don't need treatment. You should be clear about all the alternatives and their risks and benefits.

Be sure you understand everything before you leave. It's good to summarise the consultation back to the doctor, repeating the instructions

Be familiar with the tests

- **Ultrasound (also known as a USG or ultrasonogram)** is a technique that produces a moving image using soundwaves. It is very useful and accurate. The sound probe is used either on the lower abdomen, or inside the vagina with little discomfort. USG can be performed when you have your period, but you may prefer to defer it.

- **Magnetic Resonance Imaging (MRI)** is an investigation that uses a magnetic field and radio waves to get an image of internal organs. In some circumstances, such as cancer diagnosis, it is more accurate than other techniques. The woman lies on a table that slides into a large cylinder. Inside the cylinder is a magnet that, when operated, creates a powerful magnetic field. Some women find it somewhat confined or claustrophobic. Earphones are sometimes used to reduce the noise. MRI can be used in pregnancy.

- **Computer Axial Tomography (CT or CAT scan)** is an imaging technique that uses computer-processed X-rays to produce visual 'slices' of specific areas of the body. It can produce pictures of soft tissues, blood vessels and bone at the same time. The patient lies on a bed and rotating X-rays are taken, which are subsequently processed by a computer into a two- or three-dimensional image.

- **Positron Emission Tomography (PET scan)** is another imaging technique. It involves the injection of a small amount of 'positron-emitting' radioactive material. Images of the body are then taken using a PET scanner. The scanner detects emissions coming from the injected material, and the computer attached to the scanner creates two- and three-dimensional images of the area being examined. It can provide information about how an organ or system in the body is working. It is most useful in monitoring diseases such as cancer.

- **Cardiotocography (CTG)** is a means of recording and monitoring the fetal heart rate and the uterine contractions. It can be used in the antenatal period and in labour. It is one way the baby can be monitored for any signs of distress; the midwives and doctors are alerted to how the baby copes with contractions. CTG monitoring is usually done externally with a belt placed around the abdomen that measures contractions. Some gel is applied to the skin of the abdomen and a microphone is placed over the gel to record the fetal heartbeat.

and the follow-up plans. You should ask what you should do if you don't feel better. Ask for any further reading resources, if you feel this would be helpful to your understanding. Recommended reading is a better start to your research than an internet search engine.

Be sure you ask and understand the complete costs involved and what proportion of these are covered by Medicare and/or private insurance. In a public hospital there may be no costs at all or some costs for medicines and other extras. In the private sector, costing structures are complicated and dependent on what service you're receiving, whether you are on health benefits, and the level and type of your health insurance. This is hard or almost impossible for a patient to calculate, but the doctor is obliged to do so, so if it's not explained, ask. Also ask what common unexpected events would cost. Most laparoscopic procedures, for example, are day cases with no overnight stay, but minor complications such as postoperative vomiting might mean you're admitted till the next day. This has significant cost implications you might want to know about.

Get a second opinion

Finally, if you would feel more reassured by getting a second opinion, do so by asking for a recommendation or asking your doctor for a referral to a specialist for an opinion. Doctors are not offended by this and will often suggest a second opinion if they feel you can't decide whether to follow a recommendation. Alternatively, request a follow-up consultation if you need time to consider the advice.

Keep a checklist

You might find this simple 10-point checklist useful. The first five questions can be ticked off at home and the remaining five at the consultation.

	✓
1. Have I written a symptom list?	
2. Have I written and prioritised a question list?	
3. Have I written a drug list?	
4. Do I need to ask a friend to come?	
5. Do I need an interpreter?	
6. Did I ask about risks and side effects?	

7. Did I summarise the consultation before leaving?

8. Did I ask for further reading?

9. Do I understand the costs involved?

10. Do I need a second opinion?

ADOLESCENTS

Introduction

Maureen Johnson

Being an adolescent girl

Puberty refers to the time it takes for a child to become an adult, physically, hormonally and reproductively. In girls, puberty usually begins with breast development, with pubic hair, pimples and periods following soon after, and in no particular order. Puberty usually begins at around the age of nine and finishes at around 16.

Adolescence begins with the physical, hormonal and biological changes of puberty, but while the process of puberty has *usually* ended by the age of 16, adolescence is said by some psychologists to end after we have completed a number of developmental tasks and we have finally settled into independent, 'adult' roles in society. This can be as early as 16 and as late as our mid- to late 20s.

The essential difference between puberty and adolescence is that adolescence is a social construct whereas puberty is a physical one.

In richer, developed countries such as Australia, where food is more readily available and young people are generally healthy, puberty is starting earlier than in previous generations. On the other hand, adolescence is ending later because young people are delaying the traditional roles of adulthood, preferring instead to travel, to stay in the family home and to defer permanent employment, long-term relationships and children for longer than before. However, some young people are forced into early adulthood by life events, such as the death of a parent, arriving in the country as a refugee or having a baby. So, puberty can start at any time from the age of 9 to 13 and can end as young as 16; while adolescence can end at any time from 16 onwards.

Adolescence can be exciting, chaotic, overwhelming and emotion-filled. It is the time when we start to look outside ourselves and our families and explore the social world beyond. There are times during adolescence when we might feel confused and vulnerable, and times when we are at our most confident and self-assured. As adolescents we are adjusting to a rapidly developing body and learning to be comfortable in our own skin. We may feel awkward at times and embarrassed way too often, but we are equally prone to self-obsession and egocentricity. (Have you ever been accused of being selfish or the centre of your own universe?)

In adolescence we might experience love for the very first time, we might experiment with sex, we will move through an assortment of peer groups and we may be tempted by all kinds of risk-taking behaviours such as smoking, drinking alcohol and taking drugs. But at times we also crave the safety, security and relative stability of childhood. One moment we will reject our families and the next we will look to them for protection and guidance.

Adolescence may feel turbulent at times but we rarely have to get through it alone. Our friends are going through it with us and most of us will have parents, families or teachers to provide guidance and assurance, and to catch us when we fall. Health professionals can also provide support and guidance and can answer some of the many questions you are bound to have.

Young women have a very different experience of adolescence from young men. To begin with, as young women we are confronted with health and sexuality issues from a young age. Periods, pads and tampons can become a part of our lives from as young as nine and we have to be prepared and vigilant about personal hygiene. Occasionally we also have to manage some awkward social situations when our period gets in the way of playing sport or swimming.

While young men have to exercise responsibility around sex, for adolescent girls the consequences of not being responsible are far greater, such as unwanted pregnancy, followed by abortion or very early motherhood and social isolation. Sexually transmitted infections (which you can get from having oral or penetrative sex without a condom) can also be worse for young women than for young men. They can lead to problems getting pregnant when we are older and can also cause cancer.

Young women are under more pressure to look good, to have the 'right' body, and the 'right' hair, clothes and shoes, and if we don't, we can struggle to fit in with our social group, which in itself is an unpredictable creature.

But although adolescence can be a tough time for young women, it's important to remember that it's a moment-by-moment proposition.

It's a wonderful, creative and exciting time, but unarguably a roller-coaster ride. There are very good reasons for this, as you will read in the following chapters.

How this book can help

For this section we talked and listened to adolescent girls and then we asked the experts to join the conversation to answer your questions about the issues that are most important to you. This is a guide you can refer to in private that will help you to understand what is happening to your body right now and what is likely to happen as your body develops. The aim of the book is to empower you to make decisions about things that affect you, your health and your life.

In chapter 4 you will learn about your brain and about the developmental changes and milestones that are part of the normal journey towards adulthood. Chapter 5 focuses on being healthy, eating well and physical activity, and also looks at skin conditions – pimples and acne. In chapter 6 we talk about periods – when they start, how they work and what they are like. In chapter 7 we talk about sexuality and sex – the good, the bad, the ugly and the law – and we touch on contraception. Chapter 10 examines mental health and emotional wellbeing. How do we recognise when things are no longer normal? Who do we talk to and what can we do to prevent depression, anxiety and mental illness? We describe common mental health problems and discuss when extra care may be required to help manage your emotional and mental health. In chapter 11 we look at drugs and alcohol and try to provide an honest assessment of the impact of experimentation.

The information in this section has a strong focus on adolescents, but you will also find relevant and useful information in other parts of the book. For example, in chapters 17–24 in the young women's section you will find valuable information about reproduction. Chapter 16 in the young women's section also provides a comprehensive overview of contraceptive options. Chapter 29 on violence and sexual assault should be read by all women and men, at all stages of life. In the midlife section, chapter 41 talks about carers, a role anyone may have to take on, including very young women with a parent who has mental health or drug addiction problems, or a grandparent who requires care or a disabled sibling.

The lines between adolescent girls, young women, the midlife years and older women can sometimes be blurry because, after all, we are all women. Nevertheless, when we focus on the life stages, clear pictures emerge that illustrate the uniqueness of the various stages we go through physically and socially.

Your changing body

Evolution has created a mismatch between when we are physically ready to make babies and when we are intellectually, socially and emotionally mature enough to make good choices about sex and parenting. A 13-year-old can become pregnant, but she does not have the emotional and social maturity to confidently negotiate sex, and she is not mature enough to manage a pregnancy or to be a parent.

Nevertheless there is no stopping the physical, biological and hormonal changes going on in our bodies. Puberty heralds the physical journey towards young womanhood and, whether or not we are ready for it, our bodies are preparing for reproduction. For some young women the physical transition will be smooth and relatively trouble-free, while for others it can take some time to settle into a steady and predictable pattern. Emotionally, some young women find this an exciting time, while others might find it a bit scary or confronting. Everyone reacts differently but an understanding of what is actually happening to our bodies at this time can almost certainly make it a lot easier to manage. In chapter 4 we demystify what is happening inside our bodies, we describe the reproductive cycle and the changes to expect, and we describe what is and what might not be 'normal' and when it might be a good idea to talk with a doctor. We even discuss how to find a doctor, and how we can start to take responsibility for our own sexual and reproductive health.

Your body image

In chapter 5 we talk about nutrition, diet, exercise and body image. This is because young women spend a lot of time talking and thinking about these issues, and because the media continues to bombard us with images of the 'ideal' woman, who has often been airbrushed and photoshopped. As women we are under a lot of pressure to look a certain way, and despite the efforts of feminists over the last century, many women still feel valued for their looks over their intelligence, talents and abilities. It's no wonder many young women continue to aspire to what they think is the physical 'ideal'.

The media also provides confusing and contradictory information about dieting and nutrition. How many diets are there? How many really work? Many of the diets we read about make the body think it's being starved and so it responds by making you want to eat more, and ultimately you end up putting on weight! Diet, nutrition and exercise have to be balanced and have to be something you can do forever, not just for a few months to look good for a special occasion. The diet, nutrition and physical exercise chapters give you a long-term and sensible approach to eating and exercising.

Finally, adolescence is a time when we can spin out of control one minute and enjoy new feelings of independence and maturity the next. It's like a big gate has opened onto the mysterious world of adulthood, and while there are a few prickly bushes to negotiate as we wander through, we can also see glimpses of the world ahead and it looks pretty good. Making informed choices about our health and relationships will certainly make the journey a whole lot easier and the road ahead much more fun.

4

Adolescence and puberty

Melissa Cameron, Maureen Johnson

The period of adolescence begins with puberty, which is when we experience the physical and hormonal changes that make us reproductive individuals. In humans there is a pretty big mismatch between the time we reach reproductive maturity and the time we are able to manage our reproductive urges emotionally. Puberty, which is discussed in more detail further into the chapter, is generally over by the time we reach the age of 15 or 16, but adolescence, which refers to our social, emotional and psychological development, can continue into our mid- to late 20s. Adolescence is said to be over when we have achieved a number of developmental tasks, which are the intellectual and social behaviours our culture has deemed normal in adults. There is general agreement among experts that the period of adolescence can be broken down into three stages: early adolescence (between the ages of 9 and 14); middle adolescence (between 15 and 17); and late adolescence (between 18 and 21, and, for some, beyond). Within each of these stages milestones will be reached, but only at the final stage will all developmental tasks be ticked off.

The developmental tasks of adolescence

As a child, you completed developmental tasks or achievements that were considered normal: toilet training, sharing toys and reading, to name a few. In adolescence, we work through a new set of tasks that represent a cultural definition of what is 'normal' for an emerging adult. For example, in our society, developing financial independence is considered a culturally normal developmental stage, whereas in another society more credence might be given to marriage.

Achievements come in peaks and troughs – 10 steps forward and five steps back – until you settle into your own adult patterns of behaviour. They generally happen simultaneously, a cascade of tasks with small achievements along the way. It is likely you will have little knowledge or awareness of the changes as they occur, beyond feeling moments of mayhem and moments of calm. We hope these pages will resonate with you and help you to understand why you are feeling certain things and responding the way you do.

The main developmental tasks that lead you to adulthood are:

- achieving independence from your parents and other adults
- developing a realistic, stable and positive self-identity
- forming your sexual identity
- achieving social competency among your peers and in intimate relationships
- developing a realistic body image
- formulating intellectual and abstract thinking, and moral and ethical values
- acquiring education and skills for economic independence

These tasks have been adapted from those drawn up by a range of different experts and are very general. They will often be described in slightly different ways by different experts, but they essentially come down to achievements in intellectual, emotional, social and sexual development, and are characterised by a strong movement away from parental and familial influence to peer group and finally to independence.

The developmental tasks of adolescence are some of the most difficult we will ever have to face, and we are often negotiating them at the same time as dealing with any number of other physical, mental and social challenges: family breakdown, physical and mental illness, caring for physically or mentally ill parents, moving to a new country, or disability. Risk-taking behaviours can also interrupt your progression towards adulthood. Drug and alcohol use, as well as early sexual experiences are all contributors to delaying your normal development. All things being equal, our progression through this period and our achievement of key tasks will be textbook and normal. But all things are not equal, and many adults will never achieve maturity in all areas.

Achieving independence from parents and other adults

The relationship with your parents or carers can represent safety, security and support, and some adolescents can find that hard to give up. Yet adulthood demands a strong sense of independence. You might vacillate between pushing boundaries to assert your independence and an ongoing desire to stay in the protective embrace of parents or carers. Efforts to be independent can often seem, to those around you, like hostility, moodiness or a lack of cooperation. This development might be characterised by conflict with family – parents in particular – but ultimately a well-developed sense of autonomy will give you great strength as you leave the family unit.

Developing a realistic, stable and positive self-identity

Before adolescence your identity was an extension of your adult carers', but as you grow older you start to recognise your own sense of individuality and uniqueness. Throughout your adolescence, you will get to know yourself a little better, though in all likelihood it will be in fits and starts. In early adolescence you will at times experience self-doubt, you may wonder about whether you are normal, you may start to develop sexual feelings and you may prefer to spend time alone (or with a private, imaginary audience). In middle adolescence you may experiment more with different kinds of friendships or risk-taking behaviours as you continue to find your comfort zone and your individual boundaries. Finally, in the later years, you will start to pursue realistic goals and begin to relate to your family as an adult. If everything goes as planned you will arrive at adulthood with a reasonably strong and positive sense of your own identity.

Forming your sexual identity

As you develop physically and sexually you will start to incorporate a set of attitudes about what it means to be a woman – often influenced by your social and familial upbringing, your peers and other sources, such as educators and the media. There is more discussion about sexual identity and sexual preferences in chapter 7.

Achieving social competency among peers and in intimate relationships

Peer interactions intensify during adolescence, particularly during the middle years. Your ability to make friends and be accepted in a peer group is a strong indicator of how well you will adjust to other social and psychological developments. In early adolescence, your peer relationships are likely to be intense, particularly with other girls, and your contact with boys is more likely to happen within the safety of your social group. During your middle adolescence your peer allegiances will be strong and you and your girlfriends are likely to engage in fad behaviours. At this time you may also start to experiment with your ability to attract a partner. You will probably be more self-obsessed and still developing the ability to see a situation through the eyes of someone else.

In your later adolescence, your social decisions will be less influenced by your peers and you will relate more to individuals than to a peer group. Maturity brings with it the ability to see another person's perspective and to consider their needs over your own, which also improves your social competence.

People whose social skills mature early are less likely to engage in ongoing dangerous or peer-driven behaviours. Early social maturity may also improve your likelihood of having safe sexual experiences.

Developing a realistic body image

At no other time in your life will your physical appearance change as rapidly and dramatically as during puberty and adolescence. You will grow quickly and your female body parts will begin to emerge and become more accentuated. Given the impact of your peer groups at this time, it is no wonder that your body image might be slightly distorted and vulnerable. When your body development conforms to social norms and expectations you are much more likely to be comfortable with it, but if not you may be less at ease with the way you look and feel in your body. Your body shape may well be very average but for any number of reasons you may have a distorted sense of how you appear.

Developing a realistic body image is also about becoming comfortable with who you are. In early adolescence you may be preoccupied with your physical changes and likely to compare yourself with a 'standard' that you and your peers consider normal. In the middle years you might be less obsessed with your changing body and more preoccupied with your physical appearance. Some young women become very physically active during this time as well as having long periods of lethargy. In the later years of adolescence you are likely to develop a more realistic body image, though many women will continue to be troubled by their appearance and will always have unrealistic notions of how they should look. There is more information on body image in chapter 7.

Formulating intellectual and abstract thinking, and moral and ethical values

Childhood thinking is characterised by black-and-white or concrete thinking. Children exist in the here and now. In adolescence you start to develop the ability to think in a more abstract way. Also during childhood, our understanding of what is right and wrong, acceptable and unacceptable comes from our parents or carers. In adolescence you will start to adopt and integrate a complex moral framework, which will increasingly be influenced by a range of sources, including peers, teachers, and traditional and social media. There will be times when you will feel conflicted about the morals and values of your peers versus those of your family, and the process of sorting through those conflicts will form the basis of your own belief system. In early adolescence, your idea of the relationship between cause and effect is underdeveloped and you still have a stronger sense of self than social awareness. In middle adolescence the ability to think in a more abstract way is starting to develop and the relationship between cause and effect is becoming clearer. Self-obsession is generally at its height at this point. In later adolescence, abstract thought is established and you are more focused on the future. You have also developed independent thinking.

Acquiring education and skills for economic independence

Arriving at a point where we are focused on and ready for economic independence is a key milestone for adulthood in our culture. As a young adolescent our vocational ambitions are changeable and possibly not very realistic, but in later adolescence you will be more forward-thinking and able to consider what you need to do to develop financial independence. This may be skill development, education or the pursuit of work and career.

The human brain is amazing, particularly during adolescence. Throughout our lives, the brain has the capacity to change, adjust and develop in response to our environment. At particular times throughout your life, your brain is adjusting to information you are taking in and the experiences you are having. This process is referred to as brain plasticity or neuroplasticity, and is a natural process that occurs at particular life stages. The brain actively prunes areas we are not using to make way for areas that we are. It is not a random or predetermined process; it is influenced by our individual environment and the activities we are engaged in, and the things we are learning, practising, hearing and doing.

Brain plasticity also occurs if the brain has been damaged. With good therapy, people can relearn skills they have lost through brain damage by training the brain to adapt and create new pathways.

Our brains receive and send information from one neuron (nerve cell) to another through a complex pathway of synapses or synaptic connections. The brain's ability to learn is in part due to changes in number, strength and kind of synaptic connections in our brain. In the first few years of life our brains grow rapidly. At birth, the cerebral cortex, which is the outer covering of the cerebrum or the area often referred to as grey matter, has around 2500 synapses. By the time we are three years old, we have around 15,000 synapses per neuron – about twice that of an adult human brain.

The brain undergoes massive changes during adolescence, and even though we cannot prove a cause-and-effect relationship between the developmental tasks of adolescents and the changes in the brain at this time, the areas of the brain that are changing during adolescence are precisely those responsible for intellectual, social and emotional development.

As recently as 20 years ago it was thought that most of our brain development happened in early childhood and then it was all over. Recently, with the introduction of new technologies such as MRI machines (see p. 58), we have learnt that the brain is very active during adolescence, too. Our brain makes important connections during this time that are influenced by our environment, the things we are doing and learning, and the skills we are developing. A lot of adults will tell you they still remember skills they developed or things they learnt in their early teens, such as the chords of a song, a language or the steps of a dance routine. The areas of our brain that are not being used during adolescence are discarded – in a phrase more commonly used for older people, 'Use it, or lose it!' While some people argue that education is a waste of time in the early teenage years (because young people are distracted and impossible to teach), scientists say that education or knowledge-building is critical during adolescence because the brain is as receptive as it will ever be.

This activity in the brain is also linked to some of the behaviours held against young people, such as risk-taking, poor impulse control and selfishness – behaviours that unfortunately may undo some of the hard work the brain is doing to prepare you for adulthood. The front of our brain, called the prefrontal cortex, is sometimes referred to as the 'social brain'. It is responsible for decision-making, considering the needs and feelings of others, and self-control, and is very active during adolescence. Our 'emotional brain' is also very active at this time. This area is responsible for the feelings we get when we are excited or the feeling of reward we get when we take risks. You can understand, with these parts of the brain adjusting and changing throughout adolescence, why as teenagers we might get ourselves into trouble sometimes.

The adolescent brain doesn't necessarily reach its final maturation until the mid- to late 20s. (See the Resources section at the end of this book for more information on the adolescent brain.)

The contemporary adolescent

The physical, hormonal and neurological changes of adolescence may never change, but the contemporary adolescent girl in our society has her own particular challenges – no better or worse than those faced by adolescents past and future but certainly unique.

Adolescent girls and boys are under increasing pressure to succeed at school and to have some idea of their future careers long before they are ready to make such decisions. They are more likely to live in an urban environment where employment and housing are under increasing pressure. Adolescents have access to much more information (which is both good and bad) on TV, radio, a variety of print publications, the internet and social media. Adolescents are exposed to wider and more global influences than their parents and grandparents, who as teenagers only saw the world through newspapers, books, radio and limited TV. For many adolescents, their first encounters with sex are on the internet, where they can be exposed to sexual behaviours that are violent and degrading, particularly to women. Parents are less able than they were in previous generations to keep track of the many and varied influences that come in and out of their children's lives and are therefore less able to guide them.

Social media may have extended our social circles but it also allows schoolyard politics and even bullying into our bedrooms. Nowadays we can be 'rated' on social media sites, our photos can be instantly sent to hundreds of peers, we can easily be the subject of sexually explicit text messages or 'sexting', and rumours can be spread in the blink of an eye. Of course it is illegal for anyone to take, send or even possess a naked image of someone under the age of 18, and young people who do it, even 'for fun', can end up on the Sex Offender Register. But it happens and it can be very hard to deal with. In fact, managing all of this stuff can be hard work on our own, so it is important that we maintain strong relationships with our parents and teachers, or an adult we can trust who can provide guidance through some of the more difficult times.

Puberty

Puberty is the time of your life when you change from being a child to an adolescent and eventually to an adult. It is an important process in the growth and maturation of the sexual and reproductive organs such as the uterus and ovaries. It is a time of many changes, both physical and emotional, and marks an important milestone in your life, but it can be challenging for many. Importantly, everyone's experience of puberty is unique – in when the changes occur, what changes occur and how quickly these changes happen. For some, changes seem to appear overnight, whereas for others these developments can be very slow.

The changes of puberty

During puberty you will experience many changes to your body:

- growth and maturation of the breasts
- growing taller
- skin changes such as increased oiliness and pimples
- the development of pubic hair (hair in the armpits and genital region)
- weight gain and changing to a rounder body shape
- vulvar and vaginal changes and discharge
- the onset of periods (menstruation)

Puberty is usually a gradual process, occurring over many years. In fact, many of the early changes of puberty happen well before the

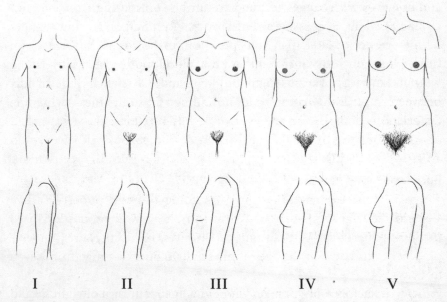

I   II   III   IV   V

Timeline of pubertal development

teenage years. The onset of puberty is influenced by many factors, including genetics, general health and the presence of other illnesses. Generally speaking, a young woman is expected to begin puberty at around the same time as her mother did. During these early years of puberty, the brain begins to send messages (hormones) to other organs of the body (such as the ovaries and adrenal glands), preparing them to make the changes essential to pubertal development. The first sign of this onset is breast development: 'budding' of the breasts may be noticed around the age of nine to 10. This is usually followed by a growth spurt and the sprouting of pubic hair. Increased body odour, oily skin and pimples may also start to appear around this time. Periods usually start within two years of the beginning of breast growth, on average around the age of 11–12 but it can begin as early as nine and as late as 15. Menstruation is one of the later signs that puberty is underway and is evidence that the ovaries are producing eggs. There is more information about periods in chapter 6.

Over the teenage years, changes continue to occur. Your breasts grow more, as does the pubic hair. The external genitals (vulva and labia) grow and become darker in colour. Your body shape also changes – the hips become rounder and wider and weight is redistributed to the hips and thighs, giving a more rounded appearance.

Puberty is often associated with marked changes in emotions. The sometimes-rapid changes of puberty can be confronting. You may feel embarrassed about or ashamed of your bodily changes. Having changes happen earlier or later than your peers can make you feel different at a time when you really just want to be like everybody else. Many young women experience various highs and lows, and may switch quite rapidly between emotions. This can be an unsettling and sometimes frightening experience – both for you and the people who care for you.

What isn't normal?

Early onset of puberty

There is some evidence that girls are going through puberty earlier. Certain racial groups, such as African-American women, appear to go through puberty earlier than others. However, in healthy girls, puberty *usually* begins between the ages of nine and 10 but can range from seven to 13.

Any of the following changes happening before the age of eight should be checked by a doctor:

- vaginal bleeding
- breast development
- pubic hair growth

In most situations no cause is found for these early changes. If a cause is found, it can include taking medication (usually accidentally taking the contraceptive pill) and, rarely, tumours in the brain, ovaries or adrenal glands. Blood tests, ultrasounds and other tests will help to rule out any serious health issues. In some cases early pubertal development will need to be stopped with medication. This will allow the body to mature at a slower rate, allowing full height to be achieved. It also allows time for the young person's emotions to catch up to deal with the changes occurring to their body.

Late onset of puberty

There are many reasons for delayed pubertal development. Most commonly it is because it's normal for you – your mother may have started her periods late, too (if you can, ask her about it!). Or, it may be because of chronic illness, or being underweight or overweight. Rarer causes include changes to the chromosomes and abnormalities of the reproductive organs, such as not having a uterus, ovarian function stopping or changes to the vagina.

Any of the following should be checked by a doctor:

- no breast development by the age of 14
- periods not beginning by the age of 16
- delay between breast development and first period of more than two years

Initially, the doctor may try to find the cause of the delay with blood tests and imaging such as ultrasound. Depending on the results of the tests, further management may be observation alone, or hormonal or surgical treatment.

Puberty ...

- makes many physical body changes happen
- can be an emotional roller-coaster
- is a unique experience for everyone
- usually begins around the age of nine or 10 with breast bud development but can start as early as seven or as late as 13
- marks the beginning of reproductive maturity

5

Food, physical activity and feeling good

Elisabeth Gasparini, Amelia Lee, Ines Rio, Margaret Sherburn, Jenny Taylor

Everyone's body shape is different. People can weigh exactly the same but have a completely different body shape. Your genes determine your body shape – that is your height, and your muscle and bone structure – and it can't be changed.

Your body image (the way you feel about how you look) may not be a reflection of what you actually look like. You may think you are thinner or fatter than you actually are, or that parts of your body are not the shape, size or colour you would like, and this can make you feel unhappy or dissatisfied.

Having a healthy body image

Lots of things can affect our body image and the way we see ourselves. Magazines often show photos of people who have a body shape that is unrealistic for a lot of people. Photos of celebrities in magazines often involve hours of hair and make-up styling by professionals and they are also digitally altered to make them look better – smoothing out lines, removing blemishes, or changing their body shape.

Also, it's easy for someone to say mean things about your body or to post or text embarrassing photos of you, all of which can affect your body image. See chapter 12 for more information on bullying and how to manage situations like this.

Having a healthy body image is important because it can affect your self-esteem, self-acceptance and your attitude towards food and exercise. Here are some ways to help improve your body image:

- Look in the mirror and focus on the things you like about yourself and the way you look, or write down the things you like about yourself.

- Don't say bad things about yourself. You can change the way you think about yourself by saying something nice.

- Focus your goals on being healthier rather than on 'fixing' things you don't like.

- Do something that makes you feel good, such as chat to a friend, put on your favourite music, get a new haircut or go for a brisk walk.

- Avoid comparing yourself to others; everyone has a different body shape.

- Be nice to others about their body shape, too. What you say can damage someone else's body image and self-esteem. Giving someone a compliment will help boost their body image and make you feel good, too.

- Put away the scales. Weighing yourself every day can put too much focus on how much you weigh rather than how healthy you are or how good you feel.

- Eat regular healthy meals. Getting the right balance of nutrients can help with improving your health and mood.

- Exercise or participate in team sports. It will keep you fit and healthy and is a great way to de-stress.

- When you read magazines, watch movies or look at advertising, remind yourself that the models and celebrities have been digitally enhanced.

- Don't worry about the size of your clothes. Different labels have different sizes that vary by up to 5 centimetres. Always try clothes on before you buy them to see how they fit.

Eating well

Why choose to eat healthily?

Eating healthy food is important at any age, but it's especially important for teenagers. As your body is still growing, it's vital that you eat enough good-quality food and the right kinds to meet your energy and nutrition needs.

Being a teenager can be fun, but it can also be difficult as your body shape changes. These physical changes can be hard to deal with if they aren't what you are expecting. There can be pressure from friends to be or look a certain way, and this might affect the foods you eat. It's not a good time to try a crash diet, as you won't get enough nutrients, and you may not reach your full potential. Following a sensible, well-balanced diet is a much better option, both for now and in the long term.

As a teenager, you'll start to become more independent and make your own food choices. You'll hang out with your friends or maybe get a part-time job so you can buy the things you like. But because you are still growing, you need some important vitamins and minerals; you should take extra care to get enough of these to feel good and be healthy.

Why do we eat?

There are many reasons why we eat, such as for our health, or social or emotional reasons. Here are some examples of why we eat:

- for good health and wellbeing
- we are hungry
- we like the taste of the food or drink
- we do lots of sports
- our friends are eating or drinking
- our parents tell us to 'finish your plate'
- we are bored
- we are upset or stressed
- we are watching a movie or the TV
- we are studying
- we like to cook
- food is offered

It may be important to be aware of the reasons why you eat because it can help you prevent overeating and gaining too much weight.

How much should I eat?

Eating three regular meals a day with some snacks will help you to meet your nutrition needs. Eating to appetite; that is, eating when you are hungry and stopping when you are full, is the best approach.

Skipping meals means you will miss out on vitamins, minerals and carbohydrates, which can leave you lacking energy or finding it hard to concentrate. Here is a guide to help you get the most value out of what you eat (see also the Australian Dietary Guidelines on pages 88–9):

1. Breads, grains and cereals contain carbohydrates that break down into glucose (sugar) to provide energy for your brain and muscles. They're

also an excellent source of fibre and B vitamins. Fibre keeps your bowels regular and B vitamins are used to convert glucose into energy and to keep your nerves working properly. Without enough carbohydrates you may feel tired and run-down. Try to include some carbohydrates at each mealtime.

2. Fruit and vegetables contain lots of vitamins and minerals, which help boost your immune system and keep you from getting sick. They're also very important for healthy skin and eyes. It's recommended to eat two serves of fruit and five serves of vegetables a day (for examples of what constitutes a serve, see the Australian Dietary Guidelines on pages 88–9).

3. Meat, chicken, fish, eggs, nuts and legumes are good sources of iron and protein. Iron is needed to make red blood cells, which carry oxygen around your body. During adolescence, you'll start to menstruate, or get your period, and this leads to loss of iron. If you don't get enough iron, you can develop anaemia, a condition that can make you feel tired and light-headed and short of breath. Protein is needed for growth and to keep your muscles healthy. Not eating enough protein when you are still growing, or going through puberty, can lead to delayed or stunted height and weight. Not enough protein is common when you go on strict diets. Include meat, chicken, fish or eggs in your diet at least twice a day.

    Fish is rich in omega-3 fatty acids, which are important for the brain, eyes and skin. Try to eat fish two to three times a week.

    If you are vegetarian or vegan and do not eat meat, there are other ways to meet your iron needs, for example, with foods such as baked beans and other legumes, pulses, nuts and seeds.

4. Dairy foods such as milk, cheese and yoghurt are the best sources of calcium and also contain some protein. Calcium helps build bones and teeth and keeps your heart, muscles and nerves working properly. You won't notice it now, but if you eat enough high-calcium foods, it will help prevent osteoporosis when you're older – a disease of the bones where they break easily. You'll need three and a half serves of dairy food a day to meet your calcium needs. In order for the body to use calcium to make bone, you also need vitamin D, which is usually made in your skin when it's exposed to sunlight.

5. Oils and fats provide your body with the fat-soluble vitamins A, D, E and K, so you should never avoid them entirely. Eating too much fat

and oil can result in you putting on weight, however, so try to use oils in small amounts for cooking or salad dressings. Other high-fat foods such as chocolate, chips, cakes and fried foods can increase your weight without giving your body many nutrients.

6. Fluids are also an important part of your diet. Drink water to keep hydrated, so you won't feel so tired or thirsty. It can also help prevent constipation. It is better not to drink flavoured waters because they add extra kilojoules, which can lead to more weight gain. Sports drinks also add extra kilojoules and are usually only needed for people who play a lot of sport or train a lot. Fruit juices and soft drinks add extra kilojoules from sugar, too, so stick to drinking these only occasionally.

Here is a sample meal plan for 12–18-year-old girls.

	Sample meal
Breakfast	1 bowl oat-based cereal with milk and banana Water
Recess or morning tea	200 g tub yoghurt and 1 cup air-popped popcorn Water
Lunch	Ham, cheese and tomato sandwich and 1 cup fruit salad Water
After-school snack or afternoon tea	¼ cup hummus dip and 3 crispbreads and 40 g dried fruit and nuts
Dinner	Chicken and vegetable stir-fry with rice Water
Evening snack (if hungry)	1–2 slices fruit bread with ricotta cheese and 1 glass milk

Why should I eat breakfast?

Breakfast is the most important meal of the day. It can help with memory and concentration at school, and give you energy to study and play. Missing out on breakfast means you'll miss out on B vitamins that keep you healthy and it can also affect your mental health. Breakfast-eaters also tend to be a healthier weight than breakfast-skippers.

Here are some healthy breakfast options:

• porridge with honey and cinnamon

• muesli with yoghurt

- fresh fruit and yoghurt
- high-fibre, low-fat breakfast cereals such as Weet-Bix, VitaBrits, Mini-Wheats, Just Right, Plus Fibre, Sustain or similar
- multigrain toast with a boiled or poached egg
- baked beans on toast
- raisin toast
- pita bread with olives, tomato and feta
- melted cheese and Vegemite on toast or an English muffin
- crumpets with Vegemite
- banana milkshake or fruit smoothie
- pancakes with yoghurt and fruit

What is a healthy school lunch?

School lunches don't have to be boring. Does your mum or dad usually make your school lunch? If you don't like what they make for you, talk to them about what you would like instead or make it yourself. Tell them what sandwich fillings you like, or what your favourite healthy snacks are.

Here are four things to think about when planning your school lunch:

1. Start with some type of sandwich bread, wrap or roll. Add a protein food, and fill the rest with salad.
2. Add a piece of fruit.
3. Add a healthy snack, for example yoghurt, nuts, dried fruit, fresh fruit, plain popcorn or vegie sticks with some dip.
4. Add water or 300 millilitres or less of milk (flavoured is okay).

Enjoy fried foods, sweet treats and soft drinks occasionally. If you want fruit juice, stick to a smaller portion, about 250 millilitres, as it's high in sugar.

Here are some healthy lunch options:

- cream cheese, chicken, grated carrot and cucumber on pita bread
- turkey, cheese and salad on multigrain bread with cranberry sauce
- vegetable and lentil soup in a thermos with a bread roll
- cream cheese, smoked salmon and salad on a bagel
- leftover pasta with lots of cooked vegetables

- quiche and salad
- cheese and salad on rye bread
- boiled egg and salad on multigrain bread with a smear of mayonnaise
- ham, cheese and spinach wrap
- cold cooked lean meat, salad and cheese quesadillas
- chicken with avocado and salad in a grainy bread roll
- beef, tomato and lettuce on sourdough bread with tomato chutney or salsa
- tuna, cheese and avocado wrap

What should I eat when I am out with my friends?

What your friends do can influence what you do and it can make a difference to your weight, mostly because you are more likely to do and eat the same things as them.

When you're out with your friends, going to a movie or sitting in front of the TV, it's easy to fall into the habit of eating, even when you're not hungry. Lots of us eat simply because it's time to, or because our friends are, or because we're used to doing it in certain situations, like buying popcorn at the movies. This is called non-hungry eating. If you are trying to watch your weight, here are some ways you can reduce your non-hungry eating:

- Share snack foods with your friends.
- Share entrees or desserts when eating out.
- Order an entree serve for your main course.
- Order a small popcorn or bring your own plain popcorn to the movies.
- Look for foods that are grilled, steamed or baked, not fried.
- If you are full, stop eating. You don't have to eat everything on your plate.
- Sit down to eat. Don't get distracted doing other things like playing on the computer, watching TV or reading.
- Drink water instead of sweet drinks such as cordial, soft drink or fruit juice.
- If you choose to drink alcohol, alternate it with water or plain mineral water, but remember that it is not recommended for anyone under 18 to drink alcohol as it affects brain development.

Eating in stressful situations

Stressful situations such as exams, competitive sports, relationship diffi-culties and mood swings can be difficult. It is often these times when you skip meals or overeat.

Eating for study

When at school or studying, your brain needs extra energy. Eating healthy foods is also linked to better concentration. Here are some tips for eating healthier when studying and during exams:

- Eat small, frequent meals to keep your blood sugar levels stable. Low blood sugar can leave you feeling light-headed and prone to losing concentration easily.

- Easy and convenient nutritious meals include frozen dinners, tinned soups, peanut-butter sandwiches, breakfast cereal, cheese sandwiches, tuna or chicken and salad sandwiches, baked beans or eggs on toast.

- Choose your snack foods carefully – snacks such as chips and savoury biscuits can be very high in fat and salt, while sugary snacks such as lollies and chocolate can send your blood sugar shooting up and crashing down, leaving you feeling grumpy, irritable and low in energy. Try healthier snacks such as yoghurt, nuts, dried fruit, fresh fruit, plain popcorn or vegie sticks with dip.

- People use caffeine for a pick-me-up, to feel more awake or alert. Too much caffeine from coffee, tea, cola and energy drinks can disrupt your sleeping patterns, send your heart racing, make it difficult to focus and/or cause nervousness in some people. Try sticking to one or two cups of coffee or tea a day, or try decaffeinated coffee or herbal teas as an alternative. Enjoy cola or energy drinks only occasionally as they have too much sugar and little nutritional benefit.

- Drink plenty of water. Thirst can be confused with hunger. When you are dehydrated you can feel tired.

- Eat only when you are hungry. Be aware of your hunger signals, like stomach pangs, grumbling guts, dry mouth, and so on. If you are not hungry, do you need a study break, are you trying to waste time, or are you feeling stressed? Instead of grabbing food, try a drink of water or go for a walk.

- Regular exercise helps improve your blood circulation, which keeps oxygen and nutrients flowing to your body and brain, helping you concentrate better.

Eating for play

Eating good foods before exercise can help boost stamina and endurance. Look for foods that contain carbohydrates and some protein and are low in fat, such as:

- breakfast cereal with milk and fruit
- dried fruit and nuts
- yoghurt and fruit
- an English muffin with peanut butter and honey
- a banana and peanut-butter sandwich
- a fresh fruit smoothie with milk and/or yoghurt
- a low-fat muesli bar
- small muffins made with oats or wholemeal flour and fruit or vegetables
- low-fat custard and fruit
- raisin toast and cream cheese
- sushi hand rolls
- fruit scones
- trail mix with dried fruit, nuts, seeds and some choc chips

Achieving a healthy weight

Food gives our bodies energy. When we eat too much food, there is too much energy and the body stores this as fat. Being careful about how much food we eat and how many sweet drinks we drink can help us maintain a healthy weight.

It is easy to grab biscuits, potato chips, cakes, sausage rolls, pies, doughnuts or chocolate bars when you're hungry, but regularly choosing those foods will make it easier to stack on the weight. Enjoy these kinds of convenience foods, and takeaway and fried foods occasionally only.

Instead of ...	Try this ...
Chocolate bar (50 g)	Low-fat chocolate milk (250 ml)
Lollies	Dried fruit
Large latte or cappuccino	Small latte or cappuccino
Ice-cream	Low-fat frozen yoghurt or sorbet

Instead of ...	Try this ...
High-sugar breakfast cereal	High-fibre breakfast cereal, e.g. Weet-Bix or All Bran
Hot chips	Baked potato
Large soft drink	Small soft drink, diet soft drink or water with lemon or lime
Chicken schnitzel	Barbecue or roast chicken
Burger meal deal	Burger and water, or small soft drink or diet drink
Doughnut	Fruit scone
Fried egg and bacon sandwich	Poached egg and ham in an English muffin

Other things to look out for are drinks with lots of sugar, such as fruit juice, cordial, soft drinks and energy drinks.

250 ml drink	Each teaspoon is equal to 5 g sugar
Low-fat milk	🥄🥄🥄
Sports drink	🥄🥄🥄🥄 (3½)
Orange juice	🥄🥄🥄🥄
Iced tea	🥄🥄🥄🥄
Diluted cordial	🥄🥄🥄🥄 (4½)
Cola	🥄🥄🥄🥄🥄
Energy drink	🥄🥄🥄🥄🥄

Moving around lets your muscles burn the extra energy you eat and helps you stay within your healthy weight range. You can get active by joining a sports club, going for a walk or a swim, going dancing or dancing in your room, throwing a frisbee, kicking a ball around, or even doing some housework.

Australian Dietary Guidelines for girls aged 14–18

Food group	Vitamins and minerals	Number of serves per day	Example of a serve
Breads and cereals	B vitamins Magnesium Zinc Fibre	7	1 slice of bread ½ medium roll or flat bread ½ cup cooked rice, pasta or noodles ½ cup cooked porridge or polenta ⅔ cup breakfast cereal flakes ¼ cup muesli 3 crispbreads 1 crumpet, English muffin or scone ½ cup cooked barley, buckwheat, semolina, polenta or quinoa
Fruit and vegetables	Fibre Folic acid or folate Beta-carotene Vitamin C Magnesium Potassium	2 fruit 5 vegetables	1 piece fruit, e.g. apple, banana, orange 2 pieces small fruit, e.g. apricots, kiwifruit, plums 1 cup diced, cooked or canned fruit ½ cup 100% fruit juice 30 g dried fruit ½ cup cooked vegetables 1 cup raw vegetables 1 small potato

Food group	Vitamins and minerals	Number of serves per day	Example of a serve
Meat, eggs, nuts and legumes and pulses	Protein Iron Zinc Vitamin B12	2½	½ cup of lean mince 2 small chops 2 slices of roast meat 1 small can of fish 2 eggs 1 cup cooked dried beans, lentils, chickpeas, split peas or canned beans 170 g tofu 30 g nuts or seeds or nut or seed paste (e.g. peanut butter)
Dairy foods	Protein Calcium Magnesium Zinc Potassium	3½	250 ml (1 cup) milk 200 g yoghurt 40 g (2 slices) hard cheese (e.g. cheddar) 120 g ricotta cheese
Oils and fats	Vitamin A Vitamin D Vitamin E Vitamin K	Use in small amounts	Vegetable oils Margarine spreads Butter

The importance of physical activity

Physical activity is important throughout our lives. As an adolescent, particularly in the middle years of adolescence, there may be times when you feel very active and other times when you feel particularly lethargic. It is quite common for teenage girls to drop out of organised sport, which can impact on their activity levels into their adulthood. So why is activity so important?

Physical activity helps to:

- maintain normal weight for age by increasing the proportion of lean body tissue to fat
- develop healthy internal organs by decreasing the amount of fat that surrounds them
- stimulate growth and repair of tissues, including bone, by increasing circulation throughout the body

Bone health

Bone growth and bone density (how solid or dense your bones are) are also stimulated by exercise. Most of us don't really think about our bone health in our teenage years, but it is an important thing to be aware of. Because our bone density declines after menopause, the higher the bone density we achieve in adolescence and young adulthood, the lower our risk of having thin, or chalky bones (osteoporosis), and bone fractures in later life. Many people do not know they have low bone density until they have a fracture, often from a minor knock or fall.

Around 60–80 per cent of our peak bone density is determined by our genes; the rest comes from our lifestyle. The critical factors in a woman's lifestyle that stimulate bone growth are:

- weight-bearing exercise
- good nutrition, which includes adequate calcium and vitamin D (see chapter 31 for more on vitamin D)
- not smoking
- low alcohol consumption
- the hormone oestrogen

The best period of life to stimulate bone growth is a narrow critical period around puberty. Around 60 per cent of our bone density is gained between the ages of 10 and 14. Exercise during childhood and adolescence produces much higher gains in bone density than does exercise in adulthood. Even moderate levels of exercise (30 minutes of weight-bearing exercise and muscle strengthening, three times per week) during adolescence can produce a 10 per cent increase in bone density. This amount of exercise is enough to halve the risk of fracture if continued into adult life.

How to look after your bone health
There are a couple of easy ways for you to look after the health of your bones in your teenage years.

1. Participate in a variety of high-impact activities. Bone growth is stimulated by engaging in a variety of activities rather than repeating the same exercise. This means you should try to participate in many different activities during your school years, such as running, skipping, gymnastics or ballet, throwing sports, basketball and netball, tennis and other bat and ball games, trampolining and dancing.
2. Decrease 'sitting time' to two hours outside of school or work time. Avoid long periods at the computer or watching TV during these critical years. Reducing sitting time has positive effects on bone health in particular, and also on general health.

Medical conditions related to bone health

Female athlete triad

Too much exercise in female adolescents can lead to problems when the exercise intensity is enough to cause menstruation to cease. This condition is called the female athlete triad. The three main symptoms are amenorrhoea (no periods) or oligomenorrhoea (irregular periods), low bone density and eating disorders.

In competitive teenage athletes, this triad can lead to lifelong serious health disorders such as low fertility, low oestrogen circulating in the body, which affects the long-term health of many internal organs, and irreversible low bone density. Treatment for this condition must be a team approach and involves education about the lifelong effects of low energy intake and no menstruation, taking hormonal medication such as the oral contraceptive pill, and addressing the obsessive component of highly competitive athletes.

Polycystic ovarian syndrome (PCOS)

PCOS is often diagnosed in late adolescence and is associated with irregular or no menstrual cycles, infertility, acne and obesity. While this is a disease of unknown cause, it is known to have long-term health risks related to high blood sugar and the risk of developing type 2 diabetes. The Australian guidelines for the management of PCOS state that lifestyle change should be the first form of therapy, with the aim of losing around 5 per cent of body weight. For more on PCOS, see chapter 24.

How to become more active

Most children and adolescents are naturally active. Encouraging this natural love of physical activity may establish good habits for life and avoid conditions arising from a sedentary lifestyle, such as obesity and type 2 diabetes. Children also learn by example, so family activity patterns play a part in children's long-term health. When girls become teenagers, their physical activity levels drop for many reasons, so at this time your parents and school should provide ongoing support and encouragement for you to remain physically active.

For many people, obesity and type 2 diabetes can be prevented by lifestyle choices, begun early and sustained throughout adulthood. The guidelines are simple – 60 minutes of moderately intense physical activity per day – but this is often not so easy to attain. Most people know that being physically active and eating healthily are the right things to do, but they just can't make the choices needed. This is partly due to the abundance of food available, providing the temptation to overeat, but also because it is easier not to exercise than to make the time to go out and be active.

Here are some ways to help you achieve the recommended physical activity levels:

- Increase incidental exercise – climb the stairs instead of taking the lift, walk or cycle to work or school, walk the dog each day, go to the beach with friends (but don't forget to 'slip, slop, slap, seek and slide') rather than to the movies.
- Use a pedometer and aim for 10,000 steps per day.
- Set exercise goals (maybe to enter a fun run or a walk) and keep a diary of your physical activity.
- Ask for support from your family or a good friend to help you achieve your exercise goals, or join a group of people who exercise together.
- Be regular with your exercise; don't give up on the first cold or wet day. Rug up and keep to your schedule.
- Truthfully examine your excuses to avoid activity – are they real?
- Choose activities you like and will continue with.

One final word about food and exercise: remember that the choices you make in your teenage years can affect your health for the rest of your life, so it helps to find someone you can talk with honestly about these choices and who can help you with them. Even when you have chosen healthy options, there will be times when you feel like flopping on the couch, or are stressed with exams or the break-up of a relationship. That's when you need your friends, family or mentor to help you get back on track. As long as there are more ups than downs, your teenage years will be healthy.

Activity recommendations for teenage girls

- A *minimum* of 60 minutes per day, which can be spread through the day.
- Activity level: moderate to intense, enough to feel moderately puffed-out and sweaty.
- Limit TV and computer time to two hours per day outside of school or work.

Sleep

The amount of sleep needed varies from person to person and depends on various factors – especially age. Most healthy adults need between seven and nine hours of uninterrupted sleep per night to function at their best.

Factors that may affect how many hours of sleep you need include the following:

- **Age** – one of the most important factors. As the table below shows, children and teenagers need more sleep than adults, between eight and 11 hours each night. In addition, there is evidence that around the time of becoming a teenager, there is a shift in the sleep–wake cycle, making you sleepy later in the evening with a preference for waking later. Despite the notion that our sleep needs decrease with age, the requirement for sleep remains constant throughout adulthood. Ageing affects the quality and quantity of sleep in older adults, and on average they get up to one hour less sleep than younger adults. While older people generally do not have problems getting to sleep, they may have difficulty staying asleep or going back to sleep when they wake up.

Age group	Recommended amount of sleep
Infants	14–15 hours
Toddlers	12–14 hours
Children	10–11 hours
Teenagers	8–10 hours
Adults	7–9 hours

- **Pregnancy** – during which women generally need more sleep, typically 8–10 hours a night.
- **Sleep deprivation** – for example, after a run of late nights and early mornings, shift work or a new baby – after which the best way to recover is increased sleep. Sleep deprivation is usually not a problem for teenagers, but can be severe for young mothers.
- **Sleep quality** – which is just as important as the amount of sleep you get. Sleep quality is affected by how restful it is and how often it is interrupted. Caffeine intake, alcohol, medications, stress and illness are some of the factors that affect sleep quality.
- **Genetic variation** – which can influence sleep requirements and timing.

- **Other** – such as cultural, environmental and behavioural factors that influence when and how much we sleep. For example, many people living in hot climates have an afternoon siesta to avoid activities in the midday sun, and consequently sleep for shorter times at night. The amount of sleep people obtain may also be affected by medical disorders and medicines.

Technology and sleep

Many young people go off to bed with an electronic device. There are a couple of reasons why this might not be a good idea. There is some evidence (though the jury is still out) that the back lighting on your device might affect your ability to fall asleep. Even more worrying, though, is the fact that adolescents enjoy the freedom of being able to contact their friends or check in with their peers throughout the night, which can play havoc with your sleep cycle. Even if you are woken only momentarily by the sound of a text message or an email arriving, it can be enough to break the cycle and deprive you of the sleep you need. Young people often use the excuse that they need their device as an alarm clock, but there are much better and cheaper clocks that let you sleep until morning – try it, and you'll feel a whole lot better.

Your skin

Your skin is your largest organ and one of the most important parts of your body. It protects you against injury and infection, helps control your temperature and water loss and is involved in producing vitamin D. Skin has a variety of nerve endings that respond to heat and cold, touch, pressure, vibration and injury. Different parts of your skin have different concentrations of these nerve endings, which is why a burn on your fingertips hurts more than the same burn on your back. The thickness of skin also varies in different parts of the body, with the thickest skin on the palms of the hands and the soles of the feet, and the thinnest skin around the eyes. This is why around the eyes is one of the first areas to show signs of ageing, such as crow's feet and wrinkles.

Importantly, your skin is a reflection of what's going on inside your body and what you have been exposed to, and therefore contributes a lot to the way you look. Healthy skin is an important part of and reflection of a healthy you, and there is a lot you can do to keep your skin healthy and looking good. Remember, a healthy body, mind and skin are all part and parcel of the same thing – a healthy you!

Sun damage

The colour of your skin is mainly due to the presence of melanin, a pigment (or colour) produced by cells in your skin. Melanin is also largely responsible for your eye and hair colour. People with naturally darker skin have more melanin in these skin cells. The production of melanin can also be stimulated by the sun's ultraviolet (UV) rays and by artificial UV rays (e.g. in a solarium) – that is, by tanning.

Melanin is the body's natural defence against the sun. It protects your skin cells against much of the potential damage of the sun, as it is good at absorbing the sun's harmful UV radiation and changing it to heat. While some sun exposure is good for you as it assists in the production of vitamin D, too much sun exposure is bad for you as it can result in damage to the DNA in skin cells, causing skin cancers and contributing to premature ageing of the skin.

The amount of sun exposure you should aim for in order to produce sufficient vitamin D yet not damage your skin depends on where you live, the season and your skin. The UV Index is an international standard measurement of the strength of UV radiation from the sun at a particular place on a particular day. UV levels are lower in the early morning as the sun comes up, gradually increase to a peak around the middle of the day when the sun is at its highest, and then decrease slowly as the sun gets lower in the sky.

To avoid damage, most Australians need sun protection when the UV Index is three or above. The UV level on a particular day can be found in most newspapers and on weather websites.

Solariums are never safe. Several Australian states have recognised this and are in the process of banning solariums, with more likely to follow.

Skin may show evidence of damage from exposure to UV radiation (from both sun or solarium), in any of the following ways:

- uneven and mottled pigmentation. This occurs when the body produces either too much or too little melanin or does so in an uneven way. Skin appears either lighter or darker than normal, and there may be blotchy, uneven areas, patches of brown, or yellow to grey discolouration.

- freckles

- skin thickening

- destruction of collagen and elastin fibres in the skin, causing lines, wrinkles, decreased elasticity and decreased skin strength

- capillary damage: dilation and damage to the small blood vessels under the skin
- mutations and toxicity in skin-cell DNA, which can lead to skin cancer and benign tumours

It makes sense that all of the above are more common in the most unprotected sun-exposed areas of the body, such as the back of the hands, forearms, chest and face. Although some of these sun effects may not be visible when you are young, they will become obvious as you age if you have had too much sun exposure.

Sunburn

Sunburn is a skin burn resulting from exposure to too much ultraviolet (UV) radiation, which damages the skin's cells. It can occur in less than 15 minutes, although the sunburn is often not immediately obvious.

After the exposure, skin may turn red and hot to the touch in as little as 30 minutes, but most often takes two to six hours, with pain usually at its worst six to 48 hours after exposure. The burn continues to develop for 24–72 hours, sometimes followed by peeling skin three to eight days later. Peeling and itching may continue for several weeks.

Extreme sunburn can be painful to the point of debilitation; pain and tenderness can make it difficult to move the affected area, to sleep and to function normally. Severe sunburn may also be associated with dehydration and being very unwell, occasionally requiring hospital care. In extreme cases it can be life-threatening.

Treatment for sunburn

The most important aspects of sunburn care are to avoid exposure of the affected area to the sun while it is healing and to prevent future burns. The best treatment for most sunburn is time: most sunburns heal completely within a few weeks.

Home treatments that help manage the pain or assist the healing process include cooling the area (placing wet cloths on the sunburnt areas, and taking frequent cold showers or baths), applying soothing lotions that contain aloe vera to the sunburnt areas and drinking lots of water.

Steroid creams (such as 1 per cent hydrocortisone cream) may also help with sunburn pain and swelling, and non-steroidal anti-inflammatory drugs (e.g. ibuprofen) may reduce the pain. There are also over-the-counter creams that may relieve the itching.

Interestingly, diet may influence both susceptibility and recovery from sunburn, with foods containing Vitamin C, E and A perhaps being beneficial.

Keeping your skin healthy

There is much you can do to keep your skin healthy. Good skin care and healthy lifestyle choices can help prevent various skin problems and delay the natural ageing process. You should do the following.

Protect yourself from the sun

One of the most important ways to take care of your skin is to protect it from the sun. A lifetime of sun exposure can cause wrinkles, age spots and other skin problems, as well as increasing the risk of skin cancer.

For sun protection, follow the advice of the Cancer Council: 'Slip, slop, slap, seek and slide'.

- *Slip* on some sun-protective clothing that covers as much skin as possible.
- *Slop* on broad-spectrum, water-resistant SPF30+ sunscreen. Put it on 20 minutes before you go outdoors and every two hours afterwards. Sunscreen should never be used to extend the time you spend in the sun.
- *Slap* on a hat. Choose one with a broad brim or legionnaire style to protect your face, head, neck and ears.
- *Seek* shade. Avoid the sun when the sun's rays are strongest.
- *Slide* on some sunglasses. Make sure they meet Australian standards.

Don't smoke

Smoking makes your skin look older and contributes to the development of wrinkles. It narrows the tiny blood vessels in the outermost layers of skin, which decreases blood flow. This reduces the amount of oxygen and nutrients reaching the skin. Smoking also damages the collagen and elastin fibres that give your skin its strength and elasticity. In addition, the repetitive facial expressions you make when smoking, such as pursing your lips and squinting your eyes to keep out smoke, can contribute to the development of wrinkles.

If you smoke, ask your GP for tips or treatments to help you quit. (See also chapter 11.)

Treat your skin gently

Daily cleansing can take a toll on your skin. Be gentle to your skin by:

- Limiting bath time. Hot water and long showers or baths remove oils from your skin. Limit your bath or shower time, and use warm, rather than hot water.

- Avoiding strong soaps. Use a mild, non-drying soap, and avoid scrubbing or repeated skin washing.

- Moisturising dry skin. If your skin is dry, use a moisturiser that fits your skin type. It doesn't need to be expensive. On sun-exposed areas, consider using a moisturiser that contains an SPF30+ sunscreen.

- Eating a healthy, balanced diet. Include plenty of fruits, vegetables, whole grains and lean proteins, and keep well hydrated.

- Maintaining a healthy body weight. Constantly gaining and losing weight is bad for your skin. When the skin frequently expands and contracts, it eventually loses its elasticity, which causes lines and wrinkles.

See also the information on page 100 about the relationship between diet and acne.

Manage stress

It's possible that stress may make your skin generally more sensitive and trigger acne breakouts and other skin problems. To encourage healthy skin – and a healthy mind – take steps to manage your stress in a positive way (see chapter 2).

Get enough sleep

During sleep, the time when most cellular repair and turnover occurs, collagen production in the skin seems to be accelerated. Collagen firms the skin and increases skin hydration. Conversely, lack of restful sleep suppresses the immune system, which can lead to skin-related problems such as rashes. Teenagers need between eight and 10 hours' sleep a night.

Exercise regularly

Exercise improves the circulation of blood, therefore increasing the delivery of oxygen and vital nutrients to your skin. This makes the skin better nourished and better able to repair itself, and increases the removal of harmful products.

Don't drink alcohol

Alcohol causes blood vessels to dilate, especially those small ones near the skin's surface, causing flushing and redness. After some time this can result in permanent facial redness. It also dehydrates the skin. It is strongly advised that people under the age of 18 should not drink any alcohol, as this can interfere with your growing brain. If you are 18 or over, only drink alcohol in moderation (see chapter 2).

Don't pick your pimples

Picking pimples can force bacteria deeper into the skin, causing greater inflammation, and can lead to scars and pigmentation.

Acne

Acne vulgaris (common acne or pimples) is the most common skin condition known, affecting about 85 per cent of people at some time between the ages of 13 and 20 and affecting people of all skin colours and types. It's also a problem for 5–10 per cent of adults and pre-teens.

It most commonly starts during adolescence, and for most people it diminishes over time and usually disappears, or at the very least substantially decreases by the age of 25. Some people, however, continue to get acne after this age, and it can develop for the first time at any age.

Acne mostly affects the skin that has the densest population of follicles. A follicle contains a hair and an oil gland (sebaceous gland), which produces oil (sebum) that helps remove old skin cells and keeps your skin soft. These areas include the face and shoulders, the upper part of the chest, and the back, but acne can also occur on the trunk, arms, legs and buttocks.

Acne is a general term for a number of skin problems, including seborrhoea (scaly red skin), comedones (blackheads and whiteheads), papules (small pimples), pustules (classic pimples), nodules (large papules and cysts), and sometimes scarring. Acne scars are the result of the body trying to heal an acne wound by putting too much collagen in one spot.

Aside from this occasional scarring, which is sometimes a different colour from the surrounding skin, acne's main effects are psychological, such as reduced self-esteem, and it can contribute to or cause depression, especially in young people. If this is the case for you, please talk to your parents and doctor.

What causes acne?

Acne occurs as a result of blockages in follicles. At puberty, in both genders, a normal increase in the level of hormones causes the sebaceous glands to increase and produce more sebum. Acne occurs when the pore becomes blocked with this sebum and with dead skin cells. The blockage is called a plug or comedo. If the top of the plug is white, it is called a whitehead. If the top of the plug is dark, it is called a blackhead. In these conditions, it is thought that the natural bacteria on our skin, which don't usually cause any problems, can cause inflammation, leading to papules, pustules, nodules and cysts. The process of acne development takes many weeks.

Why some people get acne, some don't and some get it worse than others is largely unknown. We do know that:

- Hormonal changes can trigger or worsen acne. This includes those that occur at puberty, during different parts of the menstrual cycle (acne is usually worse just before a period), during pregnancy, when taking some oral contraceptive pills, when suffering from polycystic ovarian syndrome or, more rarely, when there is an overproduction of hormones (e.g. Cushing's syndrome, where there is overproduction of steroids).

- Certain medicines can also worsen acne (such as steroids, testosterone, oestrogen, and the antiepileptic drug phenytoin).

- Acne tends to run in families, so there is a genetic component to it.

- Substances or conditions that increase the blocking of the pores can affect acne. These include greasy or oily cosmetics and hair products, and high levels of humidity and consequent sweating.

While the connection between acne and stress is not clear, it is likely that acne can be worsened by stress. This may in itself cause more stress and therefore can be self-perpetuating to some extent. If acne is being treated effectively, however, stress is not likely to have much impact for the majority of people.

The association between diet and acne isn't clear, although some research suggests that diets high in sugar, refined carbohydrates and other foods with a high glycaemic index (GI; i.e. that raise your blood sugar level quickly after eating) and milk may be related to worsening acne, while a diet rich in vitamin C and low in refined sugars, carbohydrates and other high-GI foods, and unhealthy fats might promote younger-looking skin.

There is no evidence from research that chocolate, nuts, salt or greasy foods cause acne. Foods that contain chocolate and salt are, however, often combined with other high-GI ingredients.

Acne treatment

Even without treatment, acne usually goes away after the teenage years, but it may last into midlife or appear for the first time during menopause, and there is no way to predict how long it will take to disappear entirely.

People have been treating acne since Egyptian times, and most care for acne is still self-care. As a comedo (pimple) takes so long to develop, acne usually takes six to eight weeks to respond well to treatment, and may still flare up from time to time.

Personal care
There are a number of steps you can take to look after your skin to avoid and/or treat acne:

- Clean your skin gently with a mild soap substitute (e.g. Cetaphil, QV Wash) once or twice a day, including after exercising, in order to reduce clogging of pores.
- Remove all dirt and make-up thoroughly. Look for water-based, oil-free or 'noncomedogenic' cleansers (they should have been tested and shown not to clog pores and/or cause acne).
- Keep your hair clean and out of your face.

There are also some things it's best not to do:

- Avoid scrubbing your skin or washing it repeatedly.
- Avoid touching your face with your hands or fingers.
- Do not squeeze, scratch, pick or rub pimples. Although it might be tempting, this can lead to skin infections and scars.
- Avoid wearing headbands, baseball caps and other hats that fit tightly, as this can cause rubbing of the skin of your forehead; oils can transfer from your skin and hair onto these surfaces and back to your skin.
- Avoid greasy cosmetics or creams.

A small amount of sun exposure may improve acne a little, but mostly it just hides the acne. Too much exposure to sunlight or UV rays is not recommended because it increases the risk of skin cancer and the risk of acne scars, and may worsen the side effects of acne treatments (see below).

Over-the-counter treatments
If the steps above do not control your acne sufficiently, you could try one of the many over-the-counter acne medications you apply directly to your skin. (If you suffer from allergies, be sure to check that the one you use will not cause any problems.) They act in a number of ways to help control your acne and include:

- **Keratolytics** (peeling agents or exfoliants) – salicylic acid preparations (e.g. Clearasil Pimple Cream and Pimple Clearing Cream, DermaVeen Acne Cleansing Bar) and sulfur-based treatments (sometimes made up by pharmacies when prescribed by doctors) act as keratolytics, unblocking pores and decreasing clogging of the follicle by promoting the shedding of skin cells. Sulfur also helps suppress the bacteria associated with acne.

- **Antibacterials** – benzoyl peroxide (e.g. Benzac AC Gel and Wash, Brevoxyl, Oxy, Clearasil Ultra) acts as both a keratolytic and an antibacterial by increasing the rate of removal of skin cells and suppressing the bacteria that contribute to acne. These products come in varying strengths (from 2.5–10 per cent), but, if too strong (usually greater than 5 per cent), they may cause redness or peeling of the skin. For this reason it is better to start with a lower strength; although stinging and skin redness may occur initially, it often settles. If applied at night, much of the redness caused by the treatment will have gone by morning. Also, during treatment, beware of too much sun exposure, and use sunscreen to prevent sunburn. Azelaic acid (e.g. Finacea) is another acne preparation that has both antibacterial and keratolytic properties. Like benzoyl peroxide, it can cause skin dryness and redness, especially at first. Tea-tree oil also acts as an effective antibacterial against acne-causing bacteria.

- **Antiseptic washes and bars** – some of these may also be helpful (e.g. Phisohex, Oxy Skin Wash, Sapoderm, Gamophen).

Some people find natural therapies useful, although the scientific evidence for their effectiveness varies. Options include: egg oil, which contains antioxidants and immunoglobulins, and may have antibacterial and anti-inflammatory properties; and fish oil tablets, aloe vera, turmeric, papaya, nicotinamide (vitamin B3) and zinc supplements, all of which may have combinations of antibacterial and anti-inflammatory properties.

Prescription medicines
If pimples are still a problem after several months, your acne is severe (e.g. you have a lot of redness around the pimples or you have cysts or scars) or getting worse, it's a good idea to visit your GP. If necessary, they can prescribe stronger medicine and discuss other options with you. Your GP may recommend stronger prescription formulas, combinations of over-the-counter medicines, or antibiotics (either topical, i.e. applied to the skin, or oral, i.e. taken by mouth).

Some of the medicines you might be prescribed are:

- **Antibiotics** – which both decrease the bacteria in the pores and can reduce inflammation. These can be topical or, in more severe cases, your doctor may recommend you take a course of antibiotics by mouth. The oral forms are reserved for more severe cases, since they are becoming less effective as a result of increased bacterial resistance. They are often used in combination with topical benzoyl peroxide and other over-the-counter acne medicines.

- **Retinoid creams** – tretinoin (Retin-A), adapalene (Differin) and isotretinoin (Isotrex) – a group of medicines related to vitamin A that influence cell development in the follicle lining, helping to prevent follicle blocking. They can cause significant irritation of the skin and often cause an initial flare-up of acne and facial flushing, which usually settles.

- **Hormones** – such as the oral contraceptive pill, which may help for women whose acne is caused or made worse by hormones. In some cases, though, it makes acne worse. It is usually a case of trial and error, as some pills sometimes have more effect than others.

- **Cosmetic procedures** – chemical skin peeling, removal of scars by dermabrasion, or removal, drainage or injection of cysts with cortisone or a laser procedure called photodynamic therapy.

If you have very bad acne that cannot be controlled or cystic acne, your GP may decide to refer you to a dermatologist, who may suggest trying an oral medicine called isotretinoin (e.g. Roaccutane, Accutane). This oral form of vitamin A is usually taken for four to six months, is generally very effective and can lead to long-term resolution or reduction of acne. Isotretinoin has many potential side effects, however, some of which are very serious, such as liver damage, and birth defects if you become pregnant while taking it. It therefore requires close medical supervision by a doctor and extremely effective contraception methods, as it is vital you do not become pregnant while taking it.

6

Periods

Catarina Ang, Melissa Cameron, Fiona Judd

Getting their period is a sign for many girls that they are finally growing up. Periods are something every girl has, although the age at which they start varies.

In the months before the start of your periods you may notice an increase in vaginal discharge or mucus. This discharge is normally clear or white in colour. It is not particularly smelly and should not be associated with any itch. It is a sign that your hormones are active and are encouraging the ovaries to begin releasing eggs.

Your periods won't start until you have experienced some other signs of puberty, such as breast development and the growth of pubic hair (see chapter 4). The whole purpose of having a period is tied to reproduction and having babies, because a period indicates that you have started to ovulate. The process of ovulation is covered more thoroughly in chapter 15. In short, it is the process of the ovary releasing an egg so it is ready to be fertilised by sperm so that you become pregnant. As this is a pretty special stage of a girl's life, it has a special name – menarche – just as when periods stop, there is also a special name – menopause (see chapter 33).

Where do periods come from and why do we have to have them?

Your period is also known as your menstrual cycle, menstruation or menses. During your menstrual cycle, an egg within one of your ovaries matures and is released into the fallopian tube. At the same time the lining of the uterus, or womb, is growing to prepare for a possible pregnancy. If the egg is not fertilised by sperm there will be no pregnancy, so your endometrium, or the lining of the uterus, breaks down and the blood and fluid come out of the uterus, through the cervix, and out the vagina.

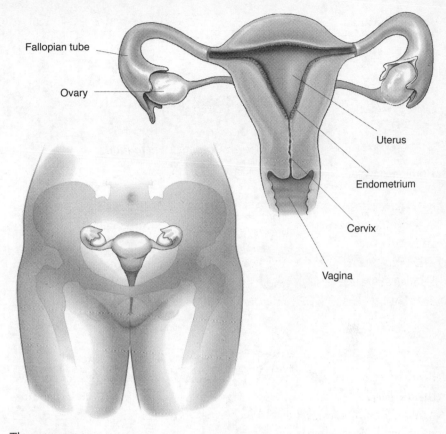

Fallopian tube

Ovary

Uterus

Endometrium

Cervix

Vagina

The uterus

Any abnormalities in the anatomy of any of these parts can delay the onset of periods (see chapter 28). If this is the case for you, it may be something you will need to discuss with your doctor.

Your periods occur approximately once a month. The timing is regulated by your ovaries talking to two other glands in your body called the hypothalamus and the pituitary gland. The monthly cycle is divided into different phases that describe what's happening at that particular stage. You can consider the menstrual cycle from the perspective of the ovary or from the endometrium, the lining of the uterus or womb.

The ovary has four phases: the phase before you ovulate, ovulation, the phase after ovulation has happened, and menstruation – your period. The phase before ovulation is called the follicular phase. The ovary's hormones increase and make the ovary concentrate on developing little cysts or follicles. Eventually, the ovary favours one follicle, and that is the one that is chosen to release the egg (ovulate). After that happens,

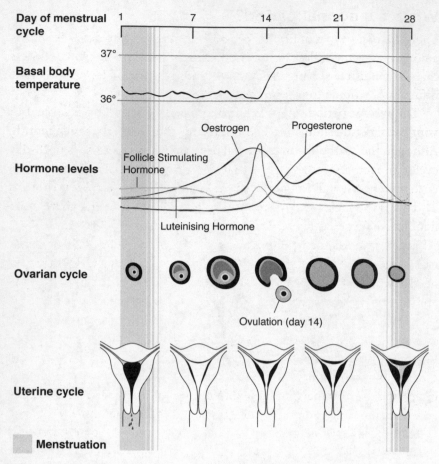

Day of menstrual cycle

Basal body temperature

Hormone levels

Oestrogen

Progesterone

Follicle Stimulating Hormone

Luteinising Hormone

Ovarian cycle

Ovulation (day 14)

Uterine cycle

Menstruation

Menstrual cycle

that follicle is given a special name, corpus luteum. The corpus luteum produces the hormones that support your pregnancy very early on if you do conceive. The phase after ovulation is called the luteal phase.

From the viewpoint of the endometrium, if you do not conceive and get pregnant, then the corpus luteum will essentially disintegrate and be absorbed into the body, triggering many internal signals that result in you getting your period.

After all the bleeding has stopped, the endometrium has to build up again. This is known as the proliferative phase, and it matches the ovary's follicular phase. The endometrium builds up until ovulation occurs, then it prepares itself for a potential conception. This is known as the secretory phase. It you don't conceive, then a series of signals between your ovary and your endometrium tells your body it's time to start the period again.

What is a normal period?

There are many types of normal period, so it is difficult to describe what is a normal amount of flow for a period. It used to be said that anything less than 80 millilitres was normal, but the amount of blood lost can be quite difficult for women to measure precisely.

The average period can be as short as two days or as long as seven, but your usual period should last about the same number of days each month. Although the 'textbook' time interval between periods is 28 days (a 28-day cycle), in fact, research suggests that only 15 per cent of women experience this cycle length in their lifetime. Your usual cycle can be as short as 21 days or as long as 35 days and still be normal. Some women have quite light bleeding, and others have quite heavy bleeding.

Every now and then, your period might come earlier or later, it might end sooner or later or it might be lighter or heavier than usual. There's no need to worry about occasional changes in your periods. The most important thing is to be aware of your usual periods and speak to your doctor if they change dramatically or something seems particularly unusual.

When you first start having periods, it is quite common for them to be irregular for the first couple of years as your brain and ovaries are still establishing connections. These cycles are often referred to as anovulatory cycles because you may not be ovulating in all of them, and your ovaries and brain are not yet doing a good job of regulating your cycle.

The period flow is made up of blood, some mucus, some water and other cells. So it is like passing a thick, bright blood that usually starts light, then becomes heavier. After that, it again becomes lighter and brownish as it finishes. You may even see little pieces of the endometrium. Occasionally clots (lumpy collections of blood) are passed. This is quite normal, but if they are large and there are many of them, this can indicate that the bleeding is abnormally heavy. Women worry about the colour of their period blood becoming darker until it is almost black. The darker colour is simply a reflection of the length of time the menstrual flow has taken to come out of the vagina. As the flow slows down, it takes longer to pass through the vagina and is exposed to more oxygen. This is called oxidation. When this happens, the blood becomes darker, and so the slower and lighter the flow, the more time it spends getting oxidised.

Some women also worry that their flow stops and starts. They may say, for instance, that they have a heavy flow for the first couple of days, that it slows down on the third and fourth day to the point where they think their period is almost finished, but then it becomes heavy again for another day or so. Some women also have a very light loss of blood or spotting before their period begins. All of this is normal.

Cramps and pain

It is quite common to experience some pain with your period, such as a cramp in your belly and/or a mild backache, often on the first one to two days of the period. You may wish to take a simple painkiller from the chemist or supermarket if it bothers you. Some women say they know when their period is coming because their period pain starts before the period does. All of these symptoms are normal, too.

Premenstrual syndrome (PMS)

Many women will also experience other typical symptoms before their period. For instance, hormonal changes are very common before and during your period. You may feel quite moody, even teary, and your family may say your temper is particularly bad just before your period. The name for this is PMS or PMT, which stands for premenstrual syndrome or premenstrual tension. Some women suffer so badly from PMS that it stops them doing their usual activities or working. Skin changes are also very common before a period. You might notice you break out and have a few pimples before your period, even when you are no longer a teenager.

How do women manage their periods?

There are many different sanitary products (panty liners, pads and tampons) on the market – so many that sometimes it's difficult to know what to choose. Most women will use a combination of pads and tampons during their period. There are pros and cons to both.

Panty liners are thin, light pads. Some women choose to wear them to manage vaginal discharge, whereas others do not find them necessary. They are usually not absorbent enough to deal with menstrual blood unless the flow is very light.

Sanitary pads are designed to be used during menstruation. A pad or sanitary liner is a large strip of cotton or similar material that absorbs your menstrual flow. There are many different brands and types: regular, super (increased absorbency), long pads, light pads, pads for night-time (with increased absorbency and often longer), maternity pads (large pads to accommodate the increased flow that occurs after childbirth), pads with 'wings' to keep them in place on your underwear, and pads that come with individual wrapping. You should choose ones that you find comfortable to wear and that do the job for you.

Pads usually need to be changed every few hours. You will need to change them more frequently if your menstrual flow is heavier, or leakage will occur.

The advantages of pads are that they are very simple to use, easy to change, and quite easy to carry about, even in a small handbag. Women whose period can start unexpectedly can wear them just in case before their period actually starts. You can't wear them to go swimming, however, if you wear tight clothing they may show up as a lump, and some women find them uncomfortable when the pad starts to absorb more blood.

This is where the tampon comes in. The tampon is a thin cylinder of dense cotton or similar synthetic material attached to a string. You put it inside the vagina to absorb the menstrual flow before it comes out of the vagina. There are different sizes available for different levels of flow, and some come with plastic or cardboard applicators to make them easier to insert. The advantages of tampons are that they are completely hidden except for the string, which is usually very small. Many women find them more comfortable than pads, and you can go swimming while using them. You won't feel them at all if you have inserted them correctly. Many women like tampons because they are so invisible; they don't feel like they are having their period. The downside is that they can be hard to insert until you get used to it. It should not be painful to insert a tampon, and you do have to be comfortable with your own body and feeling yourself 'down there'. If you can put your finger into your vagina comfortably, you can definitely wear a tampon.

When you first start out using tampons you may find it easier to use the smallest (or mini) tampons. Try them on a day when your period is a little heavy, as they are easier to insert when there is more blood and therefore more lubrication. Always remember good hygiene and wash your hands before and after inserting the tampon. When inserting a tampon it is important to remember that the vagina is on an angle, pointing towards the coccyx (tailbone); it does not run straight up and down vertically. Place the tampon at the entrance to the vagina and insert it in the direction of your coccyx. Insert the tampon completely, so there is no tampon outside the vagina. If the tampon is in correctly, and far enough inside the vagina, you should not be able to feel it. You cannot lose a tampon in the vagina – the cervix (opening to the uterus) is too small to allow a tampon to pass any further. Once in place, the tampon

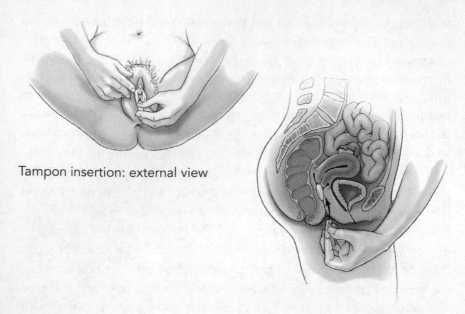

Tampon insertion: external view

Tampon insertion: side view

should not move. The string of the tampon sits outside of the vagina to allow for removal.

Some girls and their mothers worry about breaking the hymen when inserting a tampon, and whether or not they will still be virgins if they use them. The hymen is a section of tissue just at the entrance of the vagina. It is important to remember that it doesn't cover the vagina completely; otherwise, your period flow wouldn't be able to come out when you are a virgin. There is a condition called 'imperforate hymen', where a girl has a hymen that completely closes up the vagina, but this is not normal. Girls with this condition may wonder when their periods are going to start, especially if they are getting some cramps each month. These girls usually need a small operation to make a gap in their hymen.

When a girl first has intercourse, the hymen will often break and bleed, but a tampon won't break the hymen because it is quite stretchy. You are still a virgin if you have not had sexual intercourse. Even if you use tampons, or even if you have some operation or procedure where instruments had to be put in the vagina, you are still a virgin.

Tampons are even smaller than pads, and some are quite small. Even when your flow has just started and it is very light, you can carry them around and start using them. It is important to remember, though, that tampons, just like pads, should be changed regularly, even if they don't look or feel like they need changing. This is because of a condition called toxic shock syndrome, which can develop if you leave a tampon in too long and can make you very sick. Generally, it is recommended that you change your tampons every six to eight hours, and every three to four hours when your flow is heavy. Many women leave their tampons in overnight. If you are going to do so, insert a fresh tampon just before you go to bed and change it first thing in the morning. There are usually some other factors or problems that contribute to developing toxic shock syndrome, so don't worry if you slip up and forget by an hour once in a while.

Apart from that, there is very little you can't do when wearing a tampon. If you have a very heavy discharge, you may wish to use panty liners as well. You can even have sexual intercourse during your period, but remember to take your tampon out first. You can use tampons if you have an intrauterine contraceptive device (IUD) or a contraceptive vaginal ring. For more information on these contraceptives, see chapter 16.

Menstrual management kit

Although many women have regular and predictable periods, you may occasionally get a period when you least expect it. Or you may completely forget that it is due (there are several apps that can help you remember). You may find it handy to have an emergency kit stashed at school or work or in your handbag or schoolbag. This could contain:

- a few pads or tampons
- a spare pair of underpants
- some pain relief

What is an abnormal period?

To help you work out what is normal, it's easiest to describe what is definitely abnormal.

Heavy periods

During heavy menstrual bleeding, it is not normal to consistently:

- pass multiple large clots (larger than a 50-cent coin)
- have such a heavy flow that during the day you are having to change your pad or tampon every hour because it is getting soaked and perhaps staining your clothes

- have to get up more than once every night to change your pad or tampon, or to have to put a towel in your bed or use large maternity pads because the flow is so heavy

It is not normal to become low in iron levels because your periods are so heavy. Your blood contains traces of iron, which carries oxygen around your body. Your period flow also contains some blood (but it is not all blood), so if your periods are very, very heavy, you may lose more iron than your body can make up for. The symptoms of iron deficiency or having low iron stores include getting tired more easily and feeling weak. Some women's iron stores become so low due to heavy periods that they become anaemic. This means their blood count is low. Anaemic people might complain of feeling dizzy, being short of breath, or even having chest pain. Usually if a woman has been having heavy periods for a long time, though, she might not notice any of these symptoms and just feel tired. Of course, there are a lot of reasons to feel tired that have nothing to do with heavy periods, but if you have concerns, you should see your doctor.

Painful periods

Many women experience period pain at some time in their life. This often happens soon after you start getting your periods. Period pain is usually mild and goes away with simple measures like using hot packs or gentle painkillers. In many cases it improves over time. If you are experiencing pain that doesn't go away, gets worse or does not get better after taking pain relief, you should see a doctor for advice.

Period pain can result from the effects of many chemicals your body produces around the time of your period. These chemicals are commonly called prostaglandins (among others). Non-steroidal anti-inflammatory drugs (NSAIDs, such as aspirin, naproxen and ibuprofen) are effective at reducing these chemicals, and they work best if you take them as soon as the pain begins rather than waiting until the pain is at its worst. They work even better if you take them before a period actually arrives. As there are a number of NSAIDs, you might need to try a few before you find the one that suits you best.

Although a bit of period pain is normal, it is not normal to have such bad period pain that you have to take time off work or study, that it wakes you up at night, that you need to go to the emergency department at your local hospital, or that you have to take painkillers regularly during the day to be able to do your job. See chapter 15 for more information.

Unusual bleeding

It is generally not normal to have bleeding between your periods, unless you are using some sort of hormonal contraception or other hormones. This is called intermenstrual bleeding, whether it happens randomly between your periods or at the same time of the cycle between periods. Occasionally a woman gets thoroughly tested and the doctor cannot find anything wrong; if the bleeding is something new, however, you should have it checked out.

Sometimes women start bleeding between periods when they are using some sort of hormone. This may be the combined oral contraceptive pill, the minipill, the contraceptive implant that goes into your arm, a contraceptive vaginal ring, or an intrauterine contraceptive device. Your doctor may call this 'breakthrough bleeding'. The period you have when you are using the combined oral contraceptive pill isn't a true period. It is called a 'withdrawal bleed' because it usually happens when you withdraw or stop taking the active pills in your packet of contraceptives. For more information on contraception, see chapter 16. Whatever form it takes, if you have bleeding between your periods for more than three to six months, you should see your doctor.

Importantly, if you have bleeding that is so heavy that you are starting to feel weak, dizzy or short of breath, you should see a doctor immediately or go to the emergency department of your nearest hospital.

It is not normal to have ongoing problems with bleeding after sexual intercourse. This is called post-coital bleeding or PCB, and should be investigated by your doctor. You can ignore a one-off episode, but sometimes bleeding after sex is a sign that something needs to be checked. For instance, we know that women with PCB who have had normal Pap tests have a 10–15 per cent chance of an abnormality in their cervix when they are tested further.

Late periods

There are many causes for late periods. If you are sexually active, it is very important to make sure it's not because you are pregnant, even if you are using contraception. Other potential causes for late periods include stress, medications, changes in diet, weight or lifestyle, and various illnesses.

It is uncommon for your periods not to come back straight after stopping the Pill, but your periods can be delayed or quite irregular for several months after stopping the Depo Provera contraceptive injection. It is normal to have no periods or infrequent and irregular periods when using a hormonal intrauterine contraceptive device.

Irregular periods

It is not normal to have very infrequent periods. This is called oligomen-orrhoea. Occasionally a woman might have regular periods that are six weeks apart. If this is the case, you should see a doctor to have it checked. Women with a condition called polycystic ovarian syndrome (PCOS) often have infrequent and irregular periods (see chapter 24).

It can also be abnormal to have irregular periods. This can happen to women in their 30s and 40s, and it may only be a matter of a few days' difference. If your periods have been more irregular than a few days, let's say seven days' difference, for three to six months, you should see your doctor for a check-up.

Sometimes you can experience abnormal periods for a couple of cycles and then go back to normal. Sometimes the symptoms make you particularly anxious or are particularly severe. You can always go to see your doctor if that happens. They will send you to a specialist gynaecologist or gynaecology clinic if that's what they think you need.

If you used to have normal periods and then they stopped for more than six months, you should go and see your doctor. This is called secondary amenorrhoea. If you have never had your period and you are aged 16 or more, it is worthwhile going to see your doctor to be checked. Some women can be very late to start, but there are other medical reasons for this that can be treated or fixed.

Don't forget that if you have had a sexual encounter in which sperm might have reached the vagina, there is also the possibility that you could be pregnant. See chapter 7 for more information.

When should I see a doctor?

It is difficult to say in exactly what circumstances you should see your doctor about your periods, as it depends on the symptoms and the condition. You should see your doctor sooner rather than later if you have experienced any of the problems described above and any of the following apply:

- you have had the same problem before
- you have other medical problems such as diabetes, previous cancers, a thyroid condition, or are very overweight
- you take any medications that thin your blood or make you more likely to bleed

If you consult your doctor about an issue with your periods, they may want to perform a pelvic examination. You may also need a Pap test or an examination with a speculum. A speculum is a metal or plastic device the doctor inserts gently into the vagina and opens up so they can get a better look at the cervix and the vagina.

Typical initial tests your doctor will ask you to do include blood tests and an ultrasound. The blood tests may look at your blood count, your iron stores, and your levels of vitamins such as folic acid or vitamin B12. Sometimes your doctor will ask for hormonal blood tests.

The pelvic ultrasound is a very common test to have. It is quite simple, doesn't hurt, and enables your doctor to obtain an image of your uterus and ovaries. In an ultrasound, radio signals are aimed at your lower abdomen, and variations in strength of the signals that bounce back make a black-and-white image of your uterus and ovaries. If you have not been sexually active before, the scanner, called the probe, is placed on your tummy. If you have been sexually active, the scanner is placed inside your vagina. This can obtain even better imaging since it is placed much closer to your reproductive organs. There is no radiation or needles involved. Common important things that might be found in an ultrasound are fibroids, polyps, adenomyosis, ovarian cysts, polycystic ovaries, thickened endometrium and pregnancy.

For more on abnormal periods, see chapter 15.

Period-related mood disorders

Premenstrual mood changes are very common. These feelings range from mild and brief feelings of depression lasting for a day or two before the onset of your period to a more clearly defined premenstrual syndrome (PMS) and the less common and more severe premenstrual dysphoric disorder (PMDD).

Premenstrual disorders (PMDs) are characterised by a mix of physical and psychological symptoms that recur regularly in the luteal phase of the menstrual cycle, typically a week or so before menstruation, and resolve (disappear) during or shortly after menstruation. This is followed by a clear symptom-free period between the end of menstruation and the approximate time of ovulation. Up to 90 per cent of women experience normal physiological premenstrual symptoms. In addition, 30–40 per cent of women experience more severe symptoms that interfere with daily functioning; these are known as premenstrual syndrome (PMS).

Premenstrual syndrome (PMS)

The most common symptoms of PMS are emotional and behavioural irritability; moodiness; a depressed mood; anxiety; impulsiveness; feelings of loss of control; an inability to concentrate; and physical symptoms such as bloating, breast swelling and tenderness, and general aches.

Mild symptoms are common but do not cause major interference with day-to-day activities and function. If you experience the more severe symptoms of PMS, however, your social and work performance is likely to be significantly impaired, with reduced productivity at work, high rates of absenteeism, and an inability to participate in family and social activities and hobbies.

The symptoms of PMS usually start from the onset of your periods and, despite their interference in daily life, they are tolerated by many women for years before they seek help. This usually occurs when they also experience heavy or irregular menstrual bleeding or pelvic pain, or at a time of great stress or difficulty in their lives. If you do experience cyclic symptoms related to your period, ask your GP about PMS. Often simple things such as starting or changing the oral contraceptive you take can help.

Premenstrual dysphoric disorder (PMDD)

PMDD occurs in up to 8 per cent of women. This disorder is at the severe end of the spectrum of premenstrual disorders, and can be debilitating. Women with PMDD suffer from mental symptoms, not only physical complaints, and the condition is of such severity that it interferes significantly with their work or study, their usual social activities, and their relationships with others.

PMS and PMDD both occur only if you are ovulating, and are thought to be due to an abnormal response to a normal hormonal environment. If your doctor thinks you might be suffering from either of these conditions, they will ask you to keep a record of your daily symptoms across at least two menstrual cycles. This will involve you rating how you feel on a daily basis and noting when your period starts and stops. This record will be analysed to help make a diagnosis. Once the diagnosis is confirmed, there are a number of effective treatments available.

The most common treatment is one of the SSRI antidepressants (e.g. Sertraline) taken either during the luteal phase alone (the seven to 10 days before your period) or continuously. These medications increase the level of serotonin, a neurotransmitter in the brain, which affects the way your hormones influence your mood. This medication can reduce or stop the monthly mood changes. The medication is often taken for a period of approximately 12 months. Symptoms commonly return, however, and ongoing medication can be required. This medication is not addictive, has few side effects, and can be safely continued for a number of years if necessary.

Cognitive behaviour therapy, a structured psychological treatment, usually involving around 10 sessions with a clinical psychologist, is also commonly recommended for treatment of PMS and PMDD. This involves examining how your thoughts influence your emotions and behaviour, and changing your thinking style to improve your mental wellbeing.

The third common way of treating the symptoms of PMS and PMDD is hormonal therapies. This usually means you will be prescribed a particular type of oral contraceptive pill. Sometimes, if other therapies are not effective, your doctor may suggest a medication that will suppress ovulation. If your symptoms have not responded to an SSRI antidepressant, cognitive behaviour therapy or the oral contraceptive pill, ask for a referral to a specialist for advice on taking medication to suppress ovulation.

Other premenstrual disorders

In addition to these defined premenstrual disorders, many women find that a longstanding disorder such as anxiety or depression, or non-psychiatric disorders such as migraine and epilepsy, get worse before their period. (See chapter 15 for more information on menstrual headaches.) It is important to distinguish these from PMS and PMDD as the treatment should focus on the underlying psychiatric or medical problem rather than follow the course of treatments described above.

Rarely, premenstrual disorders may happen when women take tablets containing the hormone progesterone. This most often happens when a woman takes the combined oral contraceptive pill, which contains both oestrogen and progesterone. The only way to know if premenstrual syndromes are due to the progesterone is by trial and error – i.e. by excluding the progesterone and seeing if the symptoms disappear.

7
Sexuality in adolescents

Susan Carr, Maureen Johnson

Sexuality is a term used to describe a person's sexual identity, sexual orientation, and sexual knowledge, attitudes and behaviour. Your sexuality is an inherent part of you, from conception to the grave. Some aspects of your sexuality will change during your lifetime and others will not. Human sexuality describes an enormous spectrum of behaviours, identities and attitudes. There is no such thing as 'normal'; each individual is unique in their sexual life.

Your sexuality defines who you are and your sexual life. It will sometimes make you happy and sometimes sad. Understanding the different parts of your sexuality can help you cope with confusing feelings.

Sexual identity

Your sexual identity is who you are in relation to your gender: whether you feel you are male or female. About half the population is male and about half female. A tiny proportion of the population is transsexual, which means they feel as if they have been born into the wrong body. From as early as the age of four they identify as the opposite gender from their biological identity, and can suffer many confusing and unhappy years until they understand what is happening. Most people are aware of their sexual identity from birth; they know they are a boy or girl. This is knowledge that you carry throughout your life and accept as an integral part of who you are. Being male or female defines your anatomy and your reproductive expectations.

In some societies, particularly in the past, your sexual identity defined your role in society, with females frequently being assigned to traditional domestic roles. While these gender expectations still apply in some cultures and religions, for many modern societies, anything is possible for males and females.

Sexual orientation

Your sexual orientation defines to whom you are attracted sexually. This might be males, females, both or neither. The majority of people are heterosexual, feeling attraction to the opposite sex. Somewhere between 5 and 10 per cent of the total population are males who are sexually attracted to other men, generally known as homosexuals, and up to 2 per cent of the population are lesbian, that is women who are attracted to women. About 8 per cent of the population identify as bisexual; that is, they are attracted to both males and females.

Many young people struggle with coming to terms with their sexual orientation. It is quite natural to go through confusing phases of feeling different types of attraction to different people. It can be quite frightening to think you might be gay or lesbian, especially in some cultures where this is forbidden. Fortunately, there is now a lot of positive recognition of and pride in gay people in countries such as Australia, which may make it easier for you to acknowledge your sexual orientation openly, though many people still find it a difficult thing to come to terms with. Your sexual orientation is at least partially inborn, and it is accepted that your patterns of sexual attraction are probably set by the age of four.

Coming to terms with your sexual orientation

Sexual orientation begins to develop in childhood, when it is influenced by genetics and environmental factors, and becomes more established during adolescence. Sexual orientation can be both innate and fluid throughout life and includes the gender that one is attracted to and fantasises about, and with whom one ultimately engages in sexual relations.

It is very natural to have different forms of sexual feelings, particularly for adolescents. Sexuality is confusing, so allowing your feelings to form gradually without leaping into experimental relationships is best. As most people mature, their sexual orientation becomes clearer to them. All sexual orientations and identities are equally valid.

The most important thing is that through the journey to self-discovery, a young person should feel supported and able to discuss openly questions about their sexual orientation, and ultimately be able to express their sexuality without fear of harassment. It is well known that depression, substance abuse, social isolation, harassment and violence, suicidal thoughts and sexual risk-taking behaviour are all increased in lesbian, gay, bisexual and transgender (LGBT) youth compared to their heterosexual peers. This is largely due to lack of support and feelings of isolation.

As society becomes more educated and more tolerant, it is hoped that such experiences will become less common. It is important to know that there are many support groups with caring, experienced members, and health professionals who may assist during these times. See the Resources section at the end of this book for more information.

Sexual knowledge and attitudes

Sexual attitudes are generally shaped by the five Ps: parents, peer groups, publications, politics and professionals.

Where you are born, your parents and family, culture, religion and social circumstances will have a profound influence on your sexual attitudes. Some societies and some families are very open in discussion of sexual matters, and some are the opposite. Women from the most protected and loving backgrounds, for example, often find it hard to talk about sex because they have been so sheltered from it.

Peer groups are also enormously important in shaping your ideas of sex, and your friends might be very eager to pass on information – whether or not it is accurate. There is often great excitement and a sense of naughtiness about sex talk among teenagers, but there can also be pressure to have sex or to engage in risky sexual behaviour, which many young people are not ready for. Any form of taunting or bullying of a young woman with regard to sex can leave lasting negative sexual attitudes that can be hard to reverse. (See chapter 12 for more on bullying.)

The media and social media have an enormous impact on the sexual attitudes of the day. There is news about and information on sex from all over the globe, along with massive overexposure of individuals' intimate sexual lives, which makes it challenging for any young woman to find her own comfort level in the sexual world. While some degree of openness can be very positive, most people prefer some privacy when it comes to their sexual lives, and this is something everyone is entitled to.

Remember, the web is not private; it is a global space, so be very careful what you write and who you communicate with. Strangers on the web may try to trick you into sharing sexual information or meeting for sex. Please be very cautious, and tell someone if you become scared or suspicious.

Professional influence on sexual knowledge comes in the form of sex education in schools, the quality of which is enormously varied and inconsistent. Good, non-judgemental and well-taught sex education can form the basis for a safe, happy and healthy sexuality throughout your lifetime. It can also be good to talk to your parents or another adult you respect about anything you find confusing or puzzling.

Sexual behaviour

Sexual behaviour describes not only sex itself, but also encompasses your sense of self-esteem, your enjoyment of sex, and your relationships.

Sexual behaviour can start with kissing, touching and caressing, which may lead to a lot of sexual pleasure. Sex does not always have to mean vaginal penetration with a penis, neither does it have to involve oral sex (head jobs) with a man or a woman, both of which can lead to the transmission of STIs. Engaging in other forms of sexual behaviour suits many couples well, especially in the early stages of a relationship. Other sexual activities can also be emotionally exciting and physically enjoyable, while avoiding the complications of unwanted pregnancy, sexually transmitted infections or loss of self-esteem. If you choose to have sex involving penetration with a penis or oral sex with either a man or a woman, it is important to always be aware of unwanted outcomes and to use condoms together with good contraception.

Many forms of sex give pleasure, but anything you do should be agreed on by both partners, with no coercion. If your partner asks you to do anything that makes you feel uncomfortable, you have the right to say no.

Masturbation is a very useful form of sexual expression. It provides sexual pleasure, often to orgasm, without the need for a partner. It is private, free and harmless. It can also be carried out with a partner, giving sexual satisfaction to both. Some cultures disapprove of masturbation, but no health problems have ever been shown to be caused by it.

Sex and adolescents

Sex can be fun, it can be pleasurable and exciting, but only when you are ready for it and you are mature and confident enough to negotiate what you want. It is also important that you and your sexual partner respect each other enough that you both feel able to tell the other what feels good and what doesn't. Most of all, you need to be able to tell your partner when you want it to stop. Only then will sex be a truly pleasurable activity.

Sex is only legal if both parties agree to it. Sex without consent is called sexual assault. Sexual assault is a crime and the offender can be prosecuted. For a lot more information about sexual assault, see chapter 29.

There are also legal age restrictions about when you are able to consent to sex. The law says there is an age when you are too young to agree to have sex and therefore the older person is committing a crime if they have sex with you. The age restrictions are there to protect young people from being exploited by people who are older and have a degree of power and influence over them. It can be very confusing for a young person when someone they respect or admire wants them to do something that feels strange or uncomfortable. It can also be very difficult for a young person to say no to someone who is in a position of authority.

The age restrictions can often be a bit confusing and are slightly different in each state. Generally speaking if you are under 18 – even if you agree – a person who is more than two years older than you or in a position where they are meant to be caring for you (such as a teacher or a coach) cannot:

• have sex with you

• touch you in a sexual way

• perform sexual acts in front of you

It makes no difference if the person is male or female; a sexual advance is a sexual advance, no matter the sex of the people involved. More specifically:

• **If you are under 12**, no one can have sex with you, touch you in a sexual way or perform sexual acts in front of you, even if you agree.

• **If you are between 12 and 15**, a person more than two years older than you cannot have sex with you, touch you in a sexual way or perform sexual acts in front of you, even if you agree. It is not considered a crime, though, if the person genuinely believed that the age difference was less than two years (for example, they were 18 and they genuinely thought you were 16) and you consented to the sex.

• **If you are between 16 and 17**, a person who is in a position of caring for you (such as a teacher, coach or foster carer) cannot have sex with you, touch you in a sexual way or perform sexual acts in front of you, even if you agree. If the person caring for you genuinely thought you were over 18 and you consented to the sex, it would not be considered a crime.

• **If you are 18 or older**, you can consent to have sex with anyone. But remember, sex without consent is a crime no matter how old you are.

Negotiating sex

It can be very confronting, embarrassing and sometimes a bit scary when you have to negotiate sex with someone. As you get older you tend to get

You decide

Having a happy and healthy sex life, which you choose, is a basic right enshrined in a document produced by the World Health Organization in 2002. It states, among other things, that everyone, free of coercion, discrimination and violence, has the right to choose their partner, to decide whether or not to be sexually active, and to pursue a satisfying, safe and pleasurable sex life.

One of the questions you may face as a young woman is whether or not to have sex. You might think all your friends are doing it, but you may still be unsure or not ready to take this step. Remember: it's okay to say NO. It's fine to stick to any beliefs or principles you have about when it's best to have sex for the first time, or for the first time in a new relationship, and if your partner is very special, they will wait until you are ready.

a little more confident, which can make it a bit easier to tell your sexual partner what you want as well as considering their needs.

If someone really wants to have sex with you but they don't care about what it means for you, there are a number of 'tricks' they might use to convince you to do what they want:

- They might threaten you by saying they won't go out with you any more, or they might call you names or threaten to tell others you are a slut or a tease.
- They might make you feel guilty by saying you made them sexually aroused and you should let them have sex with you to make them less frustrated.
- They might tell you how much they love you and make unrealistic promises.

This kind of emotional blackmail can make you feel very conflicted, but it is not a good reason to allow a person to have sex with you. If you are in doubt, pull out. You may feel a little embarrassed if you stop things from progressing, but having sex for someone else's benefit can make you feel a whole lot worse (particularly if that someone is so disrespectful of you).

Sometimes the pressure to have sex with someone can come from your peer or social group. The person who wants to have sex might be popular and charming. If you have been feeling socially isolated or awkward, it's easy to believe that having sex with this person might make you popular too. It's also easy to think that if you don't agree to sex you might be unpopular among your peers. Having sex with someone because your peers think you should is a bad idea. It is more likely that your friends will lose respect for you. Unfortunately and unacceptably, in male–female sexual encounters, it is usually the female who is poorly judged by her peer group, no matter what decision she makes. Trust your own feelings and listen to your own warnings bells. Do what you feel is the right thing to do, and only if you feel ready and safe, and it feels right with this person.

> ### Go at your own pace
> Your first experience does not have to involve full penetrative sex. You can both explore what feels good and what you both like. Your sexual relationship can grow and develop just like the other parts of your relationship. It's okay to take it slowly and to enjoy.

How to enjoy sex

Be ready

Only agree to sex if you have genuine respect for yourself and you believe that your sexual partner respects you too. Be certain that your sexual partner will respect your wishes, no matter how you feel or when you want it to stop. If you and your sexual partner have equal say in what happens and how it happens, then you will both find it a much more positive and enjoyable experience.

Remember, any pressure on you to have sex, whether it is physical or emotional, is sexual assault.

Questions to ask yourself

- Am I really ready?
- Does this person really care about me?
- Will this person be understanding and caring if I change my mind?
- Do I feel like I could tell this person if something hurts or feels uncomfortable?
- Do we have a strong and respectful relationship?
- Am I old enough?
- Is the age difference between us legal?

If you can answer yes to all of those questions, you are in a good starting place to have a good sexual experience.

Contraception for under-18s

If you are under 18, you may be able to get contraception such as the Pill or a long-acting reversible contraception (LARC) from your doctor without the consent of your parent or guardian. The doctor must believe you are mature enough to understand what you are doing and how to use the contraception properly.

You can buy condoms from supermarkets and chemists and you do not need to be over 18.

If you are under 18 and pregnant, depending on how many weeks pregnant you are and which state you live in, you can usually get an abortion without the consent of your parent or guardian. However, the doctor or abortion clinic must believe you are mature enough to understand what you are doing. There is more detailed information about abortion in chapter 23.

Be protected

If you are sexually active it is very important to talk to a doctor or another health professional about a contraceptive method that suits you.

Condoms are critical to stop the spread of sexually transmitted infections (STIs). There are both male and female condoms, but the female ones can be harder to get. If you are having oral sex with a woman, you can use a male condom by cutting both ends off and opening it up so that it is a square.

Your sexual partner may not even be aware that they have an STI, so it is not enough for them to say they don't. STIs can cause health problems for you as you get older, including infertility, which means you may find it hard to get pregnant when you want to. There is more information about STIs in chapters 8 and 26.

You also need contraception to protect you from getting pregnant. There are a number of different types, including condoms and the Pill. The most effective contraceptives are 'fit and forget' methods, or long-acting reversible contraception (LARC). These include IUDs, contraceptive implants and hormone injections (Depo Provera). A doctor or a family planning clinic can help you decide which method is best for you. There is more detailed information about contraception in chapter 16.

Teenage pregnancy can have a detrimental effect on the lives of young women. Unfortunately, even though it takes two to make a baby, the reality is that an unplanned pregnancy will have much more of an impact on your life than on the father's life. The decision to have an abortion or have a baby is yours. Other people can support you to make it, but in the end it's a decision that will affect you more than anybody else and it can be a very lonely decision to make.

If you decide to have a baby, you are most likely to be the primary carer, which can have consequences for your education and employment opportunities. It also has an impact on your social life and friendships. It can be very difficult to watch your peers enjoying their adolescence while you are already burdened with the responsibilities of adulthood. Parenting is a demanding task and some life experience and maturity helps; without it, connecting with your baby can be very hard. There are of course many people who have babies well beyond their teens and may never be emotionally ready for parenthood. There are also people who choose to have babies when they are very young and are very successful parents. But generally, waiting until you have completed your own childhood before you become a parent will give you and your baby a better chance.

Having your own doctor

You can choose to have your own doctor. Generally, everything you and your doctor talk about is confidential. The doctor can only share the information with your parents or with another doctor if you give them permission to do so.

The law requires your doctor to report information to the police if they think you are being abused or are at risk of harm. Some infectious diseases also have to be reported to authorities: these include chlamydia, donovanosis, gonorrhoea, HIV and syphilis. In this case your identity is kept private.

You may need to pay to see a doctor but some doctors bulk bill, in which case you won't need to pay anything. Some charge a fee, most of which you can have reimbursed by Medicare. You may need to check what is expected before you go to the doctor. You will also need to take a Medicare card. You can use your parents' card, which will have your name on it, or, if you are over 15, you can apply at a Medicare office to get your own card.

Sexual difficulties

There are a number of sexual difficulties you might experience as a young woman. The most common of these are discussed below. Such difficulties often mask your discomfort with your sexual identity or orientation. You might avoid having sex because, without realising it, you don't really want to have sex with that particular individual, either because of their gender or because of them as a person, or just because you're not ready to have sex. If you are experiencing any kind of sexual difficulty, it's important to talk to someone about it, preferably your partner or a GP if you are really worried. The vast majority of sexual difficulties in adolescents are social and emotional. It would be extremely rare for anything to be physically wrong.

Vaginismus (involuntary vaginal spasm)

Vaginismus is involuntary spasm of the vaginal muscles. It doesn't indicate any disease, but it's a condition caused by a deep-seated emotional inability to relax the vaginal muscles in order to allow penetration. In almost all cases, the vulva and vagina are completely healthy.

Primary vaginismus, where nothing has ever entered the vagina, not even a tampon, is common among girls who have had a very loving but sometimes over-protective background. They find it hard to overcome the well-meaning but powerful taboos around sex that have surrounded them. Some women who experience vaginismus just think sex is painful, or that they can't have sex.

Treatment in both cases involves a combination of specialist counselling, often combined with help from a physiotherapist to use vaginal dilators or 'trainers'. These trainers are plastic tubes that allow women to learn to insert something into their vagina, under their own control. They should only be used under professional guidance. Treated appropriately, more than 80 per cent of women will overcome this distressing condition.

Marissa, aged 20, went to her GP to change her contraceptive prescription. She had been married for two years and had been on the contraceptive pill for four years. In the course of their conversation, the GP discovered that Marissa had never had a Pap test. Marissa said she was menstruating and would make an appointment to have it done at a later date.

Eighteen months later it still hadn't been done, and Marissa's GP offered to do it. Marissa hesitated and burst into tears. She explained that she had never had sex and had been too embarrassed to tell anyone.

The GP then said she wouldn't do the test, and asked Marissa to talk about the problem instead. Following their discussion, the GP referred Marissa to the psychosexual service at the Women's, where she worked with a psychosexual doctor who diagnosed vaginismus, and a physiotherapist who helped her with the aid of vaginal trainers.

Eighteen months later she went back to her GP and had her first Pap test, and confirmed she was now able to have sex with her husband.

Dyspareunia (pain during sex)

Dyspareunia is a term used to describe pain during sexual intercourse. If you suffer from this kind of pain, it is important when describing it to your doctor to distinguish between pain deep inside and pain at the beginning of sex on the outside. Sometimes the latter is due to a degree of vaginismus (see above), especially in young women, where unsuccessful attempts at penetration are painful. Internal pain may be due to a penis or sex toy touching the neck of the womb or ovaries, and having sex in a different position may help. If the pain persists, a gynaecological check should be done to exclude any gynaecological problems.

Any problems such as skin disorders, herpes infections or thrush can make intercourse very uncomfortable and/or painful. More unusually, in a condition called vulvodynia a specific area seems very tender. This condition can be difficult to treat, and is more fully described, along with other skin disorders such as eczema, in chapter 26.

There is always an emotional component to any sexual problem, whether cause or effect, and that aspect should be acknowledged by your doctor.

Dora, a 19-year-old student, had been in a partnership with Babs for the past year. They had a good relationship, but after Babs had been away on a business trip, Dora found that any time Babs touched or tried to penetrate her vagina it was painful.

Dora, who'd had an episode of herpes when she was 16, was worried that it had returned, and went for a sexual health screen. All test results came back negative. Babs was becoming increasingly upset that her sexual advances to Dora were being repelled, and the relationship was under strain.

They read about a psychosexual clinic, and made themselves an appointment to go together to try to solve the problem. After a few appointments, it became apparent that Dora was worried Babs might have met someone else on the business trip and had sex with her. This caused her to subconsciously draw back from any sexual contact with Babs. They were able to discuss these issues with the counsellor, their sex life gradually improved and the pain disappeared.

Loss of libido (loss of interest in sex)

A loss of libido describes a loss of interest in sex. There are no physical signs or symptoms; in young women it is purely an emotional condition, and there is no drug treatment available for this. Appropriate treatment involves psychosexual counselling, in which the counsellor, by listening and reflecting back to you, tries to help you understand why you feel this way, and to help you reconnect with your sexual feelings.

At any age, loss of sexual feelings can be related to problems in the past, possibly unconnected to your present partner. It can also be caused by problems within your current relationship. You only need professional help if the problem continues for a long time.

Eighteen-year-old Kylie was very happy with her new boyfriend, Jonno. They had been together for a year. At first sex was 'amazing', but over the last few months, Kylie had become uninterested in sex. She couldn't understand this, as she loved Jonno and still found him very attractive. She started to avoid sexual situations with him and it was affecting their relationship.

Kylie found the name of a sexual counsellor on a website. She didn't tell Jonno, as she felt she wanted to talk to someone on her own. After a few sessions with the counsellor, Kylie revealed that when she was 16 she'd had a very abusive and violent partner for a few months, and she had never talked about it with anyone. She found the counselling sessions emotionally draining, but dealing with the past abuse helped her put her current relationship back on track.

Making the link between past experiences and the present is not obvious to many people, who will say they have put the past behind them. That is why talking to a trained professional can be very helpful, and gives them the ability to reflect on their problem in a positive way.

Anorgasmia (inability to achieve orgasm)

The female orgasm is either clitoral, vaginal or both. The function of the female orgasm is purely pleasure, and how it is achieved in any individual may differ. In the vast majority of cases of anorgasmia there is no physical problem.

Many young women find it hard to reach any kind of sexual climax with their partner, yet they can easily orgasm by themselves. A simple solution to this problem is to try different things sexually with your partner, even if it seems embarrassing at first. It is not necessary to have simultaneous orgasm with your partner; every couple is different and each couple simply needs to find a sexual rhythm that suits them both.

Some women have never experienced an orgasm at all, either during sexual intercourse or through masturbation. If this is the case for you, or if you have never masturbated, it's a good idea to get to know your genital anatomy and try different masturbation techniques. It is fine to use a vibrator, either on your own or with a partner, if that gives you sexual pleasure, and this may help stimulate orgasm.

Where to get help for a sexual problem

One of the main issues with having a sexual problem is that it can be difficult to talk about. You might be very embarrassed and don't want to waste your doctor's time. On the other hand, a busy doctor may not give you the time or opportunity to talk about anything related to sex. This may be because the doctor is unaware of your distress in this area, or they may feel uncomfortable with the topic themselves. Young people are often anxious about confidentiality, and are sometimes concerned that the doctor may say something to another family member. This, of course, does not happen: any consultation with a doctor is private, but your doctor should reassure you of this. You can also use websites or young people's helplines if you want confidential advice.

8
Genital irritations and infections

Chris Bayly, Suzanne Garland, Yasmin Jayasinghe

Discharge from the vagina and irritation in the genital region are quite common in young women. Sometimes they may be an indication that there is an infection or inflammation that requires treatment, and at other times discharge may be normal and not require treatment. Sometimes infections in the genital region may be silent; that is, the infection may be present in the genital region but you may not notice anything untoward. That is why we recommend that if you have had a new partner or have had more than one sexual partner in a 12-month period, you should have a check-up with your doctor or health nurse even if you're feeling fine. And it is always best to see someone if you are experiencing any unusual symptoms, or anything you are concerned about.

There is no need to feel embarrassed or ashamed about seeing your doctor or health nurse about these kinds of concerns, as symptoms are common: most women experience some form of irritation or infection in their lifetime. Health staff are trained professionals who will not judge you in any way and will treat you with respect and courtesy. You have the right to private and confidential health care (that is, if the doctor feels that you have a good understanding of everything after it has been explained to you, your care does not need to be discussed with anyone else). There are only two exceptions to this rule: if someone is hurting you, or if you are at risk of hurting yourself. In either of those exceptional situations, your doctor or health nurse would discuss with you the need to involve other people in your care, for your personal safety.

What is normal in the genital region?

The diagram below shows the female internal organs: the ovaries (which produce hormones and contain eggs for future pregnancy); the fallopian tubes, which transport the egg; the uterus or womb, where periods come from and a baby would develop, and the vagina. The neck of the womb

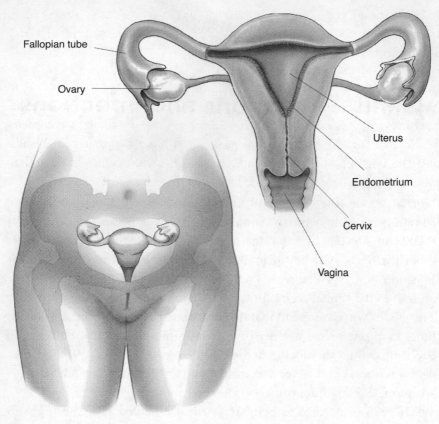

Female internal organs

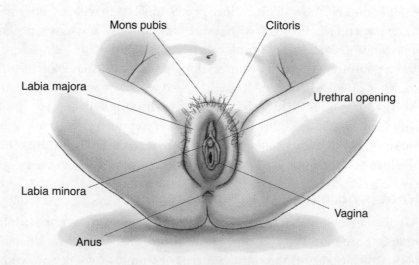

External view of vulvar area

is called the cervix. The female external organs are the labia majora and labia minora, the outer and inner lips, which can be a range of sizes, shapes and colours; the clitoris, which contributes to sexual function and pleasure; and the entrance to the vagina, otherwise known as the vestibule. The hymen is a piece of thin skin at the entrance of the vagina that has an opening in it leading into the vagina. Just outside the hymen are the openings of the Bartholin's glands, which cannot normally be seen or felt.

Normal vaginal discharge is produced by the cervix, the vaginal walls and the Bartholin's glands. It may be white, cream-coloured or transparent. It may become clearer and wetter in the two weeks after your period, due to the production of oestrogen in the ovaries, and may become thick and sticky after ovulation (after the egg pops out of the ovary, which occurs between periods) due to progesterone production. Discharge may increase during pregnancy or with use of the oral contraceptive pill. Wetness can increase during sexual arousal or during sex, whether you're aroused or not.

A lot of young women wonder if the discharge they are producing is normal or not. It is easy for a doctor or nurse to determine if there is a problem. Some women may have questions about their genital appearance (such as a perception that their labia are large or asymmetrical, which is actually normal). If you have a concern, it is best to discuss it with your doctor. It is important to understand that there are differences in genital appearance (just as there are differences between people in other parts of the body), and most often in young women everything is normal. But regardless of this, you have the right to voice your concerns without them being minimised or dismissed. See chapter 9 for further discussion regarding acceptance of differences in genital appearance.

Problems in the genital region

Non sexually transmitted causes of vaginal irritation

Bacterial vaginosis

Bacterial vaginosis (BV) is caused by an imbalance of the normal bacteria living in the vagina and produces an increased greyish vaginal discharge that may have a fishy odour. It can be detected on a vaginal swab test. While it is not considered a sexually transmitted infection (STI), it is more common in women with same-sex partners, those who douche ('clean' inside the vagina), those with new sexual partners, and where condoms are not used. It is only treated if it is causing symptoms, with antibiotic tablets or a vaginal preparation. If symptoms continue, you may be advised to use vaginal antibiotic tablets twice a week for four to six months. Condoms may reduce the risk of but not prevent a recurrence. Sexual partners do not need to be screened or treated for BV, but having BV may also increase the risk of developing an STI.

Bartholin's cyst or abscess

The Bartholin's glands sit at either side of the entrance to the vagina and normally cannot be seen or felt. They secrete fluid into the inner vagina. If the duct leading from the gland gets blocked, a cyst (a sac under the skin filled with fluid or semi-solid matter) will develop on one side of the labia, which is often painless. If they are painful, the cysts may settle if treated with repeated sitz baths (sitting in warm water with a few teaspoons of salt in it: around 1 teaspoon per litre of water). If the cyst gets infected, it can form an abscess, which can be red, swollen and tender. Treatment includes sitz baths, antibiotics and surgery, including opening up the abscess to drain and stitching the cyst wall to the skin (to keep it open). For people who have recurrent cysts or abscesses, the gland may be removed surgically. Abscesses may be due to a variety of infections, including but not limited to STIs.

Labial abscess

A labial abscess is a very tender swollen area on the labial skin, similar to a boil. It may be due to infected skin glands, an ingrown hair, or direct trauma to the skin after waxing, shaving, laser treatment or piercings. Treatment options for this condition include antibiotic tablets, but if your symptoms are severe, you may need to take antibiotics through a drip, and require incision and drainage of the abscess under sterile conditions. Complete recovery with normal appearance is the usual outcome. Simple hygiene practices may reduce the likelihood of abscess formation, such as washing the skin with soap and water before and after hair-removal procedures, never sharing razors, and using disposable razors once only. Sometimes steroid and antibiotic lotions for the skin are prescribed to prevent severe recurrent abscesses or irritations after hair-removal procedures. Some women who have problems with oily skin or increased hair growth may have problems with recurrent labial or groin abscesses not related to hair removal, and they may benefit from using the oral contraceptive pill or other hormone treatments to decrease the risk of more abscesses.

Candidiasis (thrush)

Candida or candidiasis, also known as thrush, is due to a vaginal yeast infection (scientifically known as *Candida albicans*). It can cause itchiness or soreness in the genital region, a thick white discharge, sometimes dryness and soreness in the vagina during sex, and/or burning on passing urine. Symptoms may get worse with prolonged exposure to moisture in the genital region, such as wearing tight clothing after sport; with antibiotic use; or just before your period or after intercourse. Symptoms may recur in some women, such as those with diabetes. Thrush can be detected with a vaginal swab test (by inserting a sterile cotton swab in the vagina, which is sent to a laboratory for testing), and is treated with a range of creams (e.g. Canesten vaginal cream) or pessaries (vaginal tablets) placed in the vagina. If there are recurrent symptoms, your doctor may recommend that you take long-term antifungal tablets by mouth for around three months or until symptoms resolve. There is no need to treat or routinely screen sexual partners as candida is not sexually transmitted.

Bacterial sexually transmitted infections (STIs)

Chlamydia trachomatis

Chlamydia trachomatis is one of the most common STIs, reported to occur in around 5 per cent of the population. Young women under the age of 25 have the highest rates of infection. It is important to understand that 70 per cent of women with chlamydia infection have no symptoms at all. Chlamydia may cause vaginal discharge, irregular vaginal bleeding, pelvic pain, painful periods and pain during sex. The infection can cause scarring of the fallopian tubes, and infertility (difficulty in getting pregnant) or ectopic pregnancy (pregnancy developing within a fallopian tube, requiring surgery and removal to avoid bleeding complications). Severe infection can lead to pelvic inflammatory disease (PID), which may be associated with fever and acute pain, requiring admission to hospital, antibiotics and sometimes surgery. The risk of getting other STIs is also increased. Not using condoms, a high rate of change of sexual partners, and an increased number of sexual partners all increase your risk of acquiring chlamydia. Chlamydia can also be transmitted through oral sex, and even newborn babies can get it through contact if their mother's birth canal is infected, leading to eye complications and throat and chest infections. The infectious period can last months to years if not diagnosed and adequately treated.

There are a variety of ways to test for chlamydia, including testing a first-pass urine sample, or taking a swab test, which you can collect yourself or can be collected by your doctor.

Mild infection can be treated with a single dose of antibiotics, or other antibiotic tablets taken as a seven-to-10 day course. More severe infection may require antibiotics through an intravenous drip in hospital, followed by antibiotic tablets for a further two to four weeks after being sent home. If you are diagnosed with chlamydia, it is recommended that you notify all your sexual partners over the past six months if you are comfortable with doing this, so that they can receive treatment. This is done confidentially, and you would not need to contact them personally if you did not want to; healthcare services can do that for you to maintain privacy. There are also websites with information and resources to assist you in this task, such as www.letthemknow.org.au, developed by the Melbourne Sexual Health Centre. You should avoid sex during treatment (ideally you and your partner should be treated simultaneously so that the untreated partner does not reinfect the treated partner), and safe sex (using condoms appropriately throughout sex) is encouraged from then on.

Gonorrhoea

Gonorrhoea can be transmitted through vaginal, anal or oral sex without condoms and can develop within a week of exposure from an infected person. Many women with gonorrhoea will not have any symptoms, while others may experience vaginal discharge, pelvic pain, painful periods, painful sex, pain on passing urine, or a sore throat. Gonorrhoea can also cause pelvic inflammatory disease (PID), and scarring of the fallopian tubes, which can lead to ectopic pregnancy and infertility. Testing for gonorrhoea involves a self-collected swab test or first-pass urine test. If the results are positive, you will need to have an internal examination by a doctor with possible repeat testing using a swab test to see which antibiotic will be best to treat the infection. If the infection was caught when travelling overseas or from a partner who has been overseas, the strains of gonorrhoea are more likely to be resistant to the usual antibiotics. Today most infections are treated with a single injection called ceftriaxone.

Gonorrhoea and chlamydia infections can occur together, so you will often be treated for both at the same time if the gonorrhoea test is positive. You should avoid intercourse for one week after treatment. If there is severe infection, you may need to be treated for two to four weeks, and some people may require admission to hospital and even surgery. The risk of gonorrhoea can be reduced with the use of condoms and dental dams, and decreasing the rate of sexual partner change. A repeat test is recommended at three months.

Mycoplasma genitalium
Mycoplasma genitalium is a newly recognised STI that has similar symptoms to chlamydia.

Viral STIs
Human papillomavirus (HPV)
Human papillomavirus (HPV) is the most common viral STI. Around 80 per cent of people who have ever been sexually active will get HPV at some stage of their life. It is very normal for young women to have genital HPV infections as they change sexual partners more frequently than older women (who are more likely to be in stable long-term relationships). The vast majority of HPV infections clear up on their own after a period of months to years. Most people do not know that they have an HPV infection, as it can be silent (have no noticeable symptoms). There are many different types of HPV and they are divided into high- or low-risk types.

Low-risk HPV infection (particularly types 6 and 11) can cause genital warts. Genital warts are caused by genital-skin-to-genital-skin contact, usually during sex. They may develop around six weeks to three months after exposure to the virus, which may be invisible (i.e. warts do not have to be present in your partner for you to develop genital warts). They can cause itchiness, irritation and warty lumps on the external genital region, near the anus (not only from anal sex), inside the vagina, and on the penis. Warts may actually clear by themselves over time. They can also be treated by freezing, burning, laser treatment, or a cream that works against some viruses such as HPV and by boosting the immune system (called Aldara), but they often recur. Do not use wart paint that you use on other parts of your body on genital warts. Genital warts are contagious, so avoid sex until the warts have disappeared and the skin has healed. You may be able to decrease the risk of developing warts by using condoms, but as they do not cover all of the skin that may be infected, they are not 100 per cent effective.

It is important to understand that the terms 'genital warts' and 'HPV' are not interchangeable. HPV infection is usually invisible. Genital warts are little warty lumps caused by some types of HPV. About 80 per cent of people acquire HPV as a result of having sex, whereas your lifetime risk of developing genital warts is 10 per cent (if you don't have the HPV vaccination).

HPV and cancer

For a *small number* of women (5–10 per cent) certain types of HPV can become persistent, resulting in changes in the cells on their Pap tests (see chapter 2). Generally it is persistent infection with high-risk HPVs that leads to cervical cancer; HPV 16 and 18 cause the majority (70 per cent) of cervical cancers. Smoking appears to increase the chance of persistent HPV infection and Pap test changes, so it's a good idea to avoid the habit or quit, to decrease your risk of cervical cancer.

Pap test changes are very common in women under the age of 25. We divide Pap test changes into low- or high-grade changes, depending on their likelihood of progressing further to cervical cancer. Most Pap test changes in women under 25 are low-grade and disappear on their own. Some Pap test changes are high-grade and require further examination and treatment to avoid the development of cervical cancer. But even if you have a confirmed high-grade change, it generally takes a long time (10–20 years) before a cancer would develop. It is rare for cervical cancer to develop in women under 25.

Most Pap test changes in young women are completely treatable if they follow recommended screening and treatment guidelines (see chapter 2). You should start having Pap tests at the age of 18 if you have ever been sexually active, or have a Pap test two years after the onset of sexual activity, whichever is later. For example, if you were first sexually active at 15, have your first Pap test at 18. If you were first sexually active at 21, have your first Pap test at 23. There may be some exceptions to this rule; for example, if you are a victim of childhood sexual abuse, your doctor may recommend a Pap test at 18 if you feel comfortable doing so. Now that we have the HPV vaccine, the guidelines for Pap screening, including the age of commencing screening, will probably change in the future; your doctor will be watching out for these changes and can advise you about this. Please note that even though Pap tests are not recommended until at least the age of 18, it is important to have an STI screen if you are sexually active (at least yearly or before commencing a new sexual relationship). Whenever you have a pelvic examination, it is important to clarify with your doctor if you are having a Pap test or an STI screen or both.

HPV vaccination

Two preventative HPV vaccines currently available are licensed for use in Australia: Gardasil and Cervarix. The vaccines are best received before you have ever been sexually active, before any infection with HPV. The one given free to all girls aged 12–13, Gardasil, enables the body to form anti-bodies to HPV 16 and 18 (which cause 70 per cent of cervical cancers), and 6 and 11 (which produce 90 per cent of genital warts). This vaccine can therefore prevent the majority of cases of cervical cancer and genital warts if given early. Cervarix, also licensed in Australia, enables formation of antibodies to HPV 16 and 18 only, which means it can prevent around 70 per cent of cervical cancers but will not protect against genital warts. There is new evidence to show that the vaccines are still useful (around 66 per cent effective) even if you have been sexually active in the past, and even if you have had Pap test changes before. The vaccines, however, are preventative and not a treatment for abnormalities or for removing current HPV infection. Women aged 45 and under are eligible to be vaccinated. It is still useful to get vaccinated if you are in a monogamous relationship (currently only have one sexual partner) or are in a same-sex relationship.

If you missed out on vaccination through the school system, you can receive the vaccine through your GP. It costs around $150 per injection, and you need three injections over six months. While this is expensive, it is a very good investment in your health. If you have only received one or two doses and there has been some delay in receiving the second or third dose, you don't need to start the vaccination course again: just finish the course. You will still need to have Pap tests and follow-up as per the usual guidelines. Future Pap test changes do not mean the vaccine has failed, as the changes may be due to the HPV types not covered by the vaccine or related to infections you may have been carrying before receiving the vaccine. Even though it is expected that Pap test changes will continue to be common, it is hoped that the rate of cervical cancer will reduce dramatically as a result of this vaccination. The side effects of the vaccine include pain and redness at the injection site. The vaccine is safe. Allergic reactions are exceedingly rare.

Genital herpes

Genital herpes is an STI caused by herpes simplex virus 1 or 2. It affects one in five women under the age of 50. Most infected people do not know they carry the herpes virus; it is possible, therefore, to develop herpes when your partner has never had any symptoms. Herpes can cause painful blisters and ulcers in the genital region. During the first infection some women will suffer fever and body aches, and difficulty passing urine, even requiring admission to hospital. Outbreaks can be recurrent, particularly in the first year of infection, but they usually decrease over time.

Herpes is transmitted during vaginal, anal and oral sex. It is possible to get genital herpes from cold sores after oral sex. Antiviral treatment, usually taken orally (by mouth), can reduce the frequency and intensity of an outbreak if started within three days of the onset of symptoms. Some people stay on antivirals to suppress recurrences if they are frequent. Herpes cannot be totally cured, but it is very manageable. Transmission of herpes can be reduced by consistent use of condoms, avoiding sex during an outbreak, and reducing the number of sexual partners. A doctor can diagnose herpes by looking at the sores (if they are typical) but will need a swab test from the sore to confirm the diagnosis.

HIV, hepatitis B and hepatitis C

HIV, hepatitis B and hepatitis C are infections that can be acquired during sex or via contaminated blood (such as through sharing contaminated needles during illegal drug use), or at birth from an infected mother. Testing for these infections is part of the routine screen for STIs, and also, if recommended, part of the screening blood tests done when you fall pregnant. Condoms are recommended for all sexually active young people, particularly for new encounters, to decrease the risk of these infections.

Other types of STI

Other less common STIs include syphilis, chancroid and donovanosis, all of which may be more likely acquired during overseas travel, although syphilis is also found in some areas of Australia. If you are concerned about any unusual genital symptoms especially after travelling (particularly if you had sex with someone from another country) it is best to see your doctor, remembering to mention your travel overseas.

Piercings and other genital irritation

Some women undergo genital piercing to increase sexual pleasure or as a form of personal expression. Body piercings in general have been associated with a high rate of complications such as infection, bleeding and scarring. Genital piercing can result in bleeding; nerve damage, which may cause pain or problems with sex; infection at the site of the piercing; and scarring leading to problems passing urine. Hepatitis B and C, toxic shock syndrome, kidney and brain infections have been reported from body piercings at other sites. Piercings can cause condoms to tear during sex and consequently increase the risk of pregnancy. Male piercings also increase this risk, and a second form of contraception is recommended.

Because of the associated risks, genital piercings are not generally recommended, and should be avoided particularly in women with infections such as HIV, hepatitis B and C or diabetes, and those with pre-existing heart conditions (because piercings increase the risk of an infection of the heart valves called infective endocarditis) or pre-existing skin conditions involving the genital region. You should speak to your doctor if you are considering a piercing and see your doctor as soon as possible if you have any concerns after it has been performed. If you are intent on going ahead with a piercing, it should only be performed by a qualified practitioner under sterile conditions, and careful after-care of the pierced site is important to avoid the risk of blood-borne infections such as hepatitis B and C as well as HIV.

Skin conditions of the external genitalia such as lichen sclerosus (see chapter 26) and allergic dermatitis (e.g. due to contact with irritants such as soaps), polyps inside the genital tract, or forgotten tampons can also cause irritation or a smelly discharge. There is no need to be embarrassed about a forgotten tampon, or if you're having difficulty removing a tampon after insertion. It is best to see your doctor to get it removed, and to check whether there is a reason this has occurred.

How to minimise your risk of genital infection and irritation

- Avoid fragrant soaps in the genital region, vaginal douching (vaginal washes) and feminine sprays (scented sprays for the genital area), as they can cause overgrowth of bacteria or contact irritation. Mild soap and water for the external genital area is fine.

- After going to the toilet, wipe from front to back to prevent bacteria from the bowel getting into the vagina.

- Wear cotton underwear and avoid tight clothing. Try to wash and change out of sweaty clothing as soon as possible after sport. Barrier creams that provide a layer of protection over the skin may prevent skin irritation due to moisture.

- Always use a fresh razor when shaving the genital region. Wash the area with mild soap and water before and after any hair removal. Do *not* share razors.

- Have a discussion with your doctor if you are considering any genital piercings to assess your risk, and never have piercings done by an unqualified practitioner. Be aware of the complications that can arise with genital piercings.

- Minimise the number and rate of change of sexual partners, but bear in mind that STIs can still be acquired even after only one partner or one unprotected sexual encounter.

- Be aware that STIs can be transmitted via all kinds of sex, including oral sex and anal sex. STIs cannot be transmitted via toilet seats.

- Make sure you have safe sex by using barrier protection such as condoms, female condoms or dental dams (for the mouth). They can reduce the risk of transmission of STIs if used consistently throughout the sexual act. Latex-free condoms are available for those with allergies. To use condoms appropriately, they must be worn throughout the entire sex act. Sperm may swim from the external genitalia (the vulva) into the vagina and cause pregnancy. Always check the expiry date of condoms and store them in a cool, dry place. To put on a male condom correctly, pinch the tip of the condom, then roll it down the entire shaft of the erect penis. Only use water-based lubricants (e.g. KY Jelly) with condoms. Never use spit, Vaseline or oil, as they can damage the condom. Withdraw the penis before the erection is lost, holding the base of the condom to avoid spillage.

- Get a health check and an STI screen at least once a year or before starting a sexual relationship with a new partner.

- Get the HPV vaccine if you have not already done so.

Pelvic examinations

Your doctor or health nurse will explain how the pelvic examination is performed before they start. It will generally only be performed if you have been sexually active in the past. Usually the consultation will start with a discussion of your medical history. You should be prepared to explain what medications you are on, if any; any allergies you suffer from; and if there are health issues in your family history. The doctor or nurse might ask some quite personal questions about your use of condoms, the number of sexual partners you've had, your sexuality, even any history of sexual abuse. This gives them a better idea of the risk of a problem. If there is something personal you wish to raise that the doctor or nurse has not asked, it is fine to bring it up. As mentioned earlier, all the information is confidential, unless there is a risk of harm to you. If you have not been sexually active in the past, a pelvic examination will only be performed in special circumstances.

Before the examination, you will be given some privacy while you undress (you can keep your top on), and you can cover your lower half with a sheet. You may request a chaperone at any time, and if you have a male doctor there will usually be a chaperone present. You can ask for the examination to stop at any time. During the examination, the doctor may take your blood pressure, pulse and temperature, and feel your abdomen for any tenderness or lumps. During the pelvic examination, a speculum (see below) is gently inserted into the vagina and opened so the doctor can see the cervix. It is important to relax the pelvic muscles as much as possible during that examination as it will make it more comfortable. After swabs or a Pap test are taken, the speculum is gently removed and an internal examination is performed: the doctor or nurse will insert gloved fingers into your vagina, with their other hand over your abdomen to feel for the uterus, cysts on the ovaries or tender spots.

The pelvic examination only takes about five minutes and is not painful if you are relaxed. It is normal to feel a bit embarrassed if you have not had an examination before, but your doctor is a dedicated professional who will usually have done many of these examinations. The physical pain and discomfort of untreated pelvic infections is far worse than any discomfort you will feel during the examination. It is important to be aware that just because you may have swabs taken during a speculum examination, the doctor may not necessarily perform a Pap test. It is very important that you confirm with the doctor exactly what tests were done. As mentioned earlier, some STIs can be tested with a first-pass urine test.

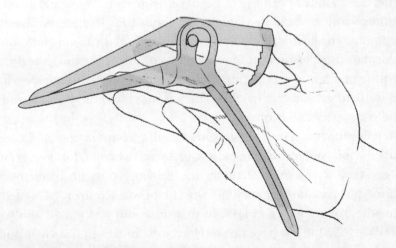

This speculum is an example of one type used, the 'duck bill'. Speculum examinations are only performed on women who have been sexually active, when required.

An STI screen

An STI screen will generally mean you have had testing for:

- Chlamydia, gonorrhoea (urine or swabs), *Mycoplasma genitalium* (swabs)
- HIV, hepatitis B and C, syphilis (blood tests)

If your test results are positive, you will be offered counselling and treatment, given information regarding safe-sex practices, advised that your sexual partners in the last six months be contacted (either by you or the Department of Health) and treated, and advised that the results will be sent (in a way that does not identify you) to the government department that collects STI statistics in your state.

Being diagnosed with an STI can sometimes be confronting, but there is no need to be embarrassed, ashamed or frightened. These infections are common, and you should be proud that you were proactive and had a check-up, and can now be treated. For many STIs it is difficult to work out exactly who you got it from, as some infections stay silent for long periods of time.

Unwanted sexual encounters and sexual abuse

Sometimes STIs are acquired through an unwanted sexual encounter, including during childhood. While it is common to have a deep sense of shame, these kinds of exposures are never your fault. We would strongly encourage you to speak to your doctor about this. If the exposures are ongoing and the doctor thinks they are abusive (e.g. if you are quite young and/or the other person is in a position of authority over you), the doctor is required by law to report this to the Department of Human Services. That is not to get you into trouble. The purpose is to keep you safe and to get help for everyone involved.

If you report a recent unwanted sexual encounter, special forensic (legal) doctors and nurses can help you. As well as doing forensic examinations, they screen for infections, and provide you with medicines to minimise the risk of pregnancy and the risk of you acquiring STIs such as chlamydia, gonorrhoea and HIV. In this situation, you should also have the HPV vaccine if you have not received it before. Even if such episodes were a long time ago, it may still be beneficial to speak to your doctor about them. They will take special care during the examinations so you don't feel scared, and they can get you the help you need. Counselling services are available in all states if you wish to speak to a counsellor regarding past experiences, see chapter 29 for more.

Female genital cutting

Female genital cutting or mutilation (FGC or FGM: see the box about terminology) refers to all procedures involving partial or total removal of the external female genitalia or other injury to the female genital organs for non-medical reasons.

It encompasses a range of procedures, from a tiny cut or 'nick' in the vulvar skin to removal of the clitoris and much of the labia (vaginal lips) with stitching to narrow the vaginal opening. It is practised in many countries in Africa, the Middle East and Asia for traditional cultural reasons, including a belief that it will increase opportunities for girls, although the actual procedures vary between communities and countries and the usual age of the girls involved varies from infancy to adolescence. FGC is harmful to girls and women and has no known health benefits. Islam scholars are clear that it is not a religious requirement, and many Muslim countries and communities do not practise it at all.

A note on terminology

The term 'female genital mutilation' or 'FGM' is used in policy discussions to acknowledge the harm caused and to support work to prevent any more girls from experiencing FGM and its consequences.

'Female genital cutting' or 'FGC' is considered more respectful when talking to affected women and communities.

Immediate problems caused by FGC include pain, severe bleeding, infection and sometimes death. Problems that may persist or occur in later life include infections of the urinary tract and reproductive system, period problems, chronic pain, pain or difficulty with sex, reduced sexual pleasure, birth complications for mother and baby and a range of psychological problems. Because the variation in procedures is wide, so is the variety of problems experienced in later life, from none at all to chronic symptoms that affect quality of life daily.

Many women in Australia have come from countries that practise FGC; girls and women who come to Australia beyond adolescence may have had these procedures done in their country of origin. On arrival in Australia they often have pressing priorities to do with settlement in a new country, and they may have a history of social and family disruption related to conflict and civil unrest in their country of origin. Help with these matters may feel more urgent than attending to health concerns that may be longstanding and accepted as a fact of life.

Many girls and women have been upset about the ways the media and sometimes health professionals talk about FGC; it can seem that we are only interested in women's genitals and that women who have had FGC are seen as mutilated. We are working to improve doctors' and nurses' knowledge and understanding of FGC, in order to provide the best possible care and to help communities stop FGC from occurring.

Health care may be very different in Australia from where you were born or grew up. Some women worry that doctors, nurses and midwives here don't know how to care for women who have had FGC, and that for instance a caesarean might be recommended for everyone who has had FGC; this is not a reason for doing caesareans, although they are commonly done in Australia for other reasons. If you have any concerns, speak with a health professional.

If you have had FGC and would like to discuss what has been done, any physical or emotional effects, or any concerns about your future health or childbirth, talk to a health professional about this. Your local doctor, community health centre, women's health centre, women's hospital or maternity service might be able to help or they might refer you to someone else with experience in this area.

If you are experiencing any of the sexual problems or other symptoms listed earlier, it's important to also consider other possible reasons for any symptoms, as health problems can have many different causes. If anything is bothering you, talk to your doctor about it and ask for a referral to a specialist service if they are not familiar with FGC.

If you have had infibulation, a type of FGC that involves narrowing of the vaginal opening by stitching, it is usually recommended that you have de-infibulation (or reversal) before or during pregnancy if possible, although it can be done during childbirth if necessary. Some women will want or need to have this done to help with period symptoms or before they establish a sexual relationship. The procedure is done with local anaesthetic to numb the area: the stitched part is then cut with surgical scissors and small stitches are used to stop any bleeding and help healing.

It is illegal to do FGC in Australia or to take a girl out of the country for this purpose, because of the harm it causes. The World Health Organization, the United Nations and many other agencies are working to end FGC around the world, and the Australian Government and the Women's support this work. It can only be achieved by working with affected communities and empowering them to take charge of the health and wellbeing of their girls and women. There is encouraging progress in many places where this approach has been taken.

The role of the Women's is to provide the best possible care for girls and women who have had FGC in the past, to support education of individuals and communities about the harm caused by FGC so that they will not seek to do it for the next generation, and to educate other health professionals to look after women who have had FGC.

The effects of FGC range from no lasting consequences to serious ongoing health problems. If you have had FGC, you should have access to responsive health care that will help you deal with any concerns or problems with your physical, mental and/or emotional health.

9

Plastic surgery in adolescence

Dean Trotter

Plastic surgery is the reconstruction or repair of part of the body through surgery, and it may be cosmetic or reconstructive. The main difference between these terms is that cosmetic surgery is generally purely elective surgery, with an aim of 'improving' appearance (cosmesis). Reconstructive surgery may also be elective surgery, but it is often part of non-elective surgery. In general it is aimed at restoring form and function, sometimes after previous surgery such as mastectomy or after injuries such as burns.

Cosmetic plastic surgery

Plastic surgery is commonly sought by young people, especially young women, who are seeking to 'improve' their appearance. The aim is to change their appearance to correct a real or perceived problem; examples are breast augmentation for 'small' breasts, rhinoplasty (a nose job) for 'unattractive' noses, or abdominoplasty (a tummy tuck) for a 'bulging' or saggy abdomen.

Adolescence and the early years beyond is a time of many changes, both physical and emotional. There are often pressures from a variety of sources such as parents, carers, friends, teachers, siblings and the media in general to look or act a certain way.

Many messages from various media (particularly the internet and women's magazines) promote an often unrealistic and unobtainable ideal of how we should look and what 'normal' is. It is sometimes difficult to determine what is real and what is fake in images in magazines. Many advertising messages further reinforce these unachievable ideals. The advertisers have the advantage of being able to alter reality to a form they think young women want.

Adolescence is a time when your self-image is maturing. It is important to remember that positive self-image is made up of many facets; it is not just about looks, but also about self-esteem and internal happiness. Your looks are not the most important thing about you; what's more important is the kind of person you are.

The decision to have plastic surgery is a serious one, and, like all surgery, it has permanent consequences. For this reason it is worthwhile discussing your issues with your GP and possibly a plastic surgeon. Some problems may in fact not be a problem at all, and a consultation may allow you to realise you are actually normal. The reverse is also true: some people are told by their family, friends and even sometimes doctors that an aspect of them is normal, when they actually do have a problem that could be improved with surgery.

Any surgery must be carefully considered and only undertaken once all the risks and potential complications have been taken into account (see chapter 3). Plastic surgery of any sort is no different. If you are considering plastic surgery you should check that your surgeon is fully trained and understands your problem. While many doctors say they perform plastic surgery, the only surgeons who are truly recognised as plastic surgeons by government and medical insurance companies are those trained by the Royal Australasian College of Surgeons. It is a good idea to check that your plastic surgeon has been certified by the Royal Australasian College of Surgeons and is a member of the Australian Society of Plastic Surgeons (www.plasticsurgery.org.au). That way you can be sure that your surgeon has undergone extensive training and has satisfactorily passed examinations checking their ability to practise plastic surgery.

Cosmetic surgery is not performed in the public hospital system. If your condition is felt to be a purely cosmetic problem, you will be advised to seek surgery outside the public health system.

Common reasons for cosmetic plastic surgery in adolescence

Breast surgery

Breast asymmetry is very common. Most women have some slight size difference between their breasts. Asymmetry of more than one cup size is less common, and when it occurs, may be profoundly psychologically troubling. Sometimes the asymmetry is part of a syndrome of abnormal development of the chest wall and upper limb (such as Poland's syndrome), or it may be simply underdevelopment of the breast (hypoplasia). Some women are also affected by tuberous breast deformity, in which varying degrees of deformity may affect the nipple and areola, the breast tissue itself, or both.

Often women with breast asymmetry are told that they will grow out of it, or it will correct itself during pregnancy or breastfeeding. While this does sometimes happen, there may be a developmental problem that neither time nor pregnancy will solve. Usually if there is still breast asymmetry once puberty has been completed, it will stay that way.

A few women develop severe psychological issues and don't realise that plastic surgery is an option. The procedures are usually reconstructive, and generally involve breast augmentation with silicone implants, or breast reduction or uplift procedures to achieve breasts of the same size. These procedures are enormously satisfying for affected women.

Wendy finished puberty when she was about 15. During puberty she noticed that her breasts were different sizes and shapes. She had hoped that as she grew older her breasts would become more similar and 'normal', but they didn't, and by the time she was 16 she was very self-conscious and concerned about the appearance of her breasts. They were not like those of her friends, and different from the pictures of breasts she saw on TV or on the internet.

Although she was slim and average height, her breasts did not seem to match the rest of her body. Her left breast was smaller than the right. It looked much like a normal breast but was quite small, only an A cup. The right breast was bigger, more like a B cup, but was quite droopy and had a much bigger nipple and areola. It seemed more tubular and elongated than a normal breast. The breasts also seemed to be separated more widely than normal and even in a bra were unable to form much of a cleavage.

Wendy discussed her breasts with her mother, who took her to her GP. The GP agreed that her breasts weren't normal and sent her to see a plastic surgeon for an opinion.

The plastic surgeon said that Wendy had an underdeveloped (hypoplastic) left breast and had a tuberous right breast. The surgeon informed her that tuberous breasts have a smaller (constricted) base than the normal breast, and a nipple and areola that tend to bulge out (are herniated) from the breast and are located closer to the fold under the breast.

Wendy was advised that the only way to try to improve her breasts was with surgery. Her right breast would need surgery to release the constriction that was making the breast tubular and improve the nipple and areola position. This would require two operations.

Wendy's first operation was to lift the right breast nipple into a better position and release the constriction. At the same time a silicone balloon containing a metal valve (tissue expander) was inserted under the breast. Over several weeks this balloon was inflated with saline by putting a needle through the skin into the valve. This stretched Wendy's skin and breast tissue so that is was no longer tight and tubular.

Six months after the first operation Wendy had the tissue expander removed and replaced with a silicone breast implant. At the same time, an implant was placed under the left breast to match the right breast.

Since the operation Wendy has renewed confidence and feels much better about herself. She now has two breasts that are similar and more proportionate for her physique. While she does have scars on her breasts, especially the right one, with clothes on it is very difficult to tell she has had surgery.

Rhinoplasty (nose surgery)

Some adolescents consider surgery to their nose, some because of problems with breathing, others simply because they do not like the look of their nose.

Surgery to the nose is not usually a straightforward procedure and like all forms of surgery needs to be carefully considered. Usually it is performed by a specialist plastic surgeon. If you are having breathing difficulties you might also need a consultation with an ear, nose and throat surgeon.

Rhinoplasty requires a general anaesthetic and usually an incision in the nose to gain access to the bones and cartilage that form the nasal skeleton. Sometimes this incision is hidden in the nostrils, but more commonly it is in the tissue between the nostrils under the tip of the nose (the columella). The bones may need to be broken and reset in a better position and the cartilage may need to be partly removed, reshaped or replaced. Usually you'll need to wear a splint for a short period after the surgery. It often involves an overnight stay in hospital and will require around two weeks off work or study.

After rhinoplasty the nose is very swollen for some time and it may take several months for all the swelling to disappear. The scar from the incision is usually very good but sometimes is visible. There is a small risk of bleeding or interfering with breathing with this surgery. Sometimes there are small lumps or bumps on the nose that can be felt but usually not seen. Some people will have minor asymmetry that is not a problem, but up to 10 per cent will need another rhinoplasty at some point to correct problems not fixed or even caused by the original procedure.

Genitoplasty (genital surgery)

Genitoplasty is surgery to alter the anatomy of the genitalia. It was initially developed for young children born with abnormal or 'ambiguous' genitalia; it is rarely performed on adolescents. The most common reason for this surgery is having uneven genitalia, particularly labia of different sizes, which is actually completely normal. Labial surgery is currently in vogue, with growing numbers of women seeking treatment. This has been partly attributed to internet pornography and increased media coverage. The vast majority actually have normal anatomy, but an extremely small number do have a genuine need for labial surgery. If the labia are especially large, some women find it uncomfortable to wear certain types of clothing, or report problems with exercise or sexual intercourse. Surgery needs to be carefully planned because sometimes the resulting scars can be painful and more problematic than the enlarged labia. It usually requires a general anaesthetic and surgery in a proper hospital facility.

Congenital (inherited) or acquired urogynaecological disorders sometimes require plastic surgery. These disorders, such as being born with abnormal genitalia or no genitalia, or suffering cancer or some other disease or trauma, are relatively rare and are best managed in a specialist gynaecological unit in consultation with a specialist plastic surgery unit. Congenital problems are usually diagnosed at a young age and fortunately cancers and other diseases in this area are fairly uncommon.

Reconstructive plastic surgery

Sometimes plastic surgery is not considered purely elective – for instance, following disease or injury or to correct congenital problems – and in these cases it is called reconstructive. The most common reason would be for breast problems (see chapter 27), but any disease or trauma that causes scarring or loss of function to any area may require plastic surgery.

You might also be offered reconstructive plastic surgery to try to rebuild or repair tissues that are affected by disease, surgery or injury.

10

Mental health in adolescence

Elisabeth Gasparini, Fiona Judd, Alessandra Radovini

Adolescence is a time of change and development. Over time this usually results in a greater understanding of who you are and your unique strengths and talents, and an increasing appreciation of the world around you and your place in it.

Times of change bring with them new opportunities and challenges that are essential for growth but can also be confusing and stressful. All this is normal and the vast majority of adolescents (and families) make this transition from childhood to young adulthood without any major hiccups.

For some young people the development of mental health problems during adolescence is not just a hiccup but can turn into a major derailment from their normal developmental path.

Better awareness of mental health problems in young people, understanding prevention strategies, early identification of problems and seeking appropriate help are the keys to good mental health for young people.

Adolescent behaviour and development

A wide range of things happens in adolescence. It is a time of experimentation, finding out who you are, and gradually becoming increasingly independent.

Some of the normal tasks of adolescents are:

- challenging your parents (and other adults)
- taking risks (and breaking rules)
- testing and demonstrating courage
- experiencing success
- recognising your feelings
- finding your voice

- developing a belief system
- becoming self-sufficient
- leaving school/leaving home
- learning to give
- recognising your mortality

Adolescence can be divided into early, middle and late stages, with different priorities or concerns for each.

Stage	Age (years)	Concern
Early	9–14	Am I normal?
Middle	15–17	Who am I?
Late	over 18	Where am I going?

Adolescence is a time of significant change and development in a number of areas: biological (physical changes), psychological (thinking) and social (increasing independence, interests). Young people become physically mature in adolescence, but we now know that brain development continues throughout adolescence and into young adulthood. Therefore adolescents have adult bodies but not yet adult brains. This 'cognitive' finetuning continues into the mid- to late 20s and explains why you might have difficulty with some of these things:

- expressing your thoughts and feelings
- regulating your emotions
- anticipating potential risks
- understanding another's point of view
- using rational thinking

The analogy is that the adolescent brain is like an engine that is fully developed and switched on, but the controls need some finetuning. This time of complex biological and social changes is what makes young people especially vulnerable to mental health issues. Having said that, most young people get through adolescence without major difficulty.

Romantic relationships

The specific age at which people develop their first romantic relationship varies widely according to culture, gender and the individual, but for most it will happen at some point during adolescence. Romantic relationships become more common and last longer as teenagers move from early to late adolescence. By mid- to late adolescence, some young people spend more time with their partner than with friends or family, and by early adulthood romantic partners may even have overtaken parents and close friends to become the primary source of support to a young person.

The challenges of developing and maintaining romantic relationships allow adolescents to achieve important milestones such as developing independence and a growing sense of who they are. They also allow adolescents to build important skills they will rely on as adults, such as the ability to manage strong emotions, develop communication and interpersonal skills (knowing how to sort out conflicts), and develop and nurture intimate relationships.

While romantic relationships are a normal and healthy part of adolescent development, they bring with them new stresses and risks. This is further amplified for young people who are same-sex attracted or questioning their sexuality or gender. If these young people experience isolation, bullying and homophobia, their risk of distress and mental health difficulties increases.

Studies tell us that relationship problems involving boyfriends/girlfriends can be one of the major stresses for adolescents, and can sometimes result in significant distress.

Some of the factors that increase vulnerability to distress when developing or maintaining a romantic relationship include:

• a first romantic relationship
• a recent break-up, especially for girls
• unhealthy relationships, which might be characterised by being very stormy and intense with extreme highs and lows, controlling behaviour or dating/partner violence

Your vulnerability increases if you are also experiencing problems in other relationships with your parents and/or peers and feel generally unsupported.

For a small number of vulnerable young people, a recent relationship break-up (in the last 12 months) appears to be one of the triggers for developing a first episode of depression during adolescence. (See later in this chapter for more on depression.)

Romantic relationships in themselves are neither good nor bad for adolescent development. Some of the positives are increased self-esteem and social status, social competence, autonomy and independence, and protection from social anxiety. Some of the negatives can include increased stress, academic difficulties, sexual health risks, unplanned pregnancy and 'dating' violence.

It can be very important to have someone to talk to about your experiences and feelings, to be able to learn the difference between healthy and unhealthy relationships, and to learn how to act respectfully towards your romantic partners and their interests.

Young people today face additional challenges that were not around a generation ago, related to social networking, social media and cyberbullying. See the Resources section at the end of the book, which can provide insight into some of these new challenges.

Dealing with a 'broken heart'

Regardless of the duration of the relationship, endings can be very difficult, distressing and messy. It is important to find ways of managing those intense feelings of sadness, anger and loss. Things that can help when you have taken a knock to your confidence include talking with a trusted person, doing things that you enjoy, going out with friends, and having the support of friends and family around you. Watch out for negative and distorted thinking, such as 'I'm ugly, nobody loves me', and remember to spend time with those who love and value you.

It is also important for you and your ex-partner to act respectfully towards each other, and know that sometimes things don't work out and it's nobody's fault. Also remember that relationships during adolescence are helping you work out who is the right person for you, and it's unlikely to be your first romantic partner.

Your body image

For many young women, body image is a key concern. Am I normal? How do I compare to my peers? These are common preoccupations. All the physical changes that occur during adolescence, along with social influences, result in our self-image changing.

Body image is how we view our physical self, including how we think and feel about our body, whether we feel we are attractive and whether we think others like how we look. Body image is closely linked to self-esteem; that is, how much we feel we are worth and how much we feel others value us. Good self-esteem and a healthy body image impact directly on whether we feel good about ourselves, which then affects our mental health and wellbeing.

The Butterfly Foundation, an organisation that provides support for those suffering from eating disorders and body-image issues, states that 'body image is the number-one concern for young Australian women aged 12–28'. Body image may not relate to actual appearance. Nearly half of all women of normal weight overestimate their size and shape, and are unhappy about how they look. Having a healthy body image means accepting and liking ourselves the way we are, having a realistic view of ourselves, knowing our strengths and weaknesses, and knowing that we are liked and appreciated for who we are.

A range of factors can contribute to the development of a poor body image: being teased as a child about one's appearance, peer pressure to go on diets and be thin, media images promoting thinness and a preoccupation with appearance, and growing up in a family where others diet or are unhappy with their body shape.

Developing a good body image is about recognising that each body is unique, no matter what shape or size it is, and focusing on being strong and healthy. It is also crucial to be clear about which aspects of appearance can realistically be changed and which can't. It's important to remember, as the Butterfly Foundation highlights, 'real people aren't perfect and perfect people aren't real'. (They are usually photoshopped.)

Illness or surgery can result in physical changes that affect body image; so can female genital cutting, a traditional practice in many African, Middle Eastern and Asian countries (see chapter 8 for more). If any of these things has happened to you, you can ask for help to understand the changes in your own body, how they might affect you and how to support a healthy body image.

Mental health problems

Mental health problems are the most common health problems in young people. Between 20 and 25 per cent of Australian adolescents will experience a mental health or substance-abuse problem in any given year. Many will experience more than one problem at the same time. Anxiety, depression and substance abuse are the leading mental health problems in young people.

Defining individuality and becoming independent, sorting out social networks, starting sexual relationships, finishing school and starting work are some of the experiences you might have as an adolescent. At this crucial stage, even relatively mild or brief mental health problems can disrupt development and have a significant impact on your life.

Mental health problems need to be taken seriously as they can have a range of negative consequences including poor academic achievement, poor social functioning, unemployment, substance abuse, self-harm and suicide. Recognising problems and getting appropriate and timely help are very important. In the first instance this might involve finding somebody to talk to, and getting some information, support and assistance to develop coping strategies. At other times it might need more specialist help.

Getting support

Young people are often reluctant to seek help when dealing with problems. Girls are generally better at seeking help than boys, but it is estimated that as many as 75 per cent of young people who need professional help do not access health care. The stigma associated with mental illness, the lack of community awareness about mental health problems that affect young people, and the lack of obviously youth-friendly services are some of the barriers to seeking help. In addition, young people might also feel reluctant or embarrassed to talk about personal issues and anxious about what sort of response they'll get, and are worried that there is something wrong with them.

The difficulties in seeking help can be even greater for young people from Indigenous or culturally and linguistically diverse backgrounds, or who are same-sex attracted. These young people are often marginalised and isolated, and while they may experience higher rates of psychological distress than the general population, they are less likely to use traditional mental health services.

Fortunately, this has been recognised and a range of youth-friendly services have been developed, and continue to expand across Australia to meet the needs of young people. This has also extended into the online environment, where a range of information and resources is available, as well as online mental health counselling and support to increase the ways young people can get help. (See the Resources section at the end of this book.)

Eating disorders

A distorted body image can lead to self-destructive behaviours such as dieting and binge-eating that predispose young women to the development of eating disorders. People with an eating disorder experience extreme disturbances in their eating behaviour and related thoughts and feelings. They have an overwhelming drive to be thin and a morbid fear of gaining weight and losing control over their eating. Eating disorders can cause serious physical and psychological problems. They are not a lifestyle choice.

Eating disorders usually start in adolescence and mainly affect young women. The two most serious eating disorders are anorexia nervosa (anorexia) and bulimia nervosa (bulimia). Anorexia is characterised by an intense fear of being fat and a relentless pursuit of thinness. Bulimia is characterised by bingeing and purging.

Symptoms of eating disorders

The symptoms of anorexia include:

- loss of weight (at least 15 per cent) as a result of restricting food intake, or in younger girls a failure to put on weight as expected developmentally (for their age and size)
- an intense fear of becoming fat and losing control
- disturbance of body image, where despite being thin, the person regards themselves as fat
- exercising excessively to lose weight
- the absence of menstrual periods

The symptoms of bulimia include:

- binge-eating involving consumption of extreme quantities of food
- feelings of loss of control, self-disgust and guilt as a result of bingeing
- purging to avoid putting on weight as a result of binge-eating, including inducing vomiting, and the misuse of laxatives or fluid tablets
- a combination of excessive exercise and restricted eating to control weight
- normal or near normal body weight

The physical and psychological effects of anorexia and bulimia are generally reversible if treated early, but they can be life-threatening if severe and untreated. It is therefore essential to identify early warning signs – such as abnormal eating patterns, ongoing loss of weight, and preoccupation with thinness and dieting – and obtain help as soon as possible.

Both anorexia and bulimia have significant physical effects on the body. These may include:

- feeling weak or dizzy and fainting
- harm to the kidneys
- dehydration, constipation and diarrhoea
- urinary tract infections
- muscle spasms or cramps and/or seizures
- erosion of dental enamel from vomiting
- intestinal and stomach problems
- growth retardation and problems with weak bones
- heart problems, which can lead to serious problems with abnormal heart rate or rhythm and in extreme cases sudden death

The psychological and emotional impact of these conditions can often be very serious and debilitating. People with anorexia or bulimia can exhibit low self-esteem, mood swings and emotional outbursts, anxiety and depression, increasing isolation and loneliness, reluctance to develop personal relationships, and fear of disapproval from others if the disorder becomes known. These kinds of effects can have a serious impact on the ability to function normally at home, school and work.

What causes eating disorders?

Biological, psychological and social factors are all involved in the development of an eating disorder. Exactly which of these factors is the most significant will vary for each young woman, but the greatest risk factor is dieting. See chapter 5 for more information on good nutrition and exercise.

Factors involved in developing an eating disorder

Biological	Those who have a mother or a sister who has had or has anorexia are more likely to develop the disorder than those who don't.
Psychological	• Perfectionism and being a high achiever • Fear of growing up and of the responsibilities of adulthood • Poor communication between family members • Stresses such as the break-up of relationships, pressure at school or the death of a loved one
Social	• Western society's obsession with body image • Media representation of thin as the ideal body shape • Media and online promotion of dieting

Treatment for eating disorders

Eating disorders can be effectively treated and, as mentioned above, the earlier the treatment the better the recovery. Families and friends often need support and assistance too, and are involved in the treatment process. Treatment is likely to include a range of approaches that cover both the medical/physical and psychological problems that occur with eating disorders.

A physical health check is essential to rule out the possible medical complications that can arise (see above). This might also include investigations such as blood tests and electrocardiographs (ECG) to assess the body's metabolic functioning: kidney, liver and heart function, and bone development.

Education about diet and healthy eating is also very important, as there is plenty of wrong or misunderstood information about food and nutrition out there.

Psychological interventions such as talking with a professional counsellor are necessary to help change thoughts, feelings and behaviours related to food and exercise, and to help deal with the stressful things that might be happening, such as relationship problems (with friends or family and/or romantic relationships), school issues (whether academic, social or related to peer group) or other things. If there are psychological complications, such as severe depression or anxiety, medications may be useful.

If you are diagnosed with an eating disorder, you are most likely to be treated in an outpatient setting or a community clinic. Those who are severely malnourished or have medical complications may need to be treated in hospital for a period of time. An important goal of treatment is to reach and/or maintain a healthy weight, develop normal eating behaviours and learn ways of managing life's stresses.

Dietary management

Dieticians who specialise in the treatment of eating disorders can assess and manage nutritional needs and give accurate nutrition education and advice. Advice on appropriate nutritional supplementation may also be needed. A dietician will often be part of the treating team.

A dietician can determine an individual's nutritional needs and set realistic short-term goals with respect to food intake, meal patterns, exercise and physical activities. They can provide education about food needed for good health, weight control and to maintain metabolism; and the physical and psychological effects of eating disorders. They will also help to correct any misinformation.

Knowing how to eat normally is a skill that will gradually need to be relearnt. Meal plans are a useful tool in this relearning process, and a dietician can help create these plans to meet individual nutritional needs. A dietician can also advise on appropriate portion sizes, and work on specific goals such as gradually introducing feared foods. Ongoing support is important to help increase confidence that reaching and maintaining a healthy weight and developing normal eating behaviours is possible.

Ultimately, the goal is for eating to become more intuitive and relaxed, with little preoccupation with food and weight. The dietician will encourage incorporation of a wide variety of foods into the diet, along with balanced meals and snacks, and practising eating spontaneously and in social situations. As recovery progresses, eating gradually becomes easier and more enjoyable.

Anxiety disorders

Anxiety is the normal feeling we have that alerts us to something dangerous, threatening or stressful. Common examples are feeling anxious before an exam or performance, or when going for a job interview or starting a new job. A certain amount of anxiety is good for us. It prepares us to face a challenge and gets us hyped up to perform at our best.

Feelings of anxiety are also common when we experience major challenges in our lives like relationship breakdowns, serious illness or the death of a loved one. These feelings are normal, appropriate and time-limited.

We experience anxiety as both physical sensations (racing heart, breathlessness, butterflies in the stomach) and worrying thoughts ('Will I be okay? Can I manage this?'), and it influences our behaviour ('I better not do that or go there').

There is a clear difference, however, between 'normal anxiety' and an anxiety disorder. When anxiety is severe, persistent, overwhelming to the degree that it stops the person from functioning properly and, importantly, out of proportion to the situation, it is likely to indicate an anxiety disorder. This kind of anxiety is like a faulty alarm that goes off when there is no danger, challenge or threat. It is usually more severe than normal anxiety and can go on for days, weeks or months.

Anxiety disorders are very common, can start at any age including childhood, and affect women more than men. In Australia one in 25 adolescents aged 13–17 will experience anxiety in any 12-month period. For 18–25-year-olds the figure is higher: one in 10.

There are six main types of anxiety disorder:

- generalised anxiety disorder
- social phobia
- specific phobia
- panic disorder
- obsessive compulsive disorder
- post-traumatic stress disorder

Symptoms of anxiety disorders

The symptoms of anxiety disorders are both physical and psychological. The physical symptoms you may experience include sweating, a racing heart, trembling, dizziness, pins and needles, breathlessness, choking, abdominal pain and nausea. These physical symptoms are usually accompanied by anxious thoughts, such as feeling out of control, that something terrible is going to happen, or that you're going to die or that you're going mad.

Types of anxiety disorders

There are a number of anxiety disorders, which are classified according to their symptoms and/or causes.

Generalised anxiety disorder

People with generalised anxiety disorder worry excessively about everyday things such as their family, friends, health or finances. They are constantly worried that something bad is going to happen and cannot be reassured otherwise. These worries are persistent, irrational and out of proportion to the situation.

Social phobia

People with social phobia worry excessively about social or performance situations. They worry they will be scrutinised and judged by others. This results in the person restricting or avoiding activities such as interacting with others, or eating or speaking in front of others.

Specific phobia

A phobia is an intense fear of a specific object (e.g. animals, spiders, snakes, water) or situation (heights, lifts, flying). People will go to extreme lengths to avoid the feared object or situation, and this can severely interfere with their lives. This intense fear can lead to a panic attack.

Panic disorder

People with panic disorder experience panic attacks whenever their anxiety gets out of hand. Panic attacks are sudden, intense, extreme anxiety symptoms that appear to come out of nowhere but are often triggered by minor things or situations that would not normally worry other people. They are accompanied by such intense physical symptoms (such as palpitations, shortness of breath, sweatiness, dizziness) that the person having them might think they are having a heart attack or going mad. This often leads such people to avoid specific situations or places and so become agoraphobic. Agoraphobia means 'fear of the market place'. People experiencing agoraphobia fear busy places, such as supermarkets, shopping centres or public transport, from which they think they might not be able to escape. When this is severe, a person with agoraphobia may consider their home the only safe place and avoid leaving their home for days, months or even years.

Obsessive compulsive disorder (OCD)

People with OCD have persistent unwanted intrusive thoughts (obsessions) that they can only manage through performing elaborate rituals (compulsions) that help to decrease the associated anxiety. For example, someone who is concerned about germs or contamination will have rituals around washing and cleanliness. These rituals can become so time-consuming that they interfere with daily living. People with OCD are often very aware that their worries are irrational and are embarrassed by their rituals, so they tend to hide them from others.

Post-traumatic stress disorder (PTSD)

PTSD can occur when people have experienced terrifying and potentially life-threatening situations of trauma, such as in wars, natural disasters, personal violence and major accidents. People with PTSD often re-experience the traumatic event through flashbacks or nightmares. They try to avoid any situations or things that might remind them of the event and trigger these distressing thoughts or images. PTSD can be extremely disabling and distressing.

What causes anxiety disorders?

Our genetic and biochemical make-up can predispose us to anxiety disorders. It can also be part of our personality (people who develop anxiety disorders tend to be 'worriers'), and can be triggered by stressful events such as bullying, family break-up or conflict, sexual abuse or the death of a significant person.

Treatment for anxiety disorders

If anxiety symptoms are severe enough to interfere with day-to-day living then help should be sought. A GP can help identify the type of anxiety disorder and the best way to manage it. This can include getting information about anxiety disorders, talking with someone about understanding possible triggers, developing better strategies to manage stress, and limiting alcohol and drug use.

It can also include structured therapies such as cognitive behaviour therapy (CBT), and relaxation and meditation techniques. CBT helps people understand the connections between their thoughts, feelings and behaviours, how these influence each other and how to change or challenge faulty or unhelpful thinking, such as 'Everyone's going to be looking at me,' or 'I'll make a mistake and it will be a disaster!'

Medication may also be prescribed in some circumstances as part of the treatment package, and this requires ongoing monitoring and evaluation.

Depression

Depression is used to describe everyday feelings of sadness as well as depressive disorders. Sadness and unhappiness are things we all experience at some point in our lives. It can sometimes be difficult to distinguish the symptoms of an emerging depressive disorder from 'normal' sadness, especially for adolescents.

We all have stressful times in our lives when we are likely to be distressed and deeply saddened, such as the death of a loved one, the break-up of a relationship, or another major loss or blow. Our normal responses to everyday life events are usually short-lived and get better on their own, and are not considered depressive disorders.

The term 'depressive disorders' describes a group of illnesses where the feelings of sadness are severe, persistent (going on for several weeks or months) and impact on the ability to function and enjoy life. In addition to the change in mood, there are changes in thoughts (overwhelmingly negative ideas) and behaviour, or in the level of interest in activities.

Depression is common, often starting in adolescence and young adulthood, and will affect one in four young people between the ages of 15 and 25. It is a serious and disabling illness that can have a significant impact on wellbeing and can even be life-threatening. Fortunately, treatment is usually very effective and safe.

Symptoms of depression

The symptoms of depression can be classified into four main types, as outlined in the table below.

The four types of depressive symptoms

Changes in mood	• Feelings of sadness, hopelessness, irritability, anxiety, guilt and helplessness
Changes in thinking	• Poor concentration • Difficulty thinking, slowed thinking, not being able to take things in, such as schoolwork • Persistent negative thoughts about oneself, one's situation and the future • Increasing thoughts about death, self-harm or suicide
Changes in behaviour	• Lack of interest and enjoyment in usual activities • Feelings of boredom • Everything feeling harder to do • Poor school performance • Becoming withdrawn, more isolated, not wanting to be with people • Increased alcohol or drug use • Self-harm
Changes in physical wellbeing	• Increased tiredness, decreased energy • Changes in appetite (commonly decreased or increased appetite, particularly for junk food) • Changes in weight (usually decreased) • Decreased sexual drive • Changes in sleep patterns (too much or too little, or trouble getting to or staying asleep)

In adolescence, depression can be easily missed, or people can dismiss symptoms of depression as just part of being a teenager. If you or a young person you know is experiencing several of these symptoms or you notice a big change in the way you or they are functioning over time, this should be checked out. This can be done by talking to a trusted adult, school counsellor or GP.

Types of depressive disorders

The common depressive disorders are classified according to their severity, duration and/or causes.

Major depressive disorder

Major depressive disorder is the most commonly diagnosed of these. It can occur following a stressful period in life or for no apparent reason.

Dysthymic disorder

When the symptoms of depression are fewer, milder but persistent (for more than two years), this is called a dysthymic disorder.

Adjustment disorder with depressed mood

When depression occurs following a defined stressful event (e.g. job loss, relationship break-up) this is sometimes referred to as an adjustment disorder with depressed mood. Usually the symptoms are not as severe and tend to be of shorter duration.

Postnatal depression (PND)

PND can occur following the birth of a baby and affects about 10 per cent of new mothers. It can be quite disabling and make it difficult for a mother to cope with the demands of everyday life and her new baby. Mothers can experience sadness, anxiety and extreme tiredness, with disrupted appetite and sleep beyond what might be usual in the postnatal period. For more on PND, see chapter 22.

Depression in bipolar disorder

Bipolar mood disorder, which used to be called manic depression, results in people experiencing episodes of depression and episodes of elevated mood (mania) that can follow each other or occur at different times in their lives. In addition to the elevated mood and elevated sense of well-being, people experience racing thoughts, rapid speech, overactivity, a decreased need for sleep, poor judgement and behave recklessly. The episodes of depression are similar to major depressive disorder.

What causes depression?

There is no single cause for depression; rather, it is the result of the interplay between an individual's risk factors or vulnerability and environmental or situational factors. Risk factors for depression that have been identified include: a family history of depression; biological vulnerability, which might cause a change in the biochemicals in the parts of the brain to do with thinking and feeling; and adverse events in childhood, such as the death of a parent or maltreatment. Other risk factors are drug and alcohol misuse, stressful life events and physical illness. Transition times have also been identified as times of increased vulnerability, such as leaving school, childbirth, menopause and bereavement.

Treatment for depression

Treatment for depression can be very effective and may involve a combination of support, education, psychological treatment, lifestyle intervention and antidepressant medication. Having support through a difficult and confusing time, having a trusted adult to talk to, and understanding the nature of depression and what is happening are very important factors in recovering from depression. Support and education for families and carers is also essential, as they too are often feeling worried and confused.

A range of psychological treatments have been found to be useful in treating depression:

- cognitive behaviour therapy (CBT), which is aimed at changing the patterns of thinking and behaviour that relate to depression
- interpersonal therapies, which aim to help people understand how their interpersonal relationships have an effect on their emotions
- improving problem-solving skills, which can help people look at problems differently and identify possible practical solutions
- lifestyle changes, such as exercising, scheduling pleasurable activities, better managing time, and limiting excessive drug and alcohol use, which can all help recovery from depression
- antidepressant medications, which may be needed for severe and persistent symptoms of depression or when other psychological interventions have not been helpful. Antidepressant medications help by relieving depressed or anxious feelings and improving sleep and appetite. They do this by changing the balance of the normal chemicals (neurotransmitters) in the brain, but they can take between two and six weeks to make a difference. Antidepressant medications usually have few side effects and are not addictive. For adolescents, doctors will usually suggest other treatments first, before antidepressant medications.

Self-harm

Self-harm is when someone deliberately injures themselves. This is also referred to as self-injury or deliberate self-harm. Some of the more common self-harming behaviours include cutting, burning and scratching. Excessive alcohol and drug misuse does not usually come under this definition. Self-harming behaviour in young people is relatively common. It often starts in early adolescence but may not be discovered for some time as it is usually kept hidden.

It can be difficult to distinguish self-harm from suicidal behaviour, as the individual's intention may be unclear or unknown. Young people who self-harm may be very distressed and overwhelmed but generally don't intend to end their lives.

Who self harms?

Self-harm is most common between the ages of 11 and 25 but is not limited to this age group. People who self-harm have usually had past or current negative experiences such as relationship breakdown, abuse (physical, sexual, emotional), significant loss, long-term family problems, bullying or serious illness or disability.

Why do young people self harm?

There are many reasons why people self-harm. Many people think self-harm is attention-seeking behaviour, but this is not the case. Most young people who self-harm keep it a secret for a long time. Some reported reasons for self-harm include:

- to cope with feelings of extreme emotional pain, such as despair, loneliness, anger, helplessness, shame, guilt and stress
- to try to gain control – some young people feel that hurting themselves gives them a sense of control (in the short term)
- to communicate distress – some young people don't know how to express their emotions verbally
- to manage feeling disconnected and isolated from others – some young people feel that hurting themselves helps them feel real
- as self-punishment – some young people hate themselves so much they believe they deserve to be punished

What to do about self-harm

Self-harm is a complex and sensitive issue. Although the intention behind the self-harm may not be for a young person to end their life, there are nevertheless many associated risks and possible complications of self-harm, ranging from significant injury to accidental death.

If you are engaging in self-harming behaviour, it is important to let someone know and not to try and manage it on your own. Talking to a trusted adult or a health professional is a good place to start.

If you are concerned that someone you know is self-harming, or you see evidence that suggests self-harm, speak to them about your concerns and offer your support and assistance in getting help. If you are unsure what to do or how to broach the topic with them, speak to your GP or to a local mental health professional such as your school counsellor.

While self-harm may not be a suicide attempt, it is still risky behaviour that can have long-term consequences for the young person and therefore should always be taken seriously.

Psychosis

The term psychosis (or psychotic disorder) refers to a group of disorders in which there is a misinterpretation of reality. The common symptoms of these disorders – disturbances in thinking and perception – reflect this.

Psychotic disorders affect one in 100 people and commonly begin in the teens to early 30s. The most common age of onset varies between women and men: women commonly experience their first episode of illness later than men. The onset of psychosis may be gradual and the symptoms non-specific. They can include a combination of suspiciousness, depression, anxiety, irritability, restlessness, a change in appetite, a sense of alteration of self or the surrounding world, social isolation or withdrawal, impairment in functioning, peculiar behaviour, deterioration in personal hygiene, and vague or disordered thinking or unusual perceptual experiences.

In many instances the symptoms may be transient and not associated with the development of illness. However, when symptoms are increasing in severity or cluster together, they may indicate developing psychosis.

Symptoms of psychosis

An acute episode of psychosis is characterised by symptoms such as delusions and hallucinations, and is usually accompanied by a loss of insight, so that many sufferers do not accept that they are ill.

Delusions are fixed false beliefs, which cannot be explained by the person's background, and which cannot be changed by logic or reason. Most commonly they involve ideas of persecution ('People are talking about me/trying to harm me', etc.) or ideas of grandiosity ('I am a world-class athlete', 'I have discovered the answer to climate change', etc.).

Hallucinations describe the experience of hearing or seeing things that are not there and that no one else can see or hear ('I can hear people talking about me/commenting on what I'm doing', etc.). They can also involve tasting, feeling or smelling things that are not there. Auditory hallucinations are the most common.

Other symptoms, such as loss of emotional expression, decreased motivation and reduced social engagement, may also occur. People who are psychotic may also have trouble paying attention or sticking to a task, show disorganised behaviour, and have speech problems such as loud, rapid and mixed-up speech. Mood disturbances can also be common, including depression or elevation of mood, or frequent and unpredictable changes of mood.

What causes psychosis?

Psychosis has a variety of possible causes, and often no one cause can be identified. Genetic make-up can predispose an individual to psychosis, but even if a person has a family member with psychosis this only means a one in 10 chance of developing a similar problem. Other factors that may increase the chance of developing a psychotic illness include one's mother having an infection such as influenza when pregnant, or experiencing trauma in early life.

Psychotic symptoms can often occur due to illicit drug use, and can accompany signs of intoxication such as confusion, disorientation and agitation. The most common drugs causing psychosis in Australia are cannabis and amphetamines.

Treatment for psychosis

Treatment for psychosis involves a comprehensive assessment to exclude medical causes for the symptoms, as well as to identify if illicit drugs have caused or worsened the symptoms.

Ensuring the safety of the person with psychosis as well as others is important. Harm to self or others can result from delusional beliefs (e.g. the belief that someone is trying to kill them, leading them to take defensive action) or hallucinations (such as a voice telling them to harm themselves), or as a result of feelings of depression leading to suicidal thoughts or actions.

If treatment is delayed, the condition is likely to have greater adverse effects on study, work, family and other relationships. Being unwell can also interfere with the normal developmental trajectory of adolescence and early adulthood, so early diagnosis and treatment is very important.

Key aspects of treatment are to stop using any illicit drugs and to start taking antipsychotic medications. These medications are effective for the treatment of delusions and hallucinations and need to be taken continuously to avoid symptoms recurring.

While medication is essential, other things are also of great importance in aiding recovery. These include psycho-education about the illness, support for families, assistance with schooling and/or work and maintaining social connections and interests.

Co-occurring problems

In adolescents it is common for mental health difficulties to occur together and either arise at the same time or as a consequence of each other. For example, depression and anxiety symptoms commonly coexist and both can be present in someone with an eating disorder. Drug and alcohol misuse, and self-harming behaviours, are risk factors for and often complicate a range of mental health difficulties. For full recovery and optimal wellbeing, it is important for each area of difficulty to be addressed appropriately.

For parents, families and carers

Looking after a young person who is experiencing mental health difficulties can be very stressful for other family members and carers. Often parents and carers feel worried, distressed and confused about what to do and how best to help a young person. Families are a very important and vital part of a young person's recovery. Young people with supportive families do better than young people without support networks.

Parents and carers looking after a young person with a mental health difficulty may find it helpful to:

- Talk with the young person about your concerns and your wish to support them in finding solutions for their current difficulties.
- Remember to be calm, non-blaming and non-judgemental.
- Remind them they are loved and valued (even though some of their behaviours might be challenging).
- Ask them what they would find helpful.
- Remember to give unconditional support.

This is a time when a young person is not functioning at their best and may not be making very good decisions, which means they need your support even more. This can also be a stressful time for you as a family member, and you may need support and assistance to deal with your own feelings and emotions as well as practical information. Your GP can give you information and refer you to local counsellors who can assist.

11

Drugs and alcohol

Ian McCahon

Drugs and alcohol are everywhere, and it's easy to find out about them. Maybe you think you know enough about alcohol and other drugs to be informed about whether they are safe to use. Maybe your friends think they know enough and have decided to try them. The only decisions that really matter about drugs and alcohol, though, are the ones you make yourself.

The information in this chapter is designed to help you to do this wisely and safely.

Things to consider

Before deciding whether to use alcohol or drugs, ask yourself:

- **Is it legal or illegal?** Alcohol and cigarettes cause the most damage to your health, but they are legal. If a drug is not legal, it may not be what the dealer says it is: it may contain other dangerous substances, or it may be weaker or stronger than you expected.

- **Is there a legal age?** You can't buy alcohol in the United States until you are 21 because it can damage your brain, but in Australia you can choose to buy, drink or possess alcohol on licensed premises when you are 18.

- **Will it damage my health or mental health?** Alcohol, methamphetamine, heroin and crack cocaine are among the most dangerous drugs. They can make you aggressive or violent. If you take them together you could have trouble breathing. If you sniff glue, paint or petrol it can stop your heart working properly. Cannabis is less dangerous, but can harm your mental health. Ecstasy, kava, khat and LSD may do the least damage but can be a gateway to other drug use.

- **Do I have a real medical reason to use this prescribed medicine?** Painkillers such as oxycodone, and benzodiazepines such as alprazolam or oxazepam are easy to start using but very hard to stop using.

National drug policy

Australia has a national drug policy that encourages people to avoid using drugs but helps them to reduce the risks if they do. It aims to reduce all types of drug-related harm to both individuals and the community. Substance abuse has many health consequences:

- Many substances are addictive and long-term use of alcohol or cigarettes causes chronic diseases.
- Substance-users have an increased risk of trauma including motor vehicle accidents and violence.
- Substance use by intravenous injection can lead to blood-borne diseases including hepatitis C and HIV/AIDS.
- Substance use increases the risk of mental health problems and suicide.
- Substance-users have an increased risk of overdose or death compared to non-users.

From the community point of view, substance use can damage relationships, and education, training and employment prospects. It also leads to increased costs for health care, social support, policing and law enforcement.

Why do people use drugs and alcohol?

People take drugs and drink alcohol for a range of reasons. Some say that:

- They drink alcohol to be social or socially accepted and do what everyone else seems to be doing.
- They drink alcohol or take drugs because there is peer pressure to do so and it is hard to resist.
- They drink before going out because they believe it will make them look and feel more confident.
- They drink to excess or take drugs as a way of coping with the impact of childhood abuse, violence or neglect, or to avoid coping with problems.
- They take drugs as a way of dealing with stress, depression or mental illness.

Why do some people not use drugs and alcohol?

Some say that:

- They do not drink alcohol because they do not like the taste or its effect on them.
- They do not drink alcohol as they have a parent or relative who is an alcoholic and they are worried they will have the same problem.
- They do not take drugs or drink alcohol because they don't see the need.
- They do not take drugs because they have seen the damaging effects on friends.
- They do not take drugs because they have previously had a psychotic episode or another type of bad experience after taking drugs.

Alcohol

The risks of drinking alcohol

- Risk of immediate damage to health, or death: LOW to HIGH if used with other drugs.
- Risk of permanent damage to health or mental health: HIGH if alcohol intake is high.
- Risk of unsafe parenting: LOW to HIGH, depending on when and how much is drunk.
- Risk of damage to the brain, physical development or long-term health of the baby if you are pregnant: LOW to HIGH, depending on when and how much the pregnant mother drinks.
- Risk of children copying parental behaviours and using this drug: HIGH.

You can decide yourself whether you want to drink alcohol and how much you would like to have. Life can be fun with only limited alcohol intake or with none at all.

There is no safe minimum amount of alcohol adolescents can drink. In some states there are laws governing drinking in private homes. Specific laws in Queensland, Victoria and Tasmania restrict to a minimum the supply of alcohol to people under the age of 18. This may mean that the parents of each person attending a party must consent individually to their son or daughter drinking alcohol while in the care of a responsible adult. A responsible adult is defined as one who is accompanying the young person and *not* consuming alcohol. In Western Australia, restrictions apply only to licensed premises, and less precise restrictions on underage drinking are defined in the laws of New South Wales, South Australia and the Australian Capital Territory.

The National Health and Medical Research Council (NHMRC) has published guidelines for safe drinking based on the latest scientific evidence:

1 **Reducing the risk of alcohol-related harm over a lifetime.** The lifetime risk of harm from drinking alcohol increases with the amount consumed. For healthy women and men, drinking no more than two standard drinks (see below) on any day reduces the lifetime risk of harm from alcohol-related disease or injury.

2 **Reducing the risk of injury on a single occasion of drinking.** On a single occasion of drinking, the risk of alcohol-related injury increases with the amount consumed. For healthy women and men, drinking no more than four standard drinks on a single occasion reduces the risk of alcohol-related injury arising from that occasion.

3 **Children and young people under 18.** For children and young people under 18, not drinking alcohol is the safest option. Children under 15 are at the greatest risk of harm from drinking and not drinking alcohol is especially important for this age group. For young people aged 15–17, the safest option is to delay the initiation of drinking for as long as possible.

4 **Pregnancy and breastfeeding.** Alcohol consumption by the mother can harm the developing fetus or breastfeeding baby. For women who are pregnant or planning a pregnancy, not drinking is the safest option. For women who are breastfeeding, not drinking is the safest option.

Adapted from: National Health and Medical Research Council, *Australian Guidelines to Reduce Health Risks from Drinking Alcohol*, NHMRC, Canberra, 2009, www.nhmrc.gov.au/ your-health/alcohol-guidelines

Standard drinks

The effect of alcohol on how you feel and on your health depends on how much you drink. Because women generally weigh less than men, the same amount of alcohol can have a greater effect on them.

If you learn how to calculate how much alcohol is in each drink, you can decide more easily how much or how little you would like to have. One way of keeping your alcohol consumption to a safer level is to limit the number of standard drinks you consume. By definition, a standard drink contains 10 grams of alcohol (i.e. 12.5 millilitres of pure alcohol).

Glasses, cans and shots of alcohol frequently contain more than one standard drink, but all bottles, cans and casks containing alcohol and produced in Australia are required by law to state on the label the approximate number of standard drinks they contain.

How much is a standard drink?

1 can or stubbie low-strength beer = 0.8 standard drink
1 can or stubbie mid-strength beer = 1 standard drink
1 can or stubbie full-strength beer = 1.4 standard drinks
100 millilitres wine (13.5% alcohol) = 1 standard drink
1 nip (30 ml) spirits = 1 standard drink
1 can spirits (about 5% alcohol) = 1.2–1.7 standard drinks
1 can spirits (about 7% alcohol) = 1.6–2.4 standard drinks

Adapted from: National Health and Medical Research Council, *Australian Guidelines to Reduce Health Risks from Drinking Alcohol*, NHMRC, Canberra, 2009, www.nhmrc. gov.au/your-health/alcohol-guidelines

---

Is alcohol harmful?

In a word, yes. There's plenty of research to show that drinking alcohol can cause serious short-term and long-term harm. Alcohol impairs normal thought processes and reflexes, and can lead to aggressive behaviour or being assaulted; to alcohol-related medical issues requiring hospitalisation; and to road accidents, either as a pedestrian, passenger or driver.

Alcohol is a drug, and like many drugs, it affects physical, social and mental health. Alcohol can affect speech, coordination, balance, vision, mood and muscle control. It can also cause nausea and vomiting and even passing out. The following day it can cause a hangover and headache that make it difficult to work or concentrate. Very high levels of alcohol intake can also cause death or serious brain damage.

Alcohol causes health problems that accumulate over a lifetime. The younger we start drinking, the greater our risk of serious health issues.

Alcohol and pregnancy

Drinking too much alcohol damages the brain and liver and, if you are pregnant, it may damage your baby.

Damage to the baby occurs mainly during the early weeks, before the mother knows she is pregnant. (Remember that many pregnancies are unplanned and that most women do not immediately know they are pregnant.) If this happens, the child may find it difficult to concentrate and learn things, and is more likely to be aggressive. In the uncommon condition fetal alcohol syndrome, the baby has an abnormal facial appearance and more severe brain damage.

Before you drink alcohol

There are several important things to think about if you do decide to drink alcohol:

- Alcohol can affect the way you think when you make decisions, including whether or not to have more alcohol, whether it is safe to drive and how you behave, including sexual inhibition.

- Drinks containing alcohol can make you dehydrated, so it is a good idea to drink plenty of water.

- Binge-drinking can make you careless with contraception and less likely to notice that you are pregnant.

- You should never leave your drink unattended. If you do leave your drink to dance or to go to the toilet, do not drink from that glass again – get a new drink. Do not risk your drink being spiked or allow the risk of date rape.

- Drinking more than the recommended amount of alcohol can lead to violence or accidents.

- You should never get into a car with a driver who has been drinking alcohol or drive yourself if you have been drinking.

How to avoid or limit drinking when you go out

Some people would rather not drink when they go out, or just don't want to drink much but feel like they have to because everyone else is doing it. Here are some strategies to help you avoid drinking:

- Plan ahead – decide if you will drink any alcohol and how much, or none at all.

- Eat some food beforehand or while you are drinking.
- Drink plenty of water.
- Hold a non-alcoholic drink such as non-alcoholic cider in a champagne glass, or cola in a tumbler.
- Be the designated driver.
- Drink mocktails.
- Join the conversation – talking with friends is more fun than drinking alcohol.
- When no one is looking, quietly pour or spit some of your alcoholic drink out in the bathroom or garden, or onto a pot plant.
- Say you are on medication that cannot be taken with alcohol, especially if this is actually the case.
- Don't try to justify why you are not drinking alcohol by discussing it.
- Avoid participating in rounds of drinks or shots.
- Plan to leave the party before too many people become affected by alcohol.

How to look after a drunk person

If someone around you has had too much to drink and is drunk, here are some things to consider:

- If they are not breathing properly, immediately call an ambulance by dialling 000.
- Turn them onto their side with their top leg and arm bent towards their head so they do not roll into the facedown position.
- Clear vomit from their mouth with your finger if necessary to clear their airway.
- Do not attempt to lift them by yourself.
- Do not give them water to drink unless they are fully awake.
- Put their car keys and wallet or purse in a safe place.

Dangers of alcohol and drugs together

Drinking alcohol while taking prescription drugs such as diazepam, alprazolam, zolpidem or oxycodone (for example, Valium, Xanax, Stilnox, Endone) can cause overdose. Taking street drugs such as cannabis or heroin with alcohol can also cause overdose, breathing problems and death.

Drinking alcohol with high-caffeine drinks, ecstasy or methamphetamine can at times cause sudden death by heart failure.

Alcohol addiction and dependence

Alcohol does not help solve problems. If you have mental health, chronic health or social issues, a support service will help you to get assistance.

If you do decide to drink, it is better to drink alcohol slowly, have water between drinks and to eat food before or with the alcohol. Binge-drinking and getting drunk may lead to alcohol dependence.

Having an alcoholic family member increases your own chances of alcoholism. Seek help if you are concerned, if you are having cravings for alcohol, if you are irritable, or if you have the shakes. You may also need help if you are drinking alone. Start taking thiamine (vitamin B1) until you get advice from your doctor or clinic – it may reduce the damage alcohol causes to nerve cells in the brain.

If you have an alcohol addiction, you may need to be admitted to a hospital or a residential care facility, depending on the severity of your addiction.

Cigarettes/tobacco

The risks of smoking

- Risk of immediate damage to health, or death: LOW.
- Risk of permanent damage to health: MODERATE.
- Risk of unsafe parenting: MODERATE.
- Risk of damage to the brain, physical development or long-term health of the baby if you are pregnant: MODERATE to HIGH.
- Risk of children copying parental behaviours and using this drug: HIGH.

Little can be said in favour of taking up smoking. Cigarettes are made from tobacco. They contain nicotine and at least 50 other chemicals that are poisonous or known to cause cancer. Chemicals found in tobacco smoke include acetone, arsenic, lead and tar. Nicotine is the addictive substance in tobacco; it is as addictive a drug as heroin and cocaine.

Cigarette smoking accounts for one-third of all cancer deaths. It is linked to an increased risk of cervical and ovarian cancers, as well as cancer of the lung, voice box, mouth, tongue, lips, nose, sinuses, throat, oesophagus, stomach, pancreas, kidney, bladder and colon, and acute myeloid leukaemia.

Smoking is also a major cause of many other serious health problems, such as heart disease, bronchitis, emphysema and stroke. It also makes many illnesses worse, such as asthma and pneumonia.

Smoking and pregnancy

Smoking can damage reproductive health and put an unborn child at increased risk. Tobacco use is linked to lower fertility, and to an increased risk of miscarriage and stillbirth. It has also been linked to a higher risk of birth defects. Smokers are three times more likely to experience preterm breaking of the waters and a premature baby, a baby who is small, or a baby who dies from sudden infant death syndrome (SIDS). A baby with a mother who smokes also has a higher risk of asthma and other chronic diseases.

Myths and misinformation about smoking

Myth 1: 'There is a safe way to smoke.' – No. All cigarettes cause damage.

Myth 2: 'Smoking fewer cigarettes is safer.' – It is actually quite hard to just smoke a few cigarettes a day, and research has found that even smoking as few as one to four cigarettes a day can lead to serious health problems, and a greater chance of dying younger.

Myth 3: 'Smoking "light" cigarettes is safer.' – This is not true. Studies have found that the risk of serious health effects is no lower in smokers of light or low-tar cigarettes.

Myth 4: 'Hand-rolled cigarettes are a healthier way to smoke.' – They are no safer than commercial brands. In fact, lifelong smokers of hand-rolled cigarettes have a higher risk of cancers of the voice box, oesophagus, mouth and throat than smokers of machine-made cigarettes.

Myth 5: 'Menthol cigarettes are safer than non-menthol cigarettes.' – This is not true. In fact, they might even be more dangerous.

Smokers are more likely to experience bleeding during pregnancy (placental abruption), which can be a danger to them as well as to the health and the life of their baby.

Passive smoking

The smoke from other people's cigarettes (called passive smoking) can also have harmful health effects on adults and children, potentially causing premature death and illness. Children who are frequently subjected to passive smoke have an increased risk of sudden infant death syndrome (SIDS), and respiratory and ear infections. Adults have an increased risk of heart disease and lung cancer.

How to give up smoking

Help is available when you decide to give up smoking. Counselling, nicotine patches and telephone support services such as the Quitline (13 7848 or 13 QUIT) can increase your chances of success threefold. Nicotine patches are safe to use in pregnancy if counselling and willpower alone are not successful.

As smoking is highly addictive, you will need to do some mental preparation, and have a solid plan and support to quit. Your GP can also help. You will need to:

- have a good reason to quit (for example, the cost, concern about your health, a planned pregnancy, exclusion from your social group, feeling embarrassed)
- have a plan, preferably written down and shared with others, which includes strategies to deal with the triggers that make you want to smoke, substitute behaviours and rewards
- put the plan into action, and engage your support person or network to help you stick to it

Other drugs

The drugs you can actually get depend on where you live and may include methamphetamine, cannabis, benzodiazepines, heroin, oxycodone, cocaine, ecstasy, GHB, volatiles, kava or khat and others. They are briefly described in the following pages.

Methamphetamine (ice)

> **The risks of methamphetamine (ice)**
>
> - Risk of immediate damage to health, or death: LOW to HIGH, depending on the amount used or if used with other substances such as GHB, opioids, alcohol or benzodiazepines.
> - Risk of permanent damage to health or mental health: HIGH. Prolonged methamphetamine use can damage your brain so that you may be unable to look after yourself and live independently.
> - Risk of unsafe parenting: HIGH.
> - Risk of damage to the brain, physical development or long-term health of the baby if you are pregnant: MODERATE.
> - Risk of children copying parental behaviours and using this drug: MODERATE. (Because of increasing parental aggression and inability to cope, it is unlikely that the children of a methamphetamine-dependent woman will live with her.)

Methamphetamine is a highly addictive stimulant that affects the central nervous system. It is a white, odourless, bitter-tasting crystalline powder that easily dissolves in water or alcohol. It can be injected or smoked.

Methamphetamine makes people restless, more alert, and more physically and mentally active. It causes increased activity and talkativeness, decreased appetite and a general sense of wellbeing. It also makes people aggressive and removes inhibitions.

Long-term use can make users anxious or depressed, and cause difficulty with sleep, memory and concentration. It can lead to 'acquired brain injury', a permanent change to brain functioning.

Methamphetamine is very dangerous if used during pregnancy: the baby may be born much too early, have a stroke and be partially paralysed, be small, or even die. Methamphetamine users are less likely than others to be safe parents.

Cannabis (marijuana, yarndi, mull, grass, hashish)

Cannabis is derived from the dried parts of the *Cannabis sativa* or hemp plant. It is usually smoked. Short-term effects of cannabis use include

The risks of cannabis

- Risk of immediate damage to health, or death: LOW.

- Risk of permanent damage to health or mental health: LOW to MODERATE, depending on the amount used.

- Risk of unsafe parenting: LOW to MODERATE, depending on the amount used.

- Risk of damage to the brain, physical development or long-term health of the baby if you are pregnant: LOW.

- Risk of children copying parental behaviours and using this drug: HIGH.

euphoria, distorted perceptions, memory impairment, and difficulty thinking and solving problems.

People who use cannabis are three times more likely to develop a mental health problem such as psychosis. They are also more likely to use other drugs, even if they are pregnant or breastfeeding.

The children of cannabis users are likely to be slow to learn in school, and more likely to develop depression.

Benzodiazepines (benzos)

The risks of benzodiazepines

- Risk of immediate damage to health, or death: LOW to HIGH if used with alcohol or heroin.

- Risk of permanent damage to health or mental health: LOW.

- Risk of unsafe parenting: MODERATE (HIGH if alprazolam taken).

- Risk of damage to the brain, physical development or long-term health of the baby if you are pregnant: LOW.

- Risk of children copying parental behaviours and using this drug: LOW. (Few users report using benzodiazepines because their parents did: they have seen how hard the medicines are to get off, that they are downers, and give only temporary relief from anxiety or panic attacks.)

Benzodiazepines are a group of drugs called minor tranquillisers. Doctors prescribe these tablets to help people with anxiety or sleep problems. They slow down the workings of the brain and the central nervous system. It is possible to become dependent on them after as little as four weeks' use.

The effects of benzodiazepines may last from a few hours to a few days, depending on the dose and type of benzodiazepines taken. They may make users feel relaxed, drowsy, confused, sleepy or really good; they may also impair judgement, cause blurred or double vision, affect memory or cause mood swings.

People who take benzodiazepines with other drugs can go into a coma or die. If they stop taking benzodiazepines suddenly, they may have fits.

Heroin

The risks of heroin

- Risk of immediate damage to health, or death: HIGH especially if used with other drugs.
- Risk of permanent damage to health or mental health: LOW. (It is possible to completely recover from prolonged heroin addiction but not from prolonged methamphetamine addiction.)
- Risk of unsafe parenting: HIGH.
- Risk of damage to the brain, physical development or long-term health of the baby if you are pregnant: LOW.
- Risk of children copying parental behaviours and using this drug: LOW to MODERATE. (Heroin users and their children often do not live together, especially if the users are having trouble with self-care.)

Heroin is a highly addictive drug derived from the morphine alkaloid found in opium. Pure heroin is a white powder with a bitter taste. It is usually 'cut' with other drugs or with substances such as sugar, starch or powdered milk. Because heroin users do not know the actual strength of the drug or its true contents, they are at risk of overdose or death. It is one of the most addictive of all drugs.

Heroin is most often injected, but it may also be smoked, snorted, used as a suppository, or taken by mouth. Injecting heroin comes with grave risks, especially if needles are shared. Heroin injectors can get hepatitis C, HIV/AIDS or endocarditis, which causes damage to the heart valves. Women whose blood type is Rhesus-negative and who share needles with someone who is Rhesus-positive, may not be able to have babies in the future.

Heroin is very addictive: it is not safe to try just once. It can affect users' ability to look after themselves. Too little or too much can lead to vomiting, which in the long term can damage teeth. It also causes constipation.

The babies of heroin users may have the jitters and irritability. This is called neonatal abstinence syndrome (NAS). NAS is treatable, however, and is unlikely to have any long-term effects on the baby.

Oxycodone

The risks of oxycodone dependency

- Risk of immediate damage to health, or death: LOW.
- Risk of permanent damage to health or mental health: LOW.
- Risk of unsafe parenting: MODERATE.
- Risk of damage to the brain, physical development or long-term health of the baby if you are pregnant: LOW.
- Risk of children copying parental behaviours and using this drug: LOW.

Oxycodone is a semi-synthetic opioid and is the active ingredient in a number of prescription pain-relief medications. As an opioid, it is similar to heroin. Some users take oxycodone to achieve a euphoric high.

Oxycodone is addictive and dangerous. Like other narcotic medications, it can impair mental and physical abilities. Other side effects include breathing irregularity or respiratory depression, headaches, nausea, dizziness, seizures, low blood pressure and heart failure. Overdose death is possible due to slowed breathing.

Cocaine (and crack cocaine)

Cocaine is a bitter, addictive pain blocker extracted from the leaves of the coca shrub, a plant that comes from the Andean highlands in South America. Cocaine has similar effects to those of methamphetamine, but it is more powerfully addictive.

The risks of cocaine

- Risk of immediate damage to health, or death: LOW (HIGH if used with alcohol).
- Risk of permanent damage to health or mental health: MODERATE to HIGH.
- Risk of unsafe parenting: HIGH.
- Risk of damage to the brain, physical development or long-term health of the baby if you are pregnant: LOW to MODERATE.
- Risk of children copying parental behaviours and using this drug: LOW to MODERATE.

It is snorted, injected or smoked, and temporarily gives the user a blissful, energetic sensation. Cocaine has a very powerful stimulating effect on the nervous system, raising levels of dopamine, a neurotransmitter linked to pleasure and movement in the brain's reward circuit. The effects generally last 15–30 minutes, or up to an hour, depending on how it is taken.

Cocaine decreases the appetite, dilates the pupils and leads to irritability. It can cause headaches, abdominal pain, nausea, high blood pressure, heart attack, stroke and respiratory arrest. Regular use can cause lost sense of smell, swallowing problems, nosebleeds, a persistent runny nose, hoarseness, severe bowel gangrene, severe allergic reactions, and paranoia or paranoid psychosis.

Researchers from the University of Sydney have found that recreational cocaine users have a significantly higher risk of a heart attack or stroke compared to those who never use the drug.

Overdosing on cocaine can lead to seizures, as well as life-threatening heart failure, cerebral haemorrhage, stroke and respiratory failure.

The babies of cocaine users are susceptible to stroke, which can cause partial paralysis or mental disability. During pregnancy bleeding can occur due to separation of the placenta, which may deprive the baby of oxygen.

Ecstasy (MDMA)

Ecstasy is a type of stimulant that also produces hallucinogenic effects. It is a 'party drug' that can give a short-term feeling of emotional warmth, awareness and mental and physical energy. It can make people shaky and sweaty and can cause them to clench their teeth a lot. It can also affect

The risks of ecstasy

- Risk of immediate damage to health, or death: LOW if used alone; HIGH if used with stimulant drinks.
- Risk of permanent damage to health or mental health: LOW.
- Risk of unsafe parenting: LOW.
- Risk of damage to the brain, physical development or long-term health of the baby if you are pregnant: LOW.
- Risk of children copying parental behaviours and using this drug: LOW.

memory and make studying difficult. Hardly anybody continues to use it for a long time.

The effect varies from person to person and depends on the amount taken. There is no safe level of use, and there is always the risk of unwanted side effects. The effects of an overdose can include floating sensations, vomiting, high body temperature, high blood pressure, increased heartbeat, hallucinations, irrational or bizarre behaviour, or convulsions.

Ecstasy has also been linked to several deaths through heart attack and brain haemorrhage. It is dangerous if taken with pep drinks containing high levels of caffeine.

GHB (gamma-hydroxybutyrate)

The risks of GHB

- Risk of immediate damage to health, or death: LOW (HIGH if used with alcohol or other depressants).
- Risk of permanent damage to health or mental health: LOW if date rape is avoided.
- Risk of unsafe parenting: MODERATE.
- Risk of damage to the brain, physical development or long-term health of the baby if you are pregnant: LOW.
- Risk of children copying parental behaviours and using this drug: LOW.

Gamma-hydroxybutyrate (GHB) is a depressant that acts on the central nervous system. It is purported to be a strength-enhancer, euphoriant and aphrodisiac, and is one of several drugs used as a 'date rape' drug. Because of its depressant effects on the central nervous system, GHB can be lethal when combined with alcohol or other depressants.

Volatile substances (sniffing petrol, glue or paint)

The risks of volatile substances

- Risk of immediate damage to health, or death: HIGH.
- Risk of permanent damage to health or mental health: MODERATE.
- Risk of unsafe parenting: HIGH.
- Risk of damage to the brain, physical development or long-term health of the baby if you are pregnant: MODERATE.
- Risk of children copying parental behaviours and using this drug: MODERATE.

Some people sniff petrol, glue or paint because these substances are easy to get and are cheap. Some use them because others in their community do. Others use them because they are not detected on urine drug screens.

They are very dangerous because they can stop the heart working properly (a condition called arrhythmia) and cause death without warning. These drugs also damage the liver, lungs and brain. The damage they cause is generally permanent.

Kava and khat

These two very different plant-based drugs are used by small populations within Australia. Kava is mostly used by people who have come from the Western Pacific, for its calming or sedative effect. Khat is a stimulant used in East Africa and the Arabian Peninsula.

In some of these communities, using these drugs may be regarded as normal and for some women they are hard to avoid. Long-term use of kava may cause a skin rash. The effects of both drugs are mainly social but they may have an effect on family and community relationships and the ability to work.

The risks of kava and khat

- Risk of immediate damage to health, or death: LOW.

- Risk of permanent damage to health or mental health: MODERATE.

- Risk of unsafe parenting: LOW to HIGH, depending on the amount used.

- Risk of damage to the brain, physical development or long-term health of the baby if you are pregnant: LOW.

- Risk of children copying parental behaviours and using this drug: MODERATE.

New psychoactive substances

These are substances that you might buy from the internet or 'head shops', as well as performance-enhancing or bodybuilding hormones and supplements.

While many of these substances are currently legal in Australia, it is worth remembering that the law in Australia and many other countries takes time to catch up with new medical findings on their use.

The fact that a substance is not banned or illegal does not make it safe or free of long-term consequences to your physical or mental health.

Think carefully before you accept the advice of others to take any of these substances and consider whether or not the recommendation is based on their own self-interest.

Important note

The information in this chapter is intended to assist you in making your own decisions about using drugs or alcohol. Your thoughtful and informed consideration will minimise any harm that you and the people around you may experience. Help is available to you at any stage and there are many in the community who will support you if you have a problem. See the Resources section at the end of this book for such organisations.

12

Bullying

Jan Davies

Bullying is deliberate and repeated intimidating behaviour from one person, or a group of people, directed towards another. It is not a single event and is not just fighting. It is a series of aggressive actions intended to humiliate, torment or harm the victim, often done in front of an audience the bully wants to impress.

Bullies can be found at all ages, in all cultures, in the home, school and workplace, on sporting fields and on social networking sites, and at all levels from schoolgirl to chief executive.

Bullying behaviours occur on a spectrum from mild teasing to more serious abuse. We usually know, at some level, when we are being bullied. Often, though, it's hard to know if it's real or whether we're being over-sensitive and it is just in our head. When mild it can also be hard to describe to other people. On the other hand, bullying can be so threatening and physical that it can be too scary to talk about or take action against.

This chapter aims to help you to recognise what bullying is, what it looks like and feels like, and how you can deal with it if it's happening to you.

Bullying can come in many different forms. Some of these include:

- **verbal bullying** – such as teasing, name-calling, insults, and personal, sexist or racist comments
- **psychological bullying** – such as threats, nasty looks and gestures, and manipulation or stalking
- **social or relational bullying** – such as spreading stories or rumours, playing deliberately mean or humiliating tricks, teasing, ridiculing or excluding someone from a group. This form of bullying is often difficult for the victim to identify because the bullying is done in a more indirect way, within a social group situation.

- **physical bullying** – such as pushing, tripping or bumping. This includes any kind of intentional damage to someone's body, clothes or belongings.
- **cyberbullying** – the use of information and communication technology such as email, mobile phones, SMS chat rooms and other social networking tools to abuse, humiliate or threaten someone

Why does bullying occur?

Bullying is a deeply unpleasant phenomenon, but understanding why it occurs can help those being bullied handle it better. It can also help them to find effective ways to stop it.

Bullies can be anyone: a friend, schoolmate, co-worker, sibling, parent, girlfriend or boyfriend, teacher, sports coach or boss. People bully others for a range of reasons and motivations. Students interviewed in a 2009 Australian study said they believed that bullying occurred 'because the person bullying didn't like the person they were bullying: found bullying fun; enjoyed bullying others; liked to feel tough and strong, in control and popular'.

One of the most common and yet complex and deep-rooted cause of bullying is when the bully has a history of being bullied or abused. They may have suffered at home, school or elsewhere, and to deal with their own pain or insecurity they take it out on those around them, especially those who appear weak or vulnerable.

Sometimes people bully others through fear of being bullied themselves. They think that by striking out first, they give off a sense of toughness and so will not be bullied by others. Another reason is to appear powerful and in control. Many bullies don't operate very well at an emotional level, and lack empathy, social values, compassion and the internal behaviour controls that would stop them from hurting others. They exhibit bullying behaviour because they just don't care about the feelings of others.

If you are bullying others, we recommend you seek help to address this behaviour and the underlying issues that might be causing it. You are not alone. Many people admit to having bullied others at some time in their lives. Nevertheless, it is dangerous to you and others and neither appropriate nor acceptable behaviour. Everyone has the right to be respected and the responsibility to respect others.

School-related bullying

Bullying happens in every school. It is likely you have experienced bullying yourself, or witnessed it happening to another person. You may even recognise some bullying tendencies in your own behaviour towards your friends or schoolmates. Examples of bullying include shouting at someone, using offensive language or insulting names that refer to a personal characteristic such as a birthmark or body shape, or simply continually staring hard at someone to intimidate them. While bullying is very common, it is never acceptable.

Just like bullying in any other place, school bullying can be verbal, physical, psychological, social or cyberbullying. It can occur in the classroom, while travelling between home and school, at sport venues, shopping centres, parties or anywhere that students come together. While traditionally the school ground has always been the most common place for bullying to occur, bullying in cyberspace is becoming increasingly common.

A 2009 Australian study found that about one in four students in years 4–9 is bullied every few weeks or more often. It can be very subtle, so that at first you may just feel confused, and perhaps imagine that you are misinterpreting events or comments. The methods of bullying vary between girls and boys. Girls are less likely than boys to use physical bullying, but more likely to use verbal abuse, such as teasing and taunting, and social isolation. Although psychological and social abuse may be less conspicuous, they are just as damaging as physical violence.

Bullying can have tragic consequences for victims. While the reasons for suicide are always complex, bullying can be a factor. An American study found that young people aged 10–17 who had been bullied by their peers in the past year were 2.4 times more likely than those who were not bullied to have suicidal thoughts.

School bullying policies

Most schools take bullying very seriously and have programs in place to create safe environments based on respect. Some schools have adopted and adapted national or international programs and others have built on their existing programs. The common components are:

- assessing the level and impact of bullying experienced by students
- raising awareness of the bullying prevention program in the school community, and engaging the students, staff and parents in its implementation and evaluation

- creating policies and rules around bullying, and disseminating and communicating these to the school community
- training staff to understand the program and to respond appropriately to bullying on every occasion
- changing the culture to one of respect, support and acceptance, and reinforcing this through all school meetings and publications
- including bullying prevention material in the school curriculum and activities

Yasmin is 15 and attends her local co-ed school. One day after a PE lesson, a group of girls approached her as she was getting changed. They took her underwear and bra and refused to give them back. When the bell for the next class sounded they threw them in the toilet. After this incident, taunts from the group increased, and one of the girls was particularly cruel and even physically abusive.

Yasmin started to fear every PE lesson. Soon she was finding excuses not to do PE, and would feel physically sick when she was around the bullies. She was constantly anxious that she would meet the group. The bullying extended to after school and weekends. She felt completely isolated. Yasmin tried to handle it by ignoring the bullies, staying in the classroom at lunchtimes and staying back in the library after school until it was safe to go home. She said that she just wanted it to stop.

At the end of term her report showed a drop in her academic performance so her parents asked her what had been happening. When she told them, they were shocked that this had been going on all term and they had not known. They experienced a range of emotions, including guilt that they had not noticed, anger that it had happened, and empathy with Yasmin and how she was feeling. They contacted the principal.

In response to their complaint, the principal called in the bullies and their parents. The main bully was suspended for five days, and banned from school excursions for the remainder of the year. But the bullying continued more covertly. Yasmin's anxiety got worse. She told her parents, who suggested she might find it helpful to see a counsellor. The family GP referred her to a child psychologist who helped Yasmin develop strategies for dealing with her feelings. He helped Yasmin ignore and reframe her negative thoughts, such as thinking she was somehow to blame for what had happened. He also gave her strategies for managing situations at school where she had to see the bullies, including visualising places where she felt safe and happy, repeating positive messages to counter the negative ones, and doing exercises to control her breathing and help her relax. Yasmin's parents engaged a solicitor who wrote to the parents of the lead bully. The bullying has stopped.

Yasmin is getting back on track. Her latest school report was good, and she has a new group of friends through her involvement in the school band. She is still wary of situations where members of the group of bullies may be present, but finds this happens less and less. Yasmin said that for her the things that kept her going were the support of her best friend and her parents.

How to prevent bullying

Bullying can happen anywhere. The best protection is to build up your emotional strength and social skills, both of which can be developed through self-awareness and good communication. A good strategy is to learn how to express what you think, how you feel and what you would like to happen. This is easier said than done, and you may need some help from your parents, a school counsellor, mentor, coach or child psychologist.

Having good friends and a wide and supportive network will help to make you less vulnerable to teasing, bullying and harassment. It's important to distinguish between friends who care about you and support you, and people who don't. While the group or people who bully others are sometimes the most powerful and popular, it is ultimately better to find friends who make you feel safe and happy, even if they are not the most popular people. Use your gut instinct to choose friends with whom you feel comfortable and avoid those who make you feel uneasy.

What you can do if you are being bullied

Just as bullies vary in their degree of mean and cruel behaviour, the targets of bullying vary in their ability to stand up to bullies. There *are* strategies that work. You may need to use several of them or get extra help by telling teachers, your parents or sometimes the police. Remember that bullying is never acceptable and it is never your fault. It is important to take action early, as bullying can get worse and continue for long periods. Having said that, it is never too late to seek help, or to put a stop to the bullying.

Schools are not liable for bullying that occurs outside school premises, including on the school bus. If someone from your school is bullying you outside school, however, you should talk to a teacher or school counsellor because they might be able to help. You can also ask your parents to talk

Tips for dealing with bullies

- Ignore the bully and walk away, if possible.

- Avoid eye contact and stay calm so the bully can't see they are affecting you – often they will get bored and give up.

- Try talking to the bully in a one-to-one conversation about their behaviour, to help them see that what they're doing is harmful and dangerous to others and to themselves. Letting the bully know this might stop them from bullying someone else in the future.

- Look and act confident in the way you walk, talk and interact with others. This sends a message to the bully that you are strong, and that their bullying tactics are not working on you. Even if you do not feel confident, pretend you are. This way the bully is less likely to pick on you.

- Stick to your views and opinions.

- If you are physically threatened, use your loudest voice and yell 'Stop!' or 'Back off!' This may also attract the attention of someone who can help protect you by calming the bully down and controlling the situation. As soon as you are in a position of safety, it is very important to seek help from someone in a position of authority (usually an adult such as a parent, teacher or boss) and tell them what has happened.

- Don't hit back, no matter what happens, as you may get seriously hurt or in trouble.

- Tell a teacher or your parents, brother, sister or another family member what is happening, or call a helpline (see the Resources section at the end of this book). Do this as soon as possible after the first event. If the bullying continues, report it again and tell the people higher up in the school hierarchy, such as your year coordinator, the deputy principal or the principal.

- Keep a record of the details of each bullying incident.

- Stay in safe areas during breaks, sit near the driver on public transport, and walk with other people when going to and from school.

- If friends ignore you or side with the bully, talk with them one-on-one and ask why they aren't supporting you. Tell them you need their support, and that when they don't defend you they are not acting like a good friend. If your friends still do not help you, then consider finding new friends who support you, and who make you feel happy and safe.

- You're probably not the only one being bullied, so you could try making friends with someone else who looks lonely. Your aim should be to find friends who really appreciate you for who you are.

- If you see someone else being bullied, defend them. This shows bullies you are strong and will not tolerate their behaviour.

to the parents of the student/s involved. Sometimes the bullying occurs at a particular place, for example at the bus stop or netball court. Ask your mum or dad to meet you there and confront the bullies directly. Often such intervention from an authority figure is effective in stopping the bullying.

What parents can do to help

- Build warm and positive family relationships, which can help protect a child from the negative effects of being bullied.
- Regularly make time to talk with your child about what is happening at school.
- Specifically ask your child about bullying at their school and whether your child has experienced it.
- If your child tells you they have been bullied, let them know you believe them, and calmly explore how they are feeling, coping and reacting. Make sure they feel safe.
- Let your child know that bullying is never acceptable and that it is not their fault.
- Let your child know that it is normal for people who are bullied to feel embarrassed, hurt or afraid.
- Be supportive and reassure your child that you will help them stop the bullying.
- Find out the circumstances of the bullying (what, when and where it happened and who was present).

- Help your child identify solutions they are comfortable with. Feeling more in control will help them rebuild confidence and self-esteem. Let them know that sometimes the solutions may include actions they are not comfortable with.

- Contact the school, if it is school-related bullying, and discuss your concerns. Find out what their policies are and how the school can help stop the bullying.

- It may be helpful to your child to disclose your own experience of bullying, if you have one, and how you stopped it. Help your child understand why bullying happens.

- Encourage your child to take up new activities and make new friends.

- Help rebuild your child's confidence by focusing on their strengths and the things they do well.

Cyberbullying

Young people enjoy access to global communication and interaction through social media. On the upside this can enrich your ability to acquire knowledge, provide positive and creative experiences, and build your friendship groups. On the downside, social networking sites are largely unregulated and can give bullies easy access to you, even in the safety of your own home. A study in 2010 found that young people aged 14–17 had the highest rate of internet use in Australia, 91 per cent of them spending time online every week.

Cyberbullying is the use of information and communication technology to abuse, humiliate or threaten someone. It can be verbal, social or psychological. The types of technology used include text messaging, email, chat rooms and social networking sites such as Facebook, MySpace, Bebo and Twitter. Instant messaging and text messages are now the most common tools used for bullying.

What does cyberbullying involve?

- Receiving anonymous demeaning or abusive text messages via mobile phone.

- Being sent nasty or threatening messages through social networking sites.

- People posting embarrassing photos or videos of you on social media pages or emailing them to other people.

- People spreading rumours about you via social media.
- People stalking, intimidating or harassing you via social media.
- People trying to stop you from communicating with others.
- People circulating your messages and emails to non-intended recipients for the purpose of embarrassing you.
- People excluding you from events or making sure you have access to information about social events you haven't been invited to.

Although the number of young people who are cyberbullied is unknown, as cyberbullying is believed to be largely unreported, research in Australia in 2010 found that 7–10 per cent of students in years 4–9 reported being the victim of cyberbullying. This is an estimate and the real incidence may be higher. The older you are, the more likely you are to have experienced cyberbullying.

The impact of cyberbullying includes feelings of isolation, embarrassment, loss of confidence and self-esteem, depression and social withdrawal. In extreme cases it can be a contributing factor in suicide.

Cyberbullying may have a far greater impact on the victim than other means of bullying. This is because of the potentially larger audience and longer lasting impact. In the past, if someone wanted to start a rumour about you, they had to do it verbally, and the impact was fairly limited. Now, a message can spread instantly around the world, and be available for months or years. This increases the feelings of humiliation, embarrassment and isolation in the victim. Another factor affecting the impact of cyberbullying is that it is harder to avoid. You may change schools but find that the cyberbullying follows you.

There are things you can do if you are the target of cyberbullying:

- If you know the person, ask them to stop. Do this in person, not via email or SMS.
- Don't respond to their messages, as this is what the bully wants and it may escalate the bullying.
- Change the settings on your computer and/or phone to block the bully.
- Turn on 'Block caller ID' on your phone so that your number is not displayed when you call someone. This way you can control who has your phone number.
- Review your privacy settings and the personal information that is available about you online. You may need to change your screen name and profile picture so you cannot be found easily.

- Contact your social media or telecommunications service provider to report the harassing behaviour.
- Keep any abusive, intimidating or other bullying messages, and record the time and date details if your phone does not automatically do this.
- Tell your parents what is happening, and show them the bullying material so that they are aware and can support you and help you stop the bullying.
- Ask a parent or other family member to answer your phone calls and warn off the bully.
- Turn off your phone and computer at night, or put them in another room where you cannot hear them.
- Change your phone number or email address, and keep them private.
- Get support through your school counsellor or a helpline (see the Resources section at the end of this book).
- Get support through positive social media site support groups, where you can access resources and share experiences with others.
- If the messages are threatening, hate-related or obscene, contact your local police.

What parents can do to prevent cyberbullying

Parents should monitor the use of social media and technology by their children. You might find the following strategies useful:

- Place computers in the family living area, so that it is easier to supervise and view what your children are sending, receiving, looking at and searching for. It is still important that your child feels some sense of privacy, however, so handle this situation carefully. When it comes to cyber safety, the most important thing is to develop an open and trusting relationship and good communication with your child. If they are on Facebook, ask for Friend status or ask to view their Facebook page. If they are on Twitter, become a follower.
- Monitor their mobile phone use, as mobile phones are the most common vehicle for bullying.
- Ensure that your children have undertaken one of the 'safe use of information and communication technology' training courses, and know how to restrict or block access from unwanted senders. Many schools run these courses. They are also available through local government

community education programs and some independent education providers. You may also find it valuable to enrol in one of these courses.

- Engage your children in other family and community activities that do not rely on social media.

Bullying at work

Many adolescents and young people have part-time or full-time jobs. Unfortunately, bullying at work is common. In an Australian study of bullying in the workplace, 6.8 per cent of respondents reported being bullied in the previous six months, and 3.5 per cent of respondents stated that the bullying had continued for more than six months.

Workplace bullying can occur between co-workers, come from a manager or supervisor to an employee, or from an employee to a manager or supervisor. The most common form of workplace bullying is verbal abuse, although all forms of bullying occur. Examples include:

- making insulting, belittling or abusive comments
- spreading rumours or undermining the employee
- setting inappropriate tasks, imposing unreasonably large workloads or giving short timelines for work completion
- withholding information or resources that are essential for satisfactory work completion
- changing work hours or place of work, without consultation, to create difficulties for the employee
- excluding the employee from work-related activities
- bumping, tripping or pushing; threatening or attacking the employee
- sexual harassment, including sexual comments
- psychological harassment; playing malevolent tricks
- intimidation, including inappropriate use of disciplinary action
- forcing the employee to undertake humiliating, dangerous or inappropriate activities as part of an initiation

Workplace bullying is also beginning to occur through online technologies, mirroring the situation in schools. The ability and legal responsibility of employers to respond to cyberbullying is currently uncertain. If you are the target of workplace bullying, you should report it to your employer immediately. This generally means the human resources department if you are in a large organisation: they have occupational health and safety and anti-harassment responsibilities. In a smaller organisation, report the bullying to your boss, unless they are the problem, in which case go higher in the organisation or report it to your state or territory work health and safety authority (see below).

The impact of bullying can extend into all areas of the victim's day-to-day life, with significant negative consequences for health and wellbeing. The effects are influenced by the nature of the bullying, its duration, how the workplace responds to the bullying, the ability of the victim to manage the bullying and the support they receive from friends and family.

Victoria is the only state with laws against workplace and cyber-bullying. Through changes to stalking laws, legislation providing jail terms of up to 10 years for bullying was introduced in Victoria in June 2011. A charge of stalking is applicable if the bullying or cyberbullying is part of a pattern of conduct likely to cause physical or mental harm, or fear of it. The legislation, called the *Crimes Amendment (Bullying) Act*, is also known as Brodie's Law. It arose from the death of a young woman, Brodie Panlock, who suicided after being bullied by colleagues at the suburban Melbourne cafe where she worked. She was only 19. There is no national law covering workplace bullying itself. The only current legislation directly addressing workplace bullying is workplace health and safety legislation.

Help and information on bullying at work

Your employer has a duty to ensure the health, safety and welfare at work of all its employees.

There are lots of resources on the internet regarding workplace bullying. The Workplace Bullying page on the Australian Human Rights Commission website provides links to the relevant state authority to contact if you're experiencing workplace bullying. See www.humanrights.gov.au/bullying/factsheets/workplace_bullying.html.

You can report workplace bullying to this authority and they will also be able to provide you with advice and help.

Bullying at home

Bullying can also occur in the home. Bullies can be parents, step-parents, siblings, carers and other relatives. Sometimes children are bullied for not meeting the academic, sporting or appearance expectations of their parents. Bullying at home can range from name-calling, labelling and extreme nagging to physical and emotional abuse, deliberate neglect, and extreme and repeated humiliation. There is a fine line between bullying and simply disciplining children. For example, parents nagging their children to do their homework is not bullying. Parents threatening or screaming at their children and calling them derogatory names if they don't do their homework *is* bullying.

Sometimes what parents see as motivation can feel like harassment, blaming and humiliation to a child. What your parents might not realise is that their behaviour can have the reverse effect or unintended consequences, such as overeating or under-eating; loss of interest in sport, music or school; and isolation, loss of self-esteem or depression. The parent–child relationship is complex. Your parents have a responsibility to care for you and provide you with a safe home environment, which forms the basis for learning, being healthy, and developing good relationships. If you feel they are not fulfilling this responsibility it can be useful to talk about it with a trusted adult outside of your home life, such as a teacher or school counsellor.

What you can do if you are bullied at home

If the bullying is coming from your parents, the first step is to tell them how counterproductive and unhelpful you find their approach. Ask them for constructive help if you do feel that you have a problem with schoolwork, friends, feelings or anything else that is affecting your physical or mental health.

If you have any concerns you feel you cannot discuss with your parents or other trusted family members, see your GP, or contact a young women's or women's health service to discuss your concerns. You can also call a kids helpline (see the Resources section at the end of this book), or see your school counsellor or pastoral care worker for support and strategies to deal with the bullying at home.

What parents can do to help

Use warmth, understanding, honesty and clear communication to talk about the issue that concerns you or your child. Be specific about the behaviour you want to change and why you are concerned. Be non-judgemental. Ask questions about the issue to understand it from your child's point of view. Help your child to identify solutions and help implement them. For example, if the issue is homework, be prepared to set time aside each evening to help.

If you are worried about the mental or physical health of your child, discuss this with them to get their views. If you are still concerned, suggest that you and your child seek professional help or advice through your GP or practice nurse or the community health centre.

If you are concerned about your child's school performance, suggest an appointment with the class teacher or counsellor to identify any problems and get specific strategies to deal with them.

The health impacts of bullying

Bullying generally leads to feelings of stress in the victim, which can be experienced as a range of physical, psychological, emotional and behavioural symptoms, particularly anxiety, difficulty getting to sleep or remaining asleep, and overwhelming fatigue. Physical symptoms include headaches, stomach aches, sweating, palpitations, changed appetite and constant tiredness.

Psychological symptoms related to bullying include panic attacks, feeling sad, depressed or anxious, finding it hard to concentrate, and fearfulness. People who are bullied may also become more emotional with bouts of crying, moodiness, irritability or anger. Facing situations where the bully might be present can induce extreme anxiety in the victim.

Bullying can also affect behaviour and personality. It can make people feel shy, lose their confidence and sense of self-worth, develop tics, lose interest in things they used to enjoy, become oversensitive to casual remarks or develop obsessive behaviours. The feelings of responsibility, fear of repercussions, humiliation and/or embarrassment it can cause can all serve to stop someone who is bullied telling anyone else what is happening.

Why people who are bullied feel the way they do

When we feel physically or psychologically threatened, our body and mind have automatic responses designed to protect us from danger. Known as the stress response or the 'fight-or-flight' response, it can be activated when we experience bullying, which is itself a form of physical or psychological threat. Different people respond with varying degrees of stress to frightening situations. When we are bullied, our level of stress will be influenced by our personality and the extent to which we feel that we have control over the situation, the predictability of the bullying behaviour, whether we perceive our circumstances to be improving, and our level of support from friends, parents, the school, the police or other professionals.

When victims of bullying are unwilling or unable to disclose what is happening to them, they are more likely to experience trauma. If they do work up the courage to disclose the issue but then those in a position of power or authority deny that there is a problem, the trauma can be exacerbated. When people who are bullied are unable to resolve the conflict or unable to express their feelings about the bullying, they may internalise these feelings, which can lead to emotional problems such as stress, anxiety and depression. When bullying is perpetrated over a long period of time, the internalised feelings may also lead to self-harm and destructive behaviour, such as abusing drugs and alcohol or attempting suicide.

Suicide is usually the result of a complex mix of factors, but the risk of suicide can be exacerbated when a young person is being bullied. We know from some highly publicised cases that a number of suicides of young people have been attributed to bullying at school or in the workplace. A report by the Queensland Commission for Children and Young People and Child Guardian found that of the 21 young people who suicided in 2010–11, six were known to be victims of bullying. Each of these deaths was preventable and unnecessary.

If you are being bullied, the most important thing is to tell someone and get help to stop the bullying.

YOUNG WOMEN

Introduction

Maureen Johnson

As adolescence draws to a close, we start to take on the many and varied roles of an adult. Starting in our 20s, we may set out on any number of journeys: experimenting and exploring, attempting to fulfil expectations, and searching for our place both socially and professionally. It is a time when strong relationships are often formed, lifelong partners are often found and the desire to settle can be strong. Young womanhood can be loosely defined as the years from 20 to 40 – our reproductive years. As with all life stages, your experience of it will vary depending on who you are, your previous life experiences and your culture.

These years can be some of our most energetic and busiest, as we juggle commitments and demands from the workplace, family and friends. We are still establishing our independence and finding the confidence to assert ourselves; we are endlessly curious, often ambitious, and almost invariably committed to large and complex groups of friends. Contemporary young women are reportedly the biggest users of social networks, which makes them more socially active and in demand than any previous generation. Social networking brings a whole range of benefits but it can also make us more socially vulnerable and more inclined to focus on the size of our friendship group rather than the quality of our friendships. Social networking can also make us more aware of social groupings, and we can easily feel excluded by friends who post the intricacies of their social lives in which we have no part. On the upside, though, social networking gives us greater opportunity to be aware of what is happening around us, and to be more connected with friends and family than ever before.

As young women we are working towards realising our dreams – experiencing, exploring and taking on roles we have fantasised about since childhood. Generally this is a time when, hopefully, we are enjoying our physical prime. Of course, many young people have to overcome poor health, poverty, or cultural issues, which can lead to significant disadvantage. Young Aboriginal women, for example, are more likely to be unemployed or dealing with teenage pregnancy or struggling with drug and alcohol issues. Young migrant women may be adjusting to a new language and, often, extreme cultural differences. Poverty, violence and lack of opportunity can hinder our growth, development and ability to enjoy and take up the opportunities of our youth.

Some young women will be obsessive about health and fitness, while for others, health and fitness will take second place to other priorities. It's not always easy to establish and build a healthy lifestyle, but any efforts to do so now will have strong implications for the future. A good diet, regular exercise, reduced alcohol and drug consumption, caring for your sexual health, and building healthy relationships and friendships will form a solid foundation for good health into the future.

How this book can help

As young women, we often leave little time to care for ourselves. It's easy to ignore our own health; after all, unless we have a prevailing illness, we generally feel pretty good during our 20s and 30s. But the lifestyle we are living now will have far-reaching consequences as we start to age. Good habits now will improve our chances of good health throughout our life.

For this section we spoke with young women in their 20s, 30s and 40s to learn about the health issues they felt were important during this life stage. High on the list of concerns were food, nutrition and staying well. In chapters 13 and 14, we focus on good food choices and exercise choices that will help young women maintain health. The diet and food industries, not to mention the tabloid press and women's magazines, owe much of their success to selling diets to women, especially those of us who feel particularly vulnerable about our body weight and appearance. In these chapters we offer realistic perspectives and achievable, sensible ways of thinking about food, nutrition and exercise.

Contraception has been described by some young women as a minefield: choosing which contraception is right for us can be overwhelming. In chapter 16, we discuss in detail our various options and why we might choose one method over another, while in chapter 23 we discuss unplanned pregnancy from a political, social and medical perspective.

There is a strong focus in this section on conception and pregnancy, and while we recognise that this is not a path all women choose or have the chance to take, it was an issue of great importance for the young women we spoke to. We discuss the options when pregnancy doesn't happen, and we explore some of the common concerns and health issues when it does. Fertility treatments and assisted reproductive technologies are discussed in chapter 24. Pregnancy is discussed in chapter 17 and birth is covered in chapter 19.

Mental health, sexual assault and family or intimate partner violence also feature in this section. These issues impact on women across their life cycle, but it is during this stage of life that women are most likely to experience violence and when mental health issues often start to emerge. Violence is of course one of the most prevalent and oppressive issues impacting on the health of all women – across all life stages. In women aged 15–44, family or intimate partner violence is responsible for more preventable death and disease than the causes *thought* to be the most common, such as high blood pressure, high cholesterol, drug and alcohol abuse, obesity or lack of exercise. Young women experiencing violence are also at a greater risk of unplanned pregnancy or abortion. For many women, violence escalates during pregnancy, leading to pregnancy complications or miscarriage. Violence takes many forms, physical and emotional, and can be so subtle and manipulative that women often feel they are responsible for it, which along with fear and stigma impacts on their ability to seek help. Chapters 29 and 30 offer in-depth information and discussion about violence against women, as well as strategies for women, as a community and as individuals. Chapter 29 also provides an understanding of sexual assault: what it is, its prevalence, community misconceptions and its impact on survivors.

This section also touches on common health problems for women as they move through their early adult years. As well as the issues that impact on reproduction such as polycystic ovarian syndrome, this may also be the first time that many women will encounter problems related to sexually transmitted infections or vaginal irritations not related to sex. Chapters 25, 26, 27 and 28 explore some of the more common psychological, physical and gynaecological conditions young women face.

Finally, plastic surgery is emerging as a major political and health issue in our society. In many ways plastic surgery has become more accessible and women are increasingly considering it a viable option when they are dissatisfied with their bodies. Unfortunately our perceptions of what is 'attractive' are persistently distorted by popular media and pornographic imagery, to which the internet has given us greater access. There are many different kinds of normal when it comes to our bodies: vaginas *and* breasts come in all shapes and sizes, and vaginas with 'dangly bits' are just as common as the neater variety. Yet women are increasingly turning to plastic surgery to enhance their breasts or neaten their genitalia, despite the enormous risks involved and the potential for surgery to lead to more problems in the future. Nonetheless, plastic surgery does play a genuine part in helping women who have physical issues that impact on their health. Like any medical procedure, the decision to go ahead with plastic surgery needs to be well considered and informed; in chapter 27 we hope to start you on that journey.

While this section of the book targets young women, you will also find information that is relevant and useful to you in other sections. Health issues will not always confine themselves to particular ages or life stages, and you may find that your particular concern or interest is discussed elsewhere.

Motherhood

For many young women – certainly not all – relationships and children are an important consideration at this time, but the decision to have a baby or not can be fraught. Women are often at the centre of a tug-of-war, with entrenched traditional and gendered values on one side, and the desire to be independent, successful and equal citizens on the other. To become a parent or not, to abort an unplanned pregnancy, to choose parenting over working, to juggle parenting and career, to put off parenting until a career is established or to put a child into childcare – these are decisions many women face at this time, and we can be damned if we do and damned if we don't.

Maternity leave (paid or not) and flexible working arrangements continue to be seen as a privilege rather than a necessity; young women's employment prospects can still be impacted by the possibility that she may get pregnant; having a sick child can influence a woman's success in the workplace. Some women will compromise their professional ambitions for family duties or vice versa and often feel, or are made to feel, dissatisfied with the choices they have made. Other women are engaged in a constant juggling act that, more often than not, is a gendered pursuit, as women still tend to take on the majority of household tasks, even when both parents are working full-time.

It is becoming increasingly common for women to wait until they are in their mid- to late 30s before attempting to get pregnant. Many women (and men) who wish to have a family will work towards establishing financial or housing security first, and – because of gender issues relating to career development – some women feel they will risk their careers if they take time out to have a baby. Alternatively, it might take a while for a woman to meet a partner with whom she wishes to have children. It is important to note that these women risk missing the window of fertility. Because of the social trend for women to have babies later in life, there is a level of comfort with putting the decision off until later, but this is a problem for biological reasons, as the number and quality of eggs we produce progressively declines with age. Fertility treatments or assisted reproductive technologies are becoming increasingly sophisticated, as you will read in chapter 24. It is even possible to have eggs preserved when we are young for use later in life, though this technology is still in its early days. But medical interventions are often stressful and expensive and not available to all women. Success rates also vary, and it can be hard for women who have invested so much to know when to stop trying.

Age is not the only barrier to fertility, of course. Younger women can face any number of physical issues that will impact on their ability to reproduce. Chapter 24 discusses how reproduction works and how seemingly easy things can go wrong. Conception is complex and the conditions need to be optimum. Sometimes it's not clear why some women conceive and others don't, or why some are suddenly successful after many years of trying. There are also some well-understood barriers to pregnancy, which are described in this section.

For many young women, parenting is a touchstone in adult life. The adjustment to parenting will vary from one person to another. It will be smooth for some and difficult for others, and it's very hard to predict how one individual may respond. With the pressures and conflicts of modern life, motherhood is placing different demands on the mental and emotional health of women than a generation ago. Chapter 21 offers a range of strategies to help you understand and enjoy your early parenting experience and to recognise when things may not be going as they should. The emotional and mental health demands of parenting are discussed, as is the importance of early bonding with your baby.

Choosing not to have children

Despite the systemic workplace discrimination against women who *do* choose to parent, choosing not to have a family, or finding that you can't have a baby for whatever reason, can also be socially very difficult for women. Despite feminism and social evolution, the expectation for young women to reproduce is strong, and the subject can be embarrassing and awkward at the least, and overtly discriminatory at worst. Women in politics who have chosen not to be mothers are still considered inadequate by some of their constituents and vocal elements of the media. Abortion continues to be stigmatised, and women who choose to abort are still labelled criminals and murderers by certain parts of society. Emergency contraception can be hard for some women to access, and religion plays a part in controlling the rights of some women to use contraception at all.

Despite the strong social and cultural overlay, as women we do have the right and the capacity to control our own reproduction. Chapter 16 provides a detailed overview of the full range of contraception methods and will help to guide you to the method that will best suit you. Despite the availability and effectiveness of contraception, unplanned pregnancies will still occur. Chapter 23 provides a comprehensive overview of abortion, including a discussion of the social and historical context, which has made abortion such a difficult decision for many women.

In our efforts to stay well, this generation of young women, more than any other, has to scale mountains of myth and misinformation, an internet maze in which the truth can be barely decipherable from fiction. It is no wonder the young women we spoke to when we were writing this book were keen on finding information provided by experts that was clear, concise and easy to follow. In these chapters, we aim to support you to understand your body, to maintain and improve your health and to explore your healthcare options. Often simple steps such as exercise, eating well, limiting your use of alcohol and other substances and building good relationships will help you to maintain your health and vitality, and prepare you for the even more interesting journey into your midlife.

13
Food and nutrition for young women

Elisabeth Gasparini, Jane Karpavicius

Nutrition is powerful – you feel better, function better and stay healthier when your diet is well balanced and you exercise regularly. It is especially important during this crucial stage of life when there is so much happening: independent living, career development, travel, establishing relationships, babies and families, among other things.

What should young women eat?

The federal government's Australian Dietary Guidelines are well founded and widely accepted pointers designed to help us choose foods for a healthy life. Use them as a basis for planning healthy meals and a healthy lifestyle:

- To achieve and maintain a healthy weight, be physically active and choose amounts of nutritious food and drinks to meet your energy needs.
- Enjoy a wide variety of nutritious foods from the five food groups every day: fruit, vegetables of different colours, legumes and beans; breads, cereals and grains (mostly whole grains); protein foods such as lean red meats and poultry, fish, eggs, tofu, nuts and seeds, legumes and beans; milk, yoghurt, cheese and/or their alternatives, mostly reduced-fat; a small amount of healthy fats and oils; and plenty of water.
- Limit intake of foods containing saturated fat, added salt, added sugars and alcohol.
- Care for your food: prepare and store it safely.

Healthy eating

Eating well as a household

Whether you live as a family unit or a blended family, in a shared household or alone, eating healthily at home can be a challenge, especially if you are working and have competing commitments or a limited budget. But it's important to eat well as a household, for more reasons than just good nutrition.

A shared meal at the table is a great way of encouraging good communication between household members. It's also more efficient and economical to organise meals for a household than for individual household members.

If you have children, you have a powerful influence on their food preferences and eating habits. If you offer only a narrow range of foods, it may be difficult for your children to be more adventurous with new foods. If it's normal in your household to eat takeaway in front of the TV most nights of the week, your children will consider this acceptable too.

Top tips for healthy household meals

1 Be organised

Prepare a weekly menu and shopping list. It may seem like a tedious task but you will reap the rewards for the rest of the week. If it gets to the end of the day when you're tired and frazzled, and you have no idea what's for dinner or what food is in the house, you're more likely to buy takeaway food. But if you know what you're having and everything is set to go, you can have a meal on the table in less time than it takes to get takeaway. Develop your own set of meal cards based on your typical meals, including everyone's favourites, plus some new meals for variety. You should end up with a good selection of meals to use as a basis for your menu plan without having to browse through recipe books.

2 Keep it varied

Make sure your menu plan and shopping list include a good variety of fruits and vegetables, wholegrain breads and cereals, low-fat dairy foods and lean meat, including fish, or vegetarian alternatives. Avoid the confectionery and snack food aisles in the supermarket unless you have extreme willpower.

3 Keep it simple

Meals don't need to be flashy and you don't need gourmet recipe books. Unless you're a real foodie, don't consider recipes that have a long list of ingredients, require rare ingredients or use complex and time-consuming cooking methods. Who needs a recipe book when you can cook barbecued lamb chops, jacket potatoes and steamed mixed vegetables with soy sauce and sesame seeds for flavour?

4 Keep it small

Plate sizes are becoming bigger, which means more food on the plate. Most people eat what's on their plate just because it's there, without thinking about whether they're full or not, so it's easy to overeat. Buy smaller plates, serve within the rim of the plate and use the 'quarter, quarter, half' rule when serving: one-quarter protein food, one-quarter carbohydrate food and one-half salad or vegetables.

5 Keep it cheap

You don't need to break the budget to have a healthy diet. Buy in bulk and freeze perishables for later. Compare supermarket prices by checking the 'price per kg' or 'price per 100 g' shelf labels. Buy fruits and vegetables in season. Use slow-cooking methods for cheaper cuts of meat. Shop at markets (especially near closing time) and look out for closing-time bargains at your local supermarket.

Understanding food labels

Food labels can be a useful guide to better food choices, but they can also be confusing. Here are some tips to help.

Ingredients list

Ingredients are listed in order of highest to lowest in quantity, and the list can also be used to identify unwanted additives.

Nutrition panel

The nutrition panel lists specific nutrients per serving size and per 100 g. The table below is an easy guide to choosing low-fat, low-salt, low-sugar and high-fibre foods.

Ingredient	per 100 g
Fat	3 g per 100 g (3%) or less
Sugars	20 g per 100 g (20%) or less
Sodium (i.e. salt)	120 mg per 100 g or less
Fibre	3 g per serve or more

NUTRITION INFORMATION
Servings per package: 8
Serving Size: 25g

	Quantity per serving	Quantity per 100g
Energy	360kJ	1440kJ
Protein	1.9g	7.6g
Fat - total	2.4g	9.6g
- saturated	0.8g	3.2g
Carbohydrate - total	15g	60g
- sugars	5.1g	20.4g
Dietary Fibre	2.3g	9.2g
Sodium	8mg	32mg

Food label with dietary information

Health claims to be wary of

Use the Heart Foundation Tick as a reliable indication of healthier products, but be cautious of misleading nutrition claims:

- **% fat-free** – if a product claims to be 93% fat-free, it still contains 7% fat, which is quite a lot. Also, many low-fat foods are high in sugar; marshmallows, for example, are 99% fat-free but 100% sugar!

- **light or lite** – this may refer to the colour or taste rather than indicating that the product is any lower in fat; 'light' olive oil, for example, is lighter in colour but no lower in fat or energy than other olive oil.

- **no cholesterol** – this doesn't mean the food is not high in other types of fat, which contain the same number of kilojoules.

- **baked not fried** – it sounds healthier, but can actually contain just as much fat.

Guidelines for nutrition claims

Certain guidelines must be met for a manufacturer to be able to make various nutrition claims:

- **no added sugar** – must not contain added sugar, but may contain natural sugars
- **fat-free** – must have less than 0.15% fat

- **low-fat** – must contain less than 3% fat for solid foods (1.5% for liquid foods)
- **reduced-fat** – should have at least a 25% reduction in fat from the original product
- **low-salt** – must contain no more than 120 mg salt per 100 g
- **reduced-salt** – should have at least a 25% reduction in salt from the original product
- **high in fibre** – must contain at least 3 g fibre per serve

Practical tips for selecting healthier foods

Compare nutritional quality
Check food labels (see above) to compare the nutritional quality of products.

Avoid packaged snack foods
Need a snack? Processed snack foods such as chips, biscuits, muffins and cakes are often high in fat, salt, sugar and kilojoules. Regular intake of these snacks can contribute to obesity, hypertension (high blood pressure) and heart disease. Here are some better options:

- fresh or dried fruits
- roasted nuts
- plain crackers with cheese or a low-fat dip
- baked pretzels
- low-fat yoghurt
- fruit smoothies made with low-fat milk
- mini cans of tuna, baked beans, corn or four-bean mix

Limit takeaway and convenience foods
It's difficult to recommend a healthy takeaway food, because most of them are high in the nutrients we don't want and low in those we do. A good rule is to avoid anything fried or covered in breadcrumbs, batter or pastry. Where lower fat, lower salt versions or smaller serves are available, choose them. Here are some better options:

- barbecued chicken (remove the skin and serve with salad)
- sushi or rice paper rolls
- a good-quality burger with salad

- pizza with a thin base, less cheese and no salami
- kebabs/souvlaki with flat bread, lean meat, salad and tzatziki
- Subway '6-inch' with less than 6 grams fat
- Asian stir-fry with rice or noodles (aim for low-fat and small serves)

Alternatively, you could use your supermarket as a 'takeaway shop': grab a fresh bread roll or bread stick, a can of tuna or sliced cheese and mixed salad leaves, and you have an instant lunch or light meal.

The large supermarket chains now have a range of good-quality frozen or freshly prepared meals that are ready to heat and eat once you're home. This would be an expensive way of eating as a family, but it's ideal for busy singles and healthier than a typical takeaway meal. These include:

- freshly prepared meals such as risotto or curry and rice
- freshly prepared soups
- healthy frozen meals such as McCain's Healthy Choice, Lite n' Easy or Weight Watchers
- quiche from the deli (just add salad)

Watch the beverages

The market is continually being flooded with new beverages, and a higher proportion of our total kilojoule intake now comes from drinks. Without a doubt, water is the best drink: it contains no kilojoules, it's the best fluid for hydrating the body and it's more or less free. Milk is also important, as it is a good source of protein and calcium; choose low-fat varieties if you have weight concerns. Most fruit juices contain similar kilojoules to soft drinks, so it is better to eat your fruit rather than drink it. Flavoured milk, smoothies, iced teas and flavoured mineral waters are all high in kilojoules and should be avoided if possible. Alcohol in moderation can form part of a healthy diet, but drinking too much can be harmful and contribute to weight gain. Current recommendations suggest that adult women drink no more than two standard alcoholic drinks per day but try to include two alcohol-free days per week. Low-carbohydrate beers and wines may be lower in carbohydrates, but they often have similar alcohol and kilojoule content to other beers and wines.

Eating out

Eating out is an important part of our social lives and can be a convenient way of eating if you have a busy lifestyle. If you eat out only occasionally, it doesn't hurt to indulge a little, but if it is a weekly occurrence, you need to be more cautious. Here are some tips to help:

- Don't overeat: do you really need an entree plus a main, or could you order two entrees instead?
- Avoid fried foods, breadcrumbs, batter, pastry and creamy sauces.
- Skip the butter or margarine on bread.
- Choose lean meats.
- Share a dessert with a friend or choose fruit instead.
- Limit alcohol: pace yourself, alternate wine and water or drink low-joule mixers with spirits.
- Avoid soft drinks (or ask for low-joule).

Nutrient-rich foods

Some foods may have components that confer special health benefits in addition to their normal nutrients. These components include:

- **Antioxidants**, which help protect against disease. Examples include vitamins C and E, zinc, selenium and phytochemicals. They are widely distributed in food, so include a variety of fruits and vegetables, wholegrain breads and cereals, nuts and seeds in your diet. Antioxidants may not have the same effect when taken as supplements.
- **Probiotics**, which contain live bacteria that can aid digestion and bowel function. The most common sources of probiotics are yoghurts with specific bacteria such as *Lactobacillus*, Yakult, or capsules containing live bacteria.
- **Phytochemicals**, which are chemicals that may protect against certain diseases such as cardiovascular disease and some cancers. Examples include lycopene, carotenoids, isoflavones and flavonols. Dietary sources include fruits and vegetables, lentils, nuts and seeds, tea and wine.
- **Organic foods**, which are foods grown without the use of pesticides and artificial fertilisers. People often prefer these foods for reasons of flavour and taste, environmental benefits or personal preference. Tests comparing organic food with food grown in the conventional way, however, show little difference in nutritional value.

'Super' foods

A number of foods have been identified as particularly nutrient-rich and especially beneficial for promoting good health or preventing disease. They tend to vary in popularity with time, and food manufacturers will often play on their popularity. Some of the current favourites include:

- green tea
- dark chocolate
- red wine
- green leafy vegetables such as broccoli, spinach and bok choy
- grains such as oats, wheat germ and quinoa
- nuts and seeds such as almonds, flaxseed (linseed) and chia

While these foods may have some nutritional bonuses, they are not essential for a healthy diet. Include them in moderation if you enjoy them, but don't force yourself to eat them if you don't.

Glycaemic index

Glycaemic index (GI) is a ranking given to food to describe how quickly the carbohydrate in the food is digested and absorbed into the bloodstream. Foods that are quickly digested and absorbed have a high GI, while those that are digested and absorbed more slowly have a low GI.

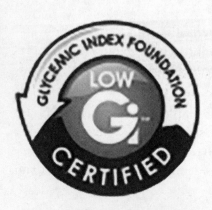

Use the low-GI symbol as your trusted guide when choosing healthy low-GI foods

Both low-GI and high-GI foods can be included in a healthy diet, but lower GI foods have several advantages. They help to control blood glucose levels, which is particularly important for people with diabetes. They also keep us feeling full for longer, therefore reducing food intake and helping us control our weight. Try to include a low-GI food with each meal, or as often as possible. See the table below for popular low-GI foods, and the Resources section at the end of this book for more information on the GI.

Some popular low-GI foods

Breakfast cereals	Weetbix, All-Bran, Guardian, Special K, porridge oats, semolina (cooked), oat bran
Breads and cereals	Wholegrain and multigrain breads, fruit loaf
Other grain products	Basmati rice, pasta, noodles (not fried), pearl barley, cracked wheat, buckwheat
Biscuits	Vita-Weat crispbreads, Ryvita Pumpkin/Sunflower Seed and Oat biscuits, Arnotts Snack Right varieties
Vegetables	Sweet corn, sweet potato
Legumes and pulses	Lentils, kidney beans, split peas, chickpeas, baked beans
Dairy	Low-fat milk, soy milk, low-fat yoghurt
Fruit	Apples, oranges, bananas, pears, grapes, stone fruit (apricots, peaches, nectarines, plums), berries

Nutrition and fertility

If you want to have children, it is a good idea to prepare your body for pregnancy so your baby has the best environment in which to grow. First, you should aim to be a healthy weight. If you are overweight or under-weight you may have trouble conceiving.

A healthy diet and exercise program is important for fertility. Your diet should be in line with the Australian Dietary Guidelines referred to at the beginning of this chapter. You should also limit your intake of alcohol and caffeine at this time. A folic acid supplement is strongly recommended if you are trying to conceive.

14

Healthy weight management for young women

Elisabeth Gasparini

Many women at some time in their life decide they are overweight and want to do something about it. Sometimes this is just a perception and their weight is actually healthy and normal, while at other times, it is a realisation that they really are overweight.

Around 60 per cent of Australian adults are now overweight or obese, and the greatest increase has been among adults aged 18–30. In most cases this is not due to lack of knowledge. Most of us know that excess energy intake and inadequate exercise are to blame, but we seem powerless to change the trend. Our lifestyle has changed, with women often working long hours, leaving little time for meal planning and food preparation. The environment has also changed, with easy access to high-fat, high-sugar takeaway and convenience foods and less opportunity for physical activity to burn off the calories. It's no wonder we're all getting fatter. For successful weight control we need not only an understanding of what is in food and how much exercise we need but also of the more complex issues that influence our eating behaviour.

Being overweight

Being overweight can increase the risk of serious health conditions such as diabetes, hypertension (high blood pressure), heart disease and some cancers. Obesity also reduces both male and female fertility and can affect emotional health and confidence. Although there are guidelines and targets for weight and health, reaching these can seem unrealistic for many people. Have you ever given up healthy eating or dieting because you thought you weren't losing enough weight or weren't losing it quickly enough? In fact, studies into weight-loss methods have shown that it is difficult to lose more than 5–10 per cent of your weight. Research has also shown, however, that this amount of weight loss can improve conditions such as diabetes, heart disease and high blood pressure. Being fit can also protect health to some degree, even if you are overweight. So don't be put off trying to improve your health because of slow progress. Eating well and regular exercise are beneficial even if that ultimate weight goal remains elusive.

What is a healthy weight?

For adults over the age of 18, the healthy weight range is calculated by measuring their body mass index (BMI). This is a measure of how heavy you should be for your height.

To calculate your BMI, you'll need to know your weight in kilograms and your height in metres. Calculate your BMI by dividing your weight by the square of your height:

BMI = weight (in kilograms)/(height in metres × height in metres)

Example: Mary weighs 65 kilograms and is 1.7 metres tall. Her BMI is therefore:

$$65/(1.7 \times 1.7) = 22.5$$

Once you've calculated your BMI, use the table below to determine what it means.

BMI classifications

BMI	Classification
less than 18.5	Underweight
18.5–24.9	Healthy weight
25–29.9	Overweight
more than 30	Obese

BMI is an internationally accepted measure and is useful for looking at populations, but it has some limitations for individuals. BMI doesn't differentiate between fat and muscle mass and may overestimate fat mass in people who have a muscular build, such as athletes. It also doesn't take into account age, gender or culture.

Health assessments commonly look at the way fat is distributed around the waist and hips. This is because carrying fat around the abdomen increases the risk of health problems more than fat around the hips. This is the case even if BMI is not high. The good news is that abdominal fat tends to be the first fat that is lost, so exercise, a healthy diet and minimising alcohol consumption can help reduce that annoying muffin top.

Abdominal fat can be measured by calculating your waist-to-hip ratio (WHR), or more simply by measuring your waist circumference. Take your waist measurement around the narrowest point between your lowest rib and your hip bones. Take your hip measurement around the point where your buttocks are widest when standing side-on.

$$WHR = \text{waist measurement/hips measurement}$$

Women should aim for a WHR of less than 0.8.

Waist circumference

Waist circumference	Risk to health
Less than 80 centimetres	Low
More than 80 centimetres	Moderate
More than 88 centimetres	High

Factors that affect body weight

Weight is affected by three key factors: genetic inheritance, food intake and physical activity.

Our shape and frame size are largely determined by genetics. Our genes also influence our metabolic rate (the rate at which we metabolise food), so that some people can eat like a horse and not gain weight while others seem to gain weight just thinking about food. Genetics can also affect our hunger and fullness signals and our fat distribution; that is, whether we are apple- or pear-shaped. We can't change our genes, but we can make the most of what we have inherited by treating our bodies respectfully with healthy food and regular physical activity.

Energy intake from food and fluids is used as fuel to maintain the body's basic functions and to meet the demands of physical activity. If the number of kilojoules we eat is greater than the number of kilojoules we use up each day through basic functions and physical exercise, then the excess energy is stored in our body as fat.

Losing weight

Losing weight is like making any other long-term life change. It requires setting a goal, having a plan and being determined.

Most overweight people opt for strategies involving lifestyle changes. These generally involve increasing exercise and changing diet; that is, reducing energy or kilojoule intake and increasing energy use. We know that changing diet alone or just exercising is less effective than using a combination of both. For many people, even small reductions in kilojoule intake or small increases in activity level can make a big difference over time. For others, overeating may be related to more complex emotional issues they need to work on before they can change their eating habits.

The problem with 'diets'

Many diets fail because they impose a meal plan. Even with a huge amount of willpower, we won't be able to maintain an eating plan that doesn't suit us. We are more likely to persist with a diet if it is based on our eating preferences than if it is very different from our usual pattern. Eating is a very personal thing, and so a healthy eating plan needs to accommodate our individual food preferences or we will never feel really satisfied. Diet plans usually don't help us recognise our body's own hunger and fullness signals, as the amount of food allowed is predetermined and may

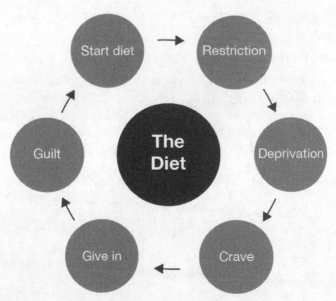

The diet cycle

not teach us how to make good food choices. The unrealistic rules of diets can leave us feeling deprived, vulnerable to temptation and then guilty if we give in (as we all eventually do). This can set up a repetitive cycle of dieting followed by overeating the foods we were deprived of when dieting, followed by more guilt and a return to dieting. It can also lead to weight gain.

Fad diets

Despite the drawbacks of diets, many people like to follow a diet plan for a while as a kickstart to a healthier lifestyle. Diets all work the same way: they have fewer calories than you normally eat. While some diets are nutritionally adequate, others are not. Fad diets are just that: a fad. They are unsustainable and often don't contain enough nutrients for good health. If the diet cuts out whole food groups such as dairy foods or contains only one food group such as vegetables, then it is a short-term fix and after a while you'll be back at square one. Examples of fad diets include the Cabbage Soup diet, detox diets and the Atkins diet.

If you hear about a new diet (and there's one coming to a magazine or website near you), look it over and ask yourself whether the diet:

- promises rapid, easy weight loss
- limits whole food groups
- allows you to eat as much as you like of any one food without putting on weight
- requires you to buy special diet pills or herbs
- allows only specific foods or foods in certain combinations
- claims to be new or revolutionary
- contains a miracle ingredient, patch or gel
- only mentions food and says nothing about exercise

If your answer to any of these questions is yes, then the diet is unlikely to be based on a healthy eating plan that will lead to sustainable weight loss and long-term healthy eating habits. Forget it!

This was not the first time Debbie had tried to lose weight. She had been to weight-loss meetings, she'd suffered through weeks of the Soup diet, and she'd even bought weight-loss shakes from the pharmacy. Nothing worked. Sure, she'd lost 5 or 6 kilograms in two weeks at one stage, but she'd piled all the weight back on again just as quickly as she'd taken it off. She was now back to 93 kilograms and miserable. Debbie knew that her ideal weight was around 66 kilograms, but thinking about this was just depressing. She just wanted to be able to pull on her size 14 jeans again.

Debbie worked in retail and her days were quite long and often frantic. She didn't eat much at all during the day because she didn't feel hungry. Usually she would have a coffee on the way to work and would only stop for lunch if she had time. Dinner was often something she'd pick up on the way home from work. She lived by herself and cooking for one was no fun.

Debbie went to see a dietician with her food diary, which showed that most of her eating was done in the evenings and on the way home from work when she was particularly hungry. She was also eating biscuits or chocolate after dinner while watching TV, even though she wasn't hungry. She also revealed that if she was stressed, she would eat more. The problem was that she didn't stop at one or two rows of chocolate; if she felt she had failed her diet, she would eat the whole block of chocolate or the entire packet of biscuits.

Debbie recognised that she was using food to feed her emotions and that it was making her weight-loss efforts very difficult. She and the dietician explored other non-food-related activities she could engage in to release her stress, such as going for a walk or calling a friend.

Ensuring Debbie ate regularly was the first step to increasing her sluggish metabolism. She began by waking 15 minutes earlier and having a wholesome breakfast. She also needed to ensure she took the time to eat lunch each day, and took an afternoon snack with her to work so she didn't stop at the shop on the way home. To reduce the amount of fat in her diet, she started taking her lunch from home and cooking her own dinner. On the weekends she cooked two different dishes and froze them in portions ready for the week. She otherwise cooked simple meat and vegetable dishes and allowed herself takeaway food once a week.

Staying up late watching TV was bad news for Debbie's weight. Her sleep quality was poor and she was mindlessly eating the equivalent of half a day's calories in front of the TV. She agreed to buy snack-sized chocolate instead of a family block, which reduced her temptation to overeat.

When Debbie went back to the dietician six weeks later, she had lost 3 kilograms. She was surprised because she felt she was eating more than before, but in fact her calorie intake had decreased and she was eating regularly rather than bingeing on sweet foods. They set a short-term goal of reaching 85 kilograms, which was more motivating than thinking about *her ideal weight. It was important for Debbie to learn that weight loss was a gradual process involving improving habits and eating behaviours. Quick fixes don't lead to sustained weight loss.*

Avoiding the diet cycle

1 Identify non-hungry eating

Food is not only sustenance. We eat for many reasons: we eat because we like nice food; we eat for social reasons; and we also use food as a comfort or to nurture ourselves, reaching for it when we're stressed and seeking it out when we are bored. We often eat mindlessly. Have you ever been eating in front of the TV and looked down to find you have finished your meal? Our busy lives see us multitasking more and eating on the run. This often means we are not concentrating on the food we are eating and sometimes we forget we have eaten at all.

Before we can look at changing our eating habits, we need to be aware of why we eat as well as what we eat. A food, hunger and mood diary (such as the eating awareness record below) can help identify whether you are eating for reasons other than hunger. If you are eating due to stress, boredom or loneliness, you may have to find alternative ways of dealing with these things before you are able to change your eating habits. Diets often fail because they do not address the real reasons why people eat.

Eating awareness record

Rate your hunger and fullness between 1 and 10, where 1 is 'starving', 5 is just right and 10 is bursting.

Time and place	Food or drink consumed	What was your trigger for eating (physical hunger or another reason)?	How hungry were you before eating?	How satisfied did you feel after eating	What other activity or food might have satisfied you more?

Everyone does some non-hungry eating, but if it's happening frequently and affecting your weight, try to stay away from situations that trigger eating and look for other ways of satisfying your emotional needs. Make a list of distracters you can try instead of eating, such as going for a walk, making time for an activity you enjoy, buying yourself a small present, doing a crossword or calling a friend. Busying your hands with artwork or knitting may also help. Often the desire to eat will pass if you wait a few minutes.

Some reasons for non-hungry eating

- Because you 'have to': pies at the football, popcorn at the movies, chocolate at the petrol station, takeaway Fridays
- Being worried about offending someone if you don't eat
- Feeling emotions like sadness, happiness, boredom, anger
- Being taught to finish off everything on your plate
- Being in places such as shops, kitchens, Mum's place, cafes
- Because it is a work break and time to eat
- Feeling full but not satisfied after a meal
- Becoming too hungry and overeating
- Eating in case you get hungry later
- Not being sure when to stop eating
- As a reward for completing tasks
- Seeing and smelling hot food
- Knowing the food tastes good
- The clock says it's mealtime
- Confusing hunger with thirst
- To have enough energy
- To have with a drink
- When others are eating
- Food advertisements
- Hormones
- Tiredness
- Habit

2 Practise mindful eating

People are less likely to overeat if they are conscious of what they are eating and enjoying it.

Practise tuning in to your body's hunger and fullness signals. Years of dieting or non-hungry eating can blunt these signals. Practise rating your hunger on a scale of 1 to 10, where 1 is 'starving' and 10 is bursting. You may need to experiment with different quantities and types of food. Aim to eat when you are peckish to hungry and stop when you're pleasantly full and have eaten enough to sustain you for the next three or four hours. Be grateful for the abundance and choice we have. Enjoy your food and avoid distractions while eating it.

Focus on the food in front of you. Savour each mouthful, aiming to extract the maximum flavour and satisfaction. Try to overcome any guilt about eating certain foods, so that you can enjoy them to the full.

Be flexible, too. Allow yourself to say 'No, thank you' when you are full or to have a little more when you are not satisfied.

Sit down to eat – don't eat while you walk or shop – and while you're retraining yourself, don't eat in front of the TV or while you read, otherwise it becomes mindless eating and you don't remember what you've eaten. If you have to eat at your desk at work, try to keep at a distance from your computer or paperwork.

3 Set realistic goals

Setting unrealistic weight-loss targets will ultimately lead to failure and feelings of frustration and poor self-worth. Recommendations for rates of weight loss vary. To be realistic, aim for a gradual weight loss of around 1–2 kilograms per month and understand that although the rate of weight loss tends to slow down and plateau over time, your weight will still gradually decrease.

Having set a realistic target, once you've reached it you can always set another one. Losing 5–10 per cent of your current weight (about 5–10 kilograms) is often enough to make a considerable difference to your health. For someone who has been steadily gaining weight, maintaining weight and avoiding further weight gain may be a good enough aim.

You should be able to eat all kinds of food. One of the reasons diets fail is that people feel deprived and start to crave foods the diet does not allow. If you know you are allowed to eat all foods, you are more likely to eat them only if you really feel like them. Foods are not 'good' or 'bad', but it can be helpful to think of them as 'everyday' foods and 'sometimes' foods. 'Sometimes' foods are higher in unhealthy fats or sugar and lower in nutrients; examples include fried foods, pastries, cakes, confectionery and sweet drinks.

Aim to eat well most of the time, and expect that you will err now and then. Don't set unrealistic food goals when it comes to giving up unhealthy foods. For some it may be best to go cold turkey with that chocolate addiction, but for others it may be more realistic to cut intake gradually or by half.

You can also try setting 'SMART' goals:

S = specific: what/where – what are you aiming to change?

M = measurable: how will you know when you've reached your goal?

A = achievable: small steps at a time

R = realistic: how practical is it to make the change?

T = time: by when?

Good habits that help with weight control

Use these tips to help you successfully manage your weight:

- Don't let yourself get overly hungry or you'll have less control over what you eat. Regular meals and snacks help stabilise blood sugar levels and prevent excessive hunger. Try not to skip breakfast or you might find yourself looking for snacks later in the day. If you can't manage to eat first thing in the morning, try a smoothie or an Up & Go drink, or eat a good morning tea.

- Eat balanced meals containing protein, carbohydrate and vegetables or salad, which increase satisfaction after eating. They also give your body the nourishment it needs and prevent cravings.

- Eat more slowly digested carbohydrates such as grainy bread, and less processed cereals such as oats, which increase the feeling of fullness after eating and help prevent the swings in blood sugar that cause hunger and sweet cravings.

- Avoid portion distortion. The portion sizes of many foods and drinks have increased over the years. Research has shown that people eat more when served a bigger portion. It can take a while for your brain to register that you have had enough to eat, and by that time you have overeaten. The increasing portion sizes of foods and drinks are

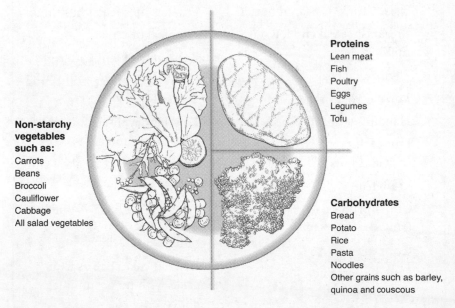

Proteins
Lean meat
Fish
Poultry
Eggs
Legumes
Tofu

Non-starchy vegetables such as:
Carrots
Beans
Broccoli
Cauliflower
Cabbage
All salad vegetables

Carbohydrates
Bread
Potato
Rice
Pasta
Noodles
Other grains such as barley, quinoa and couscous

The plate rule

significant contributors of unneeded calories. Reduce 'portion distortion' by eating slowly. Listen to your stomach and stop eating when you feel full. You don't need to finish everything on your plate. Buy the smaller size, and don't be tempted to get value for money with a bigger size. Or share with a friend or save half for later. If you work, taking lunch from home keeps you in control of portion size and fat content.

- Reduce your intake of fats and oils. They are rich in calories and can be reduced without reducing the volume of food eaten. Be careful with fats and oils used in cooking as well as with those hidden in pastries, fried foods and snack foods such as chips. Biscuits, muffins and chocolate are higher in fat and calories than many people realise.

- Watch your sugar intake. People often feel guilty about a teaspoon of sugar added to tea or coffee but may not realise their soft drink, fruit juice or commercial iced tea contains up to nine teaspoons of sugar. Soft drinks and juices can add significantly to calorie intake and can take away our appetite for more nutritious foods.

Healthy snack ideas

- Slice of grainy bread with cheese, tuna or peanut butter
- Breakfast cereal and low-fat milk
- Hard-boiled egg
- Low-fat yoghurt
- Handful of unsalted nuts
- Dried fruit or mixed dried fruit and nuts
- Fresh fruit
- Cup of fruit salad or stewed fruit
- Corn cob
- Cup of vegetable soup

- Celery or carrot sticks and low-fat dip such as hummus
- Oatmeal biscuits
- Toasted fruit loaf with a scrape of margarine or butter
- Bowl of popcorn
- Low-fat dry biscuits such as Vita-Weats and cheese
- Rice cakes or corn cakes with a spread
- English muffin or crumpet and scrape of margarine or butter
- Low-fat cake such as fruit cakes with no or minimal added fat

Active living

It can be difficult to fit in enough exercise to maintain weight and fitness, but for long-term health we need to create a pleasurable, active lifestyle. This can include a mixture of purposeful exercise and taking opportunities to increase incidental exercise such as walking up the stairs or parking further from the shops.

If you shudder at the thought of exercise, it's probably because you have never found a form of exercise you like. You don't need to be a runner or gym pro; you just need to find something you can do regularly. Brisk walking is good fat-burning exercise that most people can do. Thirty minutes a day of brisk walking will help prevent weight gain and maintain fitness. For weight loss you may need more – at least 60 minutes of walking daily. If using a pedometer (step counter), aim for at least 10,000 steps a day. This doesn't need to be done in one go.

As well as helping with weight control, regular exercise:

- clears the mind and leaves us feeling good
- improves mood and reduces stress and so can help reduce non-hungry eating
- helps us become more attuned to our appetite – evidence suggests that people who exercise may actually eat less than those who don't exercise
- improves sleep
- raises levels of the 'good' HDL cholesterol, which helps prevent heart disease
- helps prevent stroke and high blood pressure
- reduces the risk of developing type 2 diabetes and some cancers
- keeps bones strong if it's weight-bearing, such as walking

You might just need a little motivation to get started or keep going; here are some tips:

- Exercise with a friend.
- Keep an exercise diary.
- Buy some new exercise clothes and runners or comfortable shoes.
- Replace excuses with positive thoughts about how much better you will feel.

I've been exercising for ages and I'm not losing any weight!

If you've been doing the same workout for a while and your weight has plateaued, most likely your body has become used to the exercise and has adapted to cope, leaving you with no change on the scales. Your muscles can get used to an exercise routine, but changing your exercise intensity or type every few weeks can give your body the kick it needs to get weight loss going again. If you enjoy walking, for example, include short jogging bursts, or go up and down some steps along the way to fire up different muscle groups. Seeking the advice of a professional personal trainer, even for just one short session, can help you find new ways to exercise effectively.

Physical activity guidelines for Australian adults

1. **Think of movement as an opportunity, not an inconvenience.** Any form of movement of the body is an opportunity for improving health, not a time-wasting inconvenience.

2. **Be active every day in as many ways as you can.** Make a habit of walking or cycling instead of using the car, or do things yourself instead of using labour-saving machines.

3. **Aim for at least 30 minutes of moderate-intensity physical activity on five or more days of the week.** You can accumulate your 30 minutes (or more) throughout the day by combining a few shorter 10–15-minute sessions of activity.

4. **If possible, include about 90 minutes of higher intensity exercise per week in your exercise regime for extra health and fitness.**

When diet and exercise aren't enough

Sometimes, diet and exercise just aren't enough to achieve satisfactory weight loss, or there is an urgent need to lose weight quickly, such as having a very high BMI, or other significant risk factors such as diabetes, hypertension (high blood pressure) and heart disease, or there is a need to conceive without delay. In such cases, it may be appropriate to consider other, more aggressive methods of weight management that, although not necessarily ideal for long-term weight management, can achieve success in the short term.

Some of the more common alternatives for weight management are listed below, along with some of the pros and cons of each approach.

Very low-calorie diets (VLCDs)

VLCDs are commercial products (usually shakes, soups and bars, such as Optifast and Optislim) designed to be used very strictly for short periods of four to 12 weeks. They are very low in energy, with added nutrients to ensure they meet minimum nutrient requirements. These diets can help people break old eating habits and generally result in rapid weight loss, especially during the first few weeks, but they are not suitable for long-term use. Some of the problems with these types of products are:

- Some are not adequately fortified with nutrients and are therefore not safe for sole use.
- They are very limited in variety and the diets become boring, making them difficult to follow.
- For the same reason, they can result in feelings of deprivation and all the problems associated with this (see the diagram of the 'diet cycle' earlier in this chapter).
- They do not fit in with normal social eating practices and can make eating with family and friends difficult.

Meal replacement programs

These are commercially produced meals such as Lite n' Easy. They take away your need to make a decision regarding meal choices and they are convenient, since the meals can be ordered online and delivered to your door. There are several issues to consider with these types of programs, however:

- They are expensive and not suitable for family or household meals.
- They restrict food choices and, as with VLCDs (see above), can result in feelings of deprivation and all the problems associated with this (see the diagram of the 'diet cycle' earlier in this chapter).
- They make eating with family and friends difficult.
- They do not teach good menu planning, shopping or food preparation skills for the longer term.

Low-kilojoule menu plans

Many women like low-kilojoule menu plans as they take away decision-making and provide a consistent kilojoule intake. They are also more 'normal' than drinking shakes and eating bars or having meals delivered. They do have some problems, however:

- They are very prescriptive and do not take into account variations in appetite from day to day, personal food preferences or which foods are in season.

- They often require weighing, measuring and counting kilojoules, which can be tedious.

- Some do not include adequate amounts from the key food groups and so are not nutritionally safe.

- They do not teach long-term healthy eating habits.

Appetite suppressants and fat binders

Appetite-suppressant drugs are designed to reduce appetite and consequently food intake. Fat-binding drugs are claimed to soak up fat and get rid of it. Not surprisingly, these types of products sound appealing, but they can have unpleasant side effects and are not designed for long-term use. If they really worked, no one would have a weight problem.

Bariatric (weight-loss) surgery

Bariatric surgery is only an option if you are very obese, or if you are obese and have other health issues such as diabetes, high cholesterol or high blood pressure. It is an option for adults and in rare cases adolescents.

Bariatric surgery refers to four different procedures:

1. Gastric band surgery, where a band of special rubber material is placed around the stomach and then tightened to reduce the size of the stomach. This has the effect of making people feel full after a smaller amount of food.

2. Laparoscopic adjustable gastric banding (LAGB), a method of surgery that involves making a few small abdominal cuts instead of one large cut. The surgeon inserts a laparoscope (a telescope with a tiny camera) through a small cut and uses instruments through one or two other small cuts to place a band around the top of the stomach, leaving a smaller section of the stomach, or pouch, available for food. The band can be adjusted and the procedure is reversible.

3. Gastric sleeve surgery, an operation where more than half the stomach is removed, leaving a sleeve or a tube. It is more extensive surgery and is not reversible.

4. Gastric bypass, where the intestine is rerouted to bypass the stomach. This makes people digest less food, and it takes less food for them to feel full.

There are risks associated with all of these procedures, including internal bleeding, a blood clot in the leg (deep vein thrombosis) and a blood clot in the lungs (pulmonary embolism), and while these risks are avoidable and treatable, they should be considered carefully.

How does bariatric surgery work?

We don't really know exactly how it works. The surgery effectively reduces the size of the stomach and its absorptive capacity, but may also change the hormone balance and some of the metabolic processes associated with food digestion, which in turn may affect appetite and eating behaviour.

Who does bariatric surgery?

Bariatric surgery is performed by doctors who specialise in this area. As with all surgery there may be complications and these must be considered and balanced against the potential benefits. If you think it could be an option for you, you should in the first instance discuss it with your GP, who will help you decide whether it is appropriate for you.

Is bariatric surgery successful?

Bariatric surgery can be effective in producing significant weight loss in people who are very obese. It is not foolproof, however, and cannot be guaranteed to produce long-term results. Successful weight loss with bariatric surgery still requires discipline and control around food intake after surgery and should be combined with regular exercise. Most of the research into the effectiveness of bariatric surgery comes from the Swedish Obesity Study, which showed that weight loss 10 years after bariatric surgery ranged from 14 to 25 per cent, depending on the procedure. While there are some risks with bariatric surgery, there are greater health risks with remaining obese. The Swedish Obesity Study found that most people regained some weight after the surgery. To maintain the new weight and avoid possible health complications, it is necessary to adhere to the weight-maintenance strategies discussed above; that is, a restricted diet and regular exercise.

US research has found that on average people with a gastric band will lose about half their excess body weight while people with a gastric bypass will lose about two-thirds of their excess body weight.

15

Periods – normal and not so normal

Catarina Ang

Periods are also known as the menstrual cycle, menstruation or menses. Your period comes from your uterus, or womb. It is the blood and fluid formed when the endometrium, or the lining of the uterus, breaks down and comes out through the cervix and then the vagina. If you have any abnormalities in the anatomy of any of these parts, your periods may be delayed. This may be something you will need to see your doctor about.

What is a normal period?

Chapter 6 describes the many types, and differing frequencies, of a normal period. (See also p. 566 – 'Your attitude to your menstrual cycle'.)

It is quite common to experience some pain with your period, such as a cramp in your belly and/or a mild backache, often on the first one to two days of the period. You may wish to take a simple painkiller available at the chemist or supermarket if it bothers you. Some women say they know when their period is coming because their period pain starts before the period does. All of these symptoms are normal, too.

Many women will also experience other typical symptoms before their period. For instance, hormonal changes are very common before and during your period. You may feel quite moody, even teary, and your family may say your temper is particularly bad just before your period. The name for this is PMS or PMT, which stands for premenstrual syndrome or premenstrual tension. Some women suffer so badly from PMS that it stops them doing their usual activities or working. This is covered more in chapter 6.

Skin changes are also very common before a period, so you might notice you break out and have a few pimples before your period, even though you are not a teenager any more.

When should I see a doctor?

If you have been experiencing abnormal periods or symptoms as described below for more than three to six cycles, you should see your doctor. Sometimes, the symptoms might happen for a couple of cycles and then go back to normal. If they make you particularly anxious or are particularly bad, see your doctor to talk about it.

If you have bleeding that is so heavy that you are starting to feel weak, dizzy or short of breath, you should see a doctor immediately or go to the emergency department.

You should consider seeing a doctor sooner rather than later if you:

- know you have had the same problem before
- are getting older – over the age of 40
- have other medical problems such as diabetes, previous cancers, thyroid conditions, or are very overweight
- take any medications that thin your blood or make you more likely to bleed

Possible tests

Your doctor may want to perform a pelvic examination, perhaps including a Pap test or an examination with a speculum. A speculum is a metal or plastic device the doctor inserts gently into the vagina and opens up so they can get a better look at the cervix and vagina. You may have had these examinations already.

Typical initial tests your doctor will order include blood tests and an ultrasound. The blood tests may look at your blood count, your iron stores, and your levels of vitamins such as folic acid or vitamin B12. Sometimes your doctor will send off a blood sample for hormonal tests.

Ultrasound

The pelvic ultrasound is a very common test. It is quite simple, doesn't hurt, and shows a black-and-white image of the uterus and ovaries. The scanner, called the probe, is either placed on your tummy or a smaller probe is place inside your vagina. This can obtain even better imaging since it is placed much closer to your reproductive organs. There is no radiation or needles involved. It shouldn't hurt as the probe is quite small. Doctors can tell a lot of things from an ultrasound, but some women will need more tests after that.

Hysteroscopy, curettage, dilatation

Hysteroscopy is a procedure that enables a doctor to see directly inside the uterus using a fine telescope and camera. The hysteroscope can show polyps, endometrial thickening and internal fibroids that may be causing the heavy bleeding. A sample of the endometrium is usually taken at the same time for laboratory testing, and a polyp or fibroid may be removed. Hysteroscopy can be performed under local or general anaesthetic.

A curette – the removal of the uppermost layer of the uterine lining (the endometrium) – is usually performed at the same time as a hysteroscopy, and is another way to test for abnormalities. A curette alone does not improve heavy or irregular menstrual bleeding.

The word dilatation simply means that the cervix has to be opened by instruments called dilators to allow the hysteroscope or the curette instrument to go through the cervix, which is usually tightly shut. It is a bit wider in women who have delivered a baby vaginally.

Menstrual headaches

Headaches around period time are common and usually respond to simple measures, but sometimes they can be severe, difficult to control and interfere with study, work and daily living.

Women often ask the difference between a severe headache and a migraine. A migraine is characterised by its severity, is sometimes preceded by an aura (visual symptoms or altered sensations), often appears only on one side of the head, and can be throbbing in sensation.

Migraines associated with periods can be treated the same way as migraines in general: with lifestyle changes, such as reducing stress and exercising, anti-migraine medications and preventative medications, taken in consultation with your doctor. If menstrual headaches can't be controlled by lifestyle changes and by simple analgesics such as paracetamol and non-steroidal anti-inflammatory drugs (NSAIDs) such as naproxen, there are other strategies available. Some specific steps that can be taken are the use of low-dose oestrogen in the days before a period, because a contributing factor to a menstrual headache is thought to be the drop in oestrogen level that occurs in a woman's body during her premenstrual cycle. Many women prevent menstrual headache and migraine by using the oral contraceptive pill and eliminating the inactive tablets, thereby not having periods for an extended time. This is quite safe and not deleterious to health.

Note that women who suffer from migraines, whether they are associated with their period or not, should consult their doctor before they start taking the Pill. Women who have particular types of migraine have a small increased risk of having a stroke if they take the Pill.

If you feel these strategies are relevant to you, you should consult your doctor to discuss them.

What is an abnormal period?

To help you work out what is normal, it's easiest to describe what is definitely abnormal.

Period pain

Although a bit of period pain is normal, it is not normal to have such bad period pain that you have to take time off work or study, that you wake up at night or need to go to the emergency department because of the pain, or that you have to take painkillers regularly during the day to function. Please see chapter 25 for further information.

Bleeding between periods

It is generally not normal to have bleeding between your periods, unless you are taking some sort of hormonal contraception or other hormones. This is called intermenstrual bleeding, whether it happens randomly between your periods or at the same time of the cycle between periods. Occasionally a woman gets thoroughly tested and the doctor cannot find anything wrong; if the bleeding is something new, however, you should have it checked out.

Sometimes women start bleeding between periods when they are using some sort of hormone. This may be the combined oral contraceptive pill (the Pill), the minipill, the contraceptive implant that goes into your arm, a contraceptive vaginal ring, or an intrauterine contraceptive device. Your doctor may call this 'breakthrough bleeding'. The period you have when you are using the Pill isn't a true period. It is called a 'withdrawal bleed' because it usually happens when you withdraw or stop taking the active pills in your packet of contraceptives. For more on contraception, see chapter 16. Whatever form it takes, if you have bleeding between your periods for more than three to six months, you should see your doctor.

Bleeding after sex when you are not having your period

It is not normal to have ongoing problems with bleeding after sexual intercourse. This is called post-coital bleeding or PCB. You can ignore a one-off episode, but sometimes bleeding after sex is a sign that something needs to be checked. For instance, we know that women with PCB who have had normal Pap tests have a 10–15 per cent chance of an abnormality in their cervix when they are tested further.

No periods

If you used to have normal periods and then they stopped for more than six months, you should go and see your doctor. This is called secondary amenorrhoea. If you have never had your period and you are aged 16 or more, it is worthwhile going to see your doctor to be checked. Some women can be very late to start, but there are other medical reasons for this that can be treated or fixed.

It is also rare for periods not to come back straight after stopping the Pill. They can be delayed or quite irregular for several months after stopping the DMPA contraceptive injection. It is normal to have no periods or infrequent and irregular periods if using a hormonal intrauterine contraceptive device. This doesn't happen with the copper intrauterine device, though.

If your periods stop, always consider whether you could be pregnant.

Infrequent periods

It is not normal to have very infrequent periods, which is called oligomenorrhoea. It can be normal to have regular periods that are six weeks apart; nonetheless, they should be checked by a doctor. Polycystic ovarian syndrome (PCOS; see chapter 24) can involve infrequent and irregular periods.

Irregular periods

It can also be abnormal to have irregular periods. This can happen to women in their 30s and 40s, and it may only be a matter of a few days' difference. If your periods have been more irregular than a few days, let's say seven days' difference, for three to six months, you should see your doctor for a check-up.

Heavy menstrual bleeding

Heavy periods or menorrhagia is a common health complaint that affects one in five Australian women, and is the reason for many hysterectomies and other surgical procedures.

Heavy menstrual bleeding is defined as excessive menstrual blood loss that interferes with a woman's physical, social and/or emotional quality of life. It can occur alone or with other symptoms, such as pelvic pain.

During heavy menstrual bleeding, it is not normal to consistently:

- pass multiple large (around the size of a 50-cent coin) clots
- have such a heavy flow that during the day you are having to change your pad or tampon every hour because it is getting soaked and perhaps staining your clothes
- have to get up almost every night to change your pad or tampon, or have to put a towel in your bed or use large maternity pads because the flow is so heavy

It is not normal to become iron-deficient because your periods are so heavy. Your blood contains traces of iron, which carries oxygen around your body. Your period flow also contains some blood (but it is not all blood), so if your periods are very, very heavy, you lose more iron than your body can make up for.

The symptoms of iron deficiency or having low iron stores include getting tired more easily and feeling weak. Some women's iron stores become so low due to heavy periods that they become anaemic. This means their blood count is low. Anaemic people might complain of feeling dizzy, being short of breath, or even having chest pain. Some women look pale or lose some hair. Usually if a woman has been having heavy periods for a long time, though, she might not notice any of these symptoms and just feel tired. Of course, there are a lot of reasons to feel tired that have nothing to do with heavy periods.

Causes of heavy bleeding

There are multiple causes for heavy menstrual bleeding. For a long time, doctors and other healthcare professionals used a lot of Latin words for heavy menstrual bleeding, like metrorrhagia or menorrhagia, as well as phrases like 'dysfunctional uterine bleeding'. In 2011, after a great deal of discussion, the International Federation of Gynecology and Obstetrics recommended that all causes should now fall into a standard classification it had developed, called PALM-COEIN (*p*olyp, *a*denomyosis, *l*eiomyoma, *m*alignancy and hyperplasia, *c*oagulopathy, *o*vulatory dysfunction, *e*ndometrial, *i*atrogenic, and *n*ot yet classified).

On the basis of this classification, we can start to describe what this may mean for you if you have symptoms of heavy periods.

Polyps

Uterine polyps are usually non-cancerous (benign) growths of the lining of the uterus (the endometrium). They can also occur at the cervix. Polyps may cause heavy menstrual bleeding, bleeding between periods or bleeding after sexual intercourse. Occasionally, polyps can develop abnormalities, particularly in older women, so doctors will generally advise that they be removed before they become dangerous.

Adenomyosis

Adenomyosis is a common benign gynaecological problem that can cause painful and heavy periods, and can have the same symptoms as endometriosis and fibroids. It occurs when the endometrial glands grow into the smooth muscle of the uterus (myometrium). The muscle of the uterus responds by growing larger (becoming hypertrophic). As a result, the uterus grows larger, and it can be tender when examined. Adenomyosis is not easily diagnosed, as the common approaches used – ultrasound, hysteroscopy, keyhole surgery and magnetic resonance imaging (MRI) – will not pick it up all the time. Women tend to be in their 30s when they are diagnosed.

Fibroids (leiomyomas)

Fibroids are abnormal growths that form in the muscle of the uterus. They are very common and can occur in up to 80 per cent of women. They are often referred to as 'tumours', but the vast majority are not cancerous.

Fibroids can bulge from the inside or outside of the uterus. They can range in size from microscopic to the size of a grapefruit or even larger. The majority of fibroids are small and do not cause any symptoms at all.

Fibroids are more likely to cause symptoms if they are large, if there are many of them or if they push on other internal organs. Some women with fibroids experience very heavy menstrual bleeding, pelvic pressure or pain that interferes with their life, and some women have problems with fertility and pregnancy. Fibroid symptoms tend to get better after menopause, however.

The exact cause of fibroids is still unknown, although we know that fibroid growth is related to the female hormones. Some women have specific genes that make it more likely they will have fibroids. There are many other possibilities, but no one cause.

Medical or surgical treatments are available for women with fibroid-related problems such as heavy menstrual bleeding, pelvic pressure or pain, or problems with pregnancy or infertility. It depends which

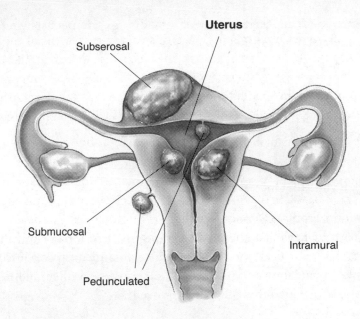

Uterus

Subserosal

Submucosal

Pedunculated

Intramural

Uterus with fibroids

symptom is the most bothersome. You do not need treatment if you have no symptoms.

The fibroids themselves cannot be removed with medications. Certain medicines can temporarily reduce their size, but surgery (called a myomectomy or fibroidectomy; see below) is used to remove them. Sometimes this can be done with laparoscopy (keyhole surgery). Hormonal medications that suppress ovulation and menstruation are used to reduce the heavy menstrual bleeding that is common in women with fibroids, and are often recommended before surgical treatments. Other medications range from pain-relief drugs such as paracetamol to non-steroidal anti-inflammatories.

The ultimate treatment for fibroids is hysterectomy – removal of the uterus that contains the fibroids. This is major surgery and means there is no possibility of further pregnancy.

Cancer (malignancy) and hyperplasia

Some women may develop an abnormally thick endometrial lining on the inside of their uterus. This condition is called endometrial hyperplasia and it may cause heavy menstrual bleeding, irregular bleeding or a blood-stained vaginal discharge. In some cases, endometrial hyperplasia may progress to endometrial cancer, a condition that is more common after menopause but can occur in younger women.

Women are at an increased risk of developing endometrial hyperplasia or endometrial cancer if they:

- are over the age of 45
- weigh more than 90 kilograms
- have never had children
- have a family history of endometrial, ovarian or bowel cancer
- have polycystic ovarian syndrome (PCOS; see chapter 24)
- carry a gene that increases their cancer risk

Coagulation problems (coagulopathy)

If you have or have had any of the symptoms described below, there is a chance that your heavy periods are related to a medical condition that affects the coagulation of your blood (such as Von Willebrand disease, which stops the blood from clotting very well):

1. Heavy menstrual bleeding since your periods started, or
2. Any one of the following:
   - losing a lot of blood after giving birth (post-partum haemorrhage)
   - bleeding related to surgery – you will need to tell your doctor so they can work out if it was connected or not
   - bleeding associated with dental work – you will need to tell your doctor so they can work out if it was connected or not, or
3. Any two or more of the following symptoms:
   - bruising once or twice per month
   - nosebleeds once or twice per month
   - frequent gum bleeding
   - a family history of bleeding symptoms

Ovulation problems (ovulatory dysfunction)

Not ovulating properly can contribute to unpredictable bleeding and possibly heavy bleeding. We don't always know why it happens, but as women grow older it seems to become more common. Some related health conditions that cause ovulation problems include underactive thyroid gland (hypothyroidism), high levels of the hormone prolactin, mental stress, weight loss and extreme amounts of exercise. Medications such as certain antidepressants or antipsychotics can also have this effect, as can certain steroids.

Endometrial problems

Sometimes if no specific cause for abnormal or heavy bleeding can be found, doctors may conclude that there is a problem in the endometrium itself. Reaching this conclusion means that all other causes need to be excluded, however.

Iatrogenic causes (causes due to medical treatments)

Some medical interventions and devices can contribute to abnormal bleeding, including the breakthrough bleeding that can occur in some women who use the Pill or have an IUS contraceptive device.

Causes not yet classified

A few causes do not fall into the other categories because they are rare, or have not been well enough studied to categorise. As we learn more, they may be moved to one of the other existing categories.

Treatments for heavy bleeding

Medical treatments are usually tried first for heavy menstrual bleeding, either on an ongoing basis, or just while tests are being performed. These include various oral medications, along with vaginal and uterine devices. They are all reversible, and most should reduce the bleeding or other symptoms within the first few weeks. They do not cure the bleeding but they can control it, and therefore usually need to be continued.

Iron deficiency due to heavy bleeding is usually treated with iron tablets, one side effect of which can be constipation. If you are severely anaemic, an iron infusion/injection or blood transfusion may be recommended. Vitamin C aids the absorption of iron, so you should take a vitamin C supplement and eat foods with plenty of iron in them, such as red meat and green vegetables.

Medical treatments for heavy menstrual bleeding can be divided into non-hormonal and hormonal options.

Non-hormonal treatments

Tranexamic acid

These tablets, which affect the way the blood clots, can be taken during bleeding to reduce the amount of blood lost. They reduce the flow by 40–50 per cent and need to be taken on the first day of bleeding. They need to be taken during every period to be effective and as many as eight tablets a day may be needed. If you have a history of stroke or clots in the family, this medication could cause problems, so be sure to mention it to your doctor.

Non-steroidal anti-inflammatory drugs (NSAIDs)

These include ibuprofen, mefenamic acid, indomethacin and diclofenac, and can be taken as tablets during bleeding. Most of them are available without prescription from the chemist, and sometimes in supermarkets. They can reduce the period flow by about a third and help with pain, but they do not change the pattern of periods. Some women experience side effects, such as an upset stomach, nausea and diarrhoea.

Hormonal treatments

IUS contraceptive device

This device, inserted into the uterus (see chapter 16), slowly releases pro-gestogen (a drug that acts like the hormone progesterone) into the lining of the uterus. It is the most effective medical treatment for heavy menstrual bleeding. The device can stay in for up to five years.

Although some progestogen is absorbed into the body, it is much less than occurs when hormone tablets are taken for heavy menstrual bleeding. It may also reduce or prevent endometrial hyperplasia.

The pros and cons of an IUS for heavy menstrual bleeding

Benefits	Disadvantages
• Reduces menstrual blood loss dramatically (by about 90 per cent) after at least three months' use • May reduce period pain • Provides reliable contraception • Daily tablets not needed • Reversible	• Commonly causes irregular bleeding or spotting, at least in the initial months of use • 20 per cent require removal because of side effects or persistent irregular spotting • May cause acne, mood changes and breast soreness • Uterine perforation can occur during insertion (but is very rare) • Not suitable if the uterus is an irregular shape, usually due to fibroids • Not suitable if the uterus is too large

Combined hormonal contraceptives

These can either be taken as the oral contraceptive pill (the Pill) or inserted as a vaginal ring.

The pros and cons of combined hormonal contraceptives for heavy menstrual bleeding

Benefits	Disadvantages
• Reduces menstrual blood loss by about 40 per cent • May reduce period pain • Helps regulate periods • Can be taken continuously to skip monthly period • Reduces the risk of ovarian and endometrial cancer by around 50 per cent	• May cause nausea, breast tenderness, headaches and changes in libido • Unsuitable for some women, such as those with a history of blood clots in the veins or smokers over the age of 30 • Requires long-term use • May cause irregular spotting

The progesterone-only pill (POP)

The minipill significantly reduces menstrual blood loss.

The pros and cons of the minipill for heavy menstrual bleeding

Benefits	Disadvantages
• Reduces menstrual blood loss by up to 87 per cent • Fast-acting and often used as short-term treatment, or with an episode of particularly heavy bleeding	• May cause bloating, mood swings and breast tenderness • May cause irregular bleeding

Medication to stop periods completely

This medication (danazol) stops the normal ovulation cycle and reduces oestrogen levels, in some women to such an extent that they stop menstruating completely. It is rarely used any more for more than a few months because it usually causes side effects such as weight gain, hot flushes and acne. It is often used for weeks to months before an operation to treat heavy bleeding.

Surgical and other treatments

Endometrial ablation

This procedure destroys the lining of the uterus. It is performed using an instrument called a hysteroscope, which is inserted into the uterus through the vagina and cervix. The ablation is performed using various methods, including heat or microwave energy. This procedure can be done under local anaesthetic, but in Australia it is still usually performed under a general anaesthetic.

Since this treatment destroys the lining of the uterus, women should have completed their family before choosing this option. Rarely, a pregnancy can still take place after endometrial ablation, but as this would invariably result in serious complications, women having this procedure will often have a tubal ligation at the same time, or consider some other permanent form of contraception.

The pros and cons of endometrial ablation for heavy menstrual bleeding

Benefits	Disadvantages
• Is a safe surgical treatment • Usually only requires a one-day hospital stay • Allows return to full activities within a few days • Reduces heavy bleeding excellently (90 per cent of women have a significant improvement and 50–80 per cent no further bleeding at all) • Does not affect hormones or pelvic anatomy • Can also remove fibroids or polyps on the inside of the uterus	• Heavy bleeding may recur in some women • May not improve pain, especially with adenomyosis • Can have major complications such as uterine perforation, bowel damage or infection (but rarely, in only one in 1000 procedures) • May be difficult to investigate future problems in the uterus, especially during and after menopause

Myomectomy
In this surgical treatment for uterine fibroids the fibroids are removed but the uterus and ovaries remain.

The pros and cons of myomectomy for heavy menstrual bleeding

Benefits	Disadvantages
• Reduces heavy menstrual bleeding • Is currently the best treatment for women who wish to remain fertile • Submucosal uterine fibroids can be removed via the vagina using a hysteroscope • May improve other symptoms caused by fibroids, such as pressure symptoms	• Has small risk of requirement for a blood transfusion or, rarely, an emergency hysterectomy • New fibroids may appear

Uterine artery embolisation

This treatment for uterine fibroids works by destroying the blood flow to the fibroid, and is performed by an interventional radiologist in consultation with a gynaecologist.

The pros and cons of uterine artery embolisation for heavy menstrual bleeding

Benefits	Disadvantages
• Usually only requires a one-day hospital stay • Reduces heavy bleeding by 60 to 90 per cent and reduces fibroid volume by 30–46 per cent	• Can be painful for some women • New fibroids may appear and heavy bleeding may recur • About 25 per cent of women need another procedure for their symptoms at a later date • May not improve pain • Can have major complications such as infection (rarely, in only one in 1000 procedures) • Is not readily available at most hospitals • May affect the ovaries and reduce fertility

MRI-guided focused ultrasound (MRgFUS)

This relatively new, non-invasive method for treating uterine fibroids uses an MRI scanner to deliver a focused, high-intensity ultrasound beam to the fibroid, heating it and causing it to shrink (though not entirely disappear).

The pros and cons of MRI-guided focused ultrasound for heavy menstrual bleeding

Benefits	Disadvantages
• Fast recovery time allows women to go home the same day • Has fewer complications than surgery	• Is not suitable for fibroids larger than 10 cm, or too close to surrounding tissues • Is not readily available at most hospitals and rarely available in the private sector • Its long-term effectiveness and safety are not yet known, including safety for future pregnancies

Hysterectomy

Hysterectomy is the removal of the uterus and may or may not include removal of the ovaries. The operation can be done in one of four ways:

1. Abdominal hysterectomy – where the uterus is removed through a cut in the abdomen.
2. Vaginal hysterectomy – where the uterus is removed through the vagina.
3. Total laparoscopic hysterectomy – where the uterus is also removed through the vagina, but the surgeon makes small cuts in the abdomen to do part of the operation.
4. Subtotal hysterectomy – where the cervix is left in place.

The type of hysterectomy a woman has depends on a range of factors, including the nature of her problem, her medical history and her preference.

The pros and cons of hysterectomy for heavy menstrual bleeding

Benefits	Disadvantages
• Is the only guaranteed way to stop menstrual bleeding • May also improve pain • Most women are highly satisfied with the procedure • Reduces the risk of uterine and of ovarian cancer (even when ovaries are retained)	• Is a major surgical procedure with potential complications and a recovery time of two to six weeks, depending on the type of hysterectomy and other factors • Results in the permanent loss of fertility • May lead to earlier menopause, even when ovaries are retained, by about a year (although this still happens gradually, not suddenly) • May increase the risk of prolapse in some women

16

Contraception

Neelam Bhardwaj, Siobhan Bourke,
Geraldine Edgley, Alexandra Marceglia

Contraception is used to protect women from an unwanted pregnancy, or, to put it another way, to allow baby-free sex. You can also use some types of contraception, such as condoms, to protect yourself from sexually transmitted infections (STIs). This is a good thing to do any time you have a new partner or multiple partners, or when you don't know if your partner has an infection.

We often need to use different forms of contraception at different times or stages of our lives, and it is important to work out which is the right contraception for you. If you are at an age where you can fall pregnant and want baby-free sex, you need to choose a method of contraception you feel comfortable with, that suits your lifestyle and that you will use reliably and honestly.

To understand how various contraceptives work, we must first understand the menstrual cycle. Each month a cascade of events occur that lead to the rise and fall of hormone levels, helping to prepare the body for a potential pregnancy each month. Your cycle is counted from the first day of a period to the start of the next period. This interval can vary between cycles in each individual – the usual range is 26–32 days.

There are several methods of contraception available in Australia, ranging from daily contraceptive options to long-term reversible options and permanent methods. Different contraceptives act at different points in the ovulation and fertilisation process, from the time the egg is released through the time the egg is fertilised by the sperm to the time the fertilised egg is ready to implant in the uterus. Each method has its positives and side effects, and some are more reliable than others.

Choose the one that suits you. Take control and be prepared.

Methods of contraception

The types of contraception are divided into the following categories: long-acting reversible contraception (LARC), hormonal contraception, barrier contraception, permanent contraception and natural contraception.

Long-acting reversible contraception (LARC)

LARC includes the etonogestrel rod (Implanon), copper intrauterine devices (IUD), and another form of IUD, the Mirena intrauterine system (IUS). These devices are all long-acting, and can stay in place for three, five or 10 years, depending upon which one you choose. You need to attend a clinic or outpatient hospital to have a doctor trained in their use to put them in, but once you have them placed, you do not need to do anything (apart from having a check-up) to make them work.

LARC is great because it offers several years of hassle-free contraception. It doesn't, however, protect you from STIs. If you change partners, have different partners or have any doubts about your partner and STIs, always use a condom.

The etonogestrel rod

Implanon is a small rod of inert plastic and hormone that goes under the skin in the upper arm. It stays for up to three years and has a failure rate of one pregnancy per 1000 insertions per year. This means if 1000 women use this contraception for one year, then one woman will become pregnant. It works mainly by interfering with ovulation. It also changes the mucus in the cervix so sperm cannot enter the uterus, and changes fallopian tube function. If you don't like it or you don't want it any more, it can easily be removed. Implanon is a good contraceptive to use if you tend to forget to take pills, if you are breastfeeding or if you cannot tolerate oestrogen for any reason.

The IUS

The Mirena IUS is a small plastic and hormone device shaped like the letter T that is placed in the uterus and stays there for around five years. It prevents pregnancy by changing the mucus in the cervix, changing the way the fallopian tubes work and making the endometrium (lining of the uterus) very thin. It has a failure rate of two pregnancies per 1000 users per year.

The Mirena will change periods, generally making them lighter. Sometimes the period may be so light it appears to have stopped. This does not mean that the IUS user is menopausal, but rather that the endometrium is not growing. This change usually happens slowly, over six to 12 months.

The Mirena can be used by women of any age, and is also safe during breastfeeding. It can be used by anyone who cannot tolerate medicine containing oestrogen. Once it is inserted, the Mirena can stay for up to five years and, depending on age, sometimes longer (towards menopause the Mirena and copper IUDs can be left in longer, because the natural decline in fertility compensates for any small reduction in the efficacy of the IUS or IUD). If you don't like the Mirena, or you want to get pregnant, it can easily be removed by your doctor.

The IUD

A copper IUD is much like a Mirena. In Australia there are three types: two of which are T-shaped and can last 10 and five years respectively; and one of which has a stem with copper wire wrapped around it and can last five years. There are no hormones in a copper IUD and you still will get your period every month. They work by causing changes in the endometrium and preventing the egg and sperm meeting. They also alter the function of the fallopian tube. Typically the failure rate is eight pregnancies per 1000 insertions per year. Copper IUDs may cause heavier and more painful periods for some women; if you already experience these things, this contraceptive may not be for you.

It is important to avoid the risk of STIs; if you have an STI when you have an IUS/IUD, it could lead to an infection in the pelvis called pelvic inflammatory disease. For this reason, an infection screen will usually be performed before an IUS or IUD is inserted.

Copper IUDs can be used by most women. They can be used after a pregnancy and also by women who cannot tolerate oestrogen. Age is no barrier to using a copper IUD, although if you have not had a baby you may experience more period pain with one of these devices. Once they are inserted by a specialising doctor, apart from check-ups, no other action is required. If you want your IUD removed for any reason, your doctor can do it easily.

Hormonal contraception

Hormonal contraception includes the combined oral contraceptive pill, the vaginal ring, the progesterone-only pill and depot medroxyprogesterone acetate injections. None of them protects against STIs.

The Pill

The combined oral contraceptive (the Pill) is a tablet you take every day. If you don't take it every day, it doesn't work. There are two hormones in the Pill: oestrogen and progesterone. Generally these are synthetic hormones (not exactly like your hormones but working like your hormones), but there are now pills that contain exactly the same hormones women make.

The Pill works by blocking ovulation. It has a typical failure rate of about nine pregnancies per 100 users per year but this can be higher in certain groups; the typical failure rate in teenagers, for example, is 15 pregnancies per 100 users per year. It is good for cycle control and managing other gynaecological problems such as dysmenorrhoea (painful periods), menorrhagia (heavy periods) and other health problems such as acne. Some women experience headaches, bloating, sore breasts or mood changes. There are lots of different pills, however, and usually your doctor will be able to find the right one for you.

Some women cannot take the Pill. They might have had a blood clot in their leg (deep vein thrombosis), have high blood pressure or have other health problems. Women who suffer from migraines are strongly advised to consult their doctor before taking the Pill, as the Pill can slightly increase the risk of stroke for women who suffer from particular types of migraine. One of the more common reasons for needing to stop taking the Pill is being a smoker over the age of 35. Smoking increases the risks of cardiovascular disease, this risk increases with age, and oestrogens worsen the effects. Make sure you talk about all your health issues with the doctor or nurse who is prescribing your Pill, so you can make an informed decision that is right for you.

The Pill has to be taken every day, and if you forget one there are special rules to manage this. Make sure you always have condoms handy so that you can have protected sex if you ever forget your Pill or you need to guard against STIs.

The vaginal ring

The vaginal ring (NuvaRing) is like the Pill, with the same types of hormones, but it is inserted into the vagina for three weeks and then removed for one week to allow a bleed to occur. A new ring is then inserted. The advantage of the ring is that you don't need to take a pill every day. If the ring is inserted high into the vagina, you should not be able to feel it. The failure rate for the vaginal ring is the same as for the combined oral pill – about nine pregnancies per 100 users per year.

The progesterone-only pill (POP)

The POP is a daily pill, also called the minipill, which has to be taken at almost exactly the same time every day (within three hours). It works by changing the mucus in the cervix, changing the function of the fallopian tube and, for a small percentage of women, disrupting ovulation. It has a typical failure rate of about nine pregnancies per 100 users per year. It can be used by women who are breastfeeding or who cannot take oestrogen for any reason. Most women will have their period on this pill and it doesn't give cycle control. Side effects might include spotting and mood changes.

Depot medroxyprogesterone acetate (DMPA)

DMPA is used infrequently nowadays. It is an injection usually given by your doctor or a practice nurse every 12 weeks (the trade names are Depo Provera and Depo-Ralovera). It consists of one hormone only, progesterone, and is the same dose for everyone. It is safe during breastfeeding and for women who cannot take oestrogen for any reason. It works by disrupting ovulation, altering fallopian tube function and changing the mucus in the cervix. The failure rate is about six pregnancies per 100 users per year, and this is often due to being late for the next injection.

Side effects include a change in periods – most women will have no period after 12 months of use. Some women will experience headaches and possibly acne and bloating.

DMPA may take a while to wear off when you stop taking it, which makes it difficult for women who experience side effects. It can take between three and 18 months for cycles to return to normal, six to nine months on average. For this reason it is best not to use DMPA for short-term contraception if you are planning a pregnancy within the next year.

Barrier contraception

Barrier contraception doesn't only protect you from pregnancy; some also give protection from STIs. Examples of barrier contraception include the male and female condom (the female condom is called a 'femidon'), diaphragms and cervical caps, which are designed to go in the vagina and provide a physical barrier between the sperm and the cervix. They all need to be used in the correct way in order to work, and diaphragms and cervical caps need to be fitted to the individual as there are different sizes. Diaphragms and caps do not protect from STIs as condoms do.

Barrier contraception may work as much as 97 per cent of the time, but in general it is around 85 per cent effective; that is, 15 women per 100 users will become pregnant using these forms of contraception.

The good things about condoms are that they are widely available (and at some places free), relatively cheap and easy to use. You can always have some on hand for when you require them. They do need to be used with a water-based lubricant (to help stop breakages).

Diaphragms, condoms and the other barrier contraceptives do not contain hormones and are therefore appealing if you have problems with hormone contraception. Anyone can use them, and there are latex-free ones if you have a latex allergy. Should a condom break or you have some other problem with your barrier contraception, then there is the option of emergency contraception.

Emergency contraception

Emergency contraception or the 'morning-after pill' is available in Australia; it is known as Levonelle-1, Levonelle-2, NorLevo, NorLevo-1, Postinor-1 and Postinor-2. It consists of high-dose levonorgestrel that is taken within 72 hours of unprotected sex (such as if your condom broke). You can buy the morning-after pill direct from any pharmacy, or you can attend your local doctor and get a prescription for it. It has minimal side effects; you might have a change in your period, either the amount of bleeding or when you bleed. You should do a pregnancy test two to three weeks after taking the tablets, as it is 85 per cent effective. The morning-after pill is *not* the RU486 'abortion pill'.

A copper IUD may also be used as emergency contraception up to five days from the time you had sex. It is important that you are not at risk of STIs, as if you have an STI when an IUD is inserted this could lead to an infection in the pelvis (pelvic inflammatory disease).

Permanent contraception

Permanent contraception is basically an irreversible operation available for women and men. Even though these operations provide contraception that lasts for the rest of your life, they have a small failure rate.

For women there are several operations available, but the two that are more widely available are an operation through the abdomen to block the fallopian tubes (laparoscopic sterilisation) or an operation through the vagina to block the beginning of the fallopian tubes in the uterus (hysteroscopic sterilisation or tubal occlusion).

Because laparoscopic sterilisation is an intra-abdominal procedure, it requires a general anaesthetic, and because of this it has a slightly higher risk, as with any procedure that involves operating on the abdomen. Most commonly two titanium clips are placed over the fallopian tubes and clipped on tight. Although a reversal procedure is offered by some hospitals, the reversal is a major operation that is generally, but not always, successful. This procedure should be considered permanent and irreversible and other methods of contraception used if there is any question that you might change your mind. It takes a few days to recover from this operation, and your periods and cycles should be normal after this. The failure rate is typically five pregnancies per 1000 operations but may increase with time.

Essure is a hysteroscopic sterilisation method where a small insert is placed inside each fallopian tube by going up through the cervix and inside the uterus. This insert eventually blocks the tube. The operation may be done under general or local anaesthetic. It is also permanent and irreversible, and takes three months to be fully effective, so another form of contraception must be used to prevent pregnancy during this time. You will need an X-ray of your pelvis or a gynaecological ultrasound after three months to ensure that the inserts are in the correct place. These are newer procedures, and the failure rate for Essure is two pregnancies per 1000 operations per year.

For a man the operation is called a vasectomy. This is a small procedure where a surgeon cuts and seals the ends of each vas deferens, the small tubule that carries the sperm from the testicles to the penis. This operation is a basic procedure and can be done under either local or general anaesthetic. It has few side effects, but can cause localised bruising and pain around the wound site that will usually go in one or two days. It will take three months to be properly effective, and another form of contraception must be used to prevent pregnancy during this time. A lot of men are worried that a vasectomy will affect their sexual function, but this is not the case, because although the vas deferens is important for fertility, it is not involved in the sexual function of the penis. The failure rate is 1.5 pregnancies per 1000 operations per year.

Before you decide to proceed with any kind of sterilisation, it is very important to consider if you would want another baby in your lifetime. People's social and financial situations often change in unexpected ways, so you must be absolutely sure that you want no more children, under any circumstances, if you choose these methods. There is no way to attempt to reverse a hysteroscopic sterilisation. Attempted reversal of a tubal sterilisation or vasectomy is a very complicated procedure and does not always work.

To access sterilisation, you will need a referral from your local doctor to an appropriate surgeon. Costs and waiting times vary depending upon where you choose to go.

Natural contraception

Natural contraception involves three different methods: withdrawal, natural family planning (NFP) and lactational amenorrhoea.

The first is withdrawal, or coitus interruptus. This is where the man pulls his penis out of the vagina during sex, before he ejaculates. This method is typically 78 per cent effective on each occasion it is used. There may be a small amount of semen in the pre-ejaculate (the lubricant a man makes when he has an erection), and this may be enough to achieve a pregnancy. It is also possible to become pregnant if a man ejaculates on the vulva or at the opening of the vagina. He must make sure to ejaculate well clear of the vaginal opening.

The second method is called natural family planning (NFP) or periodic abstinence, and involves charting your cycle using, for example, temperature charts (a woman's core temperature goes up after ovulation) and counting the days to determine when the safe times are. The Billings variation or the mucus method, teaches you to recognise the different feeling of wetness at the vulva at different times in the cycle. Mucus changes in colour, consistency and volume with hormone changes. These methods require you to learn about your cycle and to keep charts. To work as a contraceptive, these methods also require days of abstinence (no sex).

If you can use these NFP methods effectively, you can achieve a protection rate of 97 per cent, meaning only three women per 100 uses would become pregnant. It is important to know, however, that to achieve this rate you must be absolutely sure to follow the rules. The typical efficacy rate is 76 per cent. These methods can also teach a couple to identify the best time in a cycle to achieve a pregnancy. It is generally better to use them if you don't mind becoming accidentally pregnant.

The third method of natural contraception is the lactational amenorrhoea method and takes advantage of the time after having a baby when a woman doesn't get her period because she is breastfeeding. It is a safe, effective and temporary method that offers up to 98 per cent protection if the baby is exclusively breastfed, and if you have not had your first post-delivery period. It is effective until the baby is six months old or when supplementary feeds are used, whichever comes first. Once your periods return or the baby starts to take anything other than breast milk

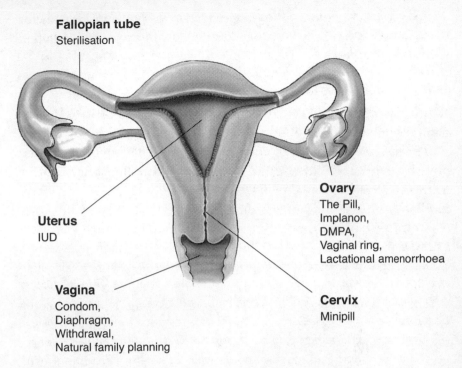

Fallopian tube
Sterilisation

Ovary
The Pill,
Implanon,
DMPA,
Vaginal ring,
Lactational amenorrhoea

Uterus
IUD

Vagina
Condom,
Diaphragm,
Withdrawal,
Natural family planning

Cervix
Minipill

Main site of action of contraceptive methods

from the breast, breastfeeding cannot be trusted to provide contraception. After this time, another form of contraception will need to be used.

Anne, a 17-year-old student, attended her GP after a pregnancy scare when her period came late. She and her boyfriend of three months had been using condoms to avoid pregnancy, but there had been the occasional episode where Anne had needed the emergency pill. When her last period did not come at the expected time, she was very worried about being pregnant and realised she was not ready to become a mother.

Her doctor discussed other methods of contraception – including the Pill; the three-year implant, Implanon; and intrauterine devices, including Mirena – as well as continuing to use condoms to prevent infections. Even though she was on the third day of her period, she had a pregnancy test (which was negative) and gave urine for a sexually transmitted infection (STI) screen.

As Anne thought it very important that she didn't get pregnant and she was not sure she could be reliable about taking a pill every day, she chose to use the etonogestrel rod for her contraception. She understood that she probably would not have a regular monthly bleed, but that her bleeding would be more unpredictable and that this was not harmful.

A few days later her GP contacted her with the results of the STI screen. All her tests were negative for infection but it was still important that Anne continued to use condoms until her partner was also tested, and with any new partner, as her negative test results did not protect her from catching infections in the future.

At Anne's review three months later, she was happy with the implant as she did not have to remember to do anything. She was bleeding for three or four days in the month and she found this acceptable. She had not noticed any side effects apart from a bruise at the site of the insertion of the implant that took about two weeks to settle. Her boyfriend had had an STI check and they had stopped using condoms.

At the age of 20, Anne returned to her GP to have her implant replaced as it was nearing the end of its three-year life. She had been happy with the protection from pregnancy that the implant offered. She had been in a new relationship for six months and thought it could be a long-term relationship. She had seen her GP three months earlier for an STI screen and Pap test when she was considering stopping using condoms.

Three years later Anne returned to have her implant removed as she was ready to try for her first pregnancy. Her doctor gave her the advice that, for most women, their fertility returns very quickly once the implant is removed, and some women even become pregnant before their first period. Anne was also given pre-pregnancy advice.

Anne returned to her GP to discuss contraception when her third child was 12 months old. She had been using condoms and was happy with this method when she was timing her pregnancies, but now it had become important not to get pregnant again. Anne didn't feel ready for a fourth child and wanted a reliable form of contraception, although she and her partner were not ready for permanent contraception. Anne had been happy with the implant in the past and was interested in it again. Her GP discussed the implant and IUDs with her. This time Anne decided to use the hormone IUS as it lasts for at least five years and leads to very light monthly bleeding. It also has the advantage of not requiring daily action.

After an infection check, her IUS was inserted at a family planning clinic as her GP did not insert IUDs. At her review six weeks after insertion, Anne was happy with her chosen method of contraception.

Contraception myths

There are many myths around contraception; some have a basis in the truth, while others are simply incorrect. Many are historical, derived from old types of contraception that are no longer used. It is important to use any method of contraception correctly, so seek advice from your doctor.

1 I can't take the Pill because ...

- **it makes you fat**. There is no evidence that the Pill makes you put on weight. You may retain a little fluid, like the feeling just before your period, but if this is a problem there are some Pill types that can help.

- **it gives you pimples**. When taking hormones some women may experience pimples or oily skin, while others may notice an improvement in these conditions. It depends on the individual. Some pills may help improve skin, but the improvement may take months.

- **it will make me moody**. The Pill can have an effect on mood and also decrease sex drive. It may be worth changing the type of Pill if this happens to you. Talk to your doctor before simply stopping the Pill, as pregnancy can affect your mood too.

- **it will change my periods**. This can be a good thing. The Pill can reduce the amount of blood loss during a period, and cramping and other premenstrual symptoms. Some women take the Pill for these very reasons.

- **it will make me infertile if I take it for too long**. When you stop taking the Pill your fertility returns to normal very quickly. If there are underlying problems with your fertility, the Pill will neither harm nor help this.

- **you need to take a break every year or so**. There is no medical reason to take a break from the Pill. When the Pill was originally made, the oestrogen (one of the hormones in the Pill) dose was three to four times higher than it is now. Women often felt nauseous on the Pill and were told to take a break every so often. Nausea is hardly ever experienced now by women who take the Pill; the most common thing that occurs when women take a break from the Pill is they get pregnant, which can also cause nausea. Don't forget that being pregnant when you don't want to be can also be risky to your health, whether you choose to continue with the pregnancy or not. You may have a medical condition that needs to be under control before you become pregnant, or you may be on medication that needs to be changed before you become pregnant.

- **it doesn't suit me**. This may be true, but if you have only tried one type of Pill there are others that might suit you. Instead of taking contraception orally (by mouth), there are other ways to deliver the hormones – for example, directly into the uterus through the Mirena IUS, directly into the vagina through the vaginal ring, or via an implant under the skin as with Implanon. Other forms of contraception have no hormones: copper IUDs, permanent contraception and barrier methods (see above). It is worth talking to your doctor about different methods of contraception that might suit you better.

- **I can still get pregnant**. Most contraception methods have a failure rate. If you take the Pill every day as directed, the likelihood of becoming pregnant is very low, less than 1 per cent.

2 If I have sex ...

- **for the first time I can't get pregnant**. If you are menstruating (getting periods), you can get pregnant the first time you have sex. It is possible you have produced an egg, and if the sperm fertilises the egg you can get pregnant.

- **during my period I can't get pregnant**. Some women ovulate (produce an egg) early in their cycle, very soon after their period finishes, and some sperm can live for several days. So if you have sex during your period and sperm is still there when an egg is produced, you can get pregnant. If, however, you are taking the Pill and you take it every day, it is just as safe to have sex when bleeding as not. It is best to take the Pill every day.

- **after missing one pill I will get pregnant**. It depends which pill you missed. Generally speaking, missing one pill in the middle of the pack is okay, but if you miss a pill near the sugar pills (the non-hormonal pills when you have your period), then the lower level of hormone created by this missed pill and the following sugar pills could mean you ovulate (produce an egg). Then it is possible to get pregnant. The best advice is not to miss pills; if you do, use condoms for extra protection until you have had seven more hormonal pills, and remember you can take emergency contraception up to 72 hours after unprotected sex (it is actually effective up to 96 hours after sex, but its effectiveness is decreased). It is better to be safe than sorry.

- **when taking the Pill I won't get a sexually transmitted infection (STI)**. The Pill protects against pregnancy, but it does not protect against STIs; condoms need to be used for that.

- **I can only take the morning-after pill the morning after unprotected sex**. You can take the morning-after pill (or emergency contraception) up to 72 hours after having unprotected sex. And you can buy it, without prescription, in most pharmacies around Australia. There is no age limit for getting emergency contraception, but some pharmacies do not like to give it to girls under the age of 16. If you need the morning-after pill and you are under 16, try asking at your local doctor, sexual health clinic or hospital, or take an adult with you to help at the pharmacy.

3 I can't have an IUD because ...

- **they are dangerous**. The IUD or intrauterine device got a bad name in the 1970s, when some IUDs caused problems for women. These IUDs are thankfully not used any more. IUDs that are used now are safe and very effective. They are easily inserted during a small procedure that takes about 15 minutes and can also be removed when no longer needed.

- **I have never had children**. IUDs can generally be used by women who have not had children. They are a very reliable form of contraception but do not prevent sexually transmitted infections (STIs); condoms need to be used to prevent STIs.

4 I can't have an Implanon implant because ...

- **it moves around the body**. When inserted correctly, the Implanon sits just below the skin on the inner surface of the upper arm. A tissue capsule forms around the implant and holds it in place. Removal of the implant is normally a simple procedure.

- **I will just bleed all the time**. Some women experience increased bleeding when using the implant and this is the most common reason for having it removed. This happens in about 23 per cent of cases. The majority of women experience less bleeding than they normally would without a form of contraception. Twenty per cent of women, though, will have no bleeding.

- **having no bleeding is bad for me**. Twenty per cent of women will have no bleeding with the implant. There is no medical reason to have your period every month. In fact, a constant level of hormone from the implant may be protective against some gynaecological cancers. If having no bleeding is unacceptable to you, choose another method of contraception.

17

Pregnancy

Shaun Brennecke, Elisabeth Gasparini, Jane Karpavicius,
Gillian Lang, Orla McNally, Jo Payne, Allison Ridge,
Penelope Sheehan, Margaret Sherburn

Australian birth statistics clearly demonstrate changing trends in birth rates and fertility. The total fertility rate in Australia for 2010 was 1.89 babies per woman, compared to 2.15 babies per woman in 1975. The other most noticeable trend is towards older first-time mothers. Until the end of the last century, women aged 25–29 had the highest fertility rates, followed by women aged 20–24. Since 2000, the highest fertility rates have been among women aged 30–34, with continually declining fertility rates in younger women. Since 2003, the second-highest fertility group has been women aged 35–39, rather than those aged 20–24.

This trend has been observed throughout the developed world. World Health Organization (WHO) data from developing countries clearly demonstrates that when education and status for women improve, fertility rates decrease. There is undoubtedly a link between declining fertility rates and older mothers. In general, fertility peaks between the ages of 20 and 35. Pregnancies after the age of 35 are associated with higher miscarriage rates and higher rates of complications. Warnings about declining fertility have become a staple of the popular press, but it is clear that in today's society, women are having babies later, after they have met their education, training, career and social goals.

Declining overall fertility has meant that women tend to place higher expectations on themselves during pregnancy, and also in many cases to have higher expectations of the pregnancy experience. Having a baby profoundly affects women, their family and their work. It is a shame when unmet expectations add a further burden. Evidence continues to emerge that factors affecting the health of the mother also affect the health of the baby, not only during the pregnancy but also possibly later in life.

Before you are pregnant

A visit to the doctor before pregnancy is absolutely essential if you have a medical condition such as hypertension (high blood pressure) or diabetes, but it is also a good idea for healthy women. At this visit, the doctor should check your immunity to illnesses that can be harmful to pregnancy, such as rubella (German measles), varicella (chickenpox) and hepatitis B. If you don't have enough immunity to any of these, you will need booster vaccinations for rubella and varicella at least 28 days before you plan to conceive. The rubella vaccine is a live vaccine and cannot be administered during pregnancy (though it can be given after delivery and is perfectly safe while breastfeeding). The risks of rubella infection for the developing baby during a pregnancy include developmental delay, congenital cataracts (blindness), enlarged liver or spleen, or death. If you are diagnosed with congenital rubella before 16 weeks gestation, your doctor may offer you the option of a termination of the pregnancy. The most dangerous time to acquire rubella is before 11 weeks gestation, which may be before you know you're pregnant. This is why if you are planning to become pregnant, it's important to ensure all your vaccinations are up to date.

Another vaccination that could be considered is a pertussis (whooping cough) booster (usually combined with diphtheria and tetanus as DTP), as whooping cough is a known cause of neonatal deaths.

A pre-pregnancy check should include a discussion of your dietary history and nutritional status. Significantly underweight women are at risk of preterm delivery and restricted growth in their baby, while obese women are at increased risk of a range of pregnancy complications including miscarriage, fetal abnormalities such as spina bifida, and hypertension (high blood pressure) and the related disorder that is unique to pregnancy, pre-eclampsia. Obese women are also at risk of complications of labour and delivery, including a higher likelihood of induced labour as a result of the pregnancy continuing past the expected due date, and a higher likelihood of a caesarean due to failed progress of labour. Markedly increased in obese women, these complications are also slightly increased in overweight women. It seems that the healthy weight range really is the ideal around the time of conception.

You should focus on eating a fresh, varied and healthy diet. Be aware that supplementing with 500 micrograms of folate daily (and possibly higher doses in overweight women) from about three months before conception has been shown to decrease the rates of fetal malformations of the spinal cord known as spina bifida. It is also recommended that women who are pregnant, breastfeeding or considering a pregnancy should take an iodine supplement of 150 micrograms per day (see chapter 32 for information on the thyroid in pregnancy). There are no proven benefits for taking any other vitamins or minerals, although iron, zinc, vitamin D and calcium are all essential nutrients and you should take supplements if there is any possibility you are deficient. Some vitamins are harmful to pregnancy when taken in high doses, such as vitamin A, so only take supplements designated as safe for pregnancy.

Some foods can also be a source of infections that can cause problems in pregnancy, such as listeriosis. Even before you become pregnant, it is a good idea to start the habit of avoiding foods with high listeria risks such as raw seafood, foods that have been left at room temperature for a length of time, delicatessen meats, leftovers, soft cheeses and pate.

Stress is often a cause of considerable concern and regret in pregnancy. A lot of women are concerned about the effect of stressful events on their pregnancy. Stress is a normal part of life but there is some evidence that significant and prolonged stress can have a harmful effect on a pregnancy due to the mother's stress hormones, which may be able to cross the placenta. Pregnancy is often a stressful event involving financial stress and career changes. Almost everybody can derive some benefit from common stress management techniques such as regular sleep, yoga and meditation. If you are experiencing more significant stress, counselling and cognitive behaviour techniques can be helpful.

Pregnancy carries a significant physical burden, with increased demands on the heart and kidneys as well as bones and muscles. Try to improve your physical fitness before pregnancy with both aerobic and weight-bearing exercise, as it will help your body to cope with the pregnancy. If you have not been exercising regularly before pregnancy, start with gentle exercise such as brisk walking or swimming. If you have an active exercise program you should be able to continue to exercise through pregnancy, with a few restrictions such as observing heart rate limits, paying careful attention to body temperature and hydration, and limiting aerobic training to low-impact exercise. Your level of athletic performance will decrease during pregnancy, but you may be able to maintain some of your previous level of fitness.

You should also visit the dentist before you become pregnant, and have any dental cavities treated. This helps to avoid transferring decay-causing bacteria to your baby (see below for more on this).

Don't forget to also speak with your health insurance company to let them know you are pregnant and the date the baby is due. You should make sure your baby is included on your health policy before they are born in case they require any special care immediately after birth.

Knowing you are pregnant

Most women recognise that they are pregnant when they miss a period. Occasionally women may continue to have bleeding at the time their period would be due, although this would usually be lighter than a regular period. You can easily confirm your pregnancy with a home pregnancy test on a urine sample. These tests have become very accurate. After a positive pregnancy test, visit your doctor to confirm the pregnancy and for referral to a pregnancy care provider.

A range of options for maternity care is available. A very fundamental choice is between the public and private system, a choice that is usually dictated by financial and insurance considerations. Private obstetric care means that both antenatal care and care throughout labour and delivery will be provided by either a single obstetrician or, more commonly, a small group of obstetricians. Antenatal visits would usually be at the obstetrician's rooms and the birth would take place at a private hospital where the obstetrician has admitting rights. Usually the choice of hospital is a shared decision between you and your obstetrician. If you would like to give birth at a particular hospital, perhaps because of location, private hospitals can provide lists of obstetricians with admitting rights.

Within the public system there are also different models of care. If you have medical problems potentially complicating your pregnancy, you will need to receive your care mostly from an obstetrician, but if you are otherwise at low risk of complications, antenatal care can be safely provided by your GP or by midwives either at the hospital, in the community, or within a one-to-one midwifery program. Antenatal care conducted by GPs or midwives outside of the maternity hospital is referred to as shared care. Typically there is a standard schedule of visits divided between the hospital and the shared care provider. Results of tests performed at the hospital will be sent to the shared care provider. You would be given a maternity record where findings related to each visit are recorded, and this forms a means of communication between the hospital and the shared care provider.

Antenatal care

In general, you can expect to have at least 10 antenatal visits during the course of a pregnancy. You should be given information regarding the scheduling of visits at the start of your pregnancy, but the schedule should still be flexible enough to accommodate your needs with extra visits available if necessary.

Traditionally, pregnancy has been divided into three 13-week periods, known as trimesters.

First trimester

A surprisingly high number of early pregnancies end in miscarriages. During the first visits, the aim of maternity care is to confirm that a pregnancy is continuing. This is usually established by an early ultrasound demonstrating the presence of a fetal heartbeat from six weeks gestation. An early ultrasound can also be helpful in establishing correct dates. An expected due date is calculated as 40 weeks from the time of the last menstrual period. Some women find it odd that due to this convention the first two weeks of a pregnancy include the time before ovulation. The reason for this is that the period forms a more obvious marker than ovulation, the signs of which can be subtle. Even the use of the last menstrual period has been found to be less accurate than an early ultrasound, however. In the early stages of a pregnancy, individual differences in growth have not had time to have an effect, so a pregnancy can be accurately dated based on the length of the embryo from the tip of its head to the end of its bottom. This is called the crown–rump length. After the first trimester, this measurement is too difficult to perform, so later measurements include the head circumference, the abdominal circumference and the length of the thigh. The later the measurements are performed, the less useful they are to determine pregnancy dates because of the influence of individual growth variation.

Your GP should identify any risks in the pregnancy to your wellbeing or that of your baby. If there are any potential problems, you should be referred to obstetric care with some urgency; otherwise, visits to obstetric care will commence later in the first trimester. In the public system, if no risk factors are identified, obstetric care may commence early in the second trimester.

Recommended first-trimester tests

A number of tests are recommended for every pregnant woman, as detailed below.

Full blood examination

This blood test can not only indicate anaemia, but also diagnose the reason for the anaemia. Low haemoglobin (the oxygen-carrying pigment in red blood cells) and small red blood cells may be due to iron deficiency. A follow-up test for iron stores may be required. Normal haemoglobin but small red blood cells may suggest thalassaemia, especially if you or your family are from an area where thalassaemia is known to be common, such as the Mediterranean countries or South-East Asia.

Women with thalassaemia produce a different type of haemoglobin that doesn't last as long as the usual kind, so they constantly have to replace their red blood cells. It is important for pregnant women with thalassaemia to be diagnosed for two reasons. First, women with thalas-saemia require extra folate supplementation during pregnancy to help them produce all the extra red blood cells required to keep up with the demands of pregnancy. The other issue involves their partner. If both parents have forms of thalassaemia, the baby can be severely affected. Rarely, this can result in a fatal form in which the baby makes no func-tioning haemoglobin at all; less severe forms mean that the baby may be dependent on regular blood transfusions throughout its life. If there is a risk of these severe forms of thalassaemia it is important that parents be properly counselled about available antenatal testing. There are a number of different types of thalassaemia and not all have consequences for the baby. If you have one of the more severe forms, your partner should also be tested.

Blood group and antibody screen

Red blood cells have marker proteins on their outer membranes. The types of marker proteins determine your blood type. This is most crucial for the Rhesus antigen because a Rhesus-negative woman is capable of forming antibodies against the red blood cells of a Rhesus-positive fetus. The mother's antibodies cause the fetus's red blood cells to be destroyed, resulting in anaemia, which may be life-threatening for the fetus. This usually only happens if the woman comes into contact with an amount of Rhesus-positive blood in a so-called 'sensitising event'. Sensitising events can be related to pregnancy, such as a miscarriage or a procedure like an amniocentesis, or may be separate, such as following a blood transfusion. Formation of antibodies is relatively rare. Most Rhesus-negative women safely deliver Rhesus-positive babies without problems.

In order to prevent the formation of antibodies, Rhesus-negative women are given injections at crucial times, such as at miscarriage or after delivery. A preventative program has been in place for some years in Australia, which includes injections at 28 weeks and 34 weeks gestation, even when the pregnancy has been completely normal. The injections can identify Rhesus-positive blood cells in the mother's circulation and coagulate them so the mother has no chance to react to them.

Other red blood cell proteins can cause similar problems, and all of these should be identified in the blood test from the first visit and the 26 week visit:

- **HIV** – in Australia, HIV is very rare in women of reproductive age. It is important that it be diagnosed in those who are HIV-positive, however, because a number of interventions can decrease the transmission of HIV to the fetus. For this reason, HIV screening is recommended for all pregnant women.

- **Hepatitis B** – transmission of hepatitis B to the fetus can be prevented by injections, which should be given at birth.

- **Syphilis** – like HIV, syphilis is relatively rare in the Australian population, but congenital syphilis results in serious developmental problems in the baby and can easily be treated by a course of penicillin during the pregnancy.

- **Rubella immunity** – if you have low levels of or lack rubella immunity, you should avoid potential risks such as young children with an undiagnosed illness accompanied by fever, as congenital rubella has serious consequences for the baby. You should be immunised after the birth.

Midstream urine screen

A midstream urine screen for asymptomatic urinary tract infections has been shown to prevent more serious urinary tract infections, preterm birth and low birth weight. If you have an infection, the test should be repeated after treatment to ensure that the infection has cleared.

Pap test

You should have a Pap test every two years, and this should still be performed during early pregnancy if it is due.

Less common first-trimester tests

Depending on your medical history, your doctor may consider other tests on your first visit.

Hepatitis C

Unlike hepatitis B, screening every woman for hepatitis C has not been recommended because it is not as common, and the same protective strategies are not available. If you have a history of intravenous (IV) drug use or your partner is an IV drug user, you have tattoos, you have been in prison, you have ever received a blood transfusion, or you have migrated from areas with high endemic rates of hepatitis C, you are at higher risk and should be tested.

Ferritin

This is the form in which iron is stored in the body. If you have any history of iron deficiency or risk factors such as a vegan diet, recent pregnancy or miscarriage, your GP might choose to investigate your iron stores immediately rather than screen with the full blood examination as above. Pregnancies require lots of iron, so storage levels well above the minimum are recommended for the start of pregnancy. Ferritin can be falsely elevated by infections so your doctor should take this into account when interpreting the result.

Vitamin D

Extremely low vitamin D levels are rare, but they can occur particularly in veiled, dark-skinned women living in temperate areas. Low vitamin D places the fetus at risk of developing neurological and skeletal disorders, as vitamin D is essential for calcium uptake.

Thalassaemia screen

As noted above, there are a number of risks associated with thalassaemia in pregnancy. If you come from an area where it is common, your doctor may order a screening test without waiting for the results of your full blood examination.

Screening for chromosomal abnormalities

Humans have a set of 46 chromosomes, which contain nearly all their genetic material (as DNA). Sperm and eggs each contain half the normal number of chromosomes, the combination of the two sets of 23 chromosomes, one set from the mother and one set from the father, during conception provides the full set of 46 chromosomes. (Note that there are 37 genes in the mitochondria, which are compartments in the cell that make energy for the body's major organs to work. Mitochondrial DNA is present in eggs but not sperm, so a person's mitochondrial DNA is passed down only from their mother.) Sometimes errors can occur during the conception process, resulting in the fetus having extra chromosomal genetic material, either a whole extra chromosome or part of a chromosome attached to another one. Chromosomes are one case where having more is not a good thing, but not having enough may also cause problems.

The most common chromosomal abnormality is trisomy 21, or Down syndrome, which occurs when there is an extra chromosome number 21. The risk of having a child with a chromosomal abnormality increases as you get older. A woman aged 37 has a one in 200 risk of having a child with Down syndrome and a similar risk of having a child with any chromosomal abnormality compared to a woman aged 28, who has a one in 1000 risk of having a child with Down syndrome. The reason for this is the subject of ongoing speculation. The father's age does not have the same impact.

There are two definitive tests for chromosomal abnormalities, chorionic villus sampling (CVS) and amniocentesis, both of which involve removing some material through a needle introduced into the womb. In CVS this material is developing placental tissue, while in amniocentesis it is amniotic fluid. Because of the invasive nature of these tests, they carry a small risk of miscarriage. The CVS procedure, which takes place around 12–14 weeks gestation, has a slightly higher risk of miscarriage, usually given as one in 100, than amniocentesis, which is performed at any time from 14 weeks gestation onwards and carries a risk of miscarriage usually given as one in 200. These invasive tests are the only way to determine whether a baby definitely has a chromosomal abnormality. Because of the risk of miscarriage, however, they are generally only offered if you have a high risk of chromosomal abnormalities – for example, if you will be aged 37 or over at the time of the baby's expected due date.

A number of non-invasive screening tests have been developed for women who are otherwise low risk but concerned about the possibility of chromosomal abnormality. The three most commonly available screening tests – the first-trimester combined screen, the nuchal translucency test (measurement of the fat pad at the back of the neck by ultrasound) and the second-trimester biochemical screening test – all give a 'high risk' or 'low risk' result rather than a definite yes or no. If a screening test result comes back with a high risk, you would be given further counselling and offered the option of a definitive test with its small risk of miscarriage. Some women choose not to have definitive testing.

Most high-risk pregnancies are actually normal, but if further testing confirms a chromosomal abnormality you may be offered a termination of pregnancy. A high-risk result causes considerable anxiety for the mother. If you have a high-risk result, you should receive appropriate counselling as soon as possible.

Although a confirmed CVS result takes approximately 10 days and a result from amniocentesis takes two weeks, a quick preliminary result may be available through the technique of fluorescence in situ hybridisation (FISH). This technique uses fluorescently labelled probes for specific common conditions such as Down syndrome to give an early indication of the result. There is an extra cost involved in having this test.

The first-trimester combined screen consists of a blood test (which is most informative if taken during the ninth week of pregnancy) and an ultrasound performed around 12–13 weeks gestation. This is the most accurate of the widely available screening tests and has the added advantage of a relatively early diagnosis, with more straightforward termination procedures if that is your choice. The ultrasound component can be performed on its own, an approach that is often used for multiple pregnancies such as twins and triplets. A number of factors can be identified during an ultrasound that increase the chance a baby might have a chromosomal abnormality. Most of these are not significant by themselves, but two or more in combination convey an increased risk; if your scan indicates these factors you should be offered definitive testing.

The second-trimester biochemical screen consists of a blood test performed between 15 and 20 weeks gestation. The biochemical markers are different from those in the first-trimester test.

Very recently, a new screening test has become available in Australia, known broadly as non-invasive prenatal testing (NIPT). It involves taking a blood sample from the mother at around nine weeks gestation and analysing small fragments of the baby's DNA that are floating in the mother's blood. The analysis is complex but the results are extremely accurate. Detection of Down syndrome has been quoted as high as 99 per cent accurate for NIPT. At the time of publication, the test is still quite expensive, but it is likely that the cost will decrease over the next 10 years. In view of its accuracy, it is likely to become the most common method of screening in the future.

Second trimester

During the second part of the pregnancy, sometimes called the 'mid' trimester, your obstetric care provider will be monitoring the baby's growth and be on the lookout for the early onset of complications such as pre-eclampsia and gestational diabetes.

Gestational diabetes

Pregnant women need two to three times more insulin than normal. If the body is unable to produce this much insulin, gestational diabetes mellitus develops. If gestational diabetes is not well looked after, it may result in problems for the baby (such as growth problems, with both small and large babies; premature birth; imbalances in blood sugar and other blood chemicals after birth; and breathing difficulties) and the mother (such as increased risk of injury at delivery; caesarean delivery; and forceps delivery). Excellent control of gestational diabetes is crucial as it decreases the risks of these problems.

While there is no one reason women develop gestational diabetes, women are at greater risk if they are older; have a family history of type 2 diabetes or gestational diabetes; are overweight; are from an Aboriginal or Torres Strait Islander, Vietnamese, Chinese, Middle Eastern, Polynesian or Melanesian background; have previously had gestational diabetes or polycystic ovarian syndrome (PCOS); or have given birth to a large baby (more than 4.5 kilograms).

Gestational diabetes occurs in 2–5 per cent of pregnancies and usually disappears after delivery. Up to about half of women affected, however, develop type 2 diabetes later in life.

The management of gestational diabetes is a team effort, involving you, your family, GP and specialists, dietician and diabetes educator, all working to maintain excellent blood sugar levels and minimise problems for the fetus and for you. Some women will require insulin injections.

Routine second-trimester tests
The following are routine during the second trimester.

Screening for gestational diabetes
A test for gestational diabetes is usually offered at around 26 weeks gestation. The test involves drinking a liquid containing a known sugar load and having blood sugar monitored either one or two hours later. In pregnancy gestational diabetes is usually managed with diet and exercise or with insulin if necessary.

Ultrasound
This test is often called the 'morphology screen', because of its role in diagnosing structural abnormalities, and is performed between 18 and 22 weeks gestation. Prospective parents have an enormous amount of faith in this test, but in reality it has a number of limitations. It is not intended to pick up chromosomal abnormalities so it is really complementary to the other screening tests, including the earlier ultrasound. Even among structural abnormalities, detection rates are better for some things than others. Spinal cord abnormalities, major cardiac abnormalities and major

brain malformations should all be detected with good accuracy, but smaller abnormalities such as cleft lip may be more difficult to detect. This test may also detect abnormalities of the placental site, such as when the placenta forms low in the womb, known as placenta praevia, a condition with a risk of bleeding and requiring a caesarean.

Third trimester

Antenatal visits in the third trimester focus on fetal growth and position, particularly whether the head is up or down. Assessment of your well-being continues, including testing for pre-eclampsia, and preparing you for labour becomes increasingly important.

Routine third-trimester tests

There are some routine tests in the third trimester, including group B streptococcus screening (GBS). About 15–25 per cent of women are thought to be carriers of GBS, a bacterium that originates in the bowel but can cross into the vagina, in neither of which sites it causes any harm. If it is present in the vagina at the time of labour, it can be transmitted to the newborn, resulting in pneumonia, septicaemia and occasionally death. The illness develops so rapidly that antibiotics given to the baby after birth may be too late. It is common to be screened close to the time of giving birth, and if you test positive you will be given antibiotics during labour. These antibiotics cross the placenta and provide the baby with protection during delivery. If you develop a temperature during labour, are delivering prematurely or have had a previous baby affected by GBS, you will usually be given antibiotics regardless of your screening results.

The standard antenatal visit

After your first visit, most antenatal checks follow a routine.

Blood pressure measurement

Your blood pressure should be recorded at every visit. Your blood pressure is considered high if it is 140 over 90 or higher. High blood pressure is one of the early signs of pre-eclampsia, a major cause of complications for mother and baby. The condition can progress rapidly. High blood pressure in pregnancy without pre-eclampsia is also associated with worse pregnancy outcomes, such as fetal growth restriction, abruption (premature separation of the placenta from the uterus) and preterm birth, so high blood pressure should be assessed by a specialist obstetrician. A diagnosis of pre-eclampsia is made when high blood pressure is accompanied by protein in the urine, swelling and fluid in feet, hands or face (oedema), liver abnormalities and clotting abnormalities on blood tests, headaches and visual disturbances or fetal growth restriction. It requires early assessment by a specialist obstetrician and, possibly, admission to hospital for the early delivery of the baby.

Measurement of the fundal height

Your baby's growth is usually checked by measuring the height of the uterus above the pelvic bone. This measurement in centimetres should be roughly equivalent to the number of weeks gestation (strange but true). If the measurement is larger or smaller than expected, an ultrasound may be required for a more accurate assessment of the baby's size. Some complications that can be detected by this method include growth restriction, too much or too little fluid around the baby, the baby being in an unusual position, and uterine abnormalities such as fibroids. For this sort of screening to work well, it is very important to have accurate pregnancy dates. Your baby's growth follows a standard pattern; the baby will grow fastest between 20 and 32 weeks gestation, which is generally equivalent to an increase of 1 centimetre in fundal height per week. After 32 weeks, the rate of growth decreases slightly. Any significant difference from the expected size should be investigated by ultrasound. A growth-restricted baby is at higher risk of death in utero as well as neurological syndromes, and extra care must be taken if you are in this situation.

Baby's position and descent into the pelvis

From about 30 weeks gestation onwards, carers should check which part of the baby is down by feeling for the fetus's head (easiest to feel as it is hard and round). Most babies have turned to be head-downward by 36 weeks. A very large international study at the end of the twentieth century showed that babies born bottom-first (known as a breech birth) were at higher risk of dying during the delivery. This finding has increased the importance of checking the baby's position. You may be offered a procedure to turn the baby around, known as external cephalic version, which is performed in the last few weeks of a pregnancy if the baby remains lying sideways or bottom-first. If the baby is found to be persistently in a breech position, you will often be advised to deliver by caesarean.

Fetal heart

Carers should listen to the fetal heart at each visit. The wide availability of Doppler ultrasound devices offers women the opportunity to hear their baby's heart beating at each visit. Many women find this the most enjoyable part of the visit!

Smoking assessment

Smoking while pregnant is associated with serious risks to the baby. No safe level of smoking has been established. Risks associated with any smoking include double the risk of growth restriction and low birth weight. The risk of sudden infant death syndrome (SIDS) is almost three times higher, and smoking while pregnant is also associated with stillbirths, premature births and spontaneous abortions.

You are identified as a smoker if you smoked at all in the year before becoming pregnant. Care providers should ask about your smoking behaviour at every visit to encourage you to reduce smoking or ideally to quit completely. You should be offered support to help prevent you from relapsing. Women often ask about nicotine replacement therapy; the risks and benefits of these various types of therapies are not clear but they may be used if the usual methods fail.

Pregnancy can be a challenging time for any woman but some women face particular challenges due to existing medical conditions. Many hospitals have special programs and services available for those with individual needs during pregnancy.

Judy attended the Women's at eight weeks into her first pregnancy. She had suffered a severe spinal injury from an accidental gunshot wound while working as a jillaroo on an outback station eight years before. Since that time, she had been a paraplegic and was only able to move around using a wheelchair. She and her partner were financially secure and the pregnancy was planned.

Judy had some ability to sense touch and temperature over the lower half of her body, but could not move her legs at all. She needed help to manage constipation and to prevent pressure sores forming on the lower half of her body. She was unable to pass urine and so she regularly used a urinary catheter to drain her bladder.

Her pregnancy required care from a team of people including an obstetrician, midwife, physician, physiotherapist and anaesthetist. This team was focused on pressure-sore prevention as the pregnancy developed and Judy gained weight, and checking her bladder and bowel function, especially to prevent urinary tract infections from the regular use of a urinary catheter. The team was also concerned about the development of a rare condition known as autonomic dysreflexia, which only occurs in people with spinal injuries above a certain point in the spine. In this condition, when the affected person experiences pain in the area affected by the spinal injury, the nerve impulses carry the message to the spinal cord but are unable to pass the site of injury. The nervous system response to these messages can cause high blood pressure, sweating and flushing, headaches and blurred vision. If not treated promptly, the consequences can include stroke, retinal bleeding and pulmonary oedema (fluid filling the lungs).

Judy had an uncomplicated pregnancy. As she approached her due date, her carers were concerned about the risk of her going into labour without realising due to her decreased sensation, and delivering the baby unexpectedly at home. After discussion, she was admitted for induction of labour at 38 weeks gestation. This planned delivery also allowed close surveillance during the labour for signs of autonomic dysreflexia, as her labour pains would be in the area affected by her spinal injury. The labour proceeded normally until the final stages, when Judy was unable to push the baby out voluntarily due to paralysis of her pelvic muscles. A 'lift out' forceps delivery (where the baby is very low in the vagina) was performed without any tears or cuts to the perineum, which was important to achieve because skin areas affected by nerve damage in spinal cord injuries heal poorly. A healthy baby boy was born weighing 2.9 kilograms.

Judy went home after a slightly longer hospital stay to establish breastfeeding, and was visited by midwives after discharge.

Molar pregnancy

This condition, which may also be called hydatidiform mole or trophoblastic disease, is a pregnancy where something goes wrong at conception. A molar pregnancy occurs in approximately one in 1000 pregnancies, and is sometimes suspected on the early ultrasound or when a woman miscarries and the tissue that is passed or removed is inspected. This rare condition may be difficult to understand, especially for couples who are experiencing such disappointment after the loss of a pregnancy.

What occurs in a molar pregnancy?

In a normal pregnancy, the woman's ovum (egg) is fertilised in the fallopian tube and about four days later the fertilised egg moves into the uterus, where it attaches to the inner wall. The outer part of the fertilised egg forms the placenta, which is made of millions of cells called trophoblasts and has many functions, including feeding the baby and removing its waste products. The inner part of the fertilised egg develops into a fetus. The placenta produces a pregnancy hormone called human chorionic gonadotropin (hCG), which causes symptoms such as morning sickness, tender breasts and lack of energy.

In a molar pregnancy, there is an abnormal overgrowth of all or part of the placenta. The placenta is abnormal, larger and contains many cysts (sacs of fluid). The woman is effectively pregnant with what is called a hydatidiform mole rather than a normally developing placenta and fetus. The first part of the name comes from the Greek word *hydatid*, meaning 'droplet'. These droplets appear to burrow into the wall of the uterus, hence the name 'mole'. This term may seem strange, but 'mole' is similarly used for a harmless growth on the skin.

In a molar pregnancy, you will have all the usual signs of pregnancy (like morning sickness or sore breasts) because the placenta continues to make the pregnancy hormone hCG. In fact, the placenta often makes higher amounts of this hormone than it would normally.

A molar pregnancy can be classed as either partial or complete, depending on the changes in the placenta. In a complete molar pregnancy, the growth stops a fetus from developing at all. In a partial molar pregnancy, a fetus develops but it will be abnormal and cannot survive.

Most of the time, a molar pregnancy is discovered in the first three months of pregnancy, often because it ends in a miscarriage (see chapter 20). If the molar pregnancy does not end spontaneously, then a D&C or 'curette', which is a minor operation to remove all tissue from the uterus, will need to be performed.

A rare condition that can arise from a molar pregnancy, or an otherwise normal pregnancy or miscarriage, is choriocarcinoma. In this very rare form of cancer, the placenta becomes malignant. Choriocarcinoma can spread throughout the body, usually to organs such as the lungs, liver and brain. It is extremely sensitive to chemotherapy and in most cases can be cured.

Why does a molar pregnancy develop?

Molar pregnancy is thought to be caused by a problem with the genetic information in an egg or sperm, but the reason a molar pregnancy develops usually remains unknown. Factors that may increase the risk of having a molar pregnancy include being over 35 or under 18, having had a previous hydatidiform mole or miscarriage, a diet low in carotene (a form of vitamin A) or being of Asian or Mexican origin.

As with skin moles, a hydatidiform mole is usually harmless. In about 10 per cent of cases, however, some of the mole cells may remain and can keep growing; if left untreated, they can bury into the organs around them, including the uterus, and even spread through the blood to other distant organs, including the lungs, liver or brain. Because the mole cells produce the pregnancy hormone hCG, doctors can discover if there are any remaining cells by monitoring hCG in the blood. This allows immediate treatment, to stop the disease before it can have serious effects.

If you have been diagnosed with a partial mole, your hCG levels will be monitored until they return to normal, when follow-up will stop. If you have a complete hydatidiform mole and your hCG levels return to normal within eight weeks from the time your molar pregnancy is ended, you will receive follow-up care for six months from the time the pregnancy ended. If your hCG levels have not returned to normal within eight weeks, monitoring will continue until they become normal, and then monthly samples will be taken for the next six months.

In about one in 10 cases the hCG level does not return to normal. This is known as persistent trophoblastic disease. When this occurs, further tests will probably be needed, perhaps followed by chemotherapy. The chances of needing treatment are slightly higher in the case of a complete hydatidiform mole than a partial hydatidiform mole, but the chance of a cure is extremely high.

After a partial mole, once your hormone levels are back to normal, you can try to become pregnant again. It is sensible to wait until you have had at least one normal period. After a complete mole, when you can try for a pregnancy again depends on what follow-up has been recommended for you. Your body will be physically ready for a new pregnancy, but it is important for you to be ready psychologically as well, which can sometimes take longer.

Doctors will recommend not using hormonal contraception methods (such as the Pill) until the levels of hCG have returned to normal but using barrier methods instead. Once hCG levels have returned to normal, it is fine to use any form of contraception.

What are the chances of another molar pregnancy in the future?

The chance of a hydatidiform mole occurring again in another pregnancy is about 1 per cent. An early ultrasound is recommended to check any new pregnancy. After the baby is delivered the placenta should be examined, and at six weeks after the delivery of the baby, one further hCG test performed.

Losing a pregnancy is devastating, and having to cope with a molar pregnancy on top of this is shattering. Grief about losing a pregnancy, combined with fear of persistent disease, mean that for most women the emotional healing takes much longer than the physical healing from surgery. Their partner, family and friends will be able to provide support. Sometimes they may also need help from a psychologist. An early pregnancy loss does not mean it will not be possible to have any more children.

The vast majority of women who suffer an early pregnancy loss have a healthy pregnancy later, but it is important that both they and their partner are emotionally healed and strong enough before they make another attempt.

Hydatidiform mole registry

In some countries women who have a molar pregnancy are registered so that their follow-up can be coordinated. In Australia, there is a Hydatidiform Mole Registry in Victoria (at the Women's) and in Queensland (at the Royal Brisbane and Women's Hospital). Following a diagnosis of hydatidiform mole, it is very important that you either have your name placed with a registry or see a gynaecologist regularly for testing if there is no registry in your state.

Nutrition for pregnancy

Eating healthily during pregnancy is important to ensure you meet the needs of your developing baby, and for your own wellbeing. Research has shown that what a woman eats can influence the development of her baby and may also have an effect on the baby's health later in life.

Pregnancy increases the need for energy and many nutrients, including protein, calcium, iron, folic acid, vitamin D and iodine. It is not difficult to meet these needs if you eat regular meals containing a variety of foods from the main food groups (see the table below).

If you follow a special diet (such as vegetarian or vegan) or feel that your diet is inadequate for pregnancy, ask for an appointment with a dietician at your hospital or antenatal clinic.

Recommended food intake for pregnancy

Food group	Serves per day	Sample serve
Protein foods	3½	65 g red meat 80 g chicken 100 g fish 2 eggs 1 cup legumes 170 g tofu 30 g nuts
Dairy foods	2½	250 ml milk or soy milk 40 g cheese 200 g yoghurt
Breads and cereals	8½	1 slice bread ⅔ cup cereal flakes ½ cup cooked porridge ½ cup rice, pasta or noodles (cooked)
Fruit	2	1 piece of medium-sized fruit (e.g. apple) 2 pieces of smaller fruit (e.g. apricots) 1 cup tinned fruit
Vegetables	5	½ cup cooked vegetables 1 cup salad 75 g starchy vegetables (e.g. potatoes)
Unsaturated spreads and oils	In small amounts but regularly	
Extra foods (e.g. containing saturated fat, added salt, added sugar or alcohol)	Only sometimes and in small amounts	

Food safety during pregnancy

There is no need to be alarmed about harmful foods during pregnancy, but there are several issues to be aware of.

Caffeine

Tea, coffee, cola drinks and energy drinks all contain caffeine. There is mixed evidence about the effects of large amounts of caffeine on a developing baby, but moderate amounts appear safe – that is, two to three

Alcohol and pregnancy

Latest guidelines advise that women abstain completely from drinking any alcohol during pregnancy. With continued heavy drinking of more than four standard drinks a day, there is a 5 per cent risk of the baby developing fetal alcohol syndrome. These babies have restricted growth before and after birth, are slow to achieve developmental milestones, have relatively small brains, have difficulties with fine movements and have particular facial abnormalities that do tend to improve as the child gets older. Alcohol intake during pregnancy has also been associated with mental retardation, behavioural abnormalities, congenital abnormalities, growth restriction, stillbirth, and neonatal deaths due to sudden infant death syndrome (SIDS).

A maximum safe amount of alcohol has not been determined, but some studies of low alcohol intake, such as less than one standard drink per week, have shown no association with fetal alcohol syndrome. Limited studies of women who stopped drinking after finding out they were less than six weeks pregnant also did not show any poor outcomes. It seems likely that there is a safe level of alcohol intake in pregnancy (which must be very low), but without any clear guidelines as to where the upper limit lies it seems best to avoid alcohol altogether.

Binge-drinking (defined as more than five standard drinks in one sitting) is associated with increased risks for the baby, including epilepsy and delayed development. Binge-drinking is more common in younger women and is of particular concern with unplanned pregnancies. Provided you stop drinking in the first six weeks of pregnancy, however, the effects are likely to be minimal. Concerns about the effects of binge-drinking on pregnancy can increase anxiety and lead women to seek a termination despite reassurance that the risk is low.

cups of coffee or five cups of tea or cola drinks per day. Don't forget cola drinks also contain large quantities of sugar. Some energy drinks can also contain large amounts of caffeine or guarana (a caffeine-like substance) and are not recommended for pregnant women.

Fish and mercury

Fish is a rich source of omega-3 fatty acids, which are important for fetal brain development. Pregnant women should eat fish several times a week, but because of possible higher levels of mercury, certain types of fish should be limited in pregnancy: shark (flake), marlin and swordfish (broadbill) should not be eaten more than once a fortnight by pregnant women. If you do eat these fish, do not eat any other fish during the fortnight. Also limit orange roughy (sea perch) or catfish to one serve per week. If you eat these fish, do not eat any other fish during the week.

Listeria

Listeria is a bacterium that can contaminate food and cause infection that can be harmful to a developing baby. Listeria infection is rare and the risk can be minimised by good food-handling practices. Here are some suggestions to help minimise the risk of listeria infection:

- Ensure good hygiene and clean utensils when preparing food.
- Thoroughly wash raw vegetables.
- Avoid foods such as pate, cold cooked chicken and sliced meats, coleslaw and salads (unless they have been freshly prepared), unpasteurised dairy products, soft cheeses (such as brie, camembert, ricotta, feta or blue cheese), soft-serve ice-cream, uncooked or smoked seafood and precooked prawns. Freshly cooked seafood is safe.
- Cook food to boiling point to kill listeria, so when reheating foods, make sure they are piping hot.

For further information about food safety during pregnancy, visit the Food Standards Australia and New Zealand website (for details see the Resources section at the end of this book).

Weight gain during pregnancy

Weight gain during pregnancy varies but should generally be between 11.5 kilograms and 16 kilograms if your pre-pregnancy weight was in the

Institute of Medicine guidelines for weight gain in pregnancy

Pre-pregnancy BMI (see page 225)	Total recommended weight gain	Rate of weight gain during second and third trimesters
less than 18.5 (underweight)	12.5–18 kg	0.5 kg per week
18.5–24.9 (healthy)	11.5–16 kg	0.4 kg per week
25–29.9 (overweight)	7–11.5 kg	0.3 kg per week
more than 30 (obese)	5–9 kg	0.2 kg per week

healthy weight range. If you were underweight at the beginning of pregnancy, you may gain more weight than average. If you were overweight, your weight gain may need to be less than average. Use the following table as a guide to your weight gain during pregnancy. If you have any concerns about your weight, ask to see a dietician at your maternity service.

Pregnancy and dental health

When you are pregnant it is important to keep your body healthy, and your teeth and gums are no exception. It is safe to visit the dentist when you are pregnant, so don't be afraid to get a check-up and treatment if necessary. You may need to be careful about X-rays, general anaesthetics and some medications, but talk to your dentist about your concerns. It is important to let the clinic know you are pregnant when you book and when you go to your appointment.

Don't put off going to the dentist because you will feel uncomfortable in the dental chair. The dental team can position you more comfortably if you remind them you are pregnant.

Morning sickness and your teeth

Many women feel sick and vomit regularly during the first three months of pregnancy. The acid in vomit can weaken teeth, so you need to take extra care of your teeth if you are experiencing morning sickness. Brushing your teeth straight after vomiting can weaken the enamel. To avoid damaging your teeth, try the following:

- Rinse your mouth out with water (or a mouth rinse) straight away.
- Rub toothpaste onto your teeth with your finger.
- Wait at least 30 minutes before brushing your teeth.
- Chew sugar-free gum to stimulate saliva, to neutralise acid and wash it away.

Gum disease (periodontitis)

Your body goes through a lot of changes when you are pregnant. If you notice that your gums are sore, puffy, red or bleeding, you may be showing signs of gum disease. Gum disease is more common during pregnancy, but you can control it.

If you think you may have gum disease, it is important to talk to your dentist. Research has shown an association between the level of gum

> **Smoking and teeth**
>
> Aside from the fact that smoking while pregnant is bad for you and your baby, smokers are more likely to develop gum disease and are at higher risk of developing oral cancers.

disease in pregnant women and preterm birth, low birth weight and pre-eclampsia.

Tooth decay and erosion

When we consume sugary or starchy food and drinks (i.e. that are high in carbohydrates), the bacteria that naturally live in the mouth and in plaque break down those carbohydrates into acids. These acids attack and dissolve the tooth enamel. If this happens often, the teeth don't get a chance to recover. Food and drinks high in acid can also soften tooth enamel, weaken teeth and make them more sensitive.

If you have a tooth cavity it is safe to have it treated during pregnancy. Treatment will reduce the likelihood of passing on the bacteria that cause tooth decay to your baby after birth. Studies show that preventing or delaying transfer of decay-causing bacteria may protect children from tooth decay later on.

After your baby is born:

- Brush your teeth every morning and before you go to bed.
- Don't clean dummies with your mouth.
- Don't share spoons when feeding your baby.

Your child should have an oral health check before the age of two. This may be carried out by a dentist, a dental therapist or a maternal and child health nurse. Regular check-ups are important approximately once every year after that (speak to a dental professional about your child's needs).

Looking after your teeth

There are things you can do to help prevent tooth decay and gum disease.

Eat well

Make healthy food choices every day. Include a variety of fruit, vegetables, grains and lean meat in your diet. Choose foods that contain calcium, such as dairy products and some soy products. Try to avoid sweet foods that are high in sugar.

Drink well

Drink lots of tap water, especially fluoridated tap water. Fluoride helps keep teeth strong and healthy and is safe for pregnant women to drink. Plain milk is also a good choice; it contains calcium, which is good for you and your baby's teeth and bones. Try to avoid sugary drinks such as cordials, soft drinks and fruit juices.

Clean well

Brush your teeth twice a day and make sure you brush where your teeth join your gums. Use a soft toothbrush and a pea-sized amount of fluoridated toothpaste. Flossing is not for everybody. Talk to your dentist about whether you need to floss.

Muscle and joint pain during pregnancy

Antenatal care aims to ensure that your growing baby is well medically, and this is obviously of vital importance. Taking care of you, the mother, is also important, especially if you have a medical condition that could affect the baby. If you have a problem that does *not* affect the health of the baby, such as muscle or joint pain, a physiotherapist is the key healthcare provider. Let your midwife or doctor know if you have any muscle or joint problems, so they can refer you to a women's health physiotherapist.

For optimal physical health for both you and your baby, get professional help for any muscle or joint problems. Don't let these common aches and pains lessen the enjoyment of your pregnancy. Exercise well, and allow time for rest and recovery. Above all, listen to your body and get the help you need as soon as you need it.

Separation (diastasis) of the rectus abdominis muscle

There are two sets of abdominal muscles, one on each side of the abdomen, joined together in the midline by a fibrous sheath that is less stretchy than the muscles. The abdominal muscles stretch over a baby as it grows. To protect the abdominal muscles from overstretching, the less stretchy midline sheath gradually widens. The widened gap in the centre of the abdomen is called a diastasis, or separation, of the abdominal muscles, and it is a protective feature rather than a dramatic injury. Stretched and separated muscles may not provide full support for the back, however, and may increase the risk of back pain and back injury.

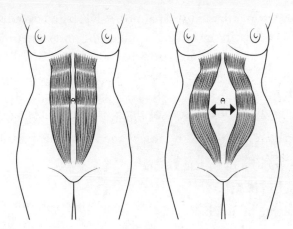

Separation of the abdominal muscles

Physiotherapy for separation of the rectus abdominis muscle

Treatment is aimed at learning how to use the abdominal muscles effectively during all activities, to relieve stretch on the muscles. If the diastasis is large, you may be prescribed a support garment to support your abdomen for the rest of the pregnancy. The support garment can also be worn after the birth, until the diastasis has healed, usually in six to eight weeks. Avoid lifting and straining with the abdomen, and sit-up exercises.

Pregnancy-related pelvic pain

Pain in the pelvic joints may develop during or after pregnancy. Pelvic pain may be due to hormonal changes that soften the ligaments of the pelvis, or to changes in posture or increased pressure on the pelvis due to the growth of the baby. These changes can place strain on the pelvic

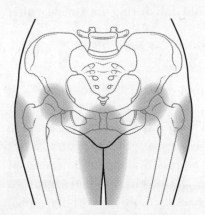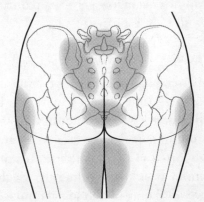

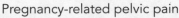
Pregnancy-related pelvic pain

joints, making them inflamed and painful. Pelvic pain is felt in the front or the back of the pelvis, in the buttocks and groin, and sometimes radiating into the thighs. An obvious sign of pelvic joint pain is walking with the 'pregnant waddle'. The shaded areas in the picture below indicate where pain commonly occurs.

Pelvic pain can be made worse by the following activities:

- prolonged or fast walking
- getting in and out of the car or bed
- rolling over in bed
- deep squatting or lunging
- going up- and downstairs
- standing on one leg (e.g. when putting on pants)
- moving from a sitting to a standing position
- high-impact exercise (such as running and jumping)

Pelvic pain lessens with relative rest rather than pushing through the pain. This means avoiding the activities that cause pain. Rest may also mean using crutches to walk, and in the most severe cases, bed rest.

Physiotherapy for pelvic pain

Treatment is aimed at learning pain-relieving strategies, such as use of an icepack, and may also involve wearing a pelvic support belt. If your buttock muscles are in spasm because of the pain, you will learn trigger-point massage and stretches. You'll then be advised to practise strengthening exercises for hip and pelvic muscles so the pelvis gains stability from the muscles surrounding the softened pelvic joints. Finally, you'll be taught tips for managing pelvic pain during labour and during the time just after your baby is born.

Lower back pain

Lower back pain is very common during pregnancy. Up to 50 per cent of pregnant women experience back pain at some time during their pregnancy, and for one-third of these women it is severe. Because it is so common, it is often seen as an inevitable part of pregnancy and so not reported to the medical team until the pain is disabling. The causes of lower back pain are mostly weight gain and postural change causing a forward drag on the spinal joints ('sway back'), combined with hormonal softening of joints, which makes them more vulnerable to strain. Fatigue and spasm of the back muscles occur as they work hard to hold up the spine and the growing baby and uterus. This muscle spasm is felt as back pain. You are more at risk of back pain in pregnancy if you have had previous back pain, have weak abdominal muscles, are overweight, do strenuous repetitive work or have joint hypermobility (unusually supple joints). It is extremely rare for lower back pain in pregnancy to be caused by a disc injury.

Physiotherapy for lower back pain
Treatment follows three pathways:

1. pain relief – through regular use of ice- or heat packs and wearing a support belt
2. postural correction – through learning postural changes and correct lifting techniques to keep the spine in best alignment and lessen the drag on spinal joints
3. strengthening back and abdominal muscles – through exercises, so that they can support the weight of the growing baby

The greatest benefit from these pain-relief strategies will come if they are incorporated into daily activities.

Upper back pain

Towards the end of pregnancy the uterus presses up under the diaphragm. This pressure makes the work of breathing harder, especially during exercise. To compensate for this, the ribs flare out to the sides as you breathe, which may cause a sharp pain under the shoulderblades that radiates around the chest. Women whose work involves sitting at a computer for long hours are often affected by this sharp upper back pain.

Physiotherapy for upper back pain
Chest pain can cause anxiety, so education about its causes will often be the first step. Pain relief can be achieved with regular use of ice- or heat packs and wearing a thoracic support to keep the upper back in alignment. The physiotherapist will also teach upper-back flexibility exercises, and advise against high-intensity exercise during the last trimester.

Carpal tunnel syndrome

Carpal tunnel syndrome is a condition that causes pins and needles, numbness or burning and stiff, painful hands. The carpal tunnel is a

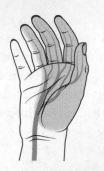

Carpal tunnel syndrome

small passage in the wrist where nerves and tendons pass from the arm into the hand and fingers. During pregnancy, hormones cause fluid retention. When this happens, the nerves running through the carpal tunnel may become squashed, and react by causing pins and needles in the fingers. The diagram indicates where in the hand symptoms may be felt. The symptoms may be worse at night and radiate back up the arm, making sleep difficult. Constant movement of the hands and heavy lifting make the condition worse. If carpal tunnel syndrome persists after birth, care must be taken when lifting and caring for the baby.

Physiotherapy for carpal tunnel syndrome

Treatment is aimed at relieving the pain, and reducing hand movements and swelling. A compression bandage or wrist splint will often be prescribed to limit hand movement and swelling, along with the application of ice or other cooling to the hand and wrist. The physiotherapist will advise elevating the arms when sitting, teach simple fluid drainage massage, and give tips for managing wrist and hand pain during labour and breastfeeding.

Incontinence

During pregnancy there is an increased risk of incontinence (bladder leakage) initially due to hormonal changes and because of increased pressure on the bladder as the uterus and baby grow. When you cough, sneeze, laugh, lift, pull or push, you increase the pressure in your abdomen, which puts an added pressure downwards on the bladder. If the pelvic floor muscles cannot hold against this extra pressure, leakage occurs. It has been shown that an intensive pelvic floor exercise program for eight to 12 weeks in the second half of pregnancy can reduce the risk of incontinence in late pregnancy and during the first year after birth.

Incontinence can also be caused by childbirth itself, especially if the second stage of labour was long, the baby is large, it is a forceps delivery, or a perineal or pelvic floor muscle tear is sustained during labour.

Physiotherapy for incontinence

Pelvic floor exercises are the main treatment for pregnancy-related incontinence (see the next chapter for how to do pelvic floor exercises). If you are unsure whether you are exercising your pelvic floor muscles correctly, see a women's health physiotherapist. One of the most common mistakes is to strain downwards instead of feeling an inward lift of the pelvic floor. You will be taught to tighten the pelvic floor before you do any activity where you feel you might leak.

Once you have had your baby, you will be encouraged to begin pelvic floor exercises within 48 hours of birth, but gently and within the limits of pain. As well as doing the pelvic floor exercises, if you have perineal swelling or pain you will be advised to use icepacks regularly until the swelling and pain have been relieved. You should also have your pelvic floor muscles checked at your postnatal six-week check-up.

18

Physical activity during and after pregnancy

Margaret Sherburn

Pregnancy is a time of great physical change to a woman's body. While many women fly through pregnancy feeling wonderfully well, with the so-called glow of pregnancy, an equal number find that carrying a baby causes physical problems that mar their experience of this otherwise exciting nine months. This chapter addresses the physical activities you can participate in safely to help you minimise physical problems during pregnancy and the postnatal period.

Physical activity

All women today benefit from being generally fit; that is, having stamina, strength and flexibility. Pregnant women in particular need to be fit specifically for pregnancy, childbirth and motherhood. Being fit makes it easier to cope with your increasing weight and the changing shape of your body, and lessens the effects of many of the physiological changes that occur during pregnancy. The best way to become fit is simply by doing regular physical activity at an intensity that pushes you to work at a moderate pace, but not to the point of being out of breath.

The benefits of exercising during pregnancy

All the research leads us to encourage pregnant women to exercise to a moderate intensity. While some women need to take more care due to

How much physical activity is good for you?
- Moderate-intensity exercise on all or most days of the week, *or*
- accumulating 150 minutes over a week, *or*
- 10,000 steps per day (measured using a pedometer)

pregnancy complications, generally speaking doing some exercise is always better than not exercising at all.

There are many benefits to continuing to exercise throughout pregnancy. Exercise will help you feel that you are contributing positively to your health, and each session of physical activity will give you an overall sense of wellbeing. If you have a higher fitness level, you will feel less tired at the end of the day and your weight gain will be easier to manage. With specific pregnancy-focused exercises, your abdominal, back and pelvic floor muscles will be stronger and more able to support your growing weight.

When you exercise regularly, your body adapts to the physiological changes of exercise. Your heart can pump more efficiently, your muscles are stronger and your body's temperature-control mechanisms are better. Best of all, you will have a greater understanding of and confidence in your body and its ability to give birth. After birth, your exercise routine will enable your body to recover faster and to get back its pre-pregnancy shape.

Many pregnant women ask whether exercise will harm their baby. As long as you undertake exercises that are safe for your level of fitness and your current stage of pregnancy, it will cause no harm at all. It is actually more risky for your baby if you become overweight during pregnancy. Research shows us that unfit women beginning exercise during pregnancy, or women doing occasional but intensive exercise during pregnancy, is less healthy for the baby than regular exercise. If certain medical conditions appear during pregnancy, however, you should exercise at a lower level or stop exercising (see box below). Seek advice from your doctor or midwife before you begin exercising for fitness if you are at all unsure of your or your baby's health status.

Exercise is a great way to prepare the body for the tasks of mothering. After all, taking care of your baby begins with taking care of yourself.

What not to do

Some forms of exercise are not recommended during pregnancy. These include:

- sports or activities where there is a risk of collision, tripping or falling, or heavy body contact
- competitive sports where you have to reach, stretch or leap beyond the safe limits of your joints and your baby, or where winning is more important than safety

Medical conditions that will generally prevent exercising during pregnancy

- Heart disease

- Ruptured membranes

- Placenta praevia in late pregnancy (see page 331)

- Pre-eclampsia (see page 280)

- Intrauterine growth retardation (the fetus is not growing well in the womb)

- Incompetent cervix (a softer and weaker cervix than is normal, or one that is abnormally short. The condition, if unrecognised, can result in a second-term miscarriage or preterm delivery.)

- Uncontrolled hypertension (high blood pressure)

- Pulmonary embolism (a blood clot in the lungs) or deep vein thrombosis (a blood clot in the leg)

- Uterine bleeding

- activities that take place in an unsafe environment, such as high temperatures – spas or hydrotherapy pools, Iyengar (hot) yoga – or those that use heavy equipment – weightlifting, water and snow skiing, and scuba or board diving

- exercise that involves repetitive high impact, lots of twists and turns, high stepping or sudden stops that may cause joint discomfort

Always listen to your body and be alert to any sign you need to stop your exercise. If you are new to exercise, start slowly and progress at your own pace and at an intensity that makes you feel good.

Signs that you may need to stop exercising include:

- vaginal bleeding

- nausea or vomiting

- feeling faint or light-headed

- strong pain, especially from the pelvis or back

- reduced movement of the baby

Exercise and body changes during pregnancy

There are both hidden and obvious changes happening within your body during pregnancy. The hidden ones are the physiological and designed to provide the right environment for your baby's development. The obvious ones are weight gain and altered posture.

Hidden changes and exercise

Cardiac changes

To meet the increasing demand for blood supply to your growing baby, your heart enlarges and also pumps faster. This means you are already doing an aerobic workout just by being pregnant. It also means your exertion during exercise should be of a moderate intensity, as there is a smaller range between your resting heart rate and the safe maximum heart rate. You are exercising at moderate intensity if you can comfortably talk, but not sing, during the activity.

Circulation changes

The volume of blood in your body increases as your baby's needs grow. A softening of the walls of your veins also occurs. Along with a heavy uterus in later pregnancy, this potentially compromises the flow of blood back to your heart, allowing blood to pool in your lower legs. You could feel light-headed if you do too many standing exercises in a row, or if you stand around at the end of an exercise session. You could wear support stockings if you have varicose veins or are prone to feeling light-headed, or do some calf raises or walking on the spot to encourage the return of blood to your heart.

After 16 weeks gestation, you should not do exercises lying on your back, as the weight of the baby can press on major blood vessels returning blood to your heart and also cause light-headedness or nausea. This means no sit-ups or bench presses, but does not mean you cannot exercise your abdominal muscles during pregnancy (see below). For the same reason, it is also recommended not to sleep on your back during the second half of your pregnancy. If, however, you wake to find yourself on your back, trust that your body has woken you in order to move to a better sleeping position.

Core temperature changes

Your body's temperature is naturally slightly higher when you are pregnant, to provide the best environment for your baby's growth. Intensive exercise may cause your core temperature to rise to an unsafe level for your baby, so take these simple precautions:

- Limit the exertion during exercise to a moderate intensity.
- Drink water before, during and after exercise.
- Wear light clothing.
- Exercise in a cool, ventilated environment (no spas or saunas).
- Don't exercise if you have a temperature or fever.

Joint changes

Pregnancy hormones cause a change in the structure of the ligaments that support your joints, making them softer. This factor, along with changes in your posture and weight gain, can increase the need to protect your joints during pregnancy, especially when you exercise. The most affected joints are those of the pelvis and lower back. Other commonly affected joints are in the upper back, feet and wrists. If any of them are causing pain and a 'waddling' gait, this can be enough to stop you exercising, but some specific muscle-strengthening around vulnerable joints can help (see chapter 17 for how these joint conditions are treated).

Here are some helpful hints to protect your joints:

- Don't take part in high-impact exercise such as netball, tennis, aerobics or running.
- Don't do dance aerobics (e.g. Zumba classes) or fast, high-impact aerobics classes.
- Change to exercise in a pool or a fitball class, rather than doing a long walk or a gym class.
- Wear supportive shoes.
- Take shorter strides when you walk.
- Bring your knees together when changing positions, and change positions in a controlled and smooth way.
- Strengthen your postural support muscles; that is, your back, hip and abdominal muscles.
- Check that you use good posture during all your exercises to avoid joint strain.

Pregnancy exercises

Even if you don't exercise for fitness, every pregnant woman should do these basic exercises for her physical wellbeing. These are essential for strengthening the abdominal, back and pelvic floor muscles.

Pelvic floor exercises

The pelvic floor muscles form the base or floor of your pelvis and support everything that sits above the floor. This includes the growing weight of the uterus, and the bladder and bowel. Because these muscles are internal and out of sight, they are often out of mind too, and not exercised as they should be. Although they form a 'floor', it has gaps to allow for the exiting passages of the organs above. If the gap widens, or the muscles don't have the strength to close the openings, symptoms occur. Often the first symptoms that the muscles are not working efficiently are bladder leakage during coughing, sneezing, lifting, pulling, pushing or doing any physical activity; or bladder urgency, the need to get to the toilet immediately. For some pregnant women, the uterus drops lower within the vagina. This is called a prolapse, and the symptoms are feeling a lump, and a heaviness or dragging sensation in the vagina.

How to do pelvic floor exercises

1. Sit comfortably with your feet and knees apart. Sit tall and relax your bottom into the chair.
2. Tighten around your vagina and anus as if you are trying to stop passing wind or urine, and lift up towards your belly button. Feel a lift upwards inside rather than a pushing down feeling. (If you feel

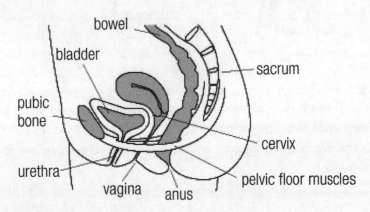

Pelvic floor muscles

yourself holding your breath or tightening your buttocks, you are not doing the exercise correctly. Relax and begin again.)

3. Hold the pelvic floor muscle tight for as many seconds as you can, up to 10 seconds.

4. Release the muscle, then repeat the exercise up to 10 times, always feeling a lift up inside your pelvis.

5. Stop when you feel fatigued, and note the number of repetitions you did. This is your training set.

6. Do your training set three times each day for maximum strengthening.

7. When this training set becomes easier to do, increase the amount of time you hold each squeeze.

8. To increase the speed at which your pelvic floor muscles can contract, also do a set of fast contractions. Lift – release – lift – release. Make sure you fully release each time, so you can lift fully on the next contraction. Do at least 10 repetitions, and up to 30 repetitions if you can.

As with any fitness training, increasing the effort over time will increase the strength of the exercised muscles, so don't become complacent and just do a comfortable squeeze. Really exercise your pelvic floor muscles to a strength-training intensity.

If you are having difficulty finding these muscles or understanding how to contract them, ask your physiotherapist, doctor or midwife to check your technique.

Exercises for the abdominal muscles

The abdominal muscles act as a natural corset to support your abdominal organs and spine. When the abdominal muscles contract they produce spinal movement so you can bend and twist, or hold the spine stable so you can stand upright; this is called 'core stability'. As the abdominal muscles stretch over the growing baby and uterus, they can become less effective at their normal support and movement tasks. And if they are not exercised at all, they can overstretch as the uterus rests forward onto them, which means they cannot return to their original length and shape after the birth.

Some women wonder if they can squash their baby by tightening their abdominal muscles. The answer is no – it's impossible, so don't allow your abdominal muscles to relax over the uterus for fear of squashing your baby. This just makes the muscles very weak and overstretched. The harm is done by *not* exercising the muscles, so that they become overstretched and cannot return to their pre-pregnancy shape.

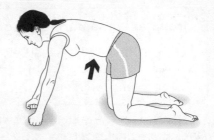

Abdominal exercises

Sit-ups or crunches are the usual exercises associated with abdominal training. These become inappropriate and ineffective during pregnancy – ineffective because the stretch on your abdominal muscles means they cannot work the way they did before you were pregnant; and inappropriate because the exercise is done lying on your back, where the baby rests on major blood vessels and may block blood flow, causing dizziness.

How to do abdominal exercises during pregnancy

The best way to exercise the abdominal muscles and gain core stability is to draw them in without moving your spine. Think of cuddling your baby with your abdominal muscles or sucking in your belly button towards your backbone.

1. Get on your hands and knees. Let your tummy relax.
2. Breathe in gently. As you breathe out, gently draw in the lower part of your stomach firmly, lifting your baby as you draw in. Hold for the count of three or more if you can. Let go.
3. Repeat this movement up to 10 times, with a few seconds' rest between each one.
4. Build up gradually until you can hold the muscles strongly for 10 seconds and repeat the exercise 10 times. Build up gradually until you can hold for 60 seconds.
5. When this exercise becomes easy, challenge yourself by alternately lifting your arms while keeping your abdominals 'switched on', then alternately lifting your legs, then your opposite arm and leg, then the same-side arm and leg. With each of these variations, build up your hold time as you did with the initial exercise.

Hint: Don't move your back at any time during the exercise. You should be able to breathe and talk as you do this exercise. You can also squeeze your pelvic floor muscles at the same time.

> ### Group exercise during pregnancy
>
> If you are exercising in a group or at a gym, choose clinical Pilates, a fitball class, aquaerobics, or a pump class (with light weights) for the best abdominal workout.

Back care and posture

As your baby grows and your baby bump becomes larger, your spine can be dragged forward with the growing weight. You then have what's known as a 'sway back'. This means the spinal joints are not in their usual alignment and they protest by causing backache or back pain. You might start to waddle when you walk to ease the pain, until even waddling begins to hurt.

Here are some simple strategies for managing back pain:

• Stand up straight so your spinal curves return to normal. Gently elongate your spine from your pelvis to the top of your head, and breathe normally as you do this.

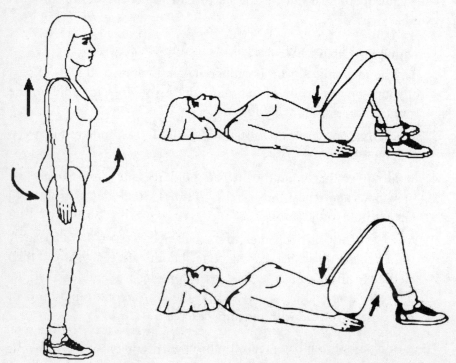

Pelvic movements

- Sit tall; don't slump.
- Draw in your abdominal muscles around your baby during all daily activities, especially when you are walking or lifting.
- Do belly dancing movements daily to retain normal flexibility in your spine.

While these strategies are simple, they do involve muscular effort. When you first start using these techniques, you will feel as though you are working quite hard to hold the new posture. Don't give up. You are getting stronger just by doing them regularly and your back pain will lessen each day. If you still experience pain after you have truly worked on these strategies, however, please seek professional advice and treatment.

Physical activity for particular needs

Obesity

If your body mass index (BMI; see chapter 14) was high (more than 30) before you became pregnant, regular physical activity can help minimise your weight gain during pregnancy. Regular exercise following the guidelines above, along with a healthy diet will help you achieve the appropriate weight gain. Consult the table in chapter 17 for the recommended weight gain during pregnancy according to your pre-pregnancy weight.

Gestational diabetes mellitus

If you have been diagnosed with gestational diabetes, you will need to change your diet immediately, begin to monitor your blood sugar and be encouraged to exercise daily. Because the exercise frequency, intensity, time and type of activity for best outcomes for women with gestational diabetes is not yet known, the best advice is to follow the normal exercise guidelines presented in this chapter. Research has shown that women with gestational diabetes who exercise need less insulin. For women who have had gestational diabetes in a previous pregnancy, exercise in the first 20 weeks of pregnancy has been shown to prevent diabetes in that pregnancy.

Returning to exercise after the birth

Once your baby is born, returning to exercise is dependent on the type of birth you had and the tissue healing that needs to take place, your fatigue level, and how overwhelmed you are by your new role as a mother. The limits imposed by your pregnancy have been lifted, but your body is still recovering from pregnancy and childbirth, and is establishing breast-feeding. Some women bounce back immediately, but for others recovery is a slower process. It is very important *not* to compare yourself with other new mothers. Everyone is different and will return to their chosen exercise at their own pace.

When to start exercising again

Immediately after the birth, women who have had a healthy, uncomplicated pregnancy and delivery can resume gentle activities, such as pelvic floor exercises, walking and a strengthening program for the back, abdominal and leg muscles, starting very gently, like an athlete returning to training after an injury.

By six weeks after the birth, more vigorous exercise programs can be resumed gradually. The emphasis is always on individual programs due to the differences in birth experiences and recovery. There is no one-size-fits-all postnatal exercise program. Bear in mind that your joints may still be lax due to the hormonal changes that occurred during pregnancy, so jerky, bouncy exercise is definitely not recommended.

The good news about postnatal exercise

Recent research shows that moderately intense postnatal exercise is beneficial for reducing postnatal depression, and for weight loss, and has no detrimental effect on breast milk supply or composition.

Postnatal exercise recommendations

- Allow time for internal healing.
- Begin your exercise slowly to prevent strain. Let the type and intensity of your chosen exercise reflect your stage of recovery. Do not expect to be back to your pre-pregnancy shape by any magical date.
- Be realistic when planning your exercise program. Allow for ligament laxity, muscle stretch and weakness, fatigue, breastfeeding, and the time it takes to mother a new baby.
- Include specific recovery exercises in your program – pelvic floor, abdominal and back retraining exercises – for both core stability and strength. (Also use these muscles correctly when you lift or carry, by maintaining a long spine and drawing in your abdomen.)

- Exercise with other mothers. Walking with a pram has been shown to be an effective way to manage postnatal depression, and can be an enjoyable social time as well.
- Exercise to feel good rather than to achieve competition-level fitness.

19

Having a baby

Maureen Johnson, Penelope Sheehan

Whether it's your first baby or your fourth, your feelings about birth may range from fear and trepidation to excitement (and maybe, for some, just a little impatience). You may also find that as soon as your pregnancy is obvious, your friends, family and total strangers will regale you with stories about their own labours and births. You will be offered a mountain of advice – much of it welcome, some of it less so – about what you can do to prepare and how you can have the perfect birth (a guarantee of that could make someone very rich!).

In this chapter we describe the process of labour and birth to help you understand what is happening during each stage; we discuss pain management throughout labour and birth; and we also talk about breastfeeding and the early days with your baby. The only thing that can be guaranteed about labour, birth and the early moments with your newborn is that the whole experience will be very powerful.

Labour

At around 30 weeks, the conversations with your doctor or midwife will turn to your baby's birth.

A birth plan

You may have particular ideas about the kind of birth you want, who you want to be there, how you would prefer to manage your pain and your preferences if things don't go as you had hoped. Many women and their partners write a birth plan, so that when you go into labour everyone involved in the birth of your baby knows what you want. Writing a birth plan is a useful exercise also because it can help you think through and prepare for a range of scenarios.

Your birth plan will be most useful if it allows for flexibility and is based on the philosophy that anything can happen during labour, and probably will. Too rigid a birth plan can lead to potential disappointment and, for some women, an unreasonable sense of failure. Unreasonable because while there are many things you can do during pregnancy to maintain your health and improve the chances of a good labour and birth, no one has complete control over how they give birth. Labour and birth are collectively a powerful, life-changing event; a unique experience where your body is in control. Generally speaking, the best you can do is to keep calm and let your body get on with it.

In most instances babies make their way into the world with little help, but sometimes the birth process doesn't work as well as it should and the baby needs some assistance. In past generations, when labour and birth didn't follow the path they should, women and babies were less likely to survive. While intervention during the birth process is not ideal, it's important to remember that it is occasionally necessary and saves the lives of women and babies who might have died in the past.

Nowadays, mainstream Australia has one of the lowest maternal and infant death rates in the world and, while some of this can be attributed to our improved living conditions, it is also because of our access to sophisticated health, midwifery and obstetric care. Unfortunately, these successes are still not reflected in Aboriginal and Torres Strait Islander communities, especially in more remote areas of the country where living conditions and other social, cultural and historical issues, as well as access to good health services, continue to differentially impact on the health of Aboriginal and Torres Strait Islander women and babies.

Support in labour

The people you have around you during your birth can actually improve your experience. In fact, research shows that having the right support people can reduce your need for pain relief, assisted vaginal birth or a caesarean birth. It is important that you have people with you who make you feel safe and free to express what you need in the moment, even if that includes you telling them to leave the room!

There are times when you will need peace and quiet, so it may be best not to have too many people around you. Your partner, mother, sister or best friend are all possible candidates. It is a good idea to talk through your birth plan with the person or people you choose to support you during your labour so they are familiar with how you would like to give birth if things go according to plan, or your alternative choices if they do not.

I got very nervous during early labour and my husband, Adam, distracted me by telling me stories about people we were watching out the window. He made me laugh but he also knew when to be quiet and not say anything at all.

There were times, later in the labour and during the more intense moments, when I swore something was wrong. He didn't try to contradict me; instead, he calmly told me that he would get the midwife to check.

I really wanted to labour and to give birth with very little medical intervention, but because I was overdue and the contractions were erratic, the obstetrician thought I might need some help. Adam helped me to weigh up the risks of waiting a little longer and advocated on my behalf. The obstetrician kept a close eye on things but did let me wait. After that, our daughter was born very quickly. I think without Adam there, medical intervention would have been inevitable.

When to go to hospital

It's not always clear whether labour has started. If you are not sure or you are worrying, call your hospital. Sometimes the process of talking through your symptoms is enough to help you to relax. Alternatively, during the course of the conversation, you and the midwife may decide it's time to go to the hospital.

The midwife will ask you how and where you feel your contractions, how often the contractions come and how long they last. This will help her to know how much your labour has progressed.

If there are strong signs of labour, such as your waters breaking, regular contractions or blood loss, it's a good idea to contact the hospital anyway.

If you are not in labour or if the labour is not yet established, depending on your situation, it is generally better to stay at home. Research has shown that women labour much better if they stay at home in the early stages.

Stages of labour

There are three distinct stages of labour and while each woman's experience is unique, there are general signs that most women experience. If you are able to recognise them (which isn't always easy), they can help you to know at what stage you are in your labour.

The first stage

This stage begins when the cervix begins to soften and to open. The first stage is complete when the cervix has opened to around 10 centimetres.

In the very early stages of labour, the cervix begins to soften and becomes quite thin. This can go on for hours; days, even. During this early stage you may feel nothing at all for some time. Eventually you might feel some pain and discomfort, but the contractions are irregular, having not settled into a pattern.

In early labour you may have:

- a blood-stained mucus discharge called a 'show'
- lower back pain
- period-like pain that comes and goes
- loose bowel motions
- a sudden gush or a slow leak of fluid from the vagina, when your waters break or your membranes rupture. The waters should be clear or slightly pink. (A greenish or bloody colour can indicate a problem with the baby so in this case you should see a doctor or contact your hospital immediately.)
- a desire to vomit (it is quite common to vomit during labour)

During this stage it's a good idea to stay at home for as long as you can. Have regular snacks, rest as much as possible and if it's night-time try to sleep. A bath or a shower can be helpful, and it's a good idea to go to the toilet regularly. Your body is preparing for birth and you can help by resting, eating for energy and emptying your bowels if you can.

Eventually, towards the end of the first stage of labour, you will start to feel a little more restless and tired, and your pain will become more intense. It will come like waves, starting small and building to a climax and then falling away again. As you move closer to the second stage, the interval between each wave will be smaller. When there is less than three to five minutes between each wave, it is time to go to the hospital.

The second stage

The second stage describes the period of time from when the cervix is fully dilated to when the baby is born.

In the second stage you may have:

- longer and stronger contractions, with a one- to two-minute break in between

- increased pressure in your bottom
- the desire or urge to push
- shaky cramps, nausea and vomiting
- stretching and burning feelings in your vagina

During this stage the best thing you can do is to concentrate on your contractions and rest in between. Try to let go and allow your body to do

Labouring and giving birth in water

These days, many hospitals are set up to allow you to labour in a bath, which can help with relaxation and pain management. Depending on the hospital, it may also be possible to stay in the bath for the birth as well. This will usually depend on whether the attending midwife or obstetrician is trained in water births and whether your birth is progressing without any problems. The midwife needs unobstructed access to your baby during the birthing process and needs to be able to get you out of the bath should anything go awry. If these are both possible, a water birth should also be possible.

When your baby is born into water, there is no risk that they will drown. The newborn has several protective mechanisms to stop them from breathing under water. When your baby is in the uterus, they receive all their oxygen through the umbilical cord, via the placenta. Your baby doesn't actually breathe inside the uterus, but they do practise breathing by moving the appropriate muscles and the diaphragm in a regular and rhythmic pattern. This happens from as early as 10 weeks.

Just before labour, hormones from the placenta cause the baby's breathing movements to slow down or stop. This is to prevent your baby from taking in fluid as they move through the birth canal.

The newborn also has fluids in their lungs, which makes it hard for the baby to breathe in water. And newborns come into the world with a 'dive reflex'. This is an automatic response that babies have up to the age of six months and it assists them with breastfeeding. The dive reflex occurs when liquid hits the back of the throat and causes the glottis to close, so that liquid is swallowed rather than breathed in.

If the birth is uncomplicated and conducted safely, there is no risk of your baby breathing before they are brought to the surface of the water.

what it needs to do. You may need to try different positions: sitting, on all fours, squatting, standing or walking. If you feel hot, a cold face washer can be very soothing. A bath or shower can also be helpful at this point. Keep up your fluids and rest when you can.

Pushing

When the urge to push arrives, it can be overwhelming. The pushing phase varies between women, but can last for up to two hours, though it is usually less if you have had a baby before. Aside from the urge to push, you are likely to feel:

- pressure, and a strong urge to go to the toilet
- stretching and burning in your vagina
- the baby's head moving down

As hard as it may seem, the best thing you can do during this phase is to try to breathe deeply, relax and follow your body's urge to push. Trust and listen to your midwife or obstetrician, who will guide you through this phase.

The third stage

The third stage begins after your baby is born and finishes when the placenta and membranes have been delivered.

In the third stage you may have:

- more contractions to expel the placenta
- a feeling of fullness in your vagina

The midwife will usually pull on the cord to deliver the placenta, but may ask you to help by gently pushing.

Managing pain in labour

Labour is painful – that goes without saying – but the way each woman experiences labour is unique to her. Pain can often be managed with relaxation techniques and trusting your body to know what to do. Fear, tension and resistance are a normal response to losing control and not quite knowing what to expect next. Paradoxically, giving over to and trusting your body will help you to relax and to manage your pain.

Your pain can also vary according to the environment in which you give birth, your support people, whether you've had a baby before, the position of your baby and the method of pain management you use.

There are a number of natural and medical methods you can use to manage your labour pain.

Natural pain relief

Active birth, or moving around and changing positions a lot, is one of the most important things you can do to manage the pain of labour and birth. Movement and the freedom to move can help you to cope with the contractions. If you stay upright, gravity will also help your baby to descend through your pelvis.

Heat and water can help to ease tension and backache in labour. Both hot and cold packs are useful, as is being immersed in water in either a shower or a bath.

Touch and massage can reduce muscle tension, as well as providing a distraction between and during contractions. Practise with your partner during your pregnancy and find out how you like to be massaged. At times during labour, you will find massage or touch useful, but at other stages you might find them irritating (an important piece of information for your support people!).

Similarly, some women use music during labour. Music is a good distraction and can be very relaxing, but it can also be suddenly and unexpectedly annoying. Be prepared for any eventuality.

Complementary therapies such as acupuncture or acupressure can also be very effective during labour, but should only be practised by qualified practitioners.

Non-medical pain relief

TENS or Trans-Electrical Nerve Stimulation
The TENS machine is a small, portable, battery-operated device that is worn on the body. The box is attached by wires to sticky pads, which are stuck to the skin. Small electrical pulses are transmitted to the body, like little electric shocks. They are said to ease the pain of labour.

While there is no harm is using a TENS machine, there is not a lot of evidence to show they are effective. However, some women say that they find them very helpful.

Intradermal water injections for back pain
Many women suffer from lower back pain, which persists throughout their labour. Midwives can use a technique involving sterile water injections into the lower back. Usually the injections are given in four different places in your lower back, just beneath the skin. The injections cause a strong, stinging sensation, which lasts for up to 30 seconds before

disappearing, along with the back pain. The injections can bring up to two hours of pain relief to your lower back, but you can still feel the contractions. Even with the back pain gone, some women will still find it hard to manage the pain of the contractions; it's not surprising then that research evidence shows that women who have intradermal injections may still need other pain relief. There are no side effects for you or your baby.

Medical pain relief

You and your carers should discuss your preferences for pain relief before you go into labour. You can also record your preferences for pain relief in your birth plan. During your labour, the midwife or obstetrician will continue to guide you and work with you, according to your expressed desires.

Gas

The gas given to women in labour is a mixture of nitrous oxide and oxygen. It is sometimes known as 'laughing gas'. It helps to take the edge off the pain during a contraction. It is inhaled during a contraction through a mask or a mouthpiece. It may make you feel a little nauseous or light-headed, and give you a dry mouth for a short time. There are no side effects for you or your baby.

Pethidine

Pethidine is a strong painkiller given by injection. It helps to reduce the severity of the pain of the contractions, but does not take it away completely. It can take up to 30 minutes to work and can make you and your baby sleepy. Sometimes pethidine may contribute to breathing problems in your baby if it is given within two hours of birth. In this case, another medication called naloxone (also injected) might be given to your baby after the birth to reverse the effects of the pethidine. Babies who have this injection need closer observation for a few hours after birth.

Due to the relatively short effect it has, pethidine is mostly helpful for women who are in well-established labour.

Epidural

An epidural is a local anaesthetic that is injected into your back (not the spinal cord). After an epidural you will have reduced or altered sensation from the waist down, so you can't walk around but you are still awake. A very thin tube will be left in your back so the anaesthetic can be topped up. Sometimes the tube is attached to a machine so that you can give yourself doses when you need them. The doses are controlled so you can't give yourself too many.

An epidural can take away the sensation to pass urine, so you will also need a urinary catheter, which is a thin tube inserted through the urethra (where your urine comes out) and into your bladder to drain your urine. You will also need an IV (intravenous) drip inserted into your hand to make sure you are getting enough fluids. A cardiotocography, or CTG machine, will continuously monitor both the baby's heart and your contractions. Your blood pressure will also be monitored closely.

The benefits of an epidural are that it actually takes away the pain of contractions, it can be effective for hours and can be increased in strength if you need to have an emergency caesarean. In a long labour, it can allow you to sleep and recover your strength. If a woman's blood pressure is high, an epidural might also be recommended for its ability to reduce hypertension.

The disadvantages of an epidural are that you are unable to move around during your labour, although you can still sit or lie on your side. Having an epidural does increase the risk that instruments will be needed to help deliver your baby: you may still feel the urge to push when you reach that stage, but the sensation is reduced.

Monitoring your baby during labour

All babies are monitored during labour, which means the midwife or obstetrician keeps a check on the baby's heartbeat and other signs that the baby might not be well. The level of monitoring will depend on your medical history, whether there are any problems with your baby or whether there are any expected problems with the birth. Monitoring can be done in the following ways:

- **Listening** – the midwife or doctor places an ear trumpet or Doppler on your abdomen and listens to the baby's heartbeat through your abdomen.

- **Continuous external monitoring** – this is when an electronic monitor is attached to a belt around your abdomen. The monitor continuously records on a paper printout the baby's heartbeat and the mother's contractions. Some monitors restrict your movement. If this concerns you, ask if there's one available that lets you move around.

- **Internal monitoring** – this involves the use of an electronic monitor that attaches a probe through the vagina to the baby's head. It is only used if the quality of the external monitoring is poor.

- **Fetal scalp lactate** – a few drops of blood are taken from your baby's scalp (like a pinprick). It gives an immediate result on the baby's condition in labour. Doctors use this test when they need to get more information than they can from continuous heart rate monitoring. The result will show if the baby has an inadequate oxygen supply and needs to be born immediately.

Assisted birth

Sometimes labour doesn't go as planned and a baby needs help to come into the world. Help can involve relatively simple procedures such as breaking the mother's membranes (waters) to more medically demanding procedures such as a caesarean birth. While some women have a preference for assisted births, others would prefer no interventions at all. From a medical perspective, interventions are only introduced when they are necessary to preserve the health of the mother or the baby.

Induction of labour

Approximately one quarter of women have an induction of labour. The most common reasons are:

- The woman has particular health concerns (such as diabetes or high blood pressure).
- There are concerns for the baby's wellbeing.
- The pregnancy has lasted more than 10 to 12 days beyond the due date and there is a risk that the placenta can no longer sustain the baby's life.
- The mother's waters have already broken, but her contractions have not started naturally.

You will only be offered an induction if your health or your baby's health is at risk.

Usually, you would make the decision to have an induction after it has been recommended by an obstetrician. Your doctor or midwife should explain to you:

- why an induction has been recommended, and the potential benefits
- the potential risks of continuing your pregnancy until labour starts naturally
- the potential risks of having an induction of labour
- what they propose to do in your particular situation

Some women choose to wait and see whether natural labour will start, but it's a good idea to make a well-informed decision and to be aware of the risks and benefits of your particular situation.

How is labour induced?

Before starting the induction, the doctor or midwife usually begins with an assessment of the cervix. The examination takes only a few minutes, but it can be a little uncomfortable. Based on this examination the doctor or midwife recommends one of the following methods of induction:

- artificially breaking the membranes or 'waters'
- artificially breaking the membranes or 'waters' and oxytocin
- prostaglandin
- a cervical ripening balloon catheter

An induction can involve one or several of these methods. While not having an induction can put the health and even the life of the baby at risk, having an induction also carries a number of risks. The doctor or midwife will explain the risks associated with your particular pregnancy.

Artificial rupture of membranes

If your waters have not broken, a procedure called an artificial rupture of membranes, or ARM, may be recommended. This is when the midwife or doctor makes a hole in the woman's membrane sac to release the fluid inside. This procedure is done through the vagina using a small instrument. Sometimes releasing the waters is enough to get things going, and labour will commence. However, most women also need oxytocin to start the contractions.

Risks and things to be aware of:

- The vaginal examination needed to perform this procedure may cause some discomfort.
- Although ARM is usually straightforward, it can increase the risk of cord prolapse, bleeding and infection.

Oxytocin

Oxytocin is the hormone that causes contractions. A synthetic version of oxytocin is given to women when the membranes are broken and contractions don't start naturally. Oxytocin is given through a drip, and enters a vein in the arm. Once contractions begin, the rate of the drip is adjusted so that contractions occur regularly until your baby is born. This process can take several hours. The baby's heart rate will be monitored throughout labour using a CTG machine.

Risks and things to be aware of:

- The ability to move around will be limited by the drip and the CTG monitor. While it will be okay to stand up or sit down, it will not be possible to have a bath or move from room to room.

- Very occasionally oxytocin causes the uterus to contract too frequently, which may affect the pattern of the baby's heartbeat. If this happens you will be asked to lie on your left side and the drip will be slowed to lessen the number and reduce the strength of the contractions. Another drug may be given to counteract the oxytocin.

Prostaglandin

Prostaglandin is a naturally occurring hormone that prepares your body for labour. A synthetic version has been developed to mimic the effect of the hormone. This is inserted into the vagina, usually in the form of a gel. It can also be inserted in the form of a pessary, which slowly releases the prostaglandin over 12 to 24 hours. When the prostaglandin is in place, you will be advised to lie down and rest for at least 30 minutes. Once the prostaglandin has been inserted you will need to remain in hospital.

When the prostaglandin takes effect, your cervix will soften and open. If you have been given the gel, you may need one, two or three doses (given every six to eight hours). When the cervix is soft and open, your body is prepared for labour. The next steps will vary from woman to woman – some might need an ARM to break their waters, and some might need oxytocin to stimulate the contractions.

Risks and things to be aware of:

- Prostaglandin sometimes causes vaginal soreness. However, there is no evidence to suggest that labour induced with prostaglandin is any more painful than a labour that has started naturally.

- A minority of women will react to the prostaglandin and experience nausea, vomiting or diarrhoea, but this is rare.

- Very occasionally prostaglandin can cause the uterus to contract too much, which may affect the pattern of the baby's heartbeat. If this happens you will be asked to lie on your left side. You may be given a medication to relax the uterus. If you have received a pessary, this may need to be removed.

Cervical ripening balloon catheter

Prostaglandin does not suit all women and there will be circumstances in which a doctor may recommend using a cervical ripening balloon catheter. This catheter is inserted into the cervix and the balloons are inflated with saline, which apply pressure to the cervix. The pressure should soften and open the cervix, preparing the body for labour.

When the catheter is in place, you will need to stay in hospital but you will be able to move around normally. Fifteen hours after the catheter has been inserted or when the catheter falls out, you will be re-examined. During this time the midwives will periodically check you and listen to your baby's heart.

What happens next will vary from woman to woman – some might need an ARM to break their waters, and some might need oxytocin to stimulate the contractions.

Risks and things to be aware of:

- The vaginal examination needed to perform this procedure may cause some discomfort.

Forceps birth

Occasionally forceps are used to help the baby out of the vagina. They may be used if you are too exhausted to push, the baby is in an awkward position or there are concerns for your baby's wellbeing. Sometimes the forceps leave a mark on the baby's cheeks, but these soon fade. You will usually need an episiotomy (see below).

Vacuum (ventouse) birth

A vacuum or ventouse is more commonly used than forceps. The vacuum cup is made of plastic and is attached to a suction device. The cup is inserted into the vagina and creates a vacuum against the baby's head. This helps the doctor to gently pull out the baby. It may cause a raised bruise on the baby's head, but this soon fades – usually within a day. You may need an episiotomy.

Episiotomy

Sometimes it is necessary to make the vaginal opening bigger, especially if you need a forceps birth or if the baby is distressed. An episiotomy is a cut made in the perineum (the tissue between the vagina and the anus). A local anaesthetic is used to numb the area and you will need stitches afterwards. The stitches will dissolve by themselves and you will be offered icepacks to reduce the swelling and pain. The swelling will usually go down after 48 hours and the pain will subside after a week.

Caesarean birth

A caesarean is a major surgical operation in which your baby is born through a cut in your abdomen and uterus. It is usually performed under a spinal or epidural anaesthesia. In some cases it is necessary to use a general anaesthetic so that you are asleep throughout.

Some caesarean births are planned in advance (an elective caesarean) because of existing problems with your pregnancy. In other cases, the decision to perform a caesarean is made during the course of labour. This is called an emergency caesarean.

An emergency caesarean is recommended for the following reasons:

- The doctors and midwives are concerned for the baby's wellbeing.
- Labour is not progressing.
- There are maternal complications, such as severe bleeding or severe pre-eclampsia.
- There is a life-threatening emergency for the mother or the baby.

What to expect if you need an emergency caesarean:

- You may be in the operating theatre for an hour or more.
- Unless you are having a general anaesthetic, in most cases your partner can be with you in the operating theatre.
- Most hospitals will ensure that a midwife stays to look after you and your baby in the theatre and the recovery area.
- Unless you have had a general anaesthetic, skin-to-skin contact with your baby will be encouraged immediately after the birth. If you have had a general anaesthetic, you will be given the opportunity to have skin-to-skin contact as soon as you are able.
- The midwife will help you with breastfeeding once you are recovered sufficiently to start feeding.
- If the baby is unwell or needs to be monitored, he or she may need to go to the special (intensive) care unit. In some cases the baby may need to go to a different hospital, which has a higher level of care.
- After surgery, you will be offered a number of different pain-relieving medications as and when you need them.

You will be encouraged to express breast milk if your baby is unable to feed from the breast. This will start as soon as possible after the birth.

There are risks and certain outcomes associated with a caesarean birth. They include:

- Side effects and complications of anaesthesia, including: nausea, drowsiness, dizziness, short-term memory loss and in rare circumstances an allergic reaction.

- Some pain. During a caesarean, several layers of body tissue are cut and then repaired, so post-surgical pain is to be expected. This can usually be managed well with medications.

- In a small number of cases, infection of the wound and bladder. This can be treated with antibiotics.

- A fever, which will usually be due to an infection.

- Blood clots, which can form after surgery. If a clot is in the lung (pulmonary embolism) it can be very serious.

Vaginal birth after a previous caesarean (VBAC)

If you have had a caesarean birth, there may be implications for your subsequent births. You will need to make a choice about whether to have another caesarean or whether to attempt a vaginal birth after caesarean birth (VBAC). Both options carry a level of risk. Another caesarean carries the usual risks, while the main risk of a VBAC is that the scar on the uterus will rupture, which can be very painful, and in some cases life-threatening. Between one and two in 200 women who attempt a VBAC will suffer a ruptured scar.

Most women who attempt a vaginal birth after a caesarean succeed (70 per cent). Thirty per cent of women who attempt a vaginal birth end up, for any number of reasons, having an emergency caesarean.

Many women who have had a previous caesarean birth find the prospect of a vaginal birth healing, particularly if the first caesarean was unplanned or traumatic. Because both paths carry a level of risk, unless there are particular health reasons why you would be advised to take a particular course of action, the decision is ultimately yours and should be based on your own preferences, desires and values. Your midwife or doctor will usually discuss this with you at around the 26-week mark. It's a good idea to ask lots of questions about the specific risks and benefits for you.

- Not being able to hold or feed your baby immediately after the birth, which may have implications for breastfeeding. This is only likely to be a problem if you have had a general anaesthetic. However, in this case, you should be able to hold and feed your baby as soon as you are more alert. It is a good idea to talk to the midwives or your obstetrician before the operation about breastfeeding, particularly if your caesarean is planned.
- Adhesions or scar tissue forming in your abdomen, which can cause ongoing pain and have implications for future abdominal surgery.
- The necessity for a hysterectomy. This is a possible but rare complication with any birth option.

After you have had one caesarean birth, the risk of complications increase with each subsequent caesarean. For example, in future pregnancies there is an increased chance of the placenta implanting into or over the scar. This condition is referred to as placenta praevia or placenta accreta.

Your newborn

After your baby is born, the most important thing is for you to spend quiet time together as a family. Skin-to-skin contact in the time immediately after the birth will help your baby to feel secure, warm and comfortable in new surrounds. It is also the first step in preparing you and your baby for breastfeeding.

When you're ready, the umbilical cord is clamped and cut. These days it has become something of a ritual for partners or support people to cut the cord. The cutting doesn't hurt either the mother or baby and the piece of cord that is left behind on the baby's belly will eventually dry up and drop off.

The midwife or doctor will assess your baby's Apgar score. This is an assessment of your baby's overall condition, including how the baby looks, breathing, heart rate, and colour. The Apgar score is taken at one minute and then five minutes after the birth and is a good measure of how well your baby has made the transition from the womb (intrauterine) into the world (extrauterine). The baby's weight is also recorded and, with your permission, your baby will have some tests and injections.

The recommended tests and medications for a newborn baby in Australia are:

- **Newborn vitamin K**. In their first eight days of life, babies can be deficient in Vitamin K, which can have serious consequences. An injection of Vitamin K ensures that your baby has adequate levels of the vitamin, which helps their blood to clot and prevents severe bleeding. If vitamin K levels are too low, even the smallest of cuts can bleed for a dangerously long time. Bleeding can happen in other parts of the body as well, such as the brain.

- **Hepatitis B**. Hepatitis B affects the liver and is spread by blood and other body fluids such as saliva. Adults don't necessarily know they are infected with hepatitis B and some people are infected even though they don't fall within the usual risk categories. This is why all babies in Australia are offered immunisation at birth and throughout their infancy until they are fully immunised at the age of four. If a parent is known to have hepatitis B, the baby will be offered an immuno-globulin injection in hospital to give them immediate protection from the virus.

Newborn neonatal screening

In Australia, it is recommended that babies are tested for a number of uncommon but very serious medical conditions. In most cases, if a baby is found to have one of these conditions, they can be treated early on and grow and develop normally. Conditions that are tested for include congenital hypothyroidism, cystic fibrosis, amino acid disorders such as phenylketonuria (PKU), fatty oxidation disorder and other rare metabolic disorders.

The test for these is usually done between 48 and 72 hours after the birth and involves making a tiny prick on the baby's heel to produce a very small amount of blood, enough to put four spots on a piece of blotting card. The blood on the card is tested and if the results are normal you will not be contacted. If your baby is found to have a medical condition you will be contacted. The card is kept in storage for future reference. Each state has slightly different arrangements for storage.

Hearing screen

With your consent, a routine hearing test is done soon after the baby is born. A small number of babies are born with hearing loss that can affect their speech and language skills. Hearing loss may not be obvious in the first few weeks but can be detected using this test.

You and your new baby

There is no right or wrong way to feel after the birth of a baby. Some women will feel exhilarated and others will worry that they are not feeling as happy or excited as they should. Sometimes the flurry of visitors and excitement around the birth of a baby can be overwhelming and some-times it is exactly what you want and need.

No matter how you are feeling, it's a good idea to give yourself some time to adjust to your new situation, and to rest and recover from the birth. We live in the age of the perceived 'super mum' and often have high expectations of how quickly we should recover and what we should be able to do, instead of taking our own time to rest, recover and care for ourselves.

Breastfeeding

You and your midwife or doctor will start talking about breastfeeding in early pregnancy. Breast milk provides all the nutrition your baby needs for the first six months of life and can give your baby most of their nutri-tion for the first year of their life and beyond. Breast milk also helps to protect your baby against a range of infections, allergies and other medical conditions.

Even if your baby is born prematurely or is ill, your breast milk is the perfect food for growth and development. Breast milk protects babies against gastroenteritis and diarrhoea, ear and chest infections, allergies, diabetes and other medical conditions. Breastfeeding is also known to reduce the risk of sudden infant death syndrome (SIDS).

Breastfeeding also has benefits for you. It causes the uterus to contract and reduces the amount of normal post-partum bleeding and the amount of lochia. Excessive bleeding after the birth can affect your iron levels and make you feel very tired for many weeks. Breastfeeding may also help you to return to your pre-pregnancy weight; and it reduces your risk of developing breast and ovarian cancer and osteoporosis in the future. It is also convenient; it costs nothing and there is very little preparation before each feed. Being able to offer your baby a breast in the middle of the night is also a lot easier than preparing and sterilising bottles!

Skin-to-skin contact immediately after the birth triggers a strong hormonal response in your body, which is linked to greater breastfeeding success. This does not mean that if you don't have skin-to-skin contact for a particular reason you won't be able to breastfeed – it is just one thing that has been shown to help you and your baby succeed.

The first few days after the birth of your baby are when you and your baby learn to breastfeed. In that time your breasts are producing the first milk, known as colostrum. Colostrum is a sticky, yellow substance and highly nutritious (although there is not a lot of it) and plays a significant role in protecting your newborn baby against disease. Your breasts are still soft during this time, but as your milk 'comes in' – that is, it changes from colostrum to mature milk, which has a more watery consistency – your breasts can become quite full and firm. This is when things may become a little more challenging for some women and their babies, though generally you will move through this time with relative ease.

We often expect breastfeeding to come easily because it is 'natural', but, like any new skill, it needs to be learnt. It requires time, patience and plenty of practice, as well as an acceptance that it may not always go as one would hope.

Like many of the decisions around pregnancy, birth and parenting, breastfeeding is subject to a range of views. No one disagrees that it is the ideal way to feed a baby and that it has great benefits for both mother and baby. Sometimes, though, the early challenges of breastfeeding can undermine the warmth and ease of the early moments with your baby – moments that are, paradoxically, key to promoting breastfeeding success. The perceived pressure to succeed at feeding your baby this way can lead to a strong sense of failure in the face of challenges and hurdles. In the case of breastfeeding, even the smallest of hurdles can lead women to quietly seek out alternative solutions too soon.

Breastfeeding is an activity around which mythologies seem to thrive – the most striking is that there are women who can breastfeed and women who can't. In fact, many women experience breastfeeding hurdles, but more often than not, and with good guidance and support, the obstacles and problems can be overcome. And while it's true there are some women who can't breastfeed, almost all can. The key is to try to relax, trust your instincts and – crucially – seek help while you are learning, or as soon as things go wrong. If you don't like the way a midwife or doctor is working with you to breastfeed, ask to see someone else. Many midwives and lactation specialists are highly skilled in the art of teaching women to breastfeed in a way that is very supportive.

There are a number of general tips most experts will give to promote successful breastfeeding in the early days:

- Feed according to your baby's need in the first days after the birth.

- Have your baby in the same room as you, both in the hospital and at home, in the first weeks to help you to recognise when your baby is hungry, tired or in need of a cuddle. This also helps you to learn when your baby needs to be fed.

- Try to set aside teats, dummies and supplementary (artificial) feeds when your baby is first learning to breastfeed, mostly because they can confuse your baby and affect your milk supply. If the baby has fluids other than breast milk they breastfeed for less time and your milk supply will decrease. Frequent, unrestricted sucking at the breast will satisfy your baby.

Initially, your baby will feed between seven and 12 times in 24 hours, just as adults need to eat and drink up to 12 times in a similar period. Remember breast milk is both food and drink for your baby, so they need to feed often. This will settle over time. Feeding when your baby wants it, feeding frequently and feeding well will help you to make enough milk for your baby's needs.

Breast milk is enough for your baby for the first six months of their life. They need no other food or drink in that time. You can be confident that your baby is getting enough food in the early weeks if they have six or more wet nappies and at least one bowel motion a day. It is also a good sign if your baby settles after most feeds.

Breastfeeding up to six months is ideal, but any breastfeeding will be good for your baby. Breastfeeding gives you an opportunity to connect with your baby in a profound and deeply satisfying way. It is a physical and emotional bond that stays with you for many years afterwards.

A small number of women are unable to breastfeed their baby and, in this case, you may have mixed feelings about not breastfeeding. It might be important to talk to your partner or a friend about how you are feeling. Formula simply isn't the same as breast milk, but formula will provide nutrition to your baby to grow well. And you can still bond with your baby, especially as you hold your baby close as they feed, and make feeding a special time for you both. Be sure, though, that you follow carefully the instructions to prepare the formula and sterilise the bottles you are using after every feed: incorrectly made formula and unclean bottles can make your baby sick.

20

Bleeding, miscarriage and stillbirth

Maureen Johnson

Most pregnancies end well, with a healthy baby. Occasionally, though, things go wrong. Some pregnancies never develop properly; others will suffer a problem along the way. Whatever the reason, a problem with pregnancy can cause great distress and sadness. The worst outcomes are when the fetus has an illness that cannot be treated, when a pregnancy ends prematurely, or when the baby is born dead (a stillbirth).

Bleeding

Reasons for bleeding during your pregnancy can include miscarriage, ectopic pregnancy, placental abruption and placenta praevia. It is also possible that you will have lots of tests and investigations but the reason for your bleeding will never be found. Many women will bleed in pregnancy but will go on to have a normal, healthy pregnancy. Any bleeding during pregnancy, however, should be investigated by a health professional.

Bleeding in early pregnancy

Bleeding in early pregnancy is quite common and does not always mean that you are having a miscarriage. One in four women will bleed in early pregnancy and many will go on to have a healthy baby.

Investigating early bleeding
The tests that you have will usually depend on how pregnant you are. You are likely to have an ultrasound or a blood test – to measure the amount of pregnancy hormone in your blood – or both.

Ultrasound
Before six weeks, the embryo is so small it can be very difficult to see the baby's heart using ultrasound, so it is not likely to give any definite

answers about the future of the pregnancy. The benefit of an early ultrasound is, however, that it can locate an ectopic pregnancy – a pregnancy growing in a fallopian tube. An ectopic pregnancy can have very serious outcomes for the mother and needs to be treated immediately.

Usually a vaginal ultrasound is used because it offers the best possible view of your pregnancy at this stage. A vaginal ultrasound is a narrow probe, which is put inside the vagina and feels much like an internal examination. It is quite safe.

If a heartbeat is found during an ultrasound, it is likely that your pregnancy will continue with no further problems. In this scenario a woman's chances of having a miscarriage are fewer than one in twenty.

Blood tests

A blood test can measure the level of pregnancy hormone hCG, which changes depending on how pregnant you are. If the pregnancy hormone is rising more slowly than is usual, it might mean that you are miscarrying or the pregnancy is ectopic. Sometimes, though, it is simply due to unusual hormonal patterns in an otherwise normal pregnancy. If the pregnancy hormone is falling, it usually means the pregnancy is ending and miscarriage is imminent.

Bleeding in later pregnancy

Placental abruption

Placental abruption is the most common cause of bleeding during the second half of pregnancy and is often associated with abdominal pain or tenderness. Placental abruption is when part, or all, of the placenta separates from the wall of the uterus before the birth of your baby. The amount of bleeding varies and the cause is not always known. Sometimes there is no bleeding but you will have sudden and severe abdominal pain. Treatment may involve monitoring you and your baby, bed rest and, in more serious cases, the birth of your baby.

Placenta praevia

This is when some or the entire placenta implants in the lower part of the uterus, instead of being attached to the top part of the uterus. When the cervix starts to open or if the uterus contracts, the mother (not the baby) can bleed from the placenta. It can be quite serious and generally you will be admitted to hospital for careful monitoring of you and your baby. In most cases you will need a caesarean birth.

Miscarriage

Miscarriage happens when a pregnancy stops growing. Eventually, the pregnancy tissue will pass out of the body. Some women will feel crampy, period-like pain and in most cases there will be vaginal bleeding.

Miscarriage is very common in the first few weeks of pregnancy. Studies show that up to one in five women who know they are pregnant will have a miscarriage before 20 weeks. Most of these happen in the first 12 weeks. The actual rate of miscarriage is even higher because some women have very early miscarriages without ever realising that they were pregnant.

If a woman miscarries it is unlikely that she will miscarry again, and it is very unusual that she would miscarry a third time. If a woman does miscarry three or more times, there is usually a reason and tests can be done to look for a cause. Testing is not usually offered to women who miscarry once or twice because it is unlikely that anything would be found.

What causes a miscarriage?

Usually no treatable cause is found for a miscarriage. Research tells us that about half of all miscarriages happen because the chromosomes in the embryo are abnormal and the pregnancy isn't developing properly. In this case, miscarriage is nature's way of dealing with an abnormal embryo. Nothing can be done to prevent miscarriage from occurring if a pregnancy is developing abnormally.

Miscarriages are more common in older women than younger women, largely because chromosomal abnormalities are more common with increasing age. They are also more common in women who smoke and in women who drink more than three alcoholic drinks per week in the first 12 weeks of pregnancy. Research also suggests that miscarriage is more common in women who drink more than 500 mg of caffeine per day; this is about three to five cups of coffee.

Some medical conditions in the mother, such as uncontrolled diabetes, fibroids or thyroid problems, can lead to miscarriage. Rare medical conditions that affect blood clotting can also cause miscarriage. Women who have three or more miscarriages in a row are likely to be checked for these conditions. Having a very high fever can also lead to miscarriage, but minor infections, such as the common cold, are not harmful.

Finally, early tests in pregnancy, such as chorionic villus sampling (CVS) and amniocentesis, carry a very small risk of miscarriage. These are tests that use a needle inserted into the uterus.

Preventing miscarriage

Miscarriages happen to the healthiest of women. Nevertheless, being healthy will increase your chances of sustaining a healthy pregnancy. Don't smoke, modify your caffeine intake, avoid alcohol and where possible avoid contact with people who have a serious infectious illness.

Diagnosing a miscarriage

Women seek medical care at different stages of a miscarriage: sometimes the miscarriage has already happened and sometimes it has only just begun. A combination of symptoms, examination findings, ultrasound and blood tests will confirm whether you have had, or you are having, a miscarriage.

After examination, your doctor can usually tell you if your miscarriage is 'complete', 'incomplete' or 'missed'.

- A miscarriage is complete when all the pregnancy tissue has passed.
- A miscarriage is incomplete when some of the pregnancy tissue has passed, but some is still inside the uterus.
- A miscarriage is missed when the pregnancy has stopped growing but the tissue has not passed and there is still a sac in the uterus.

Treating miscarriage

If a miscarriage has begun, there is nothing that can be done to stop it. Any treatment you have will be aimed at avoiding heavy bleeding and infection. You may be offered medication to help the pregnancy tissue pass, or surgery to empty the tissue out of the uterus.

You may prefer to wait for nature to take its course; this is sometimes called 'expectant management' and is usually safe to do. If it isn't, the doctor will tell you.

If the miscarriage is incomplete, with just a small amount of pregnancy tissue remaining, it's probably best to take a wait-and-see approach. But if there is heavy bleeding or signs of infection, you will need treatment.

If the tissue does not pass naturally or you have signs of infection, the doctor will recommend a dilatation and curettage (D&C). A D&C is a minor operation, usually done under general anaesthetic. There is no cutting involved because the surgery can be done through the vagina. The cervix (neck of the uterus) is gently opened and the remaining pregnancy tissue is removed. Usually the doctor is not able to see a recognisable embryo.

The actual procedure usually only takes five to ten minutes, but you will need to be in the hospital for around four to five hours recovering.

You and the doctor can discuss and decide the preferred option for you.

Waiting for treatment

If you think you are having, or have had, a miscarriage you should see a doctor or go to an emergency department for a check-up. If you have heavy bleeding with clots and crampy pain, it is likely that you are passing the pregnancy tissue. The bleeding, clots and pain will usually settle when most of the pregnancy tissue has been passed. Sometimes the bleeding will continue to be heavy and you may need further treatment.

You should go to your nearest emergency department if you have:

- increased bleeding, for instance soaking two pads per hour and/or passing golf-ball-sized clots
- severe abdominal pain or shoulder pain
- fever or chills
- dizziness or fainting
- vaginal discharge that smells unpleasant
- diarrhoea or pain when you open your bowels

After a miscarriage

Whether your miscarriage was natural, assisted with medication or treated with a D&C, the following information is important.

- It is usual to have pain and bleeding after a miscarriage. It will feel similar to a period and will usually stop within two weeks. You can take ordinary painkillers with paracetamol or codeine for the pain. Your next period will usually come in around four to six weeks after a miscarriage.
- Try and avoid vaginal sex until the bleeding stops and you feel comfortable.
- You can use sanitary pads until the bleeding stops (do not use tampons).
- Wait for at least one normal period before trying to get pregnant. This is because some research suggests that you have a higher chance of another miscarriage if you get pregnant straight away.
- All contraceptive methods are safe after a miscarriage.
- See a GP in four to six weeks for a check-up.

Anti D injection after a miscarriage

It is important to have your blood group checked. If you are RhD negative and the fetus is RhD positive this can cause problems for future pregnancies. This is because the fetus's blood cells have RhD antigen attached to them, whereas yours do not. If small amounts of the fetus's blood mix with your blood, your immune system may perceive this difference as a threat and produce antibodies to fight against the fetus's blood. Once your body has made these antibodies they can't be removed. This is unlikely to have caused your miscarriage and is more likely to affect future pregnancies. That's because the process of producing antibodies takes time. Women with a negative blood type usually need an Anti D injection, which will stop the antibodies from forming.

Feelings and reactions

There is no 'right' way to feel following a miscarriage. You may experience a range of physical or emotional reactions, or you may feel very little at all. Some degree of grief is very common, even if the pregnancy wasn't planned. Partners may react quite differently, just as people can respond differently to a continuing pregnancy. Try to take it a day at a time and to acknowledge your feelings and reactions as they arise.

Most people find it helpful to talk about their feelings; this may be with your partner, other family members or close friends. Some friends and family may not understand the depth of emotion that can be attached to a pregnancy and may unreasonably expect for you to move on before you are ready. It can also be difficult to talk to family and friends if you have chosen not to share the news of the pregnancy. You may prefer to talk with a doctor, nurse or other health professional.

Some women and their partners continue to experience feelings of loss long after a miscarriage occurs. In particular it is common to feel upset around the date of the expected birth, or the anniversary of the miscarriage. Family or close friends can be a great source of support at these times. Alternatively, you may choose to seek professional support.

When a baby dies

While miscarriage is relatively common in early pregnancy, the death of a baby later in pregnancy is fortunately much less so. Babies can die right up to the date of delivery. Some babies will die during the birthing process and others may be born unwell and die very soon after the birth. No matter how or when it happens, the death of a baby is deeply distressing for parents, and their families and friends. While there are many explanations as to why babies die, each individual circumstance is unique.

Common causes of death are:

- a fetal abnormality or birth defect
- bleeding from the placenta
- the placenta not working properly
- problems with the umbilical cord
- complications during labour
- prematurity, and complications related to this
- infections

Following the death of a baby, a number of tests may be suggested to try and find the cause of death. These tests may include:

- blood tests from the mother
- examination of the placenta
- X-rays and other imaging techniques
- post-mortem examination of the baby

More about post-mortem

A post-mortem examination or an autopsy is a medical examination of the baby, which may or may not involve surgery. A post-mortem aims to find out as much as possible about why the baby died. A specialist pathologist does the examination and even though the baby is deceased, the pathologist is trained to treat the baby as they would treat anyone having an operation, with respect and care.

Parents decide how detailed a post-mortem will be. Consent can be limited to just an external examination or permission can be given for the baby to have a surgical investigation. Parents can also express their preference about organs being removed for testing. The most information will be gleaned from a full post-mortem with organ testing but in some cases it may not be necessary. For some parents information may be less important than other issues such as a timely burial or cremation, and others simply feel uncomfortable with the notion of a surgical post-mortem.

A post-mortem can give the following information:

- the causes of death or what to exclude as causes of death
- gestational age

- sex of the baby
- time of death
- the impact of genetic or physical problems
- whether there were any complications of obstetric and/or paediatric care
- medical knowledge that will help mothers and babies in the future

Giving birth after your baby has died

If the mother is still pregnant and the baby has died, the doctor will usually recommend an induction (starting labour with medical assistance). For some women it will be possible to wait for labour to start without medical assistance, but for others there will be medical reasons as to why that is not possible.

The doctor and midwife will prepare the mother for what is going to happen during labour, how the pain can be managed, and any concerns or fears that the mother may have. The aim is to support her throughout the labour and afterwards. After the birth, the mother may need to stay in hospital for a number of days.

A caesarean will only be recommended in very specific situations. It may seem like the least unpleasant way to give birth, but caesareans can lead to longer hospital stays, more pain, and potentially more problems in future pregnancies than vaginal births.

Some women who are less than 18 weeks pregnant may have a surgical procedure called a 'termination of pregnancy'.

After the baby is born

Some hospitals are able to offer parents a private room where couples can have the baby with them. Some parents prefer that the baby is cared for in the hospital mortuary until funeral arrangements have been made. Some families want to see their baby a number of times before the funeral. Others do not wish to see their baby again. Generally, the hospital will respect and accommodate the various needs of parents.

Creating memories

How parents would like to remember their baby is a personal choice based on what's important to them and their family. The memories that parents and families create with their baby can play an important part in helping them with their grief. While in hospital there are a number of ways that parents can spend time with their baby and create memories if they wish, including:

- seeing, holding or dressing the baby
- bathing the baby
- photographs
- naming or other personal rituals
- creating a memory folder and keeping special mementoes such as teddies
- religious rituals such as baptism

Spending time with your baby

It may be useful for parents to explore this very individual decision with staff and social workers. Sometimes staff can help parents to move through some of their fears and prepare them for what they will see and experience. Some parents who choose not to spend time with their baby or may be ambivalent or undecided can regret their decision later on so it is important to try to talk through fears and concerns early on.

Your health after the birth of a deceased baby

Bleeding

After giving birth, women will generally have vaginal bleeding for five to ten days; it may be even longer if the baby was born at or close to full term. Initially, this loss will be dark red, becoming lighter over the next few days. It is recommended that women use pads rather than tampons to reduce the risk of infection.

Women need to see a general practitioner (GP) if they experience any of the following symptoms:

- prolonged or heavy bleeding
- blood clots
- severe lower abdominal pain
- changes in your vaginal discharge or offensive-smelling discharge
- fever or flu-like symptoms

Breast changes

Following the birth of your baby, you may experience some breast changes. Your breasts may show signs of producing milk in a pregnancy that ended as early as 16 to 18 weeks. Your breasts may become tender. You may notice they are larger and there may be some milk leakage. This is not unusual; it is your body responding normally to pregnancy. Your breasts will become more comfortable and softer within the first week after birth. There is no need to restrict your fluid intake or to take fluid tablets – milk production will stop as your body adjusts.

Sometimes medications are used to stop breast milk. Medications work by stopping your body from making prolactin, which is the hormone that makes milk.

If your breasts become red and sore or you develop flu-like symptoms (such as fever or body aches and pains) you may have developed mastitis. It is important to contact a doctor or the hospital to avoid your symptoms getting worse.

Grief

Every parent, couple or family will have their own reaction to a baby's death. If the baby died early in the pregnancy, it may be that they were still coming to terms with being a parent. Even when a death occurs later in a pregnancy, feelings can vary from ambivalence in one person to profound grief in another.

Society has not always acknowledged the close bond that can form between parents and their expected baby, nor the intensity of the grief that can follow. Sometimes a long-awaited pregnancy may produce a strong bond from the earliest stages of conception. As well as grieving for the loss of a baby, one may also be grieving for the loss of parenting dreams.

Grief, and the way we express it, is influenced by so many things, such as our values, beliefs, culture and upbringing. This is why people deal with their loss and grief in so many different ways. It is also why there is no right or wrong way to behave or respond. Some people find themselves overwhelmed by a number of feelings, including shock, sadness, denial, guilt and anger. Others might experience physical reactions like nausea, headaches, loss of appetite, sleeplessness, fatigue, difficulty concentrating as well as generally feeling unwell. Others again, may feel numb and unable to cry, but feel that they should.

Some people find that it takes weeks or months before they start to feel 'normal' and able to return to daily activities. Occasions such as the baby's expected birth date, the anniversary of the miscarriage or birth, a subsequent pregnancy or other significant family events, may bring back more intense feelings of grief.

It may be helpful to anticipate occasions that will remind you of your baby's death. Try putting some rituals in place with your family and loved ones so that the grief is acknowledged. Some families have a place where they can put flowers or light a candle each day; some have a special place in the garden where they can sit and remember, and others choose a time in the week where they can spend time remembering together. How people remember their baby is unique to them and their family.

If you find your grief is overwhelming or is stopping you from doing the things you need to do, or doesn't diminish with time, it may be useful for you to speak with a trained counsellor or another parent who has gone through a similar experience.

Individual differences

Many parents are concerned that their emotional and physical reactions to grief are different from their partner's. This can be especially difficult if you feel your partner doesn't understand or care about what has happened. Different people deal with grief in different ways. It can be hard to look after your relationship if you are overwhelmed by your feelings of grief and loss, but it may help to keep talking, openly and honestly about how you feel, and what both your needs are at this time. It is also important to listen; this may be very hard at first but will eventually become easier. Sometimes it is not possible for you or your partner to meet each other's support needs, and speaking with other friends, family or professional supports may be helpful.

Other children

It is often hard to know how children are affected by death because their reactions can be so different to those of adults. A child can seem upset one minute and then happy to go and play the next. It's important to remember that children use play to understand the world they live in and to make sense of things. Children's grief may come out in their behaviour: some may become more clingy or unsettled, and others may be aggressive or disruptive.

What can you do?

- Many families tell us that being open and honest with their children was helpful.
- You can include your children in activities to remember your baby. This gives them the opportunity to acknowledge the baby and respond and grieve in their own way.

- If you're not sure how to talk with your children about death, your bereavement worker can provide advice and appropriate resource material.

Reactions from family, friends and colleagues

Family and friends may respond in different ways to your loss. They may feel upset and powerless to know how to help you. Sometimes they don't know what to say or they will make comments that you find unhelpful and hurtful. Friends and family can be very helpful for the first few weeks, but some will expect you to return to normal soon. This can be very upsetting, and at this time you may need to remind them that things are still difficult for you. Professional support organisations can help, and have useful information to give to your family and friends.

Multiple pregnancy

When there has been a multiple pregnancy, parents can be divided between mourning and making funeral arrangements for the baby or babies who have died, and keeping vigil at a sick baby's cot. Sometimes joy at the birth of a healthy baby and sadness at the loss of another baby occur at the same time, which can be very confusing and distressing. Complications in a multiple pregnancy are emotionally demanding and exhausting, and parents can be left with feelings of guilt and helplessness.

The staff will support you through the day to day while you are in hospital and your bereavement worker will stay in contact with you for a time after you go home. You may have a lot of questions about what happened and why your baby or babies have died. There will be many opportunities to talk to medical staff, who will ensure that you are kept informed and involved throughout your care and the care of your babies.

When you are single

Even with a high level of support from family and friends, it can be a very isolating experience to be grieving the death of your baby on your own. It is important that you are able to share your thoughts and feelings with someone you trust. There are professional supports available to you, some of which are available 24 hours a day.

21

Motherhood and connecting with your baby

Frances Thomson-Salo

If you are lucky enough to become a mother, it can be the most wonderful thing you do, even though it may be hard at times. No other event in your life may be as momentous and life-altering as the birth of a child – particularly a first child. When you are the mother of a new baby, a cascade of change takes place emotionally as thinking of yourself as a mother becomes part of your identity. For all mothers this requires ongoing adaptation and compromise. When two people decide to raise a baby, their couple relationship evolves as they become a parental couple, but the emphasis in this chapter is on your own journey.

There are many paths to becoming a mother, both physical and psychological, and many kinds of families, including blended and single-parent families. A baby will have many meanings for you and your partner and the nine months of pregnancy provide a preparation for transition to motherhood. The tasks for this transition include beginning to bond with the baby inside you and adjusting to the new relationship with your baby, forming a threesome with your partner, and both of you beginning to see yourselves as parents. Your own experiences of being parented will influence your model of a 'good' mother and her partner; if you have to parent without having that role model, that can make it harder.

Your baby wants to be delighted in and to matter to their mother. When the relationship between you and your baby goes well, its importance for the psychological health of both of you cannot be stressed too much. What you bring of your cultural identity to parenting is important, too, and while some of the following ideas may seem to apply more to Western cultures, we think they have universal relevance. Later in this chapter, we will cover some of the difficulties that may arise.

Motherhood as a developmental stage

Your body and sense of self

Motherhood is a new developmental stage, in which an aspect of your identity is changed irrevocably; when things go well, thinking of yourself as a mother becomes a central part of your identity. There are different degrees of maternal feelings; you may have wanted to be a mother since you were little, or you may have taken time to grow into it. Mothers do the best they can, even those who have experienced great deprivation. Many of you try in the face of enormous difficulties to protect your baby from ongoing family problems (including who you choose as a partner or the coping mechanisms you develop). The rewards of motherhood usually outweigh any resentment about its demands and deprivations, and can even provide a second chance to rework difficulties from your past.

Pregnancy and birth are times of social, emotional and neurobiological change. You may welcome these or at times feel that your body has forced change on you during pregnancy. If you are anxious about the birth you are likely to find it easier if you come to accept that your body 'knows' what to do.

When you are a new mother, it can feel like you are on an emotional roller-coaster: the hormonal upheavals of pregnancy and birth; your body being exposed to strangers; the mess of your baby's urine and faeces; your leaking milk and sore breasts; the anxiety about an utterly vulnerable, unknown little baby whose life feels at times entirely dependent on you. These feelings may surface in the first few days as the transitory 'baby blues', when adjustment feels hard in the face of something as momentous as having produced a living baby.

Becoming a mother can evoke strong and continuous anxiety, and sometimes terror about how to manage. In this state you feel that you have to satisfy the urgent cries of your baby out of your own resources. The anxieties of the first weeks and months of this new responsibility may feel quite overwhelming, and having to put your own need for sleep and self-care in second place may feel overwhelming, too. You may also be sad at times about loss – of your previous body, of your pregnant body, of the baby being inside you, of your identity and sense of competence, and of your former lifestyle.

On the positive side, you will find that as you become more confident and able to calm your baby, the feelings of being lovingly attached grow. The hormone oxytocin, which helps with the birth and breastfeeding, also helps in bonding and enjoyment of your baby. Research suggests that the neurobiology of parenting and attachment shapes a mother's brain. While you may in the first few weeks feel like you will be stuck with these anxious feelings forever, they do pass, particularly as your baby grows, and you may find that you come into your own as your baby becomes slightly older. Experiences of how you were cared for as a baby are revived when you have your own baby, and often it is only when you become a mother that mixed feelings and difficulties emerge. Aspects of your personality you had not been aware of may emerge and contribute to your feeling that things have changed completely.

You may find you have three main questions: will my baby love me, will I love my baby and will I be a good mother? You may feel that you should be perfect, but you don't have to respond to all your baby's cues for most babies to develop well, which means that many mothers may feel unnecessarily guilty about being a bad mother. As you learn about your baby and gain confidence, nothing will be as reassuring as seeing your baby thrive, and being able to comfort and understand them.

Your baby

Your baby is born ready to communicate with you and wants to connect with you and other people in the family, and to feel safe and enjoyed. You may spend hours in minute observation, which is the beginning of getting to know and love your baby, whose sense of self develops in this mirroring. You may find a lot of pleasurable intimacy in caring for your baby's body, and kissing and caressing their soft skin. Breastfeeding has its own pleasure, with your baby's caresses and suckling.

Sometimes you may feel you would like to be looked after for a change; it is hard to put your wishes and needs aside 24/7. In a time of stress, it is helpful to take a temporary break from your baby in whatever way suits you; when you do this, your baby also begins to learn that small separations are manageable. And as your baby's development unfolds according to their innate maturational timetable, you are likely to find that the baby helps you respond to your changing relationship.

Your partner

While you may initially feel that your partner is very helpful, you may also come to feel that they are at times unsupportive. Developing the couple relationship requires emotional work: to keep the door of communication open between you and to facilitate your partner's relationship with your baby. You are likely to have a need for intimacy, even if you may initially be less interested in resuming a fuller sex life.

You may be raising your baby without a partner present. Most children wish to know from you the truth about their origins, however they came into the family, whether through adoption, IVF, sperm donation or some other way, and find secrecy about this extremely hard. A child whose father is not available, or where there was conflict, has a need to develop a picture in their mind of positive qualities of men in general, which is something for you to bear in mind from the moment you give birth if you are in this position.

Your mother

If you have a good relationship with your own mother you will probably find that you turn more to her for support, or else to your partner's mother or to other female friends. These relationships are vital in supporting you to be receptive to your baby. You are likely to feel that you do best when you feel that your mother is behind you and is in touch with what you feel. Without this support and if you do not feel very secure in taking care of yourself, it is harder to 'read' your baby's signals and care for your baby. Perhaps it is only to other mothers that a woman may admit that however wonderful motherhood may be, she is also dissatisfied, regretful, and at times wishes that she did not have the baby and feels guilty about that.

How your baby communicates with you

- Your baby may smile at you in pleasure from the first day onwards.
- Even on the first day your baby can reach out their hand a little way towards you.
- Your baby can copy movements you make with your face.
- Your baby will communicate when they are overwhelmed by blinking or looking away.
- A baby's crying lets you know when they feel hungry and tired or alone.

Mother–infant interaction and attachment

Bonding and attachment are important because the early social inter-actions and relationship between you and your baby have a profound influence on your baby's emotional, cognitive and neurological development. This is optimised by a supportive, nurturing relationship that is sensitive and responsive to your baby's needs. Secure attachment is protective in future life. A baby wants to be fascinating to others and if you view your baby as a person from the beginning, with their own personality and interests, your baby is more than likely to develop positively. When you hold your baby and convey to them how precious they are, they feel good about themselves, developing good self-esteem.

A surprise may be how interactive your baby is from birth, and how aware, responsive, active, curious and alert they are. For the first six weeks your baby is working out what happens in their body, and you contribute vitally to the development of their mind by making meaning of their experiences. Your baby gets more out of life by this framework you provide. Just as your baby needs your love and sensitivity for this, they also need to be kept in your mind.

When your baby feels that you will comfort them when they feel hurt, alone or distressed, and that you will 'hear' them, you are safeguarding their social and emotional development. Your baby responds to you being really 'present' and genuine in your responses. You need over time to separate your past from your baby's experiences, and still be able to respond intuitively to your baby's needs without becoming overwhelmed yourself.

It may take time to feel connected to your baby – perhaps most of the first year. Your baby is unlikely to give up hope of being able to connect with you. If you and your baby have been out of tune with each other, your baby needs you to think about it and help them surmount this challenge.

Bonding with your baby

- Smile gently at your baby from the beginning so that they feel safe and that the world is enjoyable.
- Talk to your baby – they find voices fascinating.
- Hold and touch your baby – skin-on-skin contact reduces stress for both of you and improves their breathing and heart rate.
- Spend time with your baby, just being there, and perhaps imitating their expressions.
- Soothe your baby, so they know that they matter and are not alone.
- Read stories to your baby from the beginning.

Difficulties on the path to motherhood

Transition to motherhood can be stressful and lead to crisis. Difficulties on the path to motherhood can make it harder to grow into becoming a mother. The way you were parented is likely to be the way you care for your own baby, unless you make a conscious decision to do it differently because you were unhappy. You may have a partner who is also struggling in their new role. While you may in becoming a mother resolve experiences from the past, forgiving your parents, there are many kinds of perinatal help to work through these bonding difficulties, and you should feel able to ask for help from your doctor and other health professionals as soon as possible, to change negative feelings after birth and lessen their effect on you and your baby.

You may have mixed feelings about being a mother, or you may not have wanted to be one. If you are a teenage mother you may experience great rewards in becoming a mother, but you may face considerable difficulties if you are unsupported. If your experience of being parented has been a difficult one of pain and anxiety, the fear of re-experiencing this is likely to lead you to want to avoid an intimate relationship. If you have very mixed feelings about being a mother, you face a harder task.

Other difficulties include delays in conceiving, which may affect your sense of womanhood, your intimacy with your partner, and being with your baby. Reproductive loss and miscarriages, or a difficult pregnancy and birth, can also affect bonding, but need not do so lastingly. If your baby is premature, ill or vulnerable it may be harder to read their cues, which may affect your confidence in parenting. If your baby spent some time in the neonatal intensive special care unit, you may experience post-traumatic symptoms, which may also make it difficult to feel close to your baby.

You may from pregnancy onwards experience symptoms of anxiety and depression, which may have an effect on your baby. When you feel depressed your baby may feel that he or she does not bring you joy, and may need help to feel better about themselves and their relationship with you. It is hard to face your baby's intense vulnerability while hoping that someone will recognise that you need help. (For more on postnatal depression, see chapter 22.)

If your own mother experienced postnatal depression or unresolved difficulties, these experiences may shape your parenting. If at times you have experienced serious mental illness or borderline symptoms, you should be supported as having the potential to be a capable parent.

If you have had experiences of sexual abuse, trauma or lack of support, used alcohol and drugs as a way of coping, or had experiences of violence and of non-consensual sex, these add to the difficulties of feeling connected to your baby and to provide what they need.

Your baby comes into the world wanting to bond and attach, and you may find it a rapturously wonderful experience. While it may be difficult if inner and outer experiences get in the way of the two of you enjoying each other, if you remember the pain you experienced as a child, you are unlikely to repeat it and motherhood is therefore likely to be a positive and rewarding experience.

22
Mental health and pregnancy

Tram Nguyen

Pregnancy and early motherhood can be a time of immense joy and wonder as a new life is created. Traditionally it has been considered a time of emotional and psychological wellbeing for women. Research shows that while this is true for most women, about 15 per cent of women will experience depression or anxiety during pregnancy, and an even larger number during the postnatal period. From what we know about mental health and illness, this makes a lot of sense. For most mental illnesses there is no single 'cause', but often an accumulation of multiple stresses, either emotional (bereavement), social (financial hardship, unemployment, divorce, domestic violence), and/or physical (pregnancy, medical illness, illicit drug use, chronic sleep deprivation).

The transition to motherhood is a complex rite of passage each woman will negotiate in her own unique way. The changes that inevitably occur for you as a woman (your sense of self, your changing body), in your relationships (with your partner, with your parents, with your other children) and your social circumstances (maternity leave, less available income, possible need to change accommodation) and then the arrival of your baby, can all be seen as potential stresses that leave you vulnerable in your mental health. This is particularly so if you have a pre-existing mental illness. If this is the case for you, it is advisable to speak to your professional supports if you are thinking of becoming pregnant so that a relapse management plan can be formulated and implemented.

Many women suffer unnecessarily and for prolonged periods of time with mental illness in pregnancy and the postnatal period (together called the perinatal period). For a lot of women, there is a huge sense of shame and guilt about being miserable or anxious at a time when the expectation is that it is a period of bliss. You may be unaware that there are safe and effective treatment options for depression during pregnancy and while breastfeeding. For example, a large number of antidepressant medications are classified as compatible with breastfeeding. An untreated mental illness can have potential adverse effects during pregnancy and afterwards, for you, your baby's development and your relationship with your baby. It is therefore important to get the right treatment. If you feel you are not your usual self and you are suffering, please visit your GP. From there, depending on your diagnosis, you may be referred to a psychologist and/or psychiatrist.

Baby blues

Baby blues refers to the transient mood fluctuations and heightened emotional state that commonly occur following childbirth. Baby blues are very common, affecting up to 80 per cent of new mothers. They come on three to five days after delivery, and their usual features are teariness, feeling overwhelmed, feeling anxious and moodiness. Baby blues are thought to be due to the rapid hormonal shifts that occur following childbirth, in addition to the stress of labour itself. The symptoms usually settle within a couple of days without any specific treatment other than reassurance and support. For a minority of women, however, the baby blues do not seem to go away. If this is the case for you, it is important to discuss it with your doctor, as it may be a sign of developing depression or anxiety. Depression and anxiety will need specific treatment, for your own wellbeing and that of your baby.

Depression during and after pregnancy

During pregnancy and in the postnatal period, 10–15 per cent of women will be diagnosed with depression. The first few weeks after delivery are the peak periods for the onset of depression in women. If you have had depression before, then the symptoms of depression in the perinatal period will be similar to what you have experienced previously. If you have not had depression in the past, you may not recognise it for some time. In most states of Australia, there is now standard screening for depression during and following pregnancy. This means that, as part of your antenatal care, you will be given a questionnaire to assess if you may have depression. This questionnaire will then be repeated with your maternal and child health nurse in the early weeks after your baby is born. The aim is early detection of depression, so that you can be referred to the appropriate services and your treatment is not delayed. It is therefore very important to be completely honest when answering the questionnaire.

Common symptoms and signs of depression during and following pregnancy include:

- feeling depressed or miserable for most of the day and on most days of the week
- an irritable, angry or anxious mood
- increased crying, sometimes for no apparent reason
- reduced interest in things that you would normally enjoy
- insomnia (even when your baby is sleeping) or sleeping more than usual, depending on the person
- reduced appetite or overeating, depending on the person
- excessive fatigue and tiredness
- forgetfulness and difficulty concentrating
- preoccupation with morbid thoughts or anxiety about multiple things, such as bad things happening to you, your pregnancy, your baby or your partner
- feeling disconnected from your baby, that your baby is not really yours and that you do not have a bond with your baby; this is especially distressing if it is a planned pregnancy
- excessive feelings of guilt and/or failure and that you are a 'bad mother'
- thoughts of harming yourself
- thoughts that things would be better for you and your baby if you (and your baby) were dead, leading to thoughts of suicide

In addition, you may have associated symptoms of anxiety (see also chapters 10 and 40).

What causes perinatal depression?

There is no one single cause of depression. Apart from the multiple physical, social and emotional changes associated with childbearing and mentioned above, additional factors can make you more vulnerable to developing perinatal depression, such as: a history of depression or anxiety, a family history of depression or anxiety, going through a stressful or unplanned pregnancy, having unrealistic expectations of motherhood that are not met, experiencing a traumatic or complicated delivery, relationship difficulties, a lack of social supports, and having a sick or unsettled baby. Depression and anxiety during pregnancy are a significant risk factor for postnatal depression. It is therefore important to seek professional help and treatment during pregnancy rather than leaving it until after your baby arrives.

Treatment for perinatal depression

Depression during pregnancy may affect the development of your baby. Depression following pregnancy makes it incredibly difficult for you to enjoy and care for your baby, as you would like. Being depressed and suffering from tiredness, poor concentration, irritability, difficulty coping and overwhelming anxiety makes it hard to be able to play with your child and promote their development. Getting the right treatment is important for you and your baby.

The first step to getting treatment is to see your GP. Initially, your GP may do some blood tests to rule out any medical illnesses that mimic depression, such as iron-deficiency anaemia or thyroid problems. They can then tailor a management plan according to the severity of your illness. Mild to moderate depression can be improved with psychological treatment and by increasing the supports around you.

In some cases of more severe depression, you may need to take anti-depressants. If you have been depressed in the past, it is important to consult your doctor about treatment during pregnancy and afterwards. Stopping your medication abruptly when you find out you are pregnant increases your risk of relapse during pregnancy and during the post-natal period. If you are using herbal and complementary treatments (e.g. St John's wort), it is important to discuss these with your doctor, as they may not be safe in pregnancy or may interact with other medicines.

Anxiety during and after pregnancy

Pregnancy and new motherhood are a time of change and new experiences. It is common to have some anxiety at various times throughout this journey. As many as 30 per cent of pregnant women experience anxiety symptoms, and a smaller number will have symptoms of enough duration and frequency to be diagnosed with an anxiety disorder.

There are a number of clinically classified anxiety disorders, including generalised anxiety disorder, obsessive compulsive disorder (OCD), post-traumatic stress disorder (PTSD), panic disorder, agoraphobia and social phobia (see chapters 10 and 40 for an overview of these disorders). For most women, these disorders pre-date pregnancy, though some develop symptoms for the first time during pregnancy. Some disorders, particularly panic disorder and OCD, can worsen during pregnancy. There is no single cause of anxiety. You may have a genetic predisposition, you may have been faced with an acutely stressful situation, or you may have an anxious temperament with a tendency to worry.

Some women experience pregnancy-related anxiety. This is characterised by worries about the baby's health, fears about the birth experience, and concerns about weight gain and body shape while pregnant. This type of anxiety occurs in women who have an anxious temperament, and overlaps with a general tendency to worry and symptoms of tension.

Another group of women for whom pregnancy and the birth experience may induce anxiety are those with a history of sexual abuse. Some (but not all) of these women will fulfil the diagnosis of post-traumatic stress disorder. Again, early treatment will enhance the experience of pregnancy, birth and developing a relationship with your baby.

Symptoms of anxiety disorders

There are specific symptoms for each anxiety disorder, but they all have some common characteristics: feeling worried, stressed or on edge most of the time; muscular tension and difficulty staying calm; difficulty sleeping; recurring worrying thoughts that will not go away; and panic attacks. These symptoms may lead you to avoid situations that provoke further anxiety. While this may make you feel safe in the short term, in the long term it can really limit the things you do and your quality of life. It is common to have symptoms of depression at the same time. In addition, you may try using alcohol and other drugs (including over-the-counter and prescription medication) to self-medicate in an attempt to relieve your anxiety. While this may appear to work initially, it can set you up with an addiction that creates its own significant problems, including harm to your pregnancy and baby.

During pregnancy, anxiety can lead to special problems. Sometimes the symptoms of late pregnancy, such as shortness of breath, dizziness, an increased heart rate, and feeling hot and sweaty, can be distressing as they can either mimic or precipitate panic attacks. If you experience panic attacks and/or agoraphobia, you may find it difficult to attend your antenatal care appointments. You may also be terrified of being 'trapped' at the time of delivery and of developing a panic attack during labour, even though this rarely happens. You may also find it a struggle to attend mothers' groups and appointments for your new baby. It is important to seek treatment early during pregnancy so that your experience of pregnancy and motherhood is positive rather than filled with dread, and also so that you can get quality antenatal and postnatal care for you and your baby.

Treatment for anxiety disorders

It is important to seek treatment for prolonged symptoms of anxiety and acute stress during pregnancy. Some studies have shown that if left untreated, maternal anxiety can affect the unborn baby, with increased risk of preterm labour. Anxiety continuing into the postnatal period can interfere with a mother's developing relationship with her baby; she may, for example, find that being with her baby triggers anxiety and so she avoids or minimises contact with her baby or constantly checks the baby, interrupting their sleep.

Anxiety is effectively treated with psychological therapies. These include relaxation training, cognitive behaviour therapy, and mindfulness practice. Lifestyle modifications such as stress reduction and exercise are also helpful. Sometimes, in more severe cases, medication may be required, preferably in conjunction with psychological therapies. The medicines used are anti-depressants that have been shown to work very well with anxiety.

Amy had always had an anxious temperament. She was socially anxious and particularly fearful of being the focus of attention. She would get the occasional panic attack where her heart pounded, she would get short of breath and dizzy, and feel that she was losing control. These panic attacks were usually in anticipation of either meeting new people or having to give a talk in front of others.

At university, Amy discovered alcohol. This was more than a social lubricant for her; it took away her anxiety and gave her personality. She soon began to binge-drink on the weekends, and this continued for some years into her working career.

Amy was 26 when she unexpectedly fell pregnant. She had been diag-nosed with polycystic ovarian syndrome and was under the impression that she could not fall pregnant and so she did not use contraception. Amy was initially devastated when she found out. She was not sure about the status of her relationship and felt totally unprepared. Furthermore, she had been drinking throughout early pregnancy and was worried about the effect it would have on her baby. She was also worried about how she would cope without alcohol, and the mere thought of abstinence could trigger a panic attack.

Amy spoke to her GP and was referred to a drug and alcohol service for education, counselling, and strategies to minimise her drinking and achieve abstinence if possible.

When Amy met with her midwife for antenatal care, she expressed all her concerns about fetal alcohol syndrome and also about her ongoing anxiety and panic attacks, which were now a daily event. The midwife arranged for the relevant ultrasound scans to assess the baby's development at 20 weeks. She also referred Amy for a mental health assessment.

Amy was assessed as having a panic disorder of moderate severity and associated alcohol misuse. She began some cognitive behaviour therapy to give her breathing strategies for the panic attacks and also ways to reframe her negative anxious thoughts. Amy also commenced a mindfulness group program, which she found particularly helpful and which gave her the opportunity to meet women with similar experiences.

By the third trimester, Amy's panic attacks were reduced to only one a month and her ultrasounds had shown a healthy fetus. Amy was now excited about the prospect of becoming a mother, but she was concerned about having a panic attack during labour. Amy was reassured that it was a very rare experience and that she now had the strategies to manage a panic attack. Furthermore, Amy's relationship with her partner had been consolidated by the pregnancy and Amy felt secure that he would be a support person for her during delivery.

Towards the end of her pregnancy, Amy was more settled and able to open up to her psychologist about the experience of having a mother with anxiety. Amy's mother was housebound due to panic attacks, and often pushed Amy to go out shopping and doing other chores. Amy recalled a sheltered upbringing, coloured by her mother's fear and dread of the outside world. Amy could see how this had contributed to the development of her social anxiety, and she was able to reflect on how she wanted things to be different for her own child. She imagined a life for her child without irrational fears and panic, but was unsure how she could successfully achieve this on her own. Her psychologist reiterated that managing her own anxiety was the first step, particularly in behavioural modelling for her child. Her psychologist implemented a plan to continue seeing Amy after the birth, to support her mental state, her abstinence from alcohol and any parenting issues.

Amy delivered a healthy baby girl she named Charlotte. Amy often calls Charlotte her blessing in disguise. The pregnancy was a motivating factor for Amy to abstain from alcohol and address her anxiety.

Furthermore, Amy continued to find the skills and insight she had gained through the mindfulness group and with her psychologist relevant and helpful in the postnatal period. Amy knows that escaping her lifelong struggle with anxiety and alcohol will be an ongoing challenge, but she feels optimistic for herself and for Charlotte.

Post-partum psychosis

Post-partum psychosis is a serious mental illness that starts soon after childbirth. Fortunately it is rare, occurring in only one woman per 1000 deliveries, and there are very effective treatments. It can be extremely scary, especially for someone who has never had it before, because they find it difficult to differentiate between reality and the illness playing tricks on their brain.

Psychosis essentially means a loss of reality. It usually comes on in a very quick and spectacular manner within the first few weeks after birth, but the onset can even occur within hours of delivery.

The contributing factors to post-partum psychosis include: a genetic predisposition (there is an increased risk in women with a family history of post-partum psychosis or bipolar disorder), the initial severe sleep deprivation, the rapid hormonal changes around delivery, and the physical stress of delivery – particularly if there are other medical problems. There is a relationship between post-partum psychosis and bipolar disorder. Women with bipolar disorder are at greatest risk of a relapse with psychotic symptoms soon after delivery. For some women, however, post-partum psychosis marks the first episode of a bipolar illness. Some women will have only a single episode of post-partum psychosis, while others will have an episode each time they have a baby.

Symptoms of post-partum psychosis

If you develop post-partum psychosis you may experience a range of the following symptoms:

- confusion and disorientation about the day and time and who people are
- affected concentration and the feeling that your brain is in a fog and not working properly, or that it is overloaded with too many thoughts, running very quickly through your mind
- severe physical anxiety or agitation, to the point where you cannot stay still

- variable mood, being either on a high, or irritable or depressed

- insomnia, with trouble getting to sleep or staying asleep, feeling like you need less sleep and in fact going days without sleeping

- delusions or thoughts that are not true and are often paranoid – that the hospital staff are spies, that your partner is an impostor in disguise. These thoughts may seem bizarre or silly when you are well, but in the middle of the illness it all seems real.

- hallucinations or impaired sensations – hearing, seeing or smelling things that are not there, even though they feel like they are coming from outside, including whispering, banging, people calling your name or repetitive music, smelling strange things or seeing people walk by your bed

- strange sensations that you are not really yourself and others are controlling your actions and thoughts

- thoughts of harming yourself and your baby, which may appear to you as the only solution you have. You may even start planning it, even though this is clearly not what you would want if you were well.

Treatment for post-partum psychosis

Post-partum psychosis is a psychiatric emergency requiring immediate treatment in a safe setting in a hospital. If you or anyone you know are suffering symptoms of post-partum psychosis, go to the emergency department. Immediate treatment is necessary for the safety of both mother and baby. In some states of Australia there are psychiatric mother–baby units, which specifically treat mothers with mental illness and do not separate mother from baby. If your symptoms are too severe or the facilities are not available, you will be admitted to a general adult psychiatric unit. In these circumstances, your partner, or family or friends will need to help care for your baby until you are well enough to go home. Your baby will never be taken away from you permanently, and doctors will aim to reunite you with your baby as soon as possible.

Following admission to hospital, psychiatrists will usually perform blood tests and brain scans to check before starting medication that there are no possible physical causes for the illness. Sometimes, if the episode is very severe, electroconvulsive therapy (ECT) is the fastest and most effective treatment. The medications now available are also very effective.

While the dramatic delusions and hallucinations respond fairly quickly to medication, it can take a bit longer for the brain to recover and concentration and thinking to get back on track. Be kind and patient with yourself, as you would to a friend or sister. Post-partum psychosis is not your fault; it is a biological illness and has a lot to do with all the chemicals in your body changing rapidly after giving birth and affecting your brain function.

Although the mainstay of treatment is medication, there is also a place for counselling. You may find the experience of psychosis so traumatic that you are left grieving, scared or confused about the entire event. It is often worthwhile to have counselling, either from your psychiatrist or another counsellor, to talk through your experience so you can process and make sense of it, how it has affected your life, and how you can move on from it and enjoy your family.

Bipolar disorder during and after pregnancy

Bipolar disorder is a relatively rare condition that usually emerges in the late teens or 20s. For some women, childbirth can be the trigger for a first episode of the illness. Bipolar disorder is a chronic condition that requires long-term treatment and complex medical management. Women with bipolar disorder usually have a family history of either bipolar disorder or depression.

Symptoms of bipolar disorder

Bipolar disorder is characterised by a fluctuation in mood with alternating episodes of highs (mania) and lows (depression) that are sustained over weeks to months. Everyday moodiness that changes from minutes to hours is not bipolar disorder. The depressive symptoms associated with the condition are the same as those seen with straightforward depression (see chapter 10). Some of the symptoms of mania include:

- an excessively happy mood – being high as a kite
- sometimes an irritable mood rather than happy mood, or an irritable mood mixed with an excessively happy mood
- having lots of energy and moving quickly, as though driven by an internal motor
- speaking very quickly, trying to keep up with racing thoughts
- less need to sleep; feeling energetic on little or no sleep

- feeling overly confident in looks, abilities and talents
- feeling invincible and engaging in increased risk-taking, such as dangerous driving
- increased libido that can sometimes lead to inappropriate behaviour
- having lots of plans and acting on them in a hasty and disorganised fashion
- increased spending, often on unneeded or unwanted things and resulting in debt
- behaving rashly and in ways that are out of character, such as quitting work or leaving a relationship in an abrupt and irrational manner
- increased alcohol and drug use
- in extreme cases, psychotic symptoms, meaning a loss of touch with reality

When a new mother is manic, all her energy and erratic behaviour can affect her baby. She may find that she gets caught up in her plans and neglects her baby's needs. She may take her baby along on reckless outings. She may be unaware that her manner and behaviour are too much for her baby – too loud and too fast. Newborn babies are very sensitive to over-stimulation and are easily unsettled. If this is happening to you, it is very important to get immediate treatment even though you may be feeling that the world is good and you want everything to continue as it is.

Triggers and treatment for bipolar disorder

Bipolar disorder has a lot to do with brain chemistry and there is a strong genetic component, but for lots of people, sleep deprivation is a consistent trigger for a relapse, particularly with a manic episode. Medication is the main component of treatment.

For women with a known diagnosis of bipolar disorder, pre-conception planning is recommended, as some of the medicines used to treat bipolar disorder are harmful to a fetus. Any changes to medication must be balanced with the risk of relapse during pregnancy and the post-partum period, and how this may affect the mother and her baby's wellbeing. If you are on bipolar medication and are planning to have a baby, you will need to speak to your doctor. Never cease your medicines abruptly – with bipolar disorder this significantly increases your risk of a relapse during pregnancy and after the birth, and the likelihood of needing higher doses of medication to stabilise your mental state. Your treatment should be a collaborative process between you, your partner and your treating GP or psychiatrist. You may also wish to ask for a second opinion or specialist opinion in relation to the medicines you are taking, as it is a complex area.

You are at greatest risk of a bipolar relapse in the first month after delivery, so it's a good idea to have extra monitoring from your GP or psychiatrist during this time. Some women who have had recurrent episodes may choose to start or increase medication as soon as they deliver.

Schizophrenia during and after pregnancy

Schizophrenia is a rare condition that usually emerges in the late teens or early 20s, sometimes triggered by extreme stress or drug use (hallucinogens, amphetamines and cannabis). There is often a family history or a genetic predisposition to the illness. It is a chronic condition that needs long-term management.

Symptoms of schizophrenia

The two characteristic symptoms are delusions and hallucinations. Delusions are firmly held beliefs that are not real, even though they seem real at the time of the illness. Someone with schizophrenia may believe, for example, that there is a conspiracy, or that the Mafia or government are plotting to trap them. They may believe they are being followed, monitored with cameras and talked about by strangers in the street. They may feel they have special magical powers such as mindreading, or believe that other people have control of them, their thoughts and their actions, and that their thoughts are being broadcast to the public.

Hallucinations are perceptions that are not real: when we either hear, see, feel or smell things that are not present, even though they feel like they are real to us. It is as if our ears, eyes and other senses are playing tricks on us. Someone with schizophrenia may hear people talking about them or the TV talking to them when there is no one else in the room. They may smell something burning when there is not. A pregnant woman with schizophrenia may hear her fetus talking to her in multiple languages. These experiences can be interesting, absorbing and also scary. For someone who suffers these experiences, it is often difficult for them to know who they can trust, so they may not voluntarily seek treatment; it is often others around them who notice they have changed.

In addition to delusions and hallucinations, other, more subtle symptoms can come on over time including:

- social withdrawal, often as a result of feeling paranoid and that others are not trustworthy
- difficulty organising day-to-day things such as meals, cleaning, washing and appointments
- difficulty making clear decisions due to a sense of uncertainty and ambivalence
- difficulty organising thoughts, and jumbled speech others will say they cannot understand
- reversal of the sleep–wake cycle, with sleeping during the day and being up at night

Treatment for schizophrenia

Some of the older antipsychotic medications used to treat schizophrenia tended to increase women's levels of the hormone prolactin and make it more difficult for them to fall pregnant. With the newer antipsychotics this side effect is less common. If you have been diagnosed with schizophrenia and you do not wish to get pregnant, it is important, therefore, to be aware when you are changing medications that you may be more likely to fall pregnant and that you will need to take the necessary contraceptive precautions.

When you discover that you are pregnant, it is important that not to stop your medications without consulting your treating psychiatrist or GP. The decision-making with regard to your medications is complex and will depend on your individual situation. While most women would prefer not to have to take medications during pregnancy and while breast-feeding, this desire will be weighed against the risk of relapse (and the need for hospitalisation) and how this can affect pregnancy or parenting. For most women who remain on their antipsychotic medication, the risk of relapse in the postnatal period is not significantly increased. The symptoms of schizophrenia can affect your parenting capacity, so it is important to enlist as much support as possible – from both professionals and your social network.

Eating disorders during and after pregnancy

Eating disorders most commonly occur in young women, and it is therefore inevitable that a number of pregnant women will also be suffering from an eating disorder. The three most commonly recognised eating disorders are anorexia nervosa, bulimia nervosa and eating disorders not otherwise specified (EDNOS). Anorexia nervosa involves poor body image, fear of gaining weight, severe dietary restrictions, excessive exercise and/or purging, and very low body weight, often with physical consequences. People with bulimia nervosa also have a poor body image, but tend to be in the normal weight range rather than underweight. They have periods of excessive eating (bingeing), alternating with the use of laxatives or vomiting to purge. EDNOS is the most common eating disorder. It includes a hotchpotch of people who no longer meet the criteria for anorexia or bulimia, who have milder symptoms, or who have fewer symptoms.

Pregnancy is a time when you can experience food cravings, food aversions, food restrictions, weight gain, changing body shape, and decreased mobility. All these changes can provoke panic if you are suffering from an eating disorder and feel the need to be in control. Furthermore, you will have changing nutritional needs and your body may preferentially divert nutrients to your growing baby at your expense. This means that any dietary restrictions or purging can be dangerous to you and your baby. For this reason, experts often advise women with an eating disorder to delay becoming pregnant until their eating disorder is under control or in remission. Studies show that this will lead to better outcomes for both the woman and her baby. Women who have active symptoms of bulimia nervosa have an increased risk of miscarriage. Women with active anorexia nervosa have an increased risk of small babies with smaller heads. Women with any form of eating disorder are more prone to anaemia during pregnancy, and will take longer to recover from caesarean births and any tearing or episiotomies.

Monitoring during pregnancy

Some specialists would consider a woman with an active eating disorder to be a high-risk pregnancy, requiring extra monitoring by a doctor throughout pregnancy. Ideally, a good team will be involved, including a combination of professionals, each with their specific roles: obstetrician, midwife, psychiatrist, physician and dietician. A dietician plays an important role providing information about healthy expected weight gains, nutritional requirements during pregnancy and meal plans. If the mother is not gaining enough weight or there are other signs of concern for her pregnancy, the doctors will organise extra tests to monitor her health and that of her baby. This may involve blood tests, ultrasounds and monitoring the baby's heartbeat.

After the birth

After birth, there may still be a risk of relapse, even for women who have been doing really well during pregnancy. Some women impose unrealistic expectations on themselves to lose weight after having a baby rather than being kind to themselves. The media and social pressure on celebrity mothers to lose weight have exacerbated this situation and created unrealistic expectations. Some women see the end of the pregnancy as a time when they can resume dieting, purging and exercise. This is not healthy for them or their baby. If you find yourself thinking this way, it is time to return to your professionals for more support. The time, preoccupation and energy an eating disorder consumes will take away from the precious moments you have to get to know your new baby. If you are breastfeeding, eating restrictions and exercise can affect your breast milk supply. Finally, as a mother and a role model for your baby you will want to pass on a healthy body image, good eating habits and strong self-esteem.

23

Abortion and unplanned pregnancy

Chris Bayly

To find yourself pregnant when you don't want to be may be distressing and it can take a little time to be sure how you feel. Some women are sure from the start that they can't continue a pregnancy, while others may be shocked to begin with, but are able to adjust their plans and look forward to having a baby. For some an unplanned pregnancy can be a happy surprise or accident, while others may be happy at first but as the reality sinks in may feel unable to continue.

Sometimes circumstances can change so that a pregnancy that at first was welcome or even planned becomes difficult or impossible to continue. Some reasons for this include a relationship breakdown or an illness that may damage the health of mother or baby if pregnancy continues. A diagnosis of illness or abnormality in the developing baby can lead you to decide to have an abortion if the baby can't survive or you cannot foresee good enough quality of life for them.

> 'I had always believed that abortion was wrong and I could not comprehend how people could do it. Actually experiencing an unplanned pregnancy, confronted with this as an option, helped me to understand for the first time how and why people could consider a termination and feel that this was the best option for them.'

It's been estimated that about half of all pregnancies are unplanned, and about half of those unplanned pregnancies (i.e. about a quarter of all pregnancies) end in abortion. Contraception isn't perfect, it isn't always explained or understood well, and there are lots of reasons why it may not be used some of the time.

Mixed feelings are common in early pregnancy and terms like unplanned or unwanted pregnancy often don't cover how a woman feels. You may care a great deal about the pregnancy, and your decision may be influenced by the sort of life you and your partner can see a baby having.

Research done by the University of Melbourne in conjunction with the Women's has found that women who decide to have an abortion experience it as a difficult solution to a complex problem in their lives. Reasons for abortion in the study included the effects of continuing a pregnancy on their own lives, on the lives of children they already had, on their partner and other relationships, and on the material, emotional and social needs of the potential child. Most often it was the wrong time for a baby, because they were too young, it was too soon after their last baby, they had enough children already, or there were problems in their relationship.

First steps

If you think you might be pregnant and you don't want to be, or you're not sure how you feel about it:

- Have a pregnancy test to be sure.

- Talk about it with someone you trust.

- If you think you might want an abortion, see a health professional as soon as possible so you have as many options as possible.

- See a doctor: you don't have to be sure of what you want first.

Deciding what to do

If you find that you are pregnant, there are a few options to consider:

1. You can decide to continue the pregnancy, have the baby and care for them.
2. You can decide to continue the pregnancy, have the baby and make arrangements for the baby to be adopted or placed with foster carers.
3. You can decide to have an abortion.

Probably the most important aspect of this decision is that it is your own, and you must not be pressured by others into making any particular choice.

If you think you might want an abortion, see a health professional as soon as possible, so every option is available to you and you can get as much information as you need to make decisions. You can talk to a doctor about what this might mean without having made a decision about what you want. If you are having difficulty deciding what to do, professional counselling may help you work through the things that are important to you, enabling you to choose a path you are comfortable with and to make your own decision.

Good information and a sense of being respected and in control are likely to help you feel confident about your decision, even if it feels like a crisis to begin with. If you are experiencing criticism, pressure, coercion, mental illness, emotional difficulties or conflicting values and beliefs, or if you have feelings such as anger, fear, disappointment, isolation, shame, guilt, grief or sadness, a professional counsellor may well be able to help you before and after your decision.

> 'It's very hard to go through by yourself. You know, it took me such a long time because I didn't have anyone to talk to … I guess that's the main thing: to speak to someone about it … It was so nice to have someone to talk to about it, who wasn't rushing me … She took the time to talk to me about all sorts of different things that were going on in my life.'

Adoption was more common in the past when there was less contraception, less social support available for single mothers and much greater stigma. Many women who did give up their babies in the past felt they didn't have a choice. These days, most women who decide to continue with a pregnancy will keep their baby; many say they couldn't give a baby up for adoption after a full-term pregnancy, but adoption or fostering can still be right for some women.

If you would like to consider whether adoption or fostering might be right for you, it's a good idea to talk to a social worker early on, so that you can get information and help to work through the aspects that matter to you.

A social worker can also help you find what financial and other supports are available to you in pregnancy and in raising a child if you think you will need this kind of help.

The role of your partner

It can be very helpful if an unintended pregnancy feels like a shared problem and your partner supports you in making decisions and getting your preferred health care. Partners will have their own feelings to deal with, and if you find it difficult to talk about or agree on, it may help to seek counselling or advice separately.

The research mentioned above found that 70 per cent of the women who contacted the Women's to talk about abortion had a partner who was aware of the pregnancy and supportive. For 11 per cent, the partner or father of the pregnancy was not aware of the pregnancy, while for the rest the partner was not supportive, their attitude was unknown or there may have been violence or abuse or other complex circumstances in the relationship.

If you decide an abortion is best for you

Your doctor should be able to discuss the services available nearby and refer you for an appointment. If you feel a doctor is being unhelpful or delaying referral, you can contact a family planning service for advice.

In Australia, services vary from state to state. Many services focus on providing abortion when needed, along with contraception and often other aspects of women's health care. In most states and territories the majority of abortion services are private and therefore charge fees, and public services are limited. Some gynaecologists may do abortions when needed for women who have been referred to them and some public hospitals also do abortions when needed.

Assessment for abortion

When you have a consultation about abortion, the doctor or nurse will need to confirm your decision and how sure you are about it, and to check your medical history and any health problems you may have, especially those that may affect the pregnancy or procedure. A physical check-up, an internal or vaginal examination and often an ultrasound scan may be needed to determine how far you are into your pregnancy so the right procedure can be planned. If you don't understand why an examination or test is being done, ask the doctor or nurse.

A Pap test may be done if you are due for one, and it is routine to either test for infections or to use preventative antibiotics, since unrecognised infection can be aggravated by abortion (or any procedure).

Your blood group must be checked because Rhesus-negative women will need an injection to prevent blood-group problems in future pregnancies. If you have a blood-group card, take it with you to your appointment.

If you are sure about having an abortion, you will be given information about the possible methods, and the method you choose should be discussed with you in detail, all your questions answered and informed consent obtained. This means signing a form as you would for any medical procedure. You should only sign it if you understand what it means and your questions have been answered to your satisfaction. You can change your mind at any time after you sign it up until the treatment actually begins.

Privacy and consent

All your information must be kept private, like all other health information. This applies whatever your age. If you are under 18, you are able to give consent for yourself provided the doctor believes you are mature enough to clearly understand what is being discussed and to decide for yourself. There is no requirement for any other person to be told, but it is helpful to have a supportive adult to talk to about what is happening.

Methods of abortion

Abortion can be done as a minor surgical operation or by using medicines to cause a miscarriage. Whatever method you choose, it is important you have somebody to support you and assist you should you have a problem and need medical help.

Surgical abortion

Surgical abortion is done with sedation or anaesthetic; it involves stretching the cervix (neck of the womb) and inserting instruments to remove the pregnancy and empty the uterus. The actual procedure only takes a few minutes but there is usually some waiting time beforehand and recovery time afterwards, so you are often at the treatment centre for a few hours. Sometimes medicine is required first to soften the cervix. This medicine and the anaesthetic can cause nausea and vomiting in some women, and there is usually a little pain and bleeding similar to or less than a period afterwards.

Medication abortion

Medication abortion is a different and less predictable process. The medication method became generally available in Australia in 2013, following the registration of the best drugs for this purpose by our national regulating body, the Therapeutic Goods Administration (TGA), although it has been used elsewhere, including the United Kingdom, for more than 20 years. Two different medicines are used, generally one to two days apart,

What happens in a surgical abortion

The following steps are involved in a surgical abortion:

1. Consultation, examination and tests.

2. Procedure date booked (sometimes this can be done the same day).

3. Possibly premedication a few hours before surgery to soften the cervix; this may cause crampy pain.

4. Usually a general anaesthetic or sedation; sometimes a local.

5. Surgery through the vagina to stretch the cervix and empty the uterus using suction instruments; no cutting is involved, and it usually takes a few minutes.

6. Possible insertion of a contraceptive device such as an intra-uterine device or implant, if you choose this.

7. Pain and bleeding afterwards; usually less than or about the same as a period.

to stimulate the uterus to contract and empty, rather like what happens in a miscarriage. The first tablet is taken, often at the time of consultation, and then a second dose (of four tablets) is taken one to two days later. Occasionally (in about 3 per cent of women) the abortion will happen between the two tablets. You may be able to take the second tablet at home if you prefer, if you have someone to support and assist you and if you can get to a health service if necessary. Some women prefer to be in a clinic or hospital for that support and help.

Some women experience nausea, vomiting and/or diarrhoea after taking the tablets; these symptoms are unpleasant but usually pass in a few hours. At the time of the abortion, most women experience crampy pain and bleeding heavier than a period for up to two hours, although sometimes there is rather less than this. Bleeding similar to a period may then continue for about two weeks, sometimes longer.

Follow-up is important to check that the abortion has occurred successfully.

Medication abortion after nine weeks of pregnancy

After nine weeks gestation, it is generally recommended that medication abortion, if that's what you prefer, be done in a clinic or hospital. Bleeding and pain tend to be greater because of the larger size of the fetus, and

---

What happens in a medication abortion

1. Consultation, examination and tests.
2. First medicine (a single tablet) taken, often on the same day as the consultation if you're certain about your decision.
3. Second medicine taken one to two days later as instructed by the treating doctor. There will usually be four tablets, taken by mouth, in the cheek or in the vagina according to your doctor's instructions. You may have the second tablet (and therefore the abortion) at home or in a clinic or hospital.
4. Pain and bleeding heavier than a period, which usually indicate the abortion is happening.
5. Follow-up to confirm that the abortion has been successful – this is important.
6. For one woman in 20, a curette after this treatment.

---

a curette (a minor surgical procedure that removes the contents of the uterus) is more likely to be necessary than with earlier abortions. For these reasons, more women will prefer surgical abortion if they need an abortion at this stage and many services will not offer medication abortion after nine weeks of pregnancy.

How well does abortion work?

For surgical abortion there is a very low chance of the procedure failing to end the pregnancy, but this does occasionally happen (in two or three out of 1000 cases), usually if the pregnancy is very early and therefore small and hard to find and remove.

For medication abortion, up to about nine weeks of pregnancy around 90 per cent of women will have an abortion within a few hours of taking the second tablet. In up to 5 per cent of women, the abortion does not happen until a day or more later or may be incomplete, so a curette may still be needed. In one woman out of 100 the medication abortion will not work and the pregnancy will continue.

Choosing a method of abortion

Many women have a clear preference for one particular method; sometimes there are medical reasons to recommend a particular method and not all services are able to offer both methods.

Women who prefer the surgical method tend to like the idea of a very predictable timetable and having an anaesthetic so that they are not aware of what is happening.

Those who prefer the medication method want to avoid surgery and anaesthetic and consider a miscarriage-like experience to be more 'natural'. When systems are established for this method, it can mean less waiting time, but you can't be certain when the abortion will happen and, as mentioned above, around one in 20 women will also need to have a curette, either because the tablets haven't worked or because of heavy or continuing bleeding.

Abortion after the first three months

Surgical abortion after the first three months of pregnancy requires doctors with special skills and not all services are able to offer it. It requires greater stretching of the cervix and usually for the fetus to be removed in pieces.

After 13 weeks of pregnancy, medication abortion can still be used, but the doses of drugs are different from those given in an earlier abortion. It becomes more like an induction of labour at this stage, with the passage of a recognisable fetus; around 10 per cent of women will need an anaesthetic to allow removal of retained placental material. Many services will not offer medication abortion after nine weeks of pregnancy.

Serious risks of abortion

Abortion is one of the most common medical procedures undertaken and is generally safer than continuing a pregnancy to birth. In Australia around one in 10,000 women will die in childbirth, and in Western countries about one in 100,000 women will die having an abortion.

The failure rate for surgical abortion is around two or three in 1000; for medication abortion it is around one in 100. Around two in 100 women who have a surgical abortion will need a curette afterwards, usually because of bleeding, some tissue not being removed from the womb, or continuing pregnancy, while for medication abortion around five in 100 will need a curette. The chances of needing a curette are higher after the first three months of pregnancy.

The chance of having a haemorrhage requiring a blood transfusion is around one in 1000 for both surgical and medical abortion. There is a higher chance of this occurring after the first three months of pregnancy.

Infection

Serious infection is very rare and can follow either method of abortion. Severe pelvic infection can affect future fertility, and extreme infections such as toxic shock syndrome can even be fatal. Because of this you will be tested for infection and/or have preventative antibiotics as part of your assessment before an abortion.

Complications of surgical abortion

Around one in 1000 women may suffer damage to the uterus and/or surrounding organs (bowel, bladder or blood vessels) during the procedure, requiring further surgery to repair, or in extreme cases even hysterectomy.

Up to one in 100 women may suffer a tear to the cervix, which usually requires no treatment but may need to be stitched.

Complications of medication abortion

Very rarely the medicines used may cause rupture or tearing of the uterus, which may then need surgical repair. This is very rare at any time but mainly occurs after the first three months of pregnancy.

What happens after an abortion?

In general you can expect to be physically pretty much back to normal within 24 hours of an abortion or anaesthetic. Bleeding less than a period may continue on and off until the next period. The usual advice is not to have vaginal sex or use tampons until bleeding has stopped completely, because of the risk of infection. If you usually have a four-week menstrual cycle, your next period will often start around five or six weeks after the abortion. If you are using hormonal contraception, that may alter the expected time for your next period. Pregnancy symptoms usually start to reduce quickly, but may persist for a few days.

Pain and bleeding

It is normal to experience pain and bleeding after an abortion. For a surgical abortion this is usually not more than during a period, as mentioned above, although sometimes spotting or light bleeding can continue on and off up to the next period. For a medication abortion, pain and bleeding are part of the procedure and are usually more than a period at the time the pregnancy passes. Some bleeding comparable to a period often persists for around a fortnight. You can take medication such as paracetamol or other over-the-counter pain relief, but if these are not sufficient you should seek medical advice. Severe pain occasionally indicates a problem such as serious infection or an unrecognised tubal pregnancy.

Heavy bleeding

A minority of women will experience heavier bleeding. If you soak more than two large pads per hour for more than two hours, or if prolonged bleeding worries you, you should seek medical advice. Causes can include retained placental material, infection or rare conditions such as a molar pregnancy (see chapter 17). Tests for infection, ultrasound examination and/or a curette may be needed. Around one in 1000 women will bleed enough after an abortion to need a blood transfusion; the proportion is higher if the abortion is after the first three months.

Vaginal discharge

Bleeding can be dark brown or even black. Heavier discharge that is yellow, brown or greenish and/or smells bad can sometimes indicate infection, especially if accompanied by moderate pain and/or fever. Seek medical advice, as you may need tests and/or treatment with antibiotics.

Symptoms to watch out for

You should seek medical advice if you have heavy bleeding, pain that does not respond to simple pain-relieving tablets, or a heavy, bad-smelling discharge. You should also seek help if you have fever, fainting, persistent vomiting or diarrhoea; these can be symptoms of serious infection and are signals for urgent attention.

Your feelings

Most women who have been sure of their decision feel mainly relieved after an abortion. Some feelings of sadness and loss are common, but usually pass in time. A minority of women may have more troublesome grief, feelings of guilt, or even depression. Talking about your feelings with someone you trust usually helps; if you would like some help you can talk to a counsellor or your doctor. Contact the service that performed your abortion if you need help finding someone.

Some women report positive aspects, such as:

- a sense of control over their life and personal strength to deal with a crisis

- a strengthening of their relationship with their partner if the experience is shared well
- improved knowledge of fertility and contraception
- clarification of their future wishes regarding family and children

Check-ups

You will usually be offered a follow-up appointment after an abortion, to check your physical recovery, to talk through any feelings that may concern you and to ensure you have satisfactory contraception to help you avoid pregnancy until you are ready for it.

After a medication abortion, it is also important to confirm that the abortion has been successful. This may be done in various ways, including checking the pregnancy material that passes, pregnancy tests on blood or urine, or ultrasound examination. The service treating you will advise you on the best follow-up.

Contraception

It is usually possible to get pregnant again within a couple of weeks of having an abortion, so it is important to start contraception straight away. It is best to discuss your options with the doctor or nurse before having an abortion, and consider whether there is a suitable method you can start at the time of the abortion. Women who use a long-acting reversible contraceptive (LARC; see chapter 16), such as an intrauterine device or implant, have a lower chance of another unplanned pregnancy and abortion, so it is well worth considering whether one of these methods is right for you. The LARC methods are more effective than other methods and easy to use because you don't have to worry about them once they are in place, although as with all methods there are pros and cons (as outlined in chapter 16).

If you have a surgical abortion, an implant, intrauterine contraceptive device or injection can be given at the same time. An implant or injection can also be given at the time of a medication abortion, but an additional appointment will usually be needed for the insertion of an intrauterine contraceptive device. For either method of abortion you can be prescribed the Pill or a vaginal ring to start within a few days. If using condoms or a diaphragm, you should use these from the first time you have sex after the abortion. Methods that depend on recognising the time of ovulation or counting days generally have higher failure rates and are likely to be less reliable than usual until after the next period.

Future pregnancies

An uncomplicated abortion does not appear to affect future fertility or pregnancy outcomes, with one possible exception: women who have had an abortion or miscarriage have a slightly increased risk of early birth, but what might cause this is unknown.

If you want to be pregnant again quickly, usually after an abortion for fetal abnormality, the main deciding factor is your emotional recovery and when you feel ready for another pregnancy. It is possible that there is an increased risk of miscarriage if another pregnancy happens before the first period after an abortion or miscarriage, so it is probably better to wait until after the first normal period if you do feel ready to start again.

Myths about abortion

These tend to be pushed by people who are opposed to abortion and opposed to women having choice regarding control of their reproductive health. They can make women fearful and place barriers in the way of getting good, safe care. If you hear something that worries you, ask a health professional. Even some health professionals are anti-choice, so if you are still not sure, contact a family planning organisation or women's health service.

Myth 1: 'Abortion causes breast cancer'.

Myth 2: 'Abortion causes infertility'.

Myth 3: 'Abortion causes mental health problems'.

Research does not support these links. As far as mental health problems are concerned, women who already have such problems are more likely than women without them to have further problems after either abortion or birth. For a woman who has an unplanned pregnancy, the chance of mental health problems is similar whether she has an abortion or continues the pregnancy to birth.

Abortion, history and the law

Historically, women have sought abortion when they felt unable to continue a pregnancy. Where there is no access to safe, legal abortion, the need still exists; women just use unsafe and/or illegal methods and many come to harm.

Up until 1969, the Women's had a ward that was always occupied by women with serious consequences of unsafe abortion. According to the history of the hospital, 'There was still the shock of what women in their desperation did to themselves: syringing the womb with Rinso, Persil, Dettol, copper sulphate solution, even flammable liquids … They douched themselves with hoses at high pressure. They inserted sticks, twigs, knitting needles, umbrella ribs into their cervices.' It's no wonder that women haemorrhaged, developed serious infections and died.

In many parts of the world this sadly continues. It is estimated that worldwide about 47,000 women die from unsafe abortions each year, around 13 per cent of the world's deaths from pregnancy and birth.

In most Australian states, legal changes in the 1960s and 1970s made abortion safer, but the law still varies between states and territories. In the ACT and Victoria, abortion has been removed from the criminal code, which allows it to be treated properly as a health issue. In the other states and territories either case law or specific legislation determines situations in which abortion is considered lawful.

Where abortion remains in the Crimes Act it is still possible for women and/or their doctors to be charged with a criminal offence for having or performing an abortion. In 2010 a woman faced court in Queensland, but was found not guilty.

The vast majority of the population supports access to safe abortion, and work continues to improve its legal status around the country.

24

When pregnancy isn't happening

Shlomi Barak, Alice Huang, Rachael Knight,
John McBain, Tram Nguyen, Kate Stern

Research at the Women's involving 3000 women who had kept a careful record of when they stopped using contraception and then gave birth to a baby, showed that of all babies born, 84 per cent were conceived within six months of trying. The remaining 16 per cent were conceived over the next few years.

So the first few months of trying have the highest chance of success (usually 20–30 per cent per month), and as the months pass the chance of success becomes lower and lower until it might be as low as 1 or 2 per cent per month after three years of trying.

Some people seem to get pregnant any and every month they try. While these people may not accurately recall how easy or difficult conceiving was, it is true that some people do conceive more quickly than others. Such women generally:

- are younger – human fertility is highest in women aged between 18 and 32, after which a woman's fertility declines at a rate of 5–8 per cent per year, until by the age of 40 a woman has a 50 per cent chance of being infertile just because she's 40

- have sex more often – those who have sex every night conceive four times as quickly as those who have sex once a week

- have regular ovulation cycles – while 28 days is the average, the fertile cycle length in Australian women in the 1970s was found to be between 23 and 35 days; 23 days is the lower limit of the fertile cycle. It is very difficult to get a more recent figure due to the high number of women who are now on the Pill.

- have been pregnant before – as in almost everything in life, if you've done it before you're more likely to do it again. And that goes for the man, too.

Why pregnancy might not be happening

Anyone studying human reproduction at some time experiences a feeling of wonder as to how any of us came to be born; it all seems so complicated.

The egg (or oocyte) a woman releases in any month was laid down on the outer rim of her ovaries around four or five months before she was born. The egg supply laid down at that time is to last her for all of her reproductive life, which may span from her early teen years in some countries and cultures until her mid-40s (increasingly common in some countries, such as Australia). How the eggs are retained in storage for so long is gradually being understood, and involves a hormone called anti-Müllerian hormone (AMH), which makes it difficult for resting eggs to start their growth pattern.

When sperm and eggs form in body through a process of cell division called meiosis, there is a swapping of information between chromosomes from the mother and the father, chromosomes that *they* inherited from *their* parents, which means that each child will obtain some genes from each of its four grandparents. This is the wonderful process that means we have things in common with each of our ancestors but remain a unique individual, contributing to diversity in the human race.

As women age, this process starts to go wrong and mistakes start to occur during meiosis, in the way the chromosomes are duplicated then split, then finally halved to make way for the contribution of chromosomes from the sperm. We see the outcome of such errors in women over 35, in an increasing risk of Down syndrome and of early miscarriage.

We now know that in many months where you may have thought pregnancy didn't occur, fertilisation and early embryo development actually took place but the chromosome errors were too serious for the early embryo to survive, and so your period came when you expected it or was only slightly delayed, and a home pregnancy test was negative or only faintly positive.

During the days of rapidly rising oestrogen hormone levels, before the release of the egg at ovulation, the neck of the uterus – the cervix – makes a protein-rich clear jelly that covers the top of the vagina during sex, neutralising the normal acidity of the vagina (which prevents thrush and other infections) and thus creating a suitable environment for sperm survival. The sperm rapidly swim up and into the cervix, where they may survive in that mucus for up to five days before an egg is released.

Low sperm numbers and decreased sperm vitality, which we measure as percentage motility, may make it difficult for adequate numbers of sperm to reach the site of fertilisation. Although it only takes one sperm to do it, it takes a very large number for that to happen.

The egg must find its way from the ovary into the fallopian tube to meet the sperm that have travelled up from the cervical mucus. The outermost part of the fallopian tube, the fimbriae, act like a sea anemone and catch the egg, so any past infection or surgery that has caused the delicate 'fingers' of the fimbriae to fuse together may make it difficult for them to pick up the fertile egg.

It is here in the outer part of the tube that the sperm first digest the sticky cells around the egg that helped the tube capture the egg; many sperm must attach to the outer shell and then the membrane of the egg before one can enter and fertilise the egg. One of the more common reasons for infertility is a high percentage of sperm with the wrong head shape, which means the egg does not accept those sperm. This is a more serious problem if sperm numbers and motility are also reduced.

The fallopian tube may be blocked at any part along its length by past infection or surgery (including surgery for a tubal sterilisation procedure), so the sperm and egg may never meet. Tests may show that one tube is blocked and the other open, but the infection that blocked the tube may have caused damage to the intricate inner lining and muscle organisation of the 'normal' tube. If pregnancy does occur in this situation, the embryo may remain in the tube as an ectopic pregnancy, which requires surgical removal or other medical treatment.

After fertilisation, the egg quickly becomes an embryo; the muscles and fine hair lining the tube move the embryo towards the uterus, which it enters around four days after fertilisation. The embryo must now be able to hatch from its little shell and send the correct signals to the lining of the uterus – the uterus itself must have undergone changes to allow implantation under the action of progesterone. This hormone has been made in increasing amounts by the area in the ovary where the egg grew, which is now so full of cholesterol, the building block for progesterone, that it appears yellow. It is called the corpus luteum, Latin for 'yellow body'.

The corpus luteum must now make adequate amounts of progesterone and some oestrogen. This is to support the lining of the uterus while the embryo is establishing a firm position there, sending cells to invade and colonise the very small blood vessels below the lining, and establishing a nutrient and oxygen supply for the early pregnancy.

As the pregnancy grows and invades the mother's uterine lining and blood vessels, it is sending an increasingly strong signal to the ovary, through the hormone hCG, to tell it to prolong and increase its production of progesterone. A pregnancy test measures the levels of hCG; as long as it is known when ovulation occurred, the level of hCG can be a reasonable indication of the pregnancy's wellbeing.

Possible reasons for pregnancy failure

Once implantation occurs successfully, a number of things may still go wrong that can lead to early pregnancy failure:

- The embryo may have the wrong number of chromosomes, which may mean pregnancy is not detected if the abnormalities involve the larger chromosomes, or it may cause early to later miscarriage depending upon the degree of abnormality.

- The embryo may have a normal number of chromosomes but not consume enough glucose. In laboratory studies, cells that consumed more glucose were more likely to progress normally. Failure of some embryos may be due to inefficiencies in the cell's power packs, the mitochondria, or to as-yet-unknown lethal genes on the normal chromosomes.

- The endometrium, the lining of the womb, may not have received enough progesterone for a long enough time to allow successful implantation because the period arrived fewer than 11 days after ovulation – a short luteal phase or luteal-phase defect. This is rare.

- There are other uterine or endometrial factors that are poorly understood. These factors include the natural killers cell function, which is important for remodelling the blood vessels in the endometrium; antiphospholipid antibody activity, which is a type of immune disorder; aberrant gene profiling; and thrombophilia conditions that involve blood-clotting regulation.

- Other uncommon but important factors inside the uterus that may affect the embryo's chance of successful implantation include adhesions, between the front and back wall of the endometrial cavity, and polyps, especially fibroid polyps inside the endometrial cavity. It is important to emphasise that most fibroids do not interfere with conception or pregnancy unless they are unusually large or distort the endometrial cavity.

The emotional impact of infertility

The emotional impact of infertility and its treatment is often felt before the formal diagnosis and long after the final treatment cycle. For many people, having children and creating a family are seen as central to their plans and hopes for life. When pregnancy does not happen after a few months of trying, fear, doubt and frustration can start to occur. Nonetheless, the response to hearing the diagnosis of infertility still often comes with a mix of strong emotions, all of which are normal. These include:

- shock, surprise and disbelief – these can occur even though pregnancy has not been happening for many months. Some people go into a state of denial – that none of this is really happening.
- guilt – blaming oneself for the infertility
- blame – blaming your partner for the infertility
- anger – such as thoughts of 'Why me?' or anger at others
- fear and anxiety – regarding the uncertainty and lack of control of what will happen next
- grief and loss – these losses are intangible and can be multiple: loss of identity of being female, of being a mother, a loss of purpose and the sense of losing an imagined future child

Infertility can be seen as a major crisis in life and the treatments – though effective for many – come at a financial, social and emotional cost.

Fertility treatments

Fertility drugs are so-called because when effectively used, they help women who are not producing an egg to do so and become fertile. When used in these situations they are highly effective, and you have a good chance of successful pregnancy happening over a course of treatment with these drugs if your partner's sperm are normal.

They are often used, though, by women who are already ovulating, perhaps infrequently or irregularly, or who are ovulating regularly each month. In these cases, the chance of pregnancy occurring on these drugs is low, as there are often other factors that have been stopping pregnancy and will remain a barrier to conception.

Before starting fertility drug treatment, you should have some tests to assess whether or not treatment might be useful, and to help decide which class of drug to use and which dose to start with.

You may have blood tests to check your levels of:

- **Follicle stimulating hormone (FSH)** – this hormone is essential for the fertile growth of the follicle containing the egg. In some cases the levels of this hormone will be very low, generally in women who do not have periods (amenorrhoea). In most women it will be within the normal range, but in yet others it will be above the normal range; that is generally a sign that their fertile years are over and that fertility drug treatment will not be of help.

- **Luteinising hormone (LH)** – this hormone forms the basis of most urinary ovulation tests. It may be normal or elevated in women with irregular or no periods; normal or low in women with no periods; and profoundly low in women who have lost so much weight as to place their health at risk.

- **Prolactin (PRL)** – this hormone is normally elevated during pregnancy as it plays an important role in the preparation and establishment of lactation. It may be raised in women who are not pregnant but whose periods have ceased or become very infrequent. This may be due to a small tumour in the pituitary gland, or to some classes of medication that interfere with the action of a brain hormone called dopamine. The most common medications to cause this problem are psycho-tropic medications, and any decision to stop using them should be made with the doctor who prescribed them. Rarely, elevated prolactin can be due to an underactive thyroid gland (hypothyroidism).

- **Thyrotrophin (TSH)** – the level of this hormone should be checked to see if the thyroid gland is underactive, which can first manifest as an irregular menstrual pattern.

- **Androgens** – these hormones – testosterone, dehydroepiandrosterone (DHEAS), 17-alpha-hydroxyprogesterone and sex hormone-binding globulin (SHBG) – are generally tested together to calculate a free androgen index. This index is often elevated in women with ovula-tion problems who have polycystic ovarian syndrome (PCOS) and may suffer from acne or unwanted facial hair as a consequence of the elevated androgen levels. The androgen 17-alpha-hydroxyprogester-one is measured to detect a metabolic condition called adrenogenital syndrome, which may otherwise be misdiagnosed as PCOS.

Years ago, oestrogen was measured daily in some types of fertility injection treatment, but this has mostly been replaced by ultrasound follicle measurement. This may help with the decision to use fertility drugs such as Clomid or, if the oestrogen level is very low, fertility injections of follicle stimulating hormone.

Vaginal ultrasound gives immediate and up-to-the-minute information on the state of the ovary, the target organ for fertility drug treatment. An ultrasound may allow your doctor to see and evaluate simple cysts that might interfere with treatment. It can also allow a count of the ovarian follicles less than 1 centimetre in diameter. The follicles are fluid-filled sacs containing the cells that will go on to make oestrogen to prepare the uterus for ovulation. They also contain the microscopic eggs that are released at ovulation.

If you have symptoms such as worsening period pain or significant discomfort on deep penetration during sex, or a history of recurrent pelvic infection, and particularly if your ultrasound examination suggests some pelvic problem, your doctor may consider diagnostic laparoscopy (keyhole investigation) to test fallopian tube function. Otherwise these tests are unhelpful in a woman who clearly requires ovulation treatment.

A sperm sample should also be tested, to discount a fertility issue in the man.

Fertility drugs

There are two main sorts of fertility drug: a tablet containing clomiphene citrate (Clomid), or an injection of follicle stimulating hormone (FSH; Gonal-F, Puregon). These drugs have been used for 50 years now and they remain the basis for fertility drug treatment.

Clomid affects the ovary through its action on the pituitary gland, which it forces to release more FSH and LH than it normally would. The higher hormone levels persuade some of the small follicles on the ovary to grow during and beyond the five days during which the Clomid tablets are taken. These developing follicles send a message back to the hypothalamus and pituitary glands that dampens down the stimulation message and ensures that, generally, only one or two eggs are released. The chance of twins on Clomid is around 8 per cent, and the risk of triplets is one in 200.

The Gonal-F and Puregon FSH injections come in a small pen with changeable small needles for injection under the skin. FSH acts directly on the ovary, which means there is no feedback to moderate the dose, so there is a risk of multiple follicle development and therefore multiple pregnancy. Because of this, treatment starts with the lowest dose the doctor thinks might be effective and is gradually increased by small amounts every six days until one or two follicles have reached 17–23 millimetres in diameter on an ultrasound and the endometrium, the lining of the uterus, is 8 millimetres or more thick.

At this point there will generally be a further injection of hCG to bring on ovulation, which may not otherwise occur. Following ovulation, there will be two further lower-dose injections of hCG to ensure that the second half of the cycle is long enough and progesterone levels are adequate.

Multiple pregnancy is an ever-present risk with FSH treatment, so it should not be given to someone who has a medical or obstetric reason to avoid twins. With FSH treatment, twins occur in 15 per cent of pregnancies, triplets in 4 per cent of pregnancies and quads or more in 1 per cent of pregnancies.

Where the ovulation problem is due to excessive levels of prolactin, treatment may be with the medications bromocriptine or cabergoline, which are generally fast-acting and do not increase the risk of multiple pregnancy.

In women whose ovulation failure is due to PCOS and is compounded by obesity, the loss of as little as 5–7 kilograms through exercise and dietary restriction has been found to show a rapid return to fertile ovulation. In these situations, some doctors suggest using the insulin-sensitising drug metformin. While this may work in some cases, it is no substitute for weight loss through a healthy diet and exercise.

Assisted reproduction therapy (ART)

This is treatment to get pregnant by means other than having sex. It nowadays includes intrauterine insemination (IUI) and in-vitro fertilisation (IVF) with or without intracytoplasmic sperm injection (ICSI, sperm injection directly into the egg; see 'Assisted reproductive techniques' in the 'Male infertility' section below).

Intrauterine insemination (IUI)

The success of IUI will vary depending upon the reason for choosing it as a treatment. IUI may be performed in a natural cycle without the use of medication, or in a cycle in which mild ovarian stimulation with clomiphene citrate or FSH (see above) is used to develop one or two extra ovulated eggs. A small volume of washed and concentrated sperm is placed through the cervix at the time of ovulation.

Your doctor may suggest IUI for the following reasons:

- Your partner's semen profile is normal but your cervical mucus is hostile (low pH, local sperm antibodies) or there is no mucus in your cervix to neutralise acid in the vagina – treatment is most successful in such cases.

- Your partner's semen profile is normal and your mucus is receptive to sperm – this is less successful and usually performed following mild ovarian stimulation.

- Your partner's semen profile shows a low sperm count and/or low motility – treatment is much less successful in this situation.

- Treatment is performed for social reasons; for example, if your partner is interstate or overseas – this is quite successful if his sperm freeze and thaw well.

- Donor insemination – this is quite successful if you are younger than 36.

Generally, if you do not become pregnant within the first three or four attempts, the chances of further success are low and it is time to consider IVF.

In vitro fertilisation (IVF)

The term *in vitro* is Latin for 'in glass', denoting that fertilisation has not occurred in the body, which would be *in vivo*.

The basic components of this treatment are:

- stimulation of the ovaries through daily FSH injections, with the aim of developing six to 16 mature, egg-containing follicles around 2–2.5 centimetres in diameter

- vaginal ultrasound to monitor follicle growth

- a 'trigger' injection of hCG when the scan shows the follicles to be of appropriate size and number

- day surgery admission for vaginal ultrasound-guided egg collection performed under a light general anaesthetic – there are no cuts on the abdomen, the eggs are collected through the vagina

- placing eggs and sperm together in a dish with culture fluid (standard IVF) or injecting a single sperm into the egg (ICSI) – the method used depends on how fertile the sperm were found to be before IVF treatment

- observation of early fertilisation events that identify normal fertilisation, and early breakdown of the walls surrounding the chromosomes from the egg and sperm before they mix
- transfer of generally one but possibly two embryos between two and five days after fertilisation, depending on individual circumstances
- a supplementary course of progesterone administered vaginally for two weeks from the second day after fertilisation
- freezing in liquid nitrogen any other embryos that have developed normally for later transfer. Such embryos nowadays have a 90 per cent chance of surviving freezing and thawing.

Adjuvant therapy in IVF

Many additional or adjuvant therapies before, during and after IVF cycles have been proposed and researched in an attempt to increase success. Examples of adjuvant therapies used include growth hormones, DHEAS, acupuncture, testosterone and steroids. Unfortunately, scientific research has not conclusively demonstrated a significant benefit, and the safety of many of these treatments has not yet been established. Currently there is not enough evidence from clinical studies to support the routine use of adjuvant therapies, and the possible side effects also mean that caution should be exercised as these supplements might be prescribed without evidence of benefit but in the hope that 'something might help'.

Choosing to undergo ART

Most women attempt ART several times before achieving a pregnancy and some women may never achieve a pregnancy. It is important, therefore, for you and your partner to consider carefully whether you can afford the financial, social and emotional costs of IVF before you start.

Chances of success

Overwhelmingly, the chances of success relate to the age of the woman and the genetic quality of her eggs. This means an adequate number of eggs must be retrieved, and a number of high-quality eggs need to be developed to produce good-quality embryos.

Expectations for success through IVF may be divided into two main groups: women under 36, whose chance of having a live birth from the first stimulation cycle and transfer of all of the embryos in subsequent freeze–thaw cycles is more than 50 per cent; and women over 40, whose chances are much lower, perhaps as low as 2–5 per cent per attempt by the age of 43.

Counselling and advice about options such as donor eggs or donor embryos are available at all IVF clinics.

The emotional impact of infertility and ART

With the variable success rate for any couple for any given treatment, it is likely that strong emotional responses will happen during the course of treatment. The treatments may be financially draining, physically invasive, technically challenging to understand and highly demanding of time with multiple appointments per week. Therefore it is important to be aware of how you can reduce the stress that ART can have on your life and develop your own personal set of strategies to deal with the emotional impact. These can include:

- Being with your partner (see below).

- Keeping yourself informed about the process and the options available. Get as much information as you can from the staff as well as written information (from credible sources).

- Deciding whom you will tell about your infertility and treatment. This is an individual decision. Not telling anyone can leave you socially isolated. However, telling too many people can lead to a large audience waiting for the results of every cycle. How you will tell people is another decision to make early on. For some people, face-to-face can be too confronting and they prefer social media. Others may need the opportunity to cry with someone when a cycle is not successful.

- Planning ahead to decide where and when you will be when you receive a result, as well as whom you will be with. Most people prefer not to get results at work.

- Trying to limit the stress in other aspects of your life, which may involve reducing your workload or hours, if possible. This may mean putting aside a major renovation to your house, for example, or other big stressors.

- Trying to stay active in other parts of your life that are important to your social, physical and emotional wellbeing. Continue any exercise you have been doing, your social contacts and hobbies. This prevents the process of ART taking over your life and being your one single focus.

- Trying stress management strategies: exercise, relaxation, meditation, yoga, massages and facials.

- Joining a support group and speaking with others who are going through a similar process is useful and prevents the sense of social isolation – that it's 'just happening to me'.

- Planning a review date for the ART process to decide how many cycles you will try and to plan breaks in the cycle. This can give your body a chance to recover and an opportunity for you to have a planned holiday without worrying about appointments.

Your most important support throughout this time is likely to be your partner. They may be the only other person who knows exactly what is happening. They will be invaluable in supporting you during appointments. However, sometimes relationships can suffer during the course of ART due to blame, guilt, lack of communication and the impact of ART on sexual intimacy.

It is important for you to be aware that your partner may have a very different emotional and behavioural response to infertility and the entire process. They may have either a more upbeat or a more pessimistic outlook. It is when these varying perspectives are misunderstood that conflict can occur. It is important to hear and understand each other's perspective, responses to infertility and to each stage of treatment, and each other's ideas of family and parenthood. It is also important to be aware that your partner may have different ways to cope, such as spending more time at work. Be aware of what support can be provided within the relationship and when you and your partner need extra support outside the relationship. This may be from family, friends, support groups and/or counsellors.

The process of ART is challenging in itself; however, many women find certain situations lead to additional stress. These include: seeing pregnant women (e.g. at ultrasound appointments); hearing about other people's (friends and family) pregnancies; family or social gatherings where there are babies; birthdays (for some women the knowledge of advancing age can be difficult to accept); having a miscarriage; and deciding when to stop treatment. Being aware of these potentially stressful times may allow you to plan how you might deal with them.

Most ART services will have a counselling service of varying capacity. This is a good starting point to ask about the local support services. ACCESS (www.access.org.au) is a national consumer-based independent support network for people with infertility. There might be times when women will have more prolonged or severe emotional responses that are overwhelming, and these might be an early sign of emerging anxiety or depression (see chapter 22). If you are concerned about your emotional wellbeing, your GP is a good starting point for seeking help.

Financial costs

Successive Australian governments have taken a pro-natalist approach to conception and birth through the 'baby bonus', paid maternity leave and child support. Those who are infertile for medical reasons have some of the cost of IVF paid through Medicare, but there often remain substantial out-of-pocket costs. The total out-of-pocket cost will depend on Medicare rebates, tax benefits and the Medicare safety net, the type and number of specialised tests and procedures you need, whether your partner also needs treatment, and whether you have private health insurance to cover day surgery procedures, such as egg collection and embryo transfer.

It is strongly recommended that you contact the fertility clinic you are interested in attending and ask them to explain all the fees related to your particular treatment plan before you start the IVF process. Don't forget there may be costs associated with blood collection, pathology, anaesthesia and storing embryos, too.

Preserving fertility

Medical fertility preservation

There are many young women whose fertility is threatened by cancer or other serious diseases, and by the treatment for these conditions. Medical fertility preservation refers to methods used to try to protect and preserve fertility for the future, using a variety of treatment options, including medicines to protect the ovary, freezing eggs and embryos, and freezing ovarian tissue for grafting later on if required.

Cancer treatments are nowadays very successful and most young women can expect to go on to lead normal lives and have their own family. The time of the cancer diagnosis, however, is extremely traumatic and distressing for young women and their families. Often everything feels overwhelming, especially as there is so much information to take in about the disease, its treatment options and the short- and long-term risks. While thinking ahead to the future may seem just too much to deal with, it may be very important to find out about ways to maximise future fertility.

It is now an established part of early cancer management for doctors to talk to patients about the risks of treatment, including the risk to fertility, so most young women will be referred to a fertility specialist during this time. While many young women decide to have some fertility preservation treatment, for many others, just having a discussion and becoming more informed about their reproductive future can be extremely reassuring.

Cancer treatment and the risk of fertility damage

Chemotherapy drugs can cause damage to the ovaries, and the risk increases with age. This is because as we get older, our ovaries contain fewer eggs and so are more vulnerable. The effects of these drugs can include:

- short-term ovarian failure with temporary stopping of periods, which return in three to 12 months
- immediate and permanent ovarian failure (premature menopause), which is much less common and occurs with very high-dose treatments; in this situation the ovaries stop working for good because the eggs have all been damaged
- later development of permanent ovarian failure a few years down the track, but often at the time of recovery from the cancer, when wanting to start a family

Any cancer in the pelvic area requiring radiotherapy for treatment might also damage the ovaries or uterus. These include bowel (particularly rectal), bladder, cervix, endometrium, vulva, ovary or fallopian tube cancers. Some cancers require surgery that can mean removal of the ovaries or else disturb the function of the fallopian tubes.

The table below describes the risk of permanent ovarian failure with common cancer treatments.

Cancer treatments and ovarian failure

Disease or treatment	Likelihood of premature ovarian failure
Breast cancer: • under the age of 30 • aged 30–40	less than 10% 20–40%
Sarcoma	less than 10–20%
Hodgkin's disease	less than 10% unless therapy is intensive
Non-Hodgkin's disease	10–40%
Leukaemia	less than 15%
High-dose therapy and stem-cell transplantation	more than 70%

Protection of fertility during chemotherapy

Some medicines, called GnRH analogues, may reduce the damage caused by chemotherapy drugs to the ovaries. These drugs work to keep the ovaries in a quiet, non-functioning state and suppress the normal menstrual cycle. This theoretically reduces the exposure of the eggs to the damaging effects of the cancer treatment. GnRH analogues are given as monthly injections during the time of the chemotherapy. Side effects include hot flushes, which tend to start after the second injection is given. Fortunately the side effects and the suppressing effects are only temporary, and there are no lasting effects of the analogue after the therapy finishes.

Preservation of eggs, embryos and ovarian tissue

If there is enough time before the cancer treatment starts, young women can undergo 10–12 days of hormone medications that stimulate many eggs to mature in the ovary, then have these removed in a very minor procedure under sedation (but asleep). There are no cuts on the abdomen as the entry is through the vagina. On average, 10–20 eggs are removed and frozen for use later. When needed, they can be made into embryos using the partner's sperm. For every 10 eggs frozen, we can expect to ultimately make two or three embryos. For women in long-term relationships, embryos can be created, with the retrieved eggs and partner's sperm, and then frozen after the extraction of the eggs. About 80–90 per cent of embryos will survive the thawing process.

Freezing of some ovarian tissue is also an important option. This can be considered:

- when the cancer treatment involves very high-dose chemotherapy drugs; for example, as part of a bone marrow or stem-cell transplant
- when there is not enough time for 10–12 days of hormone stimulation
- for young girls who have not yet started to have regular menstrual cycles

This process involves a laparoscopy (keyhole surgery) to remove part of the ovary, which is a day-stay procedure. As with all surgery, there are risks involved, but generally it is a very safe operation.

Grafting of the frozen and then thawed ovarian tissue is performed later if necessary to restore fertility after permanent ovarian failure. It is very important to understand that making babies from eggs that have come out of an ovarian graft is still a complex process. Even though there have been babies born after this process, we are not yet at a stage where this can be thought of as routine.

Other fertility options for the future

For some young women who may not have the opportunity to preserve fertility before cancer treatment there is the possibility later on, if their ovaries don't work, of creating a family using donated eggs. This is an established and successful treatment that offers hope to young women with permanent ovarian failure.

If the uterus is damaged or women cannot, for medical reasons, carry a pregnancy, then surrogacy, where another woman carries the pregnancy, is another possibility.

The decision to use donor eggs or a surrogate can be both emotionally and financially difficult, and also extremely legally complicated. Counselling is highly recommended, and it is vital – whether you are receiving assistance from a friend or family member or using a commercial surrogacy service overseas (only altruistic surrogacy is legal in Australia) – to be fully aware of the financial and legal implications of your choices.

Social (non-medical) fertility preservation

As we get older, we have fewer good eggs and there is a higher risk of chromosomal damage to the eggs we have left. From the mid-30s there is a progressive decline in egg number and quality.

For women who think they will not have the opportunity to start a family with a partner in their years of maximum fertility, it is now possible to freeze some eggs for the future. It is very important to understand, however, that this offers at most a limited number of opportunities to try to have a baby. Non-medical egg freezing should therefore not be relied on as a guarantee of future fertility, but more as offering a modest additional opportunity in the future.

Conclusions

Thinking about future fertility, and providing the opportunity to conserve fertility, is now an integral part of the management of serious diseases with toxic therapies. All young women in this situation should have the opportunity to discuss with their oncologist or a fertility specialist options that can genuinely increase the chances of them having their own family in the future. While we are now able to offer opportunities to maximise future fertility, because fertility declines with increasing age, and for other reasons, nothing can guarantee future fertility success.

Male infertility

In couples where pregnancy isn't happening, a problem with the male partner also needs to be considered, as it is relatively common. Infertility results solely from a problem with the male partner's sperm in 30 per cent of cases. In another 30 per cent, there is a combined contribution from both partners.

A variety of conditions can lead to infertility, including:

- problems in the testes, which occur in 30–40 per cent of cases (of which 15–25 per cent are due to genetic causes)
- a blockage in the sperm pathway caused by prior infection, which occurs in 10–20 per cent of cases
- hormonal disorders caused by conditions of the pituitary gland or hypothalamus, which occur in 1–2 per cent of cases

In 40–50 per cent of cases, however, the precise cause cannot be determined.

In the past, men with infertility had limited treatment options. Today, new tests and treatments have enabled many infertile men to father children.

Evaluation of male infertility

A comprehensive review of your partner's medical history is the first step in the process of infertility evaluation. This includes childhood growth and development, testicular descent, sexual development during puberty, sexual history, illnesses and infections, surgeries, medications, exposure to certain environmental agents (alcohol, radiation, steroids, chemotherapy and toxic chemicals), sexual performance and any previous fertility testing.

A physical examination will include examination of the scrotum and testicles. Scrotal ultrasound imaging is also commonly performed as part of the initial investigation.

Semen analysis

The most important laboratory investigation of male infertility is the semen analysis. It provides information about the volume of semen and the number, motility (movement) and morphology (shape) of sperm.

Semen may be obtained either by masturbation or during intercourse using a special non-toxic condom. Requirements of this analysis include a two-to-five-day period of abstinence from ejaculation (sex and masturbation), delivery of the sample to the laboratory within one hour of collection, and avoiding exposure to lubricants or extremes of temperature.

Because of the variability of results, several semen analyses at intervals of two or more weeks are necessary if your partner's first test shows an abnormality. Even with successful collection of samples, there will be variability in the analyses due to counting error, other technical errors, and differences in the ejaculate from day to day. These large variations need to be remembered when interpreting results of semen analysis.

The analysis tests the following:

- **Sperm antibodies** – large proteins occasionally produced by the body's immune system, which attach to sperm and can interfere with motility or cover the head of the sperm, so as to interfere with the binding to the egg and prevent fertilisation. Tests for sperm antibodies should be done routinely on all men being evaluated for infertility.

- **Variations in semen volume and appearance** – low semen volume suggests incomplete collection, a shorter period of abstinence from ejaculation than required before the test, absence or obstruction of the seminal vesicles (glands where the seminal fluid is made), or androgen (male hormone) deficiency.

- **Azoospermia** – the total absence of sperm from the ejaculate. The main causes of azoospermia are severe sperm production disorders (primary spermatogenic defect) and obstructions (obstructive azoospermia). Rarely, an illness or difficulty with collection will cause transient azoospermia.

- **Oligospermia** – sperm concentrations of less than 20 million per millilitre. There is a correlation between sperm concentration and other aspects of sperm quality. Both motility and morphology are usually poor with oligospermia.

- **Asthenospermia** – less than 50 per cent sperm motility. Spurious asthenospermia caused by exposure of sperm to latex (particularly in condoms), spermicides, extremes of temperature, or long delays between collection and examination, should be excluded.

- **Teratospermia** – a reduced percentage of sperm with normal shape, as assessed using a microscope. Abnormal shape is highly correlated with reduced binding and penetration of the sperm into the egg.

Hormone assessment

It is not necessary to perform hormone measurements routinely. However, in certain cases this kind of investigation is advised.

Follicle stimulating hormone (FSH) levels in men with azoospermia may identify whether the problem is an obstruction or a sperm production disorder. Measurement of prolactin, luteinising hormone and testosterone may also provide additional information about the state of sperm production. Prolactin should be measured in men with androgen deficiency and loss of libido.

Chromosome and genetic studies

Karyotype (chromosome analysis) is commonly performed in men with suspected sperm production disorder. If a genetic anomaly is discovered as part of an investigation into infertility, a genetic counsellor will be able to explain what it means for the man, whether assisted reproductive technologies are an option and if there are potential consequences for the children.

Klinefelter syndrome is the most common chromosomal abnormality associated with male infertility, in which there is at least one extra X chromosome, making a total of 47 chromosomes, rather than the usual 46. The result of their karyotype (the picture of their set of chromosomes) will come back as 47, XXY. These men usually have very small testicles. Although most men with Klinefelter syndrome have no sperm in the semen, some have a low sperm count, and in very rare cases are fertile. Sperm for use in IVF or ICSI can be obtained by testicular biopsy in about 50 per cent of these men.

Microdeletions (absence of small segments) in the long arm of the Y chromosome have been found in up to 15 per cent of men with severe sperm production disorders. Sons of men with these microdeletions, who have from pregnancies achieved with ICSI, have the same microdeletions, but daughters will not be affected, of course, as they do not have a Y chromosome.

The vasa deferentia are two ducts that connect the left and right epididymis (tightly coiled tubes associated with the testes) to the ejaculatory ducts, and are part of the sperm transporting system (testicles to the urethra). In some men, these ducts, or parts of them, are missing. Cystic fibrosis gene studies are important for evaluation of these men and their partners. If both partners are carriers of the cystic fibrosis gene, they have a one in four risk of having a child with cystic fibrosis. In these cases their embryos can be genetically tested before implantation.

If a genetic anomaly is discovered as part of an investigation into infertility, a genetic counsellor will be able to explain what it means for the man, whether assisted reproductive technologies are an option and if there are potential consequences for the children.

Other tests

If flow of semen into the bladder (retrograde ejaculation) is suspected, your partner will need to give a post-ejaculation urine sample.

Male infertility treatments

The treatment for male infertility depends upon its underlying cause.

Blockage of the reproductive tract

If your partner has a blockage in the ducts that carry the sperm, he can undergo surgery to correct this blockage. Another option is assisted reproductive techniques using sperm retrieved directly from the testes (see below).

Vasectomy (male sterilisation) is a specific type of blockage. Vasectomies can be reversed in up to 85 per cent of cases, but the more time that has passed since the vasectomy, the less likely vasectomy reversal is to restore fertility.

Hypothalamic or pituitary deficiency

In a small percentage of cases, male infertility is due to problems in the hypothalamus and pituitary gland (parts of the brain that regulate hormone production). In this case, your partner would be given hormone treatment with human chorionic gonadotropin (hCG) and recombinant human follicle stimulating hormone (rhFSH), also called gonadotropin treatment.

Most men will eventually develop sperm in the ejaculate, although it might take one to two years of treatment to achieve normal fertility.

Varicocele

A varicocele is a dilation of a vein in the scrotum. Many men with varicocele have a low sperm count or abnormal sperm shape. The reason a varicocele affects the sperm may be related to a higher than normal temperature in the testicles, poor oxygen supply, and poor blood flow in the testicles.

Varicocele can be treated surgically, but surgery does not always improve fertility and is not recommended for most men unless the varicocele is large. An alternative to varicocele repair, and the recommended approach, is assisted reproductive techniques, usually intracytoplasmic sperm injection (ICSI; see below).

Assisted reproductive techniques

If the semen has a low sperm count, no sperm, abnormal sperm, or sperm with poor motility, assisted reproductive techniques often help. For some infertile couples this will be the only way to achieve a pregnancy.

Intracytoplasmic sperm injection (ICSI)

ICSI is a procedure performed in conjunction with IVF. With ICSI, a single sperm is injected directly into an egg in the laboratory. This can be useful in cases of low sperm count, low motility, abnormal morphology or a combination of them, and it is the most common technique used when male infertility is the problem. Pregnancy and live birth rates are similar to that with natural conception.

Testicular biopsy

If sperm is completely absent in the ejaculate (azoospermia), it can sometimes be directly retrieved from the testicles. This is usually done using a small needle under a local anaesthetic. It might require minor surgery involving scrotal incision. If sperm can be found, it will be used for ICSI, and the fertilisation rate of the egg will be not very different from that with IVF.

Sperm harvesting using this technique is usually uneventful, with a small risk of bruising, bleeding and infection.

There is some evidence that children of couples who become pregnant after IVF or ICSI have a slightly higher rate of birth abnormalities, although these conditions are rare and the overall risk of having a child with a birth anomaly is low. If you are in this situation, your fertility specialist should discuss this potential risk with you.

Complementary and other medicines

There are various complementary or other medicines advertised as being able to treat male infertility, including various hormones and vitamins. Proper clinical trials have not yet, however, shown any of these methods to be clinically effective in treating unexplained oligospermia or azoospermia. Recommendations for using complementary and other medicines should be viewed with caution and discussed with your doctor.

When male infertility cannot be treated

Couples affected by non-treatable male infertility may consider artificial insemination using donor sperm. Donor sperm may be obtained from a sperm bank, which screens men for infections and certain genetic problems, and provides a detailed personal and family profile.

The decision to use donor sperm (from a known or unknown donor) can be complicated and difficult. Counselling may be helpful and is highly recommended.

Polycystic ovarian syndrome (PCOS)

A recent study has shown that PCOS affects up to 21 per cent of Australian women of reproductive age. Certain groups are at increased risk, including women who are overweight or from an Indigenous background.

PCOS affects reproductive health and can include a number of other important features, such as excess unwanted hair growth and acne. Longer term risks of diabetes and heart disease have been reported and some women can develop anxiety and depression as a result of the problems caused by their PCOS.

Causes of PCOS

The exact cause of this condition is still unclear, but we do know that both genetic and environmental factors play a role. Several contributing factors such as abnormalities in glucose metabolism (such as type 2 diabetes) and obesity play a strong part, as do certain cultural backgrounds, such as those of Indigenous Australians or women with a background from the Indian subcontinent.

Common symptoms of PCOS

Most commonly PCOS appears as irregular or no periods and difficulty conceiving. In two-thirds of cases this is associated with obesity, but many women with PCOS are within a healthy weight range. Those who are overweight have often tried many diets and lifestyle changes with minimal impact upon their overall weight. Other associated features include acne extending past the adolescent period, excess hair growth, mood disturbance and an increased risk of diabetes, high cholesterol and heart disease.

PCOS is a chronic (long-term) condition that often manifests as different problems throughout life. Infrequent periods or symptoms of acne and unwanted hair growth may be the first problems, followed by difficulty conceiving possibly associated with obesity, and finally diabetes or heart disease. Psychological symptoms, in particular low self-esteem, are common at any age and often fluctuate in their intensity.

Management of PCOS

The management of PCOS is best addressed as a team approach, including dieticians, fertility specialists, endocrinologists, nurses and, if possible, psychologists and exercise physiologists or trainers.

Lifestyle management remains at the forefront of treatment for women who are overweight or obese. This involves a combination of exercise and dietary modification in association with frequent support.

Irregular or absent menstrual periods are managed by lifestyle changes, followed by medication if necessary. Medication may take the form of a low-dose combined oral contraceptive pill, cyclical progesterone or the insulin-sensitising drug metformin.

Excess hair growth can be difficult to manage and will often require both hair removal and medication. Proven effective treatments for excessive hair growth in PCOS include a combined oral contraceptive pill, anti-androgen treatments such as spironolactone or cyproterone acetate or a combination of all of these treatments.

Infertility is again treated with lifestyle changes and weight loss if necessary. Stimulation of ovulation may be required and can be achieved with the fertility drugs clomiphene citrate or FSH injections (see 'Fertility drugs', above). Other common fertility treatments include IUI and IVF (see above). A healthy weight is advised before commencing fertility programs such as IVF.

Metabolic risks, such as abnormal glucose metabolism, can be modified once weight has been optimised by reducing other cardiovascular risk factors such as hypertension (high blood pressure) and elevated cholesterol. Dietary changes are advised for women with impaired glucose tolerance, to reduce the risk of developing type 2 diabetes, and the insulin-sensitising drug metformin may also be considered.

Lifestyle changes for managing PCOS

The current evidence-based guidelines for lifestyle changes to assist in managing PCOS list changes in diet and exercise as the first line of management, accompanied by other treatments only when necessary. It is important to lose weight if your BMI is 25 or higher and/or prevent weight gain. The most effective way of managing weight is to reduce the total kilojoule intake. Energy-reduced diets should be based on healthy food choices (see tips for healthy eating below). A dietician can help you formulate an eating plan that works for you.

At least 150 minutes of exercise per week is recommended; of this, 90 minutes per week should be of moderate to high intensity.

Healthy eating for PCOS

- Eat regularly and spread meals evenly over the day. Avoid long gaps between meals by including mid-meal snacks if necessary. This helps to control appetite and prevent large swings in blood sugar and insulin levels.

- Eat plenty of fruit, vegetables and salads. Include cereals, breads and grains with a low to moderate glycaemic index (GI; see chapter 13). Add some lean protein foods such as red meat, chicken, fish, dairy foods, eggs, legumes and nuts. And include small amounts of healthy fats such as mono- or polyunsaturated margarines and oils.

- Eat small portions. Each meal should contain a lean protein food, a low-GI food and some vegetables, salad or fruit. Use the 'quarter, quarter, half' rule as a guide to proportions: aim for about a quarter of your plate to be filled with lean protein foods, another quarter with low-GI carbohydrate foods and at least one-half with vegetables, salads or fruits.

- Limit high-fat, high-sugar foods that contribute to weight gain and higher insulin levels and often don't contain many useful nutrients. Be especially careful of high-fat foods such as battered, crumbed and fried foods, most takeaway foods, and snack foods, pastries, cakes, muffins and biscuits, butter, full-fat dairy foods, fatty meats, creamy

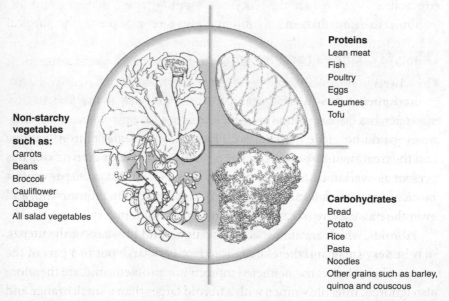

The plate rule

sauces and oily dressings. Also be wary of high-sugar foods such as sweet drinks (soft drinks, juice and flavoured milk), sweet biscuits, cakes and snack bars, desserts and ice-cream, chocolates and lollies, and sweetened breakfast cereals.

For more information on maintaining a healthy weight through diet and exercise, see chapter 14.

Reproductive surgery

Up until the 1980s, surgical repair of damaged fallopian tubes was the only option for women unable to conceive as a result of an STI that, especially if it was a repeat infection, closed the tube, stopping the sperm and egg meeting. Even with the best surgery, fewer than 20 per cent of women would then go on to have a healthy baby. This surgery is no longer offered.

Repair of tubes blocked intentionally in a sterilisation procedure, especially if a small clip has been used to block the tube rather than an electrical current to burn it, is generally successful. The results with the removal of clips and repair, using sutures smaller than a human hair, are so good that this surgery is recommended rather than IVF.

While there is a Medicare rebate available for sterilisation reversal (male and female), these operations might not be covered by a rebate or be available to public patients in all states, so check carefully before you proceed.

Over the past 20 years there has been a revolution in the surgical approach to most conditions, with minimally invasive (laparoscopic – keyhole – and hysteroscopic – through the vagina) surgery and consequent reductions in hospital stays and postoperative discomfort.

Endometriosis is a good example of a condition where the surgical approach has been revolutionised by technology. In the old days, the diagnosis would be made by diagnostic laparoscopy (keyhole investigation) and the treatment for severe cases, especially where the endometriosis was present as ovarian cysts, would be open surgery. Nowadays, 90 per cent or more of cases of endometriosis are diagnosed by vaginal ultrasound, and even the most severe of cases treated using keyhole surgery.

Fibroids, which are almost always benign, solid tumours of the uterus, may be very small and therefore ignored; or very large but in a part of the uterus where they cause neither symptom nor problem, and are therefore also ignored. Infertile women with a fibroid larger than a small orange and in the main part of the uterus, especially if it is close to or pressing on the lining of the uterus, will often be advised to have it removed. The removal process is increasingly being performed through keyhole surgery and even quite large fibroids are being removed this way by some specialists.

One exception to the practice of ignoring small fibroids is when the fibroid is partly or completely inside the lining of the uterus – a fibroid polyp in the uterine cavity. In this position it may act like an IUD, inhibiting implantation of an embryo, and would be removed by introducing a small telescope carrying a cutting device through the cervix. Other polyps, localised overgrowths of the lining of the uterus, may be treated in this way as well.

Most developmental abnormalities of the uterus are ignored, causing no delay in conception and no problem in pregnancy, although it is more common for the baby to be breech (feet-down) in these situations. Occasionally though, there may be reason to suspect that a structural, developmental abnormality in the uterus could be causing late miscarriage or preterm labour, and generally these abnormalities can be repaired using hysteroscopic surgery.

While still important and in some cases curative, surgery is performed in very few women nowadays compared to the days when IVF was relatively unsuccessful.

It is fair to say that there has been a revolution in our understanding of and ability to treat some of the major causes of infertility. Just 40 years ago, couples who were unable to conceive had virtually no options. Today many can become parents with the assistance of fertility treatment or donors. Now, one of the biggest challenges to a woman's fertility is not a medical problem, but rather the social obstacles and issues of starting a family between the ages of 18 to 32, when women are most fertile. Many women do not appreciate how rapidly fertility can decline with age, and perhaps the availability and success of medical treatments have been part of some being at ease with 'leaving children to later'.

It is important to remember that although we do have quite successful treatments for infertility, each has financial, physical, psychological and emotional costs. And these treatments will not be successful for all.

25

Responding to pelvic pain

Martin Healey, Anne-Florence Plante, Margaret Sherburn

In most situations the sudden onset of pain is a warning from the body that something is wrong. Most people respond to pain by moving the affected part of the body less, keeping still and seeking help.

When pain keeps on occurring over a long time (more than three to six months), doctors will start to describe it as 'chronic' or 'persistent'. Persistent pain can be caused by different things from short-term pain. When pain is persistent, management also changes, and aims to reduce the effect of the pain on quality of life. This means there is more of an emphasis on increasing movement and activity to a level as close to normal as possible, rather than simple pain relief.

Pelvic pain

Many women experience occasional or persistent pelvic pain. For some it is associated with the normal occurrence of periods or sexual inter-course. For others the pain may be associated with an infection, illness or condition and be localised to a specific area such as the bladder or vulvar area. It may continue over a period of weeks, months or longer. Such pain is very real and can be debilitating and depressing. The various types of pelvic pain, its causes, tests, management, treatment and likely treatment outcomes are discussed below.

Period-related pain

When we have a period, the uterus actively contracts to push the inner lining of the uterus (endometrium) and any associated blood down through the cervix into the vagina. This contracting is what we feel as cramping period pain (dysmenorrhoea). More than 70 per cent of Australian women say they experience period pain. It can vary from a mild cramp that needs no treatment to severe cramping that interferes with work or activity and requires painkillers. Most commonly, the pain is worst on the first and second day of bleeding, then settles down.

Cramping period pain often has no underlying explanation (apart from uterine contractions), but sometimes it can indicate that something is wrong. Possible causes include endometriosis, adenomyosis (see chapter 15 and later in this chapter) or the presence of a polyp inside the uterine cavity (see chapter 15).

Primary dysmenorrhoea (period pain)

Doctors will diagnosis primary dysmenorrhoea when they have excluded other causes such as endometriosis and adenomyosis. The typical symptom picture is of period pain that began with a woman's first period and has continued at the same level of severity ever since. The term 'primary' refers to it having been present from the start. It is thought that this pain is due to uterine contractions. It is not understood why uterine contractions during a period hurt some women but not others.

Endometriosis

Endometriosis is a condition where some endometrium grows outside of the uterus, usually in the pelvis, on the internal surface of the lining of the body cavity (peritoneum), including on the surface of the bladder or lower bowel, or on the ovaries. Endometrium, whether it appears in the uterine cavity or as endometriosis, grows in response to the hormones oestrogen and progesterone, which are released in cycles by the ovary. Endometriosis can cause period pain, pain during sex (dyspareunia), pain when passing bowel motions during a period, pelvic pain throughout the month, and difficulty getting pregnant (infertility). In other women endometriosis causes no symptoms at all. Once menopause occurs, the ovaries stop releasing hormones and the endometriosis shrinks, leading to the symptoms gradually settling down.

Tests for endometriosis

An ultrasound will usually be conducted when endometriosis is suspected from physical symptoms, to rule out other pelvic diseases. An ultrasound expert will recognise lumps (nodules) of suspected endometrium growing near or into the bowel and bladder. Endometriosis can only be diagnosed by taking a tissue sample during a laparoscopy (keyhole surgery of the pelvis and abdomen) and having it tested by a pathology lab to confirm that the pieces of tissue removed during surgery is in fact endometrium. There is as yet no accurate blood test that diagnoses endometriosis.

Treatment for endometriosis

Endometriosis is a benign condition (i.e. it is not cancerous) and so its management is based on the severity of the symptoms and their impact on quality of life. There are five possible options:

1. Do nothing. This is particularly sensible if there are no symptoms or they are mild and have no impact.

2. Use simple painkillers (such as paracetamol and non-steroidal anti-inflammatories such as naproxen or diclofenic).

3. Take the combined oral contraceptive pill (the Pill). This tends to reduce period pain.

4. Take hormonal medications that stop periods occurring. This usually works by also stopping ovulation. This includes taking the combined oral contraceptive pill continuously (skipping the sugar tablets), progesterone-like medications, or medications that turn off the ovaries entirely to cause a menopausal state.

5. Undergo surgery. The most obvious approach is to destroy or remove all the endometriosis tissue. Most commonly this is done as a laparoscopic operation. It becomes more complex if the endometriosis has grown into the wall of an important structure such as the bowel or bladder; in that situation, a piece of bowel or bladder will sometimes need to be removed to get all the endometriosis. Sometimes a hysterectomy (removal of the uterus) is also performed, which removes the source of new endometriosis. Sometimes doctors will also suggest removal of the ovaries, which are the source of the hormones that stimulate endometriosis to grow. Removing the uterus or ovaries is not reasonable, however, for women who still want to have children.

Adenomyosis

Adenomyosis is where endometrium grows into the muscle layer of the uterus. This seems to be more common in women in their late 30s and 40s, but can occur in some women in their 20s and even occasionally teenagers. Its symptoms include period pain, heavy periods and pain with sex. Just like endometriosis, it may cause no symptoms. It is not yet known whether adenomyosis has an impact on fertility.

Tests for adenomyosis

An ultrasound will often diagnose adenomyosis, but a normal ultrasound result does not mean adenomyosis is not there. Ultrasound is a slightly better test for adenomyosis than magnetic resonance imaging (MRI) and is substantially cheaper. The most accurate way to diagnose adenomyosis is to examine a tissue sample taken during a hysterectomy, although this is often not practicable.

Treatment for adenomyosis

Adenomyosis is a benign condition, which means that decisions regarding its treatment should be based on the severity of symptoms and their effect on quality of life. There are seven possible options:

1. Do nothing. This makes sense if there are no symptoms or they are mild.

2. Use non-hormonal drugs to reduce symptoms. Non-steroidal anti-inflammatories such as naproxen or mefenamic acid help reduce both period pain and volume of blood lost. Another drug, tranexamic acid, significantly reduces blood loss. These drugs only need to be taken during the period itself.

3. Take the combined oral contraceptive pill (the Pill). This reduces blood loss by up to 20 per cent and also tends to reduce period pain a bit.

4. Take hormonal medications that stop periods occurring. This includes taking the combined contraceptive pill (skipping the sugar tablets), progesterone-like medications (e.g. Provera), or medications that turn off the ovaries entirely to induce a menopausal state (e.g. Synarel, Zoladex).

5. Have a Mirena IUS inserted (see chapter 16). This device rests in the cavity of the uterus and steadily releases a progesterone-like drug (levonorgestrel) that provides effective contraception while reducing the volume of blood lost by 90 per cent and reducing period pain in 70 per cent of women.

6. Undergo an endometrial ablation (see chapter 15). This is an operation where some form of heat (from electricity or a hot water balloon) is used to destroy the endometrium lining the cavity of the uterus, including the deeper areas where the endometrium regrows from each month. This operation is usually performed as day-case surgery and you will often need only one or two days off work. On average the volume of blood lost per month decreases by 90 per cent, and up to 60 per cent of women will have a significant reduction in period pain.

7. Undergo a hysterectomy (removal of the uterus; see above). Because this operation means there will be no more periods, it completely stops bleeding and usually means no more period pain. The operation

involves a hospital stay of anything from one to five days, depending on the approach, and a recovery time of four to six weeks.

Cyclical pain at other times of the month

Sometimes women experience pelvic pain at other times of the month, but find that this pain gets worse in a cyclical pattern. There are two main patterns. With the first, the pain will become more severe around the period. Often this pain will start midway between periods (mid-cycle) or a few days before the period; less commonly, the pain will occur just after the period finishes. The cyclical pattern of the pain indicates that the ovarian hormones are an underlying cause. This pain is often associated with endometriosis or adenomyosis. The second pattern is pelvic pain that appears or gets worse around mid-cycle. This is usually associated with either ovulation or enlargement of an ovary (coming up to ovulation of an egg) that is trapped or stuck down with adhesions (scar tissue).

Tests for cyclical pelvic pain

A pelvic ultrasound will sometimes be of benefit in working out the cause of pain. A diagnostic laparoscopy (keyhole investigation), although more invasive, provides more information (such as whether scar tissue or endometriosis are present) and can allow immediate treatment. A third test is to fully suppress or turn off the ovaries for about three months using medications, which should significantly improve pelvic pain that is truly cyclical, under the influence of ovarian hormones. If pain does not improve with such medications, then the doctors should check for non-gynaecological causes, including bowel, bladder or back problems.

Pain during sexual intercourse (dyspareunia)

Sex is a painful experience for 14–49 per cent of women. This detracts from the pleasure normally associated with sex and can also strain a relationship; your partner may feel guilt for causing pain, or you may feel obliged to have sex for the sake of your partner even though it hurts.

There are a number of different reasons for experiencing pain with sex. These can be grouped according to where the pain is felt: deep pain or pain at the opening of the vagina.

Pain at the vaginal opening during sex

Pain at the opening is usually noticed at first penetration during sex. Sometimes this will be bad enough to abandon sex and avoid it in future.

Other times, the entry pain settles after penetration and so sex can proceed. Four main problems can lead to this symptom: skin problems, pelvic floor muscle spasm, vestibulodynia, and vaginismus (see chapter 7).

Skin problems at the vaginal entrance

One of the most common skin problems in this area is a thrush infection. The redness and irritation of the skin associated with thrush usually make sex painful. A range of other skin problems can also make initial contact of sex painful. Contact dermatitis is very common; this is where the skin is irritated by something it comes into contact with, such as additives in soap or laundry detergent, or synthetic fibres in underwear. The treatment is to avoid the irritant and use steroid ointment to settle the inflammation and soreness. Another common problem is seen in women after menopause, where the lack of oestrogen results in the skin of the vagina becoming very thin and prone to abrasions (atrophic vaginitis). This results in pain and dryness at the opening during sex. Treatment involves oestrogen cream and/or pessaries to locally thicken the skin of the vagina and opening.

Several other skin disorders, including lichen sclerosus and lichen planus (see chapter 26), can result in soreness at the opening of the vagina with sex. Treatment for these conditions should be managed by a gynae-cologist or dermatologist who specialises in this area.

Pelvic floor muscle spasm

The pelvic floor muscles are found about 3 centimetres from the entrance to the vagina. Contraction of the pelvic floor reduces the size of the vaginal entrance and can make penetration more difficult or impossible, with associated pain. A muscle that is contracted (particularly over a long time) can become tender, which means touching the pelvic floor muscle through the vagina wall can be painful.

Spasm of the pelvic wall can be triggered by a range of situations: vagin-ismus (see chapter 7), fear, previous painful experiences, or a moment of initial pain due to some other cause. The treatment involves learning to relax the pelvic floor muscles consciously, and is usually taught by physio-therapists with a special interest in pelvic floor issues.

Vestibulodynia (unexplained vaginal entrance pain)

This condition is common but can only be diagnosed after the other explanations have been excluded. The underlying problem is thought to be that the nerve fibres taking messages of pain from the entrance of the vagina have become overactive, possibly triggered by a previous pain event in the specific area or even more generally in the pelvic region.

The doctor will usually gently press at the base of the skin-tag remnants of the hymen using a cotton bud. If this produces the same type of pain as is felt with sex the diagnosis will often be vestibulodynia. Treatment aims at trying to reduce the sensitivity of the pain nerve fibres back to their original, normal level. The drug amytriptyline has been used to help in this situation; it is traditionally given as tablets but more recently has been available as cream to apply locally. Other treatments include learning to relax the pelvic floor to avoid reflex spasm using biofeedback to 'down train' the pelvic floor muscles, and using dilators of increasing diameters to gradually stretch the vaginal entrance (see below). If these treatments are not successful then surgery to cut out the strip of skin containing the overactive nerve fibres (called a vestibulectomy) can be performed.

Deep pain during sex

This pain is typically brought on by deep penetration. It may be sharp or dull. Intercourse may also stir up pelvic pain felt at other times. If the pain is more severe it may result in having to stop sex or avoid it. It is also common to have a pain or ache for some hours or even days afterwards. Sometimes a change in position during sex will stop the pain occurring or reduce it.

Causes of sudden onset of deep pain with sex include infection or inflammation involving the bladder (urinary tract infection), uterus and fallopian tubes (pelvic inflammatory disease), appendix (appendicitis) or an ovary (bleeding from ovulation). Once the cause is treated, the pain generally settles.

Longer term pain with sex is usually due to endometriosis, pelvic scar tissue or adenomyosis. Sometimes a large mass in the pelvis such as big fibroids or an ovarian cyst can also cause pain.

Tests and treatment for deep pain during sex

A vaginal ultrasound is helpful as it can show evidence of endometriosis, adenomyosis and big pelvic masses, and can also provide information on areas that are tender. The next step is a diagnostic laparoscopy (keyhole investigation) specifically to identify and treat endometriosis and scar tissue. If the only explanation for deep pain with sex is that it is coming from the uterus (in which case it will be presumed to be due to adenomyosis), then treatments will include turning off the ovaries with medications (e.g. Synarel, Zoladex), in the hope that this will make the uterus less tender, inserting a Mirena IUS or performing a hysterectomy (which is the option most likely to succeed).

Management of dyspareunia (pain during sex)
Down-training or relaxation of the pelvic floor muscles

Women with persistent pelvic, vulvar, bladder or bowel pain, also often experience sexual dysfunction. Those with persistent pelvic pain usually report deep dyspareunia (painful intercourse), while those with vulvar pain feel entry dyspareunia (pain at the vaginal entrance). Pain management for dyspareunia follows the principles described above, but there are specific extra strategies.

Just as in a fire the fire door will be closed to contain the fire, in pelvic pain the pelvic floor muscles will tense up as a guarding reflex against intercourse. Repetition of that reflex causes ongoing muscle spasm. This spasm of the pelvic floor muscles is common to all pelvic pain and can be a major limiting factor in achieving intercourse. It has been shown that the pelvic floor muscles are the first muscles to contract when we are exposed to a threat, so it is a survival response. Long-term muscle spasm can lead to pain (through the same mechanism as in a tension headache – in fact, persistent pelvic pain has been called a 'headache of the pelvis') and to bladder and bowel symptoms such as urinary urgency and constipation. Because pelvic floor muscle spasm is associated with danger or fear, learning to relax these muscles may be a slow process, especially if the pain has been present for a long time. Techniques used to assist down-training or relaxation may include looking at the perineum with a mirror, trigger-point massage, pelvic movements ('belly dancing'), relaxation strategies and graduated use of vaginal dilators.

Dilator training or graded exposure

This treatment is a home-based training program using a vaginal dilator or 'trainer'. The dilator is gradually inserted in the vaginal opening to gently stretch the tissues, while focusing on pelvic muscle relaxation. As the tissues become desensitised over time, larger diameter dilators are inserted. The aim of this treatment is to normalise thoughts and feelings about the pelvis and over time alter how the pelvis is represented in the brain. Acceptance of the use of the dilator is the first stage. Once it can be used without flinching or triggering a pain response, it should be inserted gradually in a sequential and non-threatening way. The environment plays a part in making this activity less threatening, so relaxing music, soft lighting, pleasant scents, and self-monitoring of breathing and heart rate all help reduce fear. Larger diameter dilators are sequentially used until insertion and movement of the dilator is managed easily and without causing pain. Partners are often involved at this stage, which helps regain intimacy in a graded manner. The sexual counsellor and physiotherapist work together when managing this training to treat sexual pain. (See chapter 28 for information on using vaginal dilators.)

Common reasons for persistent pelvic pain

Any structure or organ in the pelvis can be a potential source of persistent pelvic pain, so an investigation into persistent pelvic pain should include an examination of problems arising from the uterus and ovaries, bladder and lower bowel, pelvic nerves, the muscles running through the pelvis including the pelvic floor, and the bones and joints nearby, including in the lower back.

A small but significant group of women go through all the available tests and treatments but are still left with persistent pelvic pain. For these women, the focus shifts to finding ways to help them cope with the pain better and increase day-to-day activity and function. Management of this process is usually best provided by a persistent (or 'chronic') pain team, usually involving a pain specialist, a physiotherapist and a psychologist. They will initially perform an extensive assessment, and will then develop a tailored treatment program.

Typical practitioners in a pelvic pain management team

Team members	Role
Doctor (gynaecologist, gastroenterologist, urologist, anaesthetist and/or pain specialist)	Support; diagnosis; medications; surgery
Women's health physiotherapist	Support; pain education; progressive pacing of daily activities; relaxation strategies; movement and exercise (such as aerobics, yoga); normalisation of bladder, bowel and sexual function
Psychologist	Support; cognitive behaviour therapy (CBT); guided imagery; management of associated anxiety disorders or PTSD symptoms
Social worker	Social support; counselling
Sexual assault counsellors	Specialised trauma response; support; legal assistance; counselling

Management of persistent pelvic, vulvar and bladder pain

No matter what the diagnosis, treatment is aimed at relieving pain. It has been shown that the amount of pain experienced is not directly related to the amount of tissue damage that has occurred. This makes pain management complicated, because it means that pain is the body's response to many different factors or causes, not just tissue damage. All aspects of pain should be addressed for the best outcome. For instance, sleeplessness is common in people with a 'switched-on' autonomic nervous system. Relaxation or meditation training would be a good strategy to manage this symptom of persistent pain.

There is no one pathway to treat persistent pain. It is just too complex for that. Treatment for persistent pain is best when it involves a multi-disciplinary team of skilled clinicians to manage the different components of pain. Good clinicians assist their patients to master their pain, rather than cure it. They should actively listen to your story, not be judgemental, and help you rebuild resilience by offering an alternative pathway.

What causes pain to persist?

There are two main reasons why pain might persist. The first is the idea that because pain alerts you to danger, if your body thinks you are still in 'danger', you will continue to experience pain. Pain is complicated by previous experiences you may have had and that your body remembers. If pain is unpredictable, has variable symptoms, or comes from deep inside, then it can be perceived as frightening. Fear can be a large part of persistent pain. It can cause people to be extra vigilant about any minor changes in their pain, and even to exaggerate the possible impact of their pain.

The second reason is that chemical changes occur in the nerves that transmit sensation to the brain, and the nerves can become extra sensitive. This is called central sensitisation. When this happens, the nerves can either make a painful stimulus feel stronger (this is called hyperalgesia), or they incorrectly report a message of pain for a stimulus, such as touch, that did not cause pain before (allodynia). This means the brain receives a greater stimulus for pain than when pain was not persistent. Although it makes people more aware of pain, this information is not really accurate. The 'danger' or tissue damage is no greater, but the pain sensation is distorted and amplified in the brain, like turning up the volume control too much. This amplification of pain is associated with changes in other body systems such as the endocrine hormonal system, the immune system and the autonomic, or automatic, nervous systems. The whole nervous system becomes sensitised, causing symptoms other than pain, such as emotion, sleeplessness and muscle spasms.

Many people with persistent pain become, understandably, desperate to escape it. There is a real connection between physical pain and the emotional and mental anguish it produces. Women (and men) suffering from chronic pain often take up pain-escaping behaviours, such as 'doctor shopping', seeking a guru or a lawyer, taking any sort of medication from the internet, stopping work or stopping everything, to find an answer for their pain. They are willing to try anything to relieve their ongoing pain until many of them simply withdraw from active participation in life. This is known as the mind–body connection in persistent pain.

Physiotherapy in the management of persistent pelvic pain
Generally speaking, pain management begins by clearing all sources of pain that can be treated, such as infection. Then the doctor will treat the continuing pain with short-term effective medication while the physiotherapist or another pain team member will teach how pain-protective mechanisms operate. Recent research has shown that pain education can play a major role in early pain management.

The physiotherapist will then use specific treatments for localised pain. The most common of these is trigger-point massage to any back, hip and pelvic muscles that have tight, painful nodules, including internal relaxation or massage to the pelvic floor muscles.

Pacing: controlled exposure to pain triggers
The next stage is a graded program of controlled exposure training. The person experiencing the pain will make a list of feared activities or pain triggers, then they and their pain management team will develop a plan for gradual exposure to these activities in a controlled environment; this is called 'pacing', and is the part of treatment that is slow. It requires patience and persistence to avoid or manage flare-ups, or to avoid quitting for another 'quick fix'. The sensitised nervous system can put blockers in

Personal pain-control techniques

Use any or all of the following when a pain flare-up occurs:

Ice	Laughter with	Stretching
Scents	friends	Meditation
Change of position	Heat	Relaxation
Affirmations	Music	

the way if this pacing is done too quickly; it may cause reactions such as fainting or vomiting if the activity was greater than the body and mind were truly ready for. Pacing or graded movements are only effective when the person in pain remains in control and in charge of challenging themselves to just the right level. Flare-ups may occur because the nervous system is so sensitive, but with the understanding gained from pain education, these should not cause overwhelming emotional stress or lead to giving up. It is important to have personally developed active pain-control techniques if a flare-up does occur.

Bladder pain management

When pain comes from within the bladder there may also be bladder urgency and maybe bladder leakage, so treatment will target these bladder symptoms as well as the pain. This includes learning techniques to increase 'holding on' time rather than going to the toilet immediately and how to relax when there is a strong urge to go. Treatment will also include education about diet and fluid intake to lessen irritation of the lining of the bladder (including drinking plenty of water). To avoid skin inflammation on top of the other symptoms, skin care is also a part of management.

All these treatment strategies aim to enable a return to sexual intercourse with new resilience and understanding about sexual function, with either no pain or no fear of pain.

26

Genital irritations and infections

Suzanne Garland, Yasmin Jayasinghe, Sarah McQuillan, Ross Pagano

Infection or irritation in the genital region may cause confusion and embarrassment. Many women may wish to keep such concerns private or are fearful of asking for help, but just as there are normal physical variations within this region, many irritations and infections are treatable. In the following pages, we will review what is considered normal and what you should do if you develop any symptoms or are concerned.

What is normal in the external genital region?

The term 'vulva' refers to the external female genitalia – the outside parts of the genitals. This area is made up of the clitoris, labia minora and majora (inner and outer lips), and many different glands that release secretions to maintain lubrication within the vagina.

All women experience vaginal discharge of varying quantities and consistencies, depending on the stage of their individual menstrual cycle.

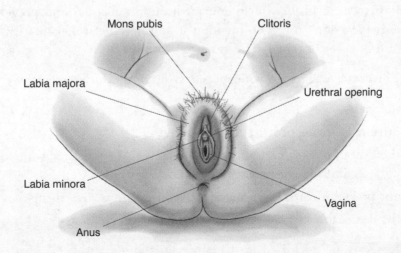

Mons pubis · Clitoris · Labia majora · Urethral opening · Labia minora · Vagina · Anus

External view of vulvar area

This is called physiological discharge and is typically an odourless secretion formed by the bacteria, cells and fluids of the vagina, excreted to clean and moisturise the vagina. The discharge is generally white or clear. Women who are tracking their menstrual cycle, for timing intercourse either as a means of contraception or in order to conceive, comment about the change in consistency of their discharge around the time of ovulation, when it becomes clearer and more stringy.

Normal discharge can irritate the sensitive skin around the vulvar area. Moisture can also be irritating, and is further exacerbated by heat and tight clothes, as well as many other stressors. Other than referring to clinical history, the only way to differentiate between normal physiological discharge and discharge caused by infection is by physical examination, or the use of a microscope to examine a sample of the discharge.

Diagnosing genital discharge and irritation

An accurate diagnosis is imperative to resolving the issue. If you have this sort of problem, the doctor may ask a series of questions about your:

- menstrual history, including the first day of your last normal period
- gynaecological history, focusing on previous sexually transmitted infections (STIs), and your last Pap test result
- obstetrics history; that is, information about any previous pregnancies and/or births
- sexual history, including new partners and pain with intercourse
- past medical history, including medications, allergies and previous surgeries; don't forget to mention if you have been diagnosed with autoimmune or skin diseases such as psoriasis

The doctor will review your specific symptoms, which may include:

- itchiness
- burning, stinging or irritation of the vulva
- the time of day or month it occurs, whether it is associated with your periods, and what helps or worsens the symptoms
- any previous treatments and your response to those treatments
- the degree to which the issue affects your daily activities

Expect your doctor to wash their hands and allow you privacy to undress from the waist down. Prior to this, the physical examination will commence with a general examination and may include measurement of your height and weight, calculation of your body mass index (BMI), and taking your blood pressure. The doctor will then examine your stomach, feeling for any abnormalities and/or pain in any potentially sensitive areas.

For the genital examination the doctor or nurse will wear gloves. You will be asked to lie on the examination table with your knees bent and feet apart so the doctor or nurse can properly inspect the external genitalia using a bright light. They will look for any changes such as redness, irritation, ulcers, discharge, infections, lice or trauma, then insert a speculum into the vagina to examine the inner walls. You may stop the examination at any time if you feel uncomfortable.

Once they have inspected the cervix, they may take specimens to rule out bacterial or viral infections and may also do a Pap test, for patients who have been sexually active for more than two years. According to the Australian guidelines, a Pap test should be done every two years to screen for cervical cancer. This is currently being reviewed, and may change in the near future to begin at around 25 years of age (currently it is from 18 years), as elsewhere in the world. By completing the Pap test every two years, we are able to detect over 75 to 80 per cent of the most common forms of cervical cancer. Should there be any obvious ulcers or lesions, your doctor may take a swab or biopsy of the affected area.

What causes genital irritations?

The causes of genital irritation are very broad, but the most common cause is a non-specific irritation (similar to a contact dermatitis).

Non-specific irritation

This is best treated by vulvar hygiene, which includes *avoiding* the following:

- irritating soaps
- sanitary napkins except while menstruating
- perfumes, deodorant products and douching
- tight synthetic clothing
- wearing underwear at night
- irritating detergents and softeners for washing clothes
- over-cleaning the vagina

To keep the genital area clean and irritation-free, we recommend:

- no cloths or sponges, only bare hands
- patting, rather than rubbing dry
- when the skin is dry, using a bland emollient to hold moisture such as sorbolene or QV cream
- perhaps using a bland barrier cream if the skin feels irritated due to moisture
- careful planning if considering a genital piercing (which can become infected)
- no douching

Finally, during sexual intercourse, we recommend:

- using small amounts of lubricants (when you use condoms it is better to use water-based glycerine lubricants and to avoid oil-based lubricants)
- switching to non-latex condoms in case of allergy to latex
- limiting the number and the rate of change of sexual partners. If you change partners, a new STI screen is necessary to protect both you and your new partner.
- perhaps abstaining from intercourse until the irritation settles down

If you have been following a conscientious regimen of vulvar hygiene and yet the genital irritation or itchiness persists, it is time to consider other causes.

Non sexually transmitted causes of vaginal irritation

Labial abscess

In very rare cases a larger collection of bacteria and pus cells beneath the skin may develop, called an abscess. Abscesses are similar to boils. The abscess will probably need to be drained, either under local anaesthetic or, rarely, under a general anaesthetic with intravenous antibiotics. Some women with oily skin or increased hair growth may have problems with recurring abscesses in the labial or groin area that are not related to hair removal; these women may benefit from taking the oral contraceptive pill or other hormone treatments to decrease the risk of recurrent abscess formation.

Bartholin's abscess

The Bartholin's glands sit on both sides of the entrance to the vagina – they cannot normally be seen or felt – and secrete fluid into the vagina. If the duct leading from the gland gets blocked, a cyst will develop on one side of the labia, which is often painless. Cysts can often be treated with repeated use of sitz baths (sitting in warm water with around one teaspoon of salt per litre). If the cyst gets infected it can form an abscess and become painful. Treatment includes sitz baths, antibiotics and surgery to drain the abscess, including 'marsupialisation' of the abscess (opening it and turning it inside out by suturing the cyst wall to the skin to keep it open). Complete removal of the gland may be required for recurrent abscesses or cysts.

Bacterial vaginosis

Bacterial vaginosis (BV) can cause a fishy-smelling, greyish discharge and occurs when there is a change in balance of the normal bacteria that live inside the vagina. This disturbance of the bacteria results in over-growth of anaerobic bacteria (i.e. bacteria that don't need oxygen), which are responsible for the smell and discharge. The exact cause of BV is unknown. BV occurs more commonly in sexually active women and does seem to be associated with sexual activity, but is currently *not* considered to be a conventional STI. It is more common in women who have sex with women. BV only needs to be treated if it is causing symptoms; in a pregnant woman with no symptoms but a history of or risk factors for preterm delivery; or before gynaecological surgery. It is generally treated with an oral antibiotic, but if the woman is not pregnant, a vaginal preparation can be used to avoid the side effects of the antibiotic.

Candidiasis (thrush)

Yeast called candida normally live in the vagina but can increase in concentration, particularly following antibiotic use, or in women with immunosuppression (for example, diabetics or HIV-positive women). Candidiasis, otherwise known as thrush, causes an intense itchiness and a cottage cheese-like discharge; it is diagnosed by swabbing the vagina. Vaginal thrush is best treated with a vaginal cream or suppository available from the chemist. If it doesn't clear up on its own, however, you should see your doctor for a prescription for an oral antifungal medication and to rule out other causes of discharge or immunosuppression. See also 'Chronic thrush of the vulva', below.

Vulvar skin conditions

Skin conditions of the external genitalia such as lichen sclerosus, allergic dermatitis, polyps inside the genital tract, or forgotten tampons may cause irritation or discharge.

Genital shaving and waxing have increased in popularity in recent years and with them has come an increase in folliculitis, an irritation or infection of the hair follicles. This occurs when bacteria get trapped below the skin in the genital region, encouraged by the high density of hair follicles being kept in the dark more than 90 per cent of the day, surrounded by heat and moisture. Folliculitis can cause pain, redness and itchiness. It is best managed by avoiding shaving and/or waxing, never using used razors, keeping the area clean, plucking the hair if the skin is infected, and using oral antibiotics if there is significant infection of the surrounding skin.

A number of benign vulvar skin conditions can affect the vulva at all ages. These are commonly referred to as a 'dermatitis of the vulva'. It is estimated that at least 50 per cent of women will develop a dermatitis of the vulva at some stage in their life; these conditions can be quite distressing and in some cases can have serious consequences if not treated adequately, such as:

1. persistent, unnecessary suffering in terms of itch, burning and pain
2. scarring, disfigurement of the vulva and restriction of sexual activity
3. possible development of cancer of the vulva

Some other conditions of the vulva, such as thrush, can mimic these skin changes, and one condition affecting the vulva, provoked vestibulodynia, causes untold distress to women by causing severe pain that prohibits sexual intercourse.

The most common skin disorders of the vulva are:

- eczema (lichen simplex chronicus)
- lichen sclerosus
- psoriasis
- lichen planus
- aphthous ulcers
- precancerous lesions (VIN)

Eczema (lichen simplex chronicus)

This is the most common skin disorder affecting the vulva; it can be quite mild and is often temporary. Eczema usually causes itching, especially of the outer, hair-bearing part of the vulva. The condition usually affects both sides of the vulva and may include a thickening of the skin and prominent skin creases. There is usually no rash apart from changes in the skin due to the trauma from scratching.

There are two main causes of eczema: emotional stress, worry or anxiety, in which case it will usually resolve when that stressful episode passes; or a contact irritant to the vulvar skin, such as sanitary pads (especially using panty liners daily), excessive soap, toilet paper, female deodorants and so on. Excessive vaginal discharge can also constantly irritate the vulva.

To treat eczema, avoid irritants. Soap can irritate the vulva, so use soap substitutes when showering, not just on the vulva but also on the rest of the body. Use tampons during periods and avoid panty liners. If protection is necessary, try using cotton terry towelling instead. Only wear cotton underwear, and only wash them in pure soap; avoid detergents, which can irritate the skin because they are never completely rinsed out. If you have excessive vaginal discharge, see a gynaecologist to have it treated. Try arranging counselling for any stressful event that could be a contributing factor.

Eczema responds well to cortisone creams, usually of a mild to moderate potency; these will need to be applied once or twice a day or as required. Long-term treatment is rarely necessary, and this condition is not regarded as precancerous.

Lichen sclerosus

This is a much more serious condition as the consequences of misdiagnosis or not treating it are significant. Lichen sclerosus is thought to be an autoimmune disorder, where the immune system wrongly targets the vulva and slowly destroys it. It can occur in women who have other autoimmune conditions, such as thyroid disorders and ulcerative colitis. It is usually a lifelong condition (except in children, where it can resolve once they reach puberty). There is no cure; although it will often go into a dormant phase where treatment is no longer required. At some point it will recur, often in response to a stressful event. It occurs in approximately one in 80 women. A doctor should be able to diagnose it from the typical appearance of the skin. A biopsy is not always required but is necessary if there is any suspicion of cancer.

Women with lichen sclerosus usually complain of a chronic itch that can be anywhere on the vulva, although it usually starts on the inner part of the vulva and then spreads outwards, often involving the skin around the anus as well. The condition was originally thought to occur only in elderly women and is certainly more common among midlife and elderly women, but young women and even children can also get it. It usually starts with episodes of itching that resolve spontaneously for a while. In the early stages, it is often self-diagnosed as thrush, especially as anti-thrush treatment appears to improve the symptoms. This improvement, however, is not due to the treatment but is just a natural progression of the condition. Each time it happens, though, more damage is done to the vulva, which is why it is vital to visit a doctor and have an examination if you experience any vulvar symptoms.

If this condition is not treated properly, it results in significant scarring of the vulva and the entrance to the vagina. The skin will often look pale, with a parchment-like crinkled appearance interspersed with thickened areas (called leukoplakia). These areas may split as a result of scratching and hence cause pain. Itching, however, is the most common symptom. With time, the skin scars, resulting in the labia minora (the skin folds around the entrance of the vagina) disappearing due to fusion with the surrounding skin and also a narrowing of the vaginal opening. This narrowing, together with burying of the clitoris, can make intercourse less satisfying and eventually impossible if the vaginal opening closes. The end result of this chronic scarring in 4 per cent of women with this condition is the development of cancer of the vulva.

Treatment consists of avoiding local irritants to the vulva as with eczema, and applying a strong cortisone ointment on a regular basis. Treatment is usually long-term; the cortisone cream will generally need to be applied on a regular preventative basis once or twice per week (or more frequently) after the initial flare-up is under control. Women are often scared to use a strong cortisone cream on the vulva because of the mistaken belief that it will cause thinning of the skin. While this is true when applied to normal skin, it is not the case with inflamed skin, and the consequences of not using it far outweigh any potential 'damage' from the treatment itself.

After the diagnosis, careful follow-up will be required in order to detect any early precancerous changes. Any skin undergoing cancerous or pre-cancerous changes will need to be surgically removed. Surgery will also be required to enlarge the opening of the vagina if it has narrowed and sexual intercourse is still desired.

Psoriasis

Psoriasis of the vulva usually occurs in conjunction with psoriasis elsewhere on the body (such as the elbows, the groin or the trunk), and only rarely occurs solely on the vulva. On the vulva, it will often cause a red rash with a distinct border, but less scaliness than in psoriasis on other parts of the body. Itchiness is the main symptom, and treatment requires a high-potency cortisone cream as required.

Lichen planus

This is another autoimmune disorder but unlike those mentioned above, it affects both the vulva and vagina. This condition is common in the mouth and often begins there before developing in the vulva. It generally causes pain and burning rather than itchiness, although it may also cause itchiness. There will be reddish brown patches on the inner part of the vulva, often extending around the urethra (the opening of the bladder).

Lichen planus is not as common as lichen sclerosus, but if not treated aggressively it can also cause scarring (especially of the vaginal canal) and possibly cancer. Treatment involves applying high-potency cortisone creams to both the vulva and vagina, as well as medication such as prednisolone (a corticosteroid) and/or methotrexate (a chemotherapy drug). It will need lifelong care and surveillance.

Aphthous ulcers

These ulcers are exactly the same as mouth ulcers. There are often many of them, with small punched-out, shallow ulcers scattered throughout the inner part of the vulva. Pain is the main symptom, and they usually erupt at the same time as mouth ulcers, commonly at times of stress. They respond well to the same treatment as for mouth ulcers: strong-potency cortisone cream applied several times a day.

Precancerous lesions

These lesions are usually single, but can also occur in multiples. They should be suspected if there is itchiness in one spot and on examination, there is a well-defined lesion in this spot, either pale or reddish. In older women, the lesion is often associated with lichen sclerosus, but younger women are more likely to have more than one lesion and it will often be associated with wart virus (HPV) infection (see below). You should always be concerned if there is a focal area of irritation anywhere on your vulva. Examination is essential and a biopsy will be necessary to confirm the diagnosis.

Treatment usually involves having the lesion surgically removed under general anaesthetic. If there is more than one lesion, laser treatment under general anaesthetic is preferable. If the lesions cannot be treated in this way, prolonged application of a special cream (imiquimod) that stimulates a local immune response can be effective. Long-term follow-up will be necessary to detect any early recurrences.

Chronic thrush of the vulva

While thrush is the most common infection of the vulva (see above), chronic thrush is a rare condition that can develop in women who have experienced multiple attacks (more than four in a year) of vaginal thrush. Women with chronic thrush often complain of a burning sensation in the vulva rather than itch and discharge. The symptoms are usually worse in the week leading up to the menstrual period and are relieved during the period. Symptoms often flare up a day or two after sex and can make intercourse uncomfortable. The condition is often confused with derma-titis and the cortisone cream prescribed can make the condition worse.

The treatment for chronic thrush involves taking an oral anti-thrush tablet (such as fluconazole) continuously for up to six months, as well as modifying diet, avoiding the contraceptive pill and avoiding stress.

Vulvodynia

This is the name used for pain, burning and discomfort of the vulva not due to any specific cause, and where the vulva looks essentially normal on examination. Some doctors may be unaware of the problem and miss the condition, deciding instead that it is a purely psychological problem. Vulvodynia can occur at all ages in adult women, but it's most common among young women who experience pain during intercourse and are often unable to have penetrative sexual intercourse at all. This type of vulvodynia is called 'provoked vestibulodynia'.

We now believe these women are born with a higher concentration of nerve endings in the vulvar vestibule (that portion of the vulva immedi-ately surrounding the opening of the vagina, approximately 1 centimetre wide) and that if these nerves are damaged, the skin becomes hyper-sensitive and any pressure on it causes pain. The damage may result from chronic thrush of the vulva, previous sexual trauma due to inadequate lubrication, tampon trauma, and even childbirth.

Treatment for vestibulodynia involves explanation and encouragement, using adequate lubrication, medications (now available in a topical cream form), physiotherapy to relax the pelvic muscles and, if all else fails, surgery to remove the tender area.

Bacterial sexually transmitted infections (STIs)

Chlamydia trachomatis

Chlamydia trachomatis (chlamydia) is the most common bacterial STI, and its rate has quadrupled in Australia over the last 10 years. Sixty to 80 per cent of infected women will have no symptoms; it does not always cause symptoms, but when it does it produces a yellowish discharge or bloody spotting after intercourse or between menstrual periods.

If left untreated, chlamydia can spread upwards into the uterus and fallopian tubes, resulting in pelvic inflammatory disease (PID), a serious infection with high fevers, abdominal pain, muscle aches, and/or a yellow–bloody discharge. It may also occur with mild symptoms such as abdominal pain and diarrhoea, or it can occur without any symptoms at all. One-third of infected women will develop blocked fallopian tubes after their first episode of PID, which increases the risk of an ectopic pregnancy (pregnancy outside the uterus; e.g. in the fallopian tube), or simply renders them infertile altogether. PID also causes persistent deep pelvic pain, and the infection may be transmitted to a partner. The only way to treat PID is to use intravenous (IV) antibiotics until there are no signs of fever for 48 hours, after which a two-week course of oral antibiotics must be taken. Uncomplicated chlamydia (without PID) is treated with one dose of oral antibiotics, followed by avoiding sex for seven days. Any partners should be treated simultaneously, to avoid reinfection.

Chlamydia is diagnosed with a urine test or a vaginal or cervical swab. All previous partners from the last six months should also be informed, so they can be treated. If you are infected, you may do this yourself, or you can use a letter from your doctor to maintain confidentiality. There are also websites with information and resources to assist you in this task, such as www.letthemknow.org.au, developed by the Melbourne Sexual Health Centre. The doctor will probably recommend testing for other STIs such as gonorrhoea, *Mycoplasma genitalium*, and blood tests for HIV and hepatitis for peace of mind.

Gonorrhoea

Gonorrhoea is the second most common bacterial STI in Australia, but it is more likely to cause symptoms, such as vaginal discharge or pain during urination. It is treated similarly to chlamydia, with either one dose of an oral antibiotic or an intramuscular antibiotic injection. As with chlamydia, gonorrhoea can lead to PID. Once again, sex should be avoided for seven days and all partners from the last six months should be contacted and treated. Unlike chlamydia, gonorrhoea can be spread by oral sex and can cause severe throat or joint infections.

Syphilis

Syphilis is a rarer bacterial STI, although some parts of the world are seeing an exponential rise in cases. In Australia, it most commonly occurs in remote communities and among men who have sex with men. Primary syphilis (i.e. the initial infection) can cause a single painless genital ulcer, which may go unnoticed. Syphilis then progresses through three more stages. Secondary syphilis is characterised by a rash on the palms of the hands or soles of the feet. The third phase is latent syphilis, meaning there are no symptoms, and finally, without treatment 40 per cent of those infected develop tertiary syphilis, which can cause organ dysfunction and/ or dementia.

Syphilis is most transmissible during the first and second phase, but most destructive during the last two phases. It is diagnosed by swabbing an ulcer or from a blood test and is readily treated with a penicillin injection, either intramuscular or intravenous, depending on the stage of the infection. Syphilis is the most worrisome bacterial STI, because if unrecognised and untreated it can be transmitted to an unborn baby during pregnancy, causing lifelong congenital anomalies or developmental delay. That is why all women are tested for syphilis when they fall pregnant, as appropriate treatment can prevent the risk of these complications.

Mycoplasma genitalium

Mycoplasma genitalium is a bacterium that has recently been discovered to be an STI. It may infect the cervix, cause discharge, spotting or pelvic pain, or cause no symptoms at all. It can be detected on a vaginal swab test and is treated with antibiotics. Screening for other STIs is recommended, and sexual partners over the last six months should be contacted and treated.

Viral STIs

Human papillomavirus (HPV)

The most common viral STI is human papillomavirus (HPV): up to 80 per cent of people who are sexually active acquire HPV at some stage of their life. It causes both genital warts (largely the low-risk HPVs, types 6 and 11) and cell changes on the cervix or neck of the womb (largely the high-risk HPVs, types 16 and 18) that can be detected with a Pap test. HPV infection is very common and does not need treatment in itself. Persistent infection with high-risk HPVs can, however, lead to precancerous high-grade cervical cell changes (called CIN2 or CIN3). High-grade changes can be treated by removing the affected tissue, surgically, by laser or by cauterisation. If it is not removed, in around 30 per cent of cases it may progress to cervical cancer in the future. This is the basis of the Pap screening program: to detect abnormal cells and get rid of them before they develop into cancerous lesions. It is worth noting that it takes decades for cancerous lesions to develop from original persistent infection. We do not understand why a proportion of women end up with persistent infection, although we do know that smoking increases the risk. Having had chlamydia or herpes, also increases the likelihood of abnormal cells due to HPV infection.

There are about 40 different subtypes of HPV that can infect the genital area, but types 16 and 18 make up the bulk (70 per cent consistently worldwide) of those causing cancer. These types, especially type 16, can also lead to some other types of cancers, such as some penile, anal and vaginal cancers. The majority of the time, our immune system can clear the virus.

The only way to prevent the most dangerous HPVs (16 and 18) is to be vaccinated with the HPV vaccine prior to any sexual contact. In Australia there are two vaccines approved for use up to the age of 45, and if you've never been in contact with the virus, they are both 100 per cent effective for protection against types 16 and 18, which means your risk of acquiring cervical cancer is decreased by 70 per cent. The vaccine being used in the government funded school-based program (Gardasil) also protects against HPVs 6 and 11, and therefore against 90 per cent of genital warts. If you decide to have one of the vaccines and you have already been sexually active, it will be of some benefit, particularly for those infections you have not had previously. In addition, some new studies show that the vaccines are effective in women who have had a previous infection, as they boost the natural immunity from that infection. The vaccines do not, however, treat current infections with HPV. The vaccines are safe and do not contain live virus, however they are currently not recommended during pregnancy. Should you fall pregnant during the three-vaccine regime, it is recommended the scheduled injections are resumed after the baby's birth.

HPV is spread by skin-to-skin contact, so condoms only protect us if the virus is located directly beneath the condom. The best way to protect yourself from cervical cancer is to have a routine Pap test every two years once you become sexually active. HPV testing on top of a Pap test is currently not done routinely in Australia, but it is expected that such testing will be included in the future. At the moment, HPV testing is only recommended to women who have had treatment for high-grade cervical changes. This is done with their yearly Pap test until they have had two negative tests in a row; after which they may return to routine screening. Unfortunately, the virus can recur, and a new infection can occur on contact with a different HPV type. Cervical cancer is easily prevented by having regular Pap tests, however.

Even if you have received the vaccine, it is important to continue having Pap tests to detect changes due to other HPV types not covered by the vaccine.

Genital herpes

Another common viral STI is genital herpes, which is caused by the same virus that gives us cold sores. There are two types of herpes simplex virus: type 1 and 2. Type 2 is more likely to infect the genital area, while type 1 often causes cold sores, but both types can mix and match sites. If type 2 infected the mouth, it is less likely to recur. Similarly, type 1 in the genital area is less likely to cause obvious recurrences.

When it infects the genitals, the virus produces genital swelling and ulcers. Genital ulcers are spread via genital, oral and/or digital (with the fingers) sexual activity. The first episode of genital ulcers is the most painful, even forcing some women to be admitted to hospital for help with going to the toilet. In the initial infection, HSV may also cause lumps in the groin, fever and difficulty passing urine.

Sometimes it is possible to have recurrent bouts of infection, with usually much milder local symptoms (such as one or a few ulcers or blisters on the vulva). Many women will have some pre-infectious (prodromal) symptoms, such as itchiness, that indicate they are about to have an infectious outbreak. It is extremely important to avoid all sexual contact during the prodromal phase or while there are active lesions, to avoid transmitting the infection to a partner.

As with many other STIs, HSV can also be transmitted even when there are no symptoms, so an individual may not know they have been infected. The virus is spread due to genital secretions, usually without any symptoms being present, so many people may have had exposure to these viruses without even knowing.

As with HPV, there is no cure for herpes, but antiviral medications lessen the side effects, decrease the transmission rate and decrease the number of recurrences a year. If you have an outbreak during pregnancy, you can be given a course of suppressive therapy starting in the third trimester at 36 weeks gestation, to prevent transmission to the baby at the time of delivery. If you have an outbreak when labour starts, your doctor may speak to you about having a caesarean to avoid the risk of contact to the baby. The risk is highest if it is your first outbreak. HSV can cause severe disease in a newborn baby, such as infection of the lungs and brain.

Hepatitis B and HIV

Hepatitis B and human immunodeficiency virus (HIV) are two viruses that are spread via sexual contact as well as bodily fluids, including transmission to babies from infected mothers. Neither is curable, and both are diagnosed by blood tests. Both are also included in the screening tests conducted at the first prenatal appointment during pregnancy.

Hepatitis B affects the liver and results in chronic liver disease, whereas HIV primarily affects the immune cells and can progress to acquired immunodeficiency syndrome (AIDS). As of 2013, there have been 6700 deaths in Australia from AIDS since it was first discovered in 1981. Disturbingly, what makes these viruses so difficult to detect is that both infections begin with relatively few symptoms or with only flu-like symptoms. Both require early diagnosis to prevent transmission to other people, as well as to avoid some of their long-term consequences. Both will require lifelong medications to keep the consequences of the infection under control.

Today, mother-to-baby transmission of hepatitis B is prevented by vaccinating all babies at birth, and the babies of mothers who are found to be carriers of the virus will also be given an injection of immunoglobulin (which provides the baby with immediate protection). Similarly, HIV-positive mothers can be treated during pregnancy with antiviral agents to make them largely non-infectious and allow delivery of healthy, uninfected infants. HIV-positive mothers cannot breastfeed an infant, as this is another form of mother-to-child transmission. For hepatitis B breastfeeding is acceptable.

Parasitic infections

Trichomonas ('trick')

Parasitic infections occur when a non-bacterial, non-viral organism attaches to the host and uses it to feed, grow and reproduce more organisms that can then be transmitted to other people. Fifty per cent of women who are infected with the organism *Trichomonas vaginalis* will have symptoms and most will develop a smelly discharge, itchiness or pain with intercourse within one week of contracting the infection through sexual intercourse. Trichomonas gives the cervix a strawberry pattern. It is diagnosed with a high vaginal swab inserted in the vagina, and is treated with a seven-day course of an antibiotic (metronidazole), which may cause some stomach discomfort or a metallic taste. Alcohol cannot be consumed while taking these antibiotics. All partners need to be treated and sexual activity should be avoided for at least seven days after treatment. As with most STIs, leaving it untreated can lead to infertility, chronic pelvic pain or an ectopic pregnancy.

Pediculosis pubis *(pubic lice or 'crabs')*

Pediculosis pubis are tiny parasites that nest in pubic hair, just like hair lice. They cause intense itchiness and occasionally tiny little lice, eggs or bluish bites will be visible. The persistent scratching can lead to a secondary bacterial infection. Pubic lice are transmitted via intimate contact, including sharing towels or bedding. The treatment includes a non-prescription special shampoo from the chemist, as well as strict hygiene (including possibly the need to shave the area) and washing in hot water all the bedding, towels, clothing and so on in your home. Partners need to follow this same regime for the infection to be eradicated.

Scabies

Scabies causes similar symptoms to pubic lice, but is caused by parasitic mites that burrow into the skin. Scabies are also transmitted both by intimate contact and sharing towels. The treatment is a special lotion from the chemist that is applied to the affected area. Treatment must be accompanied by avoiding sexual contact and cleaning all the bedding, towels and clothing in the house.

Rare STIs

A few infections are rare in Australia but occur more frequently in people who engage in sexual activity overseas, are recent immigrants from certain countries or are sex workers. These infections, such as donovanosis, chancroid and lymphogranuloma venereum, are treatable but can cause serious complications if left unattended. Your doctor will be able to advise you further if you are concerned about any of these.

STI screening

An STI screen generally involves testing for:

- chlamydia, gonorrhoea (through urine or swabs)
- *Mycoplasma genitalium* (through swabs)
- HIV, hepatitis B, hepatitis C, syphilis (through blood tests)

If any of your tests is positive, you will be offered counselling and treatment, and will be advised that your sexual partners in the last six months will be contacted (either by you or the Department of Health), and advised that the results will be sent (in a way that does not identify you) to the government department that collects STI statistics in your state.

Being diagnosed with an STI can sometimes be confronting, but there is no need to be embarrassed or ashamed. These infections are common, and you should be proud that you were proactive and had a check-up, and that now it can be treated.

Many STIs may stay silent for long periods of time, so it can be difficult to tell exactly who you got it from. It is very important to discuss your past sexual history with your partner, be tested for STIs with a doctor at least every year or every time you change partner, and use condoms *every* time you have sex. One in four women is reinfected with an STI in the first year after treatment.

Infections and prenatal care

As previously discussed, STIs can lead to infertility, chronic pelvic pain or an ectopic pregnancy. They can also cause complications for an unborn baby; your best chance for a safe pregnancy and healthy baby is through early prenatal care.

Ideally, as soon as you find out you are pregnant, you should have routine prenatal blood work, testing for your blood type, haemoglobin (as an indication of your iron levels), HIV, hepatitis B, hepatitis C, syphilis, and immunity to rubella (German measles) and varicella (chickenpox). On your first prenatal visit you should also expect to have a full medical history taken and a full physical examination, including a pelvic examination with a speculum to diagnose vaginal infections and perform a Pap test. Finally, at the end of the appointment you'll need to give a midstream urine sample. Your doctor will then arrange for you to have an ultrasound to confirm the pregnancy. If your urine sample suggests bacteria are present, you will be treated for a urinary tract infection even if you have no symptoms. This is because it is possible during pregnancy to become very ill very quickly with a urinary tract infection; the enlarging uterus causes urine to pool in the urinary system, allowing bacteria to grow quickly and spread to the kidneys. This can cause premature labour.

If the vaginal swab suggests bacterial vaginosis (BV) and if you have risk factors for a premature baby, you will be given a prescription for antibiotics and asked to repeat the vaginal swab a few weeks later to ensure the BV has been eradicated.

As mentioned earlier, HIV can easily be transmitted to the developing baby. The biggest risk for the baby is at the time of vaginal delivery, when without treatment the risk of transmission approaches 40 per cent. If you are diagnosed with HIV, you will be offered a combination of anti-retrovirals to minimise the number of HIV virus particles in your bloodstream. If your viral load continues to be high, at 38 weeks gestation you will also be offered a caesarean. If the viral load is low and you have been on a combination of anti-retrovirals, you may choose to attempt a natural vaginal delivery. Unfortunately, regardless of the mode of delivery, when you are HIV-positive, you do not have the option of breastfeeding; however, formula is an excellent alternative. Your baby will be treated immediately after birth with anti-retroviral medication for up to a year and periodically screened for HIV.

At 36 weeks gestation you will have a vaginal swab to test for group B streptococcus (GBS), a bacterium that normally lives in the vagina in about 15–25 per cent of women. If you are GBS-positive, you will need antibiotics (usually penicillin) when you go into labour or your waters break, to decrease the risk of infection in the baby. Infection with GBS in a newborn can have very serious consequences. If you are infected with GBS and you have not received intravenous antibiotics for at least four hours during labour, then the paediatric team will monitor the newborn.

27

Plastic surgery in young women

Dean Trotter

Some young women may consider plastic surgery in order to improve their appearance, while others may be forced to think about it by disease or trauma. It is not something to be undertaken without careful consideration. Most young women who seek plastic surgery want to improve their appearance or to increase their confidence and self-esteem. While these reasons are similar to those of other, older women who seek plastic surgery, many young women have a greater need to fit in with others and may not yet have a fully developed sense of self.

These operations are not minor corrective procedures and any surgery involves risk, which is discussed below. When carefully planned, however, plastic surgery can significantly improve your quality of life. The common procedures a plastic surgeon undertakes are discussed in this chapter, as are the most common plastic surgery operations in young women – those involving the breast and the nose.

For information on cosmetic surgery, see chapter 38.

Breast surgery

It is common for young women to consider breast surgery. There may be many reasons for this: to increase or reduce the size of breasts, change their shape or the position of the nipples, or reconstruct them following surgery for breast cancer.

There are four main types of breast surgery:

1. breast augmentation
2. breast reduction
3. breast uplift, and
4. breast reconstruction

Breast augmentation

Young women often seek breast augmentation (increased breast size); some have breast asymmetry or even a specific breast deformity, such as tuberous breasts (see chapter 9), while others simply believe their breasts are too small. Breast augmentation is generally relatively safe, and produces a high level of satisfaction provided there is adequate preoperative consultation and the surgeon is appropriately trained. It is, however, a medical procedure and so carries with it the potential risk of complications. These may be related to the surgery itself or to the products used for augmentation. Surgical risks include bleeding, infection, asymmetry, sensory change, pain, anaesthetic complications, deep vein thrombosis or pulmonary embolism, poor scarring and wound-healing problems.

Many women are now heading overseas for breast augmentation procedures. Sometimes the procedure is less expensive than in Australia, but the quality of the surgery and implants used varies, so complication rates are often higher than in Australia. If complications occur once back home in Australia, it is very difficult to have follow-up with the surgeon who performed the procedure. This may entail further cost and inconvenience. These factors need to be carefully considered before undergoing surgery overseas.

If you are considering breast augmentation, we strongly advise that you see a qualified plastic surgeon for a consultation before undergoing surgery. You do not need a referral to a plastic surgeon for breast augmentation from your GP but it is recommended you talk to your doctor about the surgery.

Breast augmentation with implants

Most commonly in Australia, silicone implants are used for breast augmentation. In the past, they were thought to cause a multitude of problems ranging from connective tissue disorders to chronic fatigue syndrome and even cancer. After extensive research, silicone breast implants are considered safe, and not to cause any systemic diseases. Like any foreign material implanted in the body, implants become surrounded by a sac of scar tissue (called a capsule). This scar tissue can become thick and can make the implant feel hard, change shape, or even be painful. This capsule has also been recently associated with an extremely rare form of lymphoma. A breast augmentation is therefore not something to be undertaken lightly.

Breast augmentation may be performed with saline implants rather than silicone implants, but the results are similar. Saline implants have a silicone shell filled with saline (salt solution), so they generally behave similarly to silicone-filled implants.

> ## Safety of breast implants
>
> There are two commonly used types of breast implants. They have different fillings but both have a silicone shell. Silicone implants – the most common type – are filled with a thick silicone gel. Saline implants – the other type – are filled with saline (sterile salt water).
>
> Both silicone and saline implants can rupture. The rupture rate is thought to be around 0.3 per cent per year, but this increases with time. The rupture may be due to a fault of the implant; surgical error; or if very strong force is applied to the implant. The silicone shell is quite strong and a fall or a mammogram would generally not cause the implant to rupture. If a silicone implant ruptures, the implant and any silicone gel that has spread outside it may need to be removed because the ruptured implant may cause pain, or the breast may change shape or size. A ruptured implant doesn't necessarily have to be removed, though, if it is not causing any problems. If a saline implant ruptures, the saline is absorbed naturally into the body and the silicone shell remains, but the breast will usually reduce in size or change shape.
>
> According to current research, there are no significant differences in safety between silicone and saline implants. Neither is there evidence that the spread of silicone gel from a ruptured or leaking silicone implant increases your risk of disease, including cancer or autoimmune diseases.

Breast augmentation with injections

Products such as liquid silicone and more recently hyaluronic acid have been injected into or around the breast. The results tend to be less predictable than with silicone or saline implants. Liquid silicone is to be avoided as it tends to form hard painful lumps as the body tries (unsuccessfully) to remove it from tissues.

More recently there has been a trend towards injecting fat into the breast. This is a controversial practice and needs careful consideration before going ahead with the surgery. The main concerns are that the fat may potentially cause breast cancer or make it harder to diagnose with X-rays or other tests. The fat may form hard or even painful lumps that might feel like breast cancer. Transferred fat may contain stem cells, which can possibly induce breast cancer in susceptible cells. These concerns may in time turn out to be unfounded, but at this stage the Australian Society of Plastic Surgeons, and major indemnity insurance companies only recommend fat injections for women who have previously had surgery for breast cancer. This is because these women usually have no breast tissue, which makes it safe to inject fat where the breast once was. Some do have breast tissue remaining, but it has been extensively checked to exclude cancer and often 'sterilised' with radiotherapy. Fat injection to breasts that have not had cancer might be recommended one day once more is known about the long-term outcomes of using injected fat for augmentations.

Breast reduction

Women with large breasts may seek breast reduction to reduce back, neck and/or bra-strap pain, to improve the ability to exercise or for hygiene reasons, rather than to improve appearance. Breast reduction surgery has one of the highest satisfaction rates of any surgical procedure and most women are very pleased that they underwent surgery. There are several different techniques, but in general the breast tissue is reduced, along with the overlying skin. The breast tissue is then remodelled to provide a better breast shape and the skin tailored to the new breast shape. Depending on the size of the reduction, this may result in a scar around the areola, with or without a vertical scar down the front of the breast (vertical breast reduction – the scar looks like a lollipop) and possibly another in the fold below the breast ('wise pattern' breast reduction – the scar looks like an anchor). Some techniques also involve liposuction.

If you are considering breast reduction surgery, you will need to accept that all breast reduction techniques leave some form of scar. Other complications (as with any operation on the breast) include possible bleeding, infection, asymmetry, slow wound healing, anaesthetic complications and deep vein thrombosis or pulmonary embolism. Specific complications relate to the nipple. Usually with breast reduction the nipple and areola are lifted from a lower position on the breast to a more 'ideal' position. This means that the blood and nerve supply to the nipple and areola may become compromised. Very rarely, this results in failure of the nipple and areola to survive the operation. More commonly there is some reduction or even loss of feeling in the nipple following breast reduction. Up to one-third of women will experience this. The other issue related to the nipple is that the ability to breastfeed may be affected. Not all women are able to breastfeed, so it is hard to determine exactly if a breast reduction will interfere with breastfeeding. Some women are unable to breastfeed following breast reduction, others can but have to supplement with formula, while still others can breastfeed normally.

At the age of 22, Betty's GP referred her to a plastic surgeon for possible breast reduction because she had constant neck and back pain. Betty had cup size F breasts, despite being of average height and weight. She had deep notches on her shoulders from her bra straps and found it difficult to buy bras and clothes. She was very self-conscious of her large breasts and found it difficult to exercise, even when wearing two or even three bras. Her mother and older sister also had large breasts. Her mother had a breast reduction at the age of 45 and said that it changed her life. Betty's mother had prompted her to see a plastic surgeon for an opinion.

The surgeon described her as a good candidate for surgery, noting that she was not overweight and mentioning that this meant Betty was at low risk of complications. The surgeon was also pleased that Betty had given up smoking and said that they didn't normally operate on smokers due to the significant risk of complications.

Betty wanted to be about a C cup after the operation. The surgeon explained that they couldn't guarantee a specific cup size but they would reduce the breast to a size that was about a C and in proportion with the rest of Betty's body.

The surgery took about two and a half hours and Betty stayed in hospital overnight. It was not a particularly painful operation and she felt quite comfortable with over-the-counter painkillers. By the time she saw the surgeon again about two weeks later, she had noticed a huge difference. Her neck and back pain had disappeared. By six weeks she was starting to do exercises she had not done for many years, and she has not looked back. The anchor scar on her breasts faded gradually and, although she can still see them if she looks for them, she would be happy to have the operation again or recommend it to her friends.

Breast reduction surgery is offered in public hospitals to women who meet strict criteria. These criteria exist to try to minimise the risk of women developing complications of surgery. It is known, for example, that if a woman's body mass index (BMI; see chapter 14) is higher than 30, her risk of complications increases significantly. In general, if a woman's BMI is greater than 30 she will not be considered for a breast reduction procedure, unless it is to match the other breast following breast cancer surgery. Smoking interferes with wound healing and for this reason smokers are not usually candidates for breast reduction surgery in a public hospital.

Breast uplift (mastopexy)

Women seeking breast uplift have usually breastfed their children and as a result have deflated, ptotic (droopy) breasts. These women desire an uplift to improve the appearance of their breasts and hope to restore their breasts to something approaching their pre-pregnancy state. In some cases an uplift can be effective with a silicone-implant breast augmentation alone, in others breast reduction techniques are necessary, and in many cases a combination of both techniques is required.

When a combination of both techniques is used, the risk of complications increases because the breast reduction reduces the amount of breast skin available to reshape the breast tissue itself while the implant increases the breast size. These techniques have contrary rather than complementary aims, which makes the chance of a problem much higher. To try to reduce this risk, the procedure may be undertaken as two separate operations spaced several months apart.

Breast reconstruction

Young women undergoing mastectomy commonly desire breast reconstruction. They may have undergone mastectomy due to breast cancer, but women who carry genes that put them at high risk of breast cancer commonly undergo bilateral (double) mastectomy and reconstruction. Reconstruction is either with their own tissue (flaps), most commonly from the abdomen or the back, or may be with silicone breast implants.

Breast reconstruction may be performed at the time of mastectomy (immediate reconstruction) or at a later date, once all the necessary treatment for the breast cancer has been completed (delayed reconstruction). Both techniques usually result in high satisfaction and an improvement in quality of life for women. The major benefit of immediate reconstruction is that more breast skin can be preserved and then used to reconstruct the breast – which means that the reconstructed breast is more like the original breast. If the reconstruction is delayed, a large amount of breast skin needs to be removed to ensure a good mastectomy scar. This breast skin then needs to be replaced during the reconstruction, which generally means more scarring on the chest.

Breast reconstruction with implants

Silicone breast implants are used to reconstruct the breast. Implant breast reconstruction tends to be at least a two-stage procedure. At the first stage you have the mastectomy and much of the breast skin is preserved. A tissue expander is placed under the pectoral (chest) muscles and the skin closed. The tissue expander is a silicone balloon with a metal valve on one side. When it is inserted it is usually empty, allowing the skin to heal without tension or stress. Once the skin and wound are healed, the device can be safely expanded by using the valve to fill the expander with saline (salt water) until the desired volume is reached. After a period of allowing the skin to stretch and the scar to mature (usually several months), the second stage occurs: the expander is removed and a silicone breast implant inserted. Most women will elect to have a third stage, when a nipple is reconstructed. This process is undertaken in stages to minimise the risk of complications; the most severe of these is infection. If there is any problem with the skin at the first stage, the implant may become infected and need to be removed.

The first stage of implant breast reconstruction generally requires a three-night hospital stay, while the second stage requires one night in hospital. Recovery time is usually about four to six weeks for the first stage and two to four weeks for the second. Most women do not drive for around two weeks after the first stage and one week after the second. They should avoid heavy lifting for six weeks.

Implant breast reconstruction can generally recreate the breast mound, allowing women to wear normal clothing and restoring or maintaining their self-confidence and body image. The feel of the reconstructed breast is different from the original breast and the breast tends to stay much the same over time, despite changes in weight or ageing.

Implant breast reconstruction is possible in most women but generally not recommended for those who require radiotherapy as part of their cancer treatment. This form of reconstruction tends to work best in younger women who are slim and whose breasts are not ptotic. Many women will also require surgery to the other breast to achieve better symmetry. This is particularly so in women with larger and more ptotic breasts.

The breast implant itself may develop problems. As mentioned above, the breast implant will induce scar tissue to form around it, called the capsule. Usually this is soft or a little firm, but sometimes it becomes quite hard or even painful. It may change the shape of the implant and affect the appearance of the reconstruction. This may be minor, such as 'rippling' of the skin over part of the implant, or it may be severe, with the implant moving out of position. These complications are far more likely to occur if radiotherapy is required as part of the breast cancer treatment, which is why it is not recommended for women who need radiotherapy. The breast implant itself tends to wear out with time and has a failure rate of around 0.3 per cent per year. The majority of women with breast implants will request surgery to try to correct problems related to the implant within 10–15 years of the implant being inserted.

Breast reconstruction with tissue (flaps)

It is possible to reconstruct the breast using a woman's own tissue. As discussed earlier, this can be performed in the same operation as the mastectomy or any time afterwards. There are various methods, but the most common is to use tissue from the abdomen or back to replace the breast tissue removed during the mastectomy. These methods are summarised below.

The advantage of flaps is that generally no implants are required and the breast is recreated from a woman's own tissues. The tissue is living and behaves more like a breast; it is usually softer and has similar characteristics to those of a natural breast. It will gain weight and lose weight and age with the rest of the body. Surgery to the opposite breast is less likely to be required and compared with implant reconstruction there is less chance of requiring surgery for problems with the breast in the longer term.

Tissue breast reconstruction tends to be more complex than implant reconstruction. It usually requires a hospital stay of around five days and six weeks off work. There is a very small risk that the tissue transferred will not survive and the procedure will fail completely. There is a slightly higher risk that there will be a partial failure – generally when some of the transferred fat doesn't survive and forms a hard lump (fat necrosis). The other complications are the same as for other methods of reconstruction: possible bleeding, infection, scars, asymmetry, numbness, deep vein thrombosis or pulmonary embolism, slow wound healing, fluid collection (seroma), bulging or hernia and anaesthetic complications.

Abdominal flaps

There are two types of procedure using an abdominal flap. The first is called a transverse rectus abdominis myocutaneous (TRAM) flap; the second is a deep inferior epigastric artery perforator (DIEP) flap.

In a TRAM flap, skin, fat, blood vessels and muscle from the lower abdomen are removed and transferred to the chest to recreate a breast. The tissue may be detached from the body completely and then reattached using microsurgical techniques, or it can remain connected by blood vessels and moved to the chest. This is a popular technique as the surgery to the abdomen is similar to a 'tummy tuck' procedure.

A DIEP flap is similar to the TRAM flap and uses the same skin, fat and blood vessels from the lower abdomen and transferred to the chest. Microsurgery is performed to reattach the blood vessels and restore blood flow to the tissue and a tummy tuck procedure is performed to repair the abdomen. Unlike the TRAM flap, no abdominal muscle needs to be transferred, which limits damage to the abdomen. This procedure is therefore generally considered to be the best method of breast reconstruction currently available.

Latissimus dorsi (back) flap

This flap reconstructs the breast using tissue from the back: the latissimus dorsi muscle and overlying skin and fat. The tissue remains connected to the body at all times via its blood vessels and is moved from the back of the chest to the front. It is often combined with a breast implant, as many women have insufficient tissue available on their back to reconstruct an adequately sized breast. It leaves a scar on the back, which is generally well hidden by clothing.

Transverse upper gracilis (TUG; upper thigh) flap

In this procedure the skin, fat and gracilis muscle are microsurgically transferred from the upper inner thigh to the chest, leaving a scar that is hidden near the groin crease. It is a good option for slim women who would like a tissue reconstruction and do not want a breast implant, but are unable to use an abdominal flap. Some women don't have enough fat on their abdomen to make a breast, while others may not be able to have an abdominal flap due to scars on the abdomen from previous surgeries, such as a tummy tuck.

Gluteal (GAP) flaps

These flaps are harvested from the skin and fat on the lower or upper buttocks. They are useful in women who wish to have a flap but are unable to have one of the other methods of reconstruction.

Kate was 29 when her mother was diagnosed with breast cancer. Her grandmother and aunt had also had breast cancer. She was advised to have genetic testing and it turned out that she was a carrier for one of the known breast cancer genes, BRCA1. This meant that she was at high risk for developing breast cancer too, and she was advised to consider undergoing a bilateral (double) mastectomy.

Kate decided she would like to reduce her risk of breast cancer by having surgery. She decided that once she had finished having children, she would have a bilateral mastectomy and reconstruction.

When she was 34, Kate had a bilateral mastectomy with an immediate breast reconstruction using DIEP flaps. This involved an eight-hour operation in which both breasts were removed, preserving all the breast skin except the nipple and areola. The breasts were replaced with skin and a flap from her abdomen. The removed breasts were weighed and replaced with the same amount of tissue, giving her two new breasts that closely matched her original breasts. She was in hospital for six nights. She was unable to drive for two weeks but found that she could do light exercise after about two weeks. Six weeks after the operation she was back at work part-time, as well as going to the gym.

Six months later, Kate had surgery to recreate nipples. This was a day-case operation and she was able to go back to work the next day. Three months after that, she had tattoos to recreate the appearance of the areolas. Although her new breasts aren't exactly the same as her old ones, she is pleased she had the surgery. She now doesn't fear developing breast cancer and is looking ahead to a bright future. She still has numbness on the breasts and some scars are still faintly visible, but unless she tells them, no one would know she has had a double mastectomy, even in a bikini.

Rhinoplasty (nose surgery)

Many women consider surgery to their nose. For some this is due to problems with breathing, while for others it is simply because they do not like the look of their nose.

Surgery to the nose is not usually a straightforward procedure and like all forms of surgery it needs careful consideration. Usually it is performed by a specialist plastic surgeon. If you are having breathing difficulties a consultation with an ear, nose and throat surgeon may also be required.

Rhinoplasty requires a general anaesthetic and most commonly an incision in the nose to gain access to the bones and cartilage that form the nasal skeleton. Sometimes this incision is hidden in the nostrils but more commonly it is in the tissue between the nostrils under the tip of the nose (the columella). The bones may need to be broken and reset in a better position and the cartilage may need to be partly removed, reshaped or replaced. Usually a splint will need to be worn for a short period after the surgery. An overnight stay in hospital is often necessary, followed by about two weeks off work or study.

After rhinoplasty the nose is very swollen for some time and it may take several months for all the swelling to disappear. The scar from the incision is usually very good but is sometimes visible. The surgery involves a small risk of bleeding or interfering with breathing. Sometimes there are small lumps or bumps on the nose that can be felt but usually not seen. Some people will have minor asymmetry that is not a problem, but up to 10 per cent will need another rhinoplasty in time to correct problems not fixed, or even problems caused, by the original procedure.

Genitoplasty (genital surgery)

There has been an enormous increase in women seeking cosmetic genital surgery to alter the appearance of their external genitalia. This has been attributed in part to the increased awareness of pornography. Most commonly surgery is requested to reduce the size of the labia, and less commonly vaginal rejuvenation is sought. For more on genitoplasty, see chapter 9.

28

Variations in sexual development

Yasmin Jayasinghe, Sarah McQuillan

Variations in sexual development occur in more than one in 5000 births, and involve variations in genes, and pelvic or external genital anatomy. They may also be known as 'disorders of sexual differentiation' or 'intersex'. Some women with variations in development may feel isolated or different, but in truth there is a great deal of natural diversity related to our development. Gender identity, gender role and sexual orientation are distinct entities. We now understand that these entities are diverse and may encompass a spectrum, and this is natural. Such variations do, however, pose unique challenges for these resilient women, largely because of lack of knowledge and understanding of such diversity in the wider community.

Variations in the development of the genitals

Although sex chromosomes are determined at conception, a complex interaction between genes and hormones determines the development of physical sexual characteristics. During development in utero (before birth), boy and girl babies all start off the same – they are gender neutral – and have the potential for development into either sex. In general female babies have XX sex chromosomes and undergo further development of female genital structures the uterus, vagina, vulva and gonads (ovaries), and regression of the male counterparts. It is important to understand that it is normal for females to also produce androgens (male hormones such as testosterone), but at lower levels than males. In general male babies have XY sex chromosomes, which result in development of gonads, the testes (singular testis), also called the testicles (where sperm can be stored in the future). The androgen hormones produced by an active testis result in the development of the male external genitals, and regression of female genital tract structures.

Types of variation in sexual development in women

Very rarely, variations in the normal course of these gene and hormone interactions result in differences between chromosomal sex and genital anatomy, which have been called disorders of sexual differentiation or 'DSD'. The terminology has changed and is under ongoing discussion to take into account the diversity in our development.

These variations may be identified at birth if the genitalia are of uncertain sex or 'ambiguous' (see below) or at puberty or later in life, when there is a lack of periods, infertility or sometimes other health problems.

Diversity in female development includes:

- variability in sex chromosomes, such as XO in women with Turner syndrome (see below)
- women with typical XX sex chromosomes who have been exposed to higher levels of androgens during development in the uterus, such as with congenital adrenal hyperplasia (see below)
- women with typical XX chromosomes who are born with some congenital variations in the genital tract (such as Müllerian agenesis, meaning the absence of development of one or more parts of the female genital tract, such as the vagina or uterus; see below)
- women with XY chromosomes, where androgens work less effectively, such as androgen insensitivity syndrome (see below), resulting in female external genitalia or variations in genital development and those with a combination of chromosomes and mixed tissue in the gonads

Some males have XX chromosomes, which means our chromosomes alone don't determine if we are male or female. Our gender identity is our private sense of male- or femaleness or in between. While we often refer to gender as being either male or female, some communities have accepted a third gender category. Most recently a children's book in Sweden has been published (and translated into English) with a new pronoun that means 'he or she'.

These conditions are diverse, and some may result in variations in the appearance of the external or internal genitalia at birth (sometimes referred to as ambiguous genitalia). The appearance of the genitalia itself is not the major issue, as many adults have expressed comfort and happiness with who they are and how they were born. We support and endorse this. It is important to recognise that there may be other coexisting symptoms or even later effects that may require consideration at birth or during child-hood, such as issues with metabolism and electrolyte balance in the body, problems passing urine, delayed puberty, absent periods, hormone effects in the body (such as increased acne or hair growth) and occasionally, in some very rare circumstances, development of pelvic tumours. These potential risks mean that doctors and parents may be faced with difficult decisions regarding treatment or surgery for a child at a young age.

What if my baby is born with ambiguous genitalia?

This can be a challenging time for parents, only because one of the first questions that family and friends ask is, 'Is it a boy or a girl?' There is little awareness in the general community about the diversity of sexual development, but hopefully this perception will change over time.

If your baby is born with ambiguous genitalia, the hospital staff will refer you immediately to a specialist team of doctors, allied health pro-fessionals and counsellors at the tertiary referral hospital in your state. The specialist team will undertake a complete set of tests to identify any immediate medical concerns, develop a diagnosis and provide affirmation of gender. They will evaluate the long-term outcomes for your child, and present various treatment options for you and your child as they grow up.

At some stage, the team may discuss the possibility of surgery. The decision to proceed to surgery while your child is young may be a difficult one. In principle, surgery would be recommended at a young age only to restore anatomy or reduce medical risks, and would be fully discussed with you. In some conditions where there is a Y chromosome, for example, leaving a non-functioning gonad inside the abdomen may significantly increase the risk of cancer in the future. At other times, delays in surgery may be associated with recurrent bladder or urine problems. Some sur-geries may be deferred until the child can make the decision themselves. Some people advocate no surgery, allowing the child to choose when they are old enough, but there is limited information regarding the long-term psychological impact of this approach.

If surgery is performed in childhood, it is best done in Centres of Excellence (highly specialised centres) in collaboration with clinical ethics committees. The long-term outcomes of childhood surgery are known and reported in the medical literature, so ask your doctors for the relevant articles or where to look for information.

Before making a decision, it is most important to be fully informed about the various options, and to be aware that there is some controversy both in Australia and the rest of the world regarding timing of surgery and the best surgical procedures. It is true that gender dissatisfaction may manifest later in life in a proportion of young people. This is more likely with some conditions than others, but it has prompted some healthcare professionals to seek advice from the Family Court before undertaking some types of surgery. It is hoped that when following the principles of full disclosure and gender affirmation rather than gender reassignment, gender dissatisfaction will be less likely to occur. There are generally strict ethical protocols regarding such surgery, which your healthcare team will fully discuss with you in a timely fashion as information becomes available.

Conditions causing variations in sexual development

Turner syndrome

Turner syndrome occurs in between one in 2000 and one in 5000 live births. In women with Turner syndrome, one of the X chromosomes is missing (XO in classic Turner syndrome means that there is only one X chromosome). In some women only some of the cells in their body have a missing X, while others have two X chromosomes (this is called mosaicism). There may also be mosaicism with a Y chromosome mixed in with X chromosome genetic material. In the presence of a Y chromosome, doctors would recommend removing the gonads at birth to avoid the high risk of cancerous change.

Most women are born with around 1 million eggs in the ovaries. Over time, these eggs degenerate, until the ovaries do not produce any more hormones and periods stop (at the time of menopause). In Turner syndrome, the eggs deteriorate more quickly, which means that many girls with Turner syndrome may not go through puberty, have periods or be able to have their own biological children. The ovaries do not lose their function as fast in women with mosaicism. Around 9 per cent of women with classic Turner syndrome and 30–50 per cent of women with mosaicism will go through puberty on their own, and around 2–5 per cent may spontaneously get pregnant. It is therefore important, if you have Turner syndrome, to discuss contraception with your doctor if required.

Management of Turner syndrome

For those women who do not go through puberty, it can be induced with hormone therapy started at very low doses by an experienced doctor. This will induce breast development and growth of the uterus, and eventually produce periods. Some girls with Turner syndrome will receive growth hormone to stimulate increased final height, as Turner syndrome is associated with shorter stature due to lower hormone levels.

Ongoing monitoring is important to check for any other medical issues. This can include heart monitoring with either an echocardiography (a heart ultrasound) or a heart MRI (magnetic resonance imaging); blood pressure checks (because of associated changes in development of the heart); ear and hearing tests; blood tests to check and monitor for diabetes, thyroid changes and coeliac disease; and bone density tests (to monitor the strength of the bones). Women with Turner syndrome will frequently be cared for by a team of health professionals, including endocrinologists, gynaecologists and social workers, with referrals to other services as well (such as cardiology and orthopaedics).

Turner syndrome and fertility

Fertility may be an issue that is very important to young women with Turner syndrome. They may make use of adoption, or use donor eggs (using someone else's eggs to achieve pregnancy through IVF) to carry a pregnancy in their own uterus. An experimental method of freezing ovarian tissue for possible use later in life exists, but this is a controversial area because the procedure may need to be considered before puberty, when a child cannot fully consent the way an adult can. To date, no pregnancies have been reported in women with Turner syndrome using this method.

It is very important to understand that for women with Turner syndrome, carrying a pregnancy may be associated with significant medical risks. The most important of these is death due to a sudden rupture of the aorta (the large blood vessel from the heart), which is reported in 2 per cent of women with Turner syndrome. There may be other medical risks, such as the possibility of a caesarean due to a small pelvis, miscarriages, and sometimes chromosomal changes in the offspring. If you have Turner syndrome and are considering pregnancy, it is very important to have a full discussion with your doctors (including a high-risk obstetrician). If you are in a relationship and do not wish to get pregnant, you should consider contraception because of the small chance of spontaneous ovulation and unexpected pregnancy.

Congenital adrenal hyperplasia (CAH)

CAH is a genetic condition affecting the production of adrenal hormones that occurs in one in 14,500 babies. Babies are often diagnosed after birth with ambiguous genitalia, or high blood pressure and blood electrolyte disturbances. The first few weeks of life can require intense investigations with a prolonged hospital stay for correction of electrolyte disturbances; failure to diagnose and treat this condition can be associated with dire risks.

In CAH a normal uterus and ovaries are present. More than 90 per cent of women with CAH identify as female. The condition is usually treated with corticosteroids to replace the lack of steroids produced by the infant, which are then increased to higher doses during times of stress or illness. Some young females with ambiguous genitalia might be considered for surgery before six months of age, but this will depend on the centre in which she is being treated, her specialist's opinion and, of course, her family's views.

Some women with classic CAH report narrowing of the vaginal entrance (whether they have had surgery as a baby or if surgery has been delayed) and sometimes discomfort with intercourse, and may have anxieties about sexual performance. Follow-up studies suggest that only a small proportion of women may require a revision operation at an older age after their childhood surgery. If there is vaginal narrowing, more women manage this by using vaginal dilators (see later in this chapter) than surgery. The timing of these procedures is guided by the young person in question.

A rarer, late-onset form of CAH can occur in later childhood or adolescence. These young women have normal genitalia, but may have irregular periods, acne or facial hair growth, thinning of scalp hair, and sometimes delays in falling pregnant. Teenagers with late-onset CAH will generally go through pubertal development normally but develop these symptoms later on. Late-onset CAH is usually only diagnosed through blood test investigations that find an abnormally high increase in androgen hormones and steroids and can be managed with hormonal treatment alone.

Androgen insensitivity syndrome (AIS)

Women with AIS have XY chromosomes. AIS occurs in one in 20,000 to one in 64,000 XY births and is due to the body not recognising androgen hormones, resulting in female external development. There are two forms: complete (CAIS) and partial (PAIS). In CAIS, the body does not recognise the androgens, whereas in PAIS, there is partial androgen activity.

Women with CAIS are born without a uterus, their vagina may be shortened and they may have sparse or no body hair, but apart from this they have typical female features (such as breasts and vulvar tissue). Most women with CAIS identify as females. Previously, gonads would be removed at birth, but the risk of cancer at a young age is low if the gonads are not in the abdomen (2–3 per cent), so some prefer to leave the gonads in until after puberty, as they will produce hormones that induce puberty and allow for normal breast development. After puberty, oestrogen therapy is recommended to assist with maintaining healthy bone acquisition. Options for having children may include adoption.

Those with partial AIS may be born with ambiguous genitalia and may identify as male or female. Women with PAIS do not have a uterus. They may notice some body hair due to the partial circulation of androgens, but this is very variable. If the gonads are inside the abdomen, they are usually removed at diagnosis to decrease the risk of cancer. Hormone replacement therapy and gender affirmation surgery are utilised in management.

Women with complete or partial AIS may have normal sexual relationships. They can dilate the vagina through sexual activity alone, or most commonly with the use of vaginal dilators (see the box below, and chapter 25, for more information on using vaginal dilators), and occasionally surgery, which in most cases would still require vaginal dilation afterwards.

Surgery to create a larger vagina would only be performed if dilators have not worked. Dilators or a vaginal mould may be required after

---

Using vaginal dilators

Vaginal dilators or 'trainers' are only used when women are comfortable with their own body, emotionally mature enough and motivated to use them. They are best used when you are nearly ready for sexual activity. We recommend finding a quiet, private time to use the dilators; some like to use them in the bath. There are different sizes of dilator you can use, but you would always start with the smallest. The doctor will initially demonstrate how the dilators may be used. The use of lubricant or numbing cream may make the dilation more comfortable.

Apply gentle pressure along the angle of the vagina (downwards and backwards if you are lying down). The dilators can be used for any length of time – we usually say around 15–20 minutes a day, but it is up to you. The skin gently inverts over time, and you may obtain normal vaginal length over two to six months. You should wash the dilator in soapy water after each use.

surgery. The mould stays in the vagina all the time for the first four to six weeks and then can be used daily, for those who are not sexually active, for a period of six months to a year or possibly longer.

Müllerian agenesis

Müllerian agenesis, also called Mayer-Rokitansky Kuster-Hauser syndrome or MRKH, occurs in one in 5000 women. If you have MRKH, you have typical XX chromosomes with normal ovaries but no uterus, and you may have shortening of the vagina. Commonly it is diagnosed in the teenage years when periods do not begin. Sometimes there may be very small, rudimentary uterus structures inside the pelvis that may cause intermittent pain. You will usually have normally functioning ovaries, so options for having children include adoption or surrogacy with a gestational carrier (where your ovaries are stimulated to produce eggs, and the eggs are collected and fertilised by sperm to make an embryo before being placed inside a trusted female's uterus). Normal sexual relationships are common. Sometimes the vagina may need to be lengthened with the use of vaginal dilators (see above), or sexual intercourse itself, and very rarely surgery.

Other conditions

Other variations of changes in the female reproductive tract are far rarer. These include a rudimentary uterine horn, cervical agenesis, transverse vaginal septum, and the more common imperforate hymen (which occurs in one in 1000 women).

The uterus can sometimes develop to look heart-shaped (bicornuate uterus). Sometimes half of the heart-like structure can be blocked (a rudimentary horn) or absent (unicornuate uterus). This can cause period pain or problems during pregnancy such as recurrent miscarriages or preterm delivery, so rudimentary horns are often removed before childbearing. If the other horn of the uterus is normal, it is possible to get pregnant but the risk of preterm delivery is still increased.

In other cases, two entire uterine horns and cervices (the neck of the womb) can develop, resulting in a uterus didelphis, which means a double uterus. If you have a complete double uterus your Pap tests will need to sample both cervices. It is best to speak to your doctor, who can explain if this is relevant for you.

In cervical agenesis there is a blockage at the neck of the uterus (due to failure of the cervical canal to develop), causing blockage of periods and retention of the blood inside the uterus. This can be managed in a variety of ways, including surgery to reconnect the uterus to the vagina. The most important side effect is infection, which can be very serious.

A transverse vaginal septum occurs in one in 70,000 women. It is basically a layer of skin (of variable width) in the vagina obstructing the flow of period blood. This requires surgery by an experienced doctor to decrease the risk of the vagina closing over again. The surgery is generally done at a time of emotional maturity, as vaginal dilators may need to be used afterwards. Until then, periods may be suppressed with hormones such as the Pill for months to years, thereby decreasing pain.

An imperforate hymen is a more common condition where there is a thin layer of skin blocking the entrance of the vagina. Usually the hymen has a small hole in it, allowing passage of period flow. The first indication of imperforate hymen is usually difficulty inserting a tampon or with sexual activity. If blood builds up in the vagina, it can cause pain or difficulty passing urine. It is easily treated with day surgery.

Gender and sexuality

Having a variation in sexual development does not imply that there is a variation in gender identity or sexual orientation. All of these things are quite distinct.

Gender identity refers to a person's internal sense of being male or female or other. Those with variations in sexual development are not transgender (where gender identity or expression does not conform to biological sex at birth).

Gender identity and sexual orientation are not the same. Sexual orientation refers to a person's enduring romantic, physical and emotional attraction to a particular sex (or sexes in the case of bisexuality). As discussed in chapter 7, sexual orientation begins to develop in childhood and becomes more established during adolescence and into adulthood. Sexual orientation can be both innate and fluid throughout life and includes the gender one is attracted to and fantasises about, and with whom one ultimately engages in sexual relations.

Through the journey to self-discovery, a young person should feel supported and able to discuss questions about their sexual orientation openly, and ultimately be able to express their sexuality without fear of harassment. It is well known that depression, substance abuse, harassment and violence, suicidal thoughts and sexual risk-taking behaviour are all increased in lesbian, gay, bisexual and transgender (LGBT) youth compared to their heterosexual peers. This is largely due to lack of support and feelings of isolation. As society becomes more educated and more tolerant, it is hoped that such experiences will become less common. It is important to know that there are many support groups with caring, experienced members, and health professionals who may assist during these times. See the Resources section at the end of this book for more information.

Leading a normal life

Variations in sexual development are more common than you might think. There are many other variations too numerous to list here. It is important to recognise that as human beings, we are diverse. As well as seeing a specialist who has expertise in the field, it is really important to have a good relationship with a family doctor or GP so that the usual preventative health checks that most people have are kept up to date. Most young women with variations in sexual development lead productive, happy lives and are in caring relationships. There is no reason why you cannot have the same.

29
Violence against women: sexual violence and sexual assault

Jill Duncan

Intimidating and/or unwanted sexual behaviour from another person can have wide-ranging harmful effects on a woman's health.

Sexual assault is a powerful force used against women and children; it is a component of a broader phenomenon known as violence against women. Sexual violence affects women across all age groups, and from all cultural, racial and economic backgrounds, including women with disabilities, lesbians and transgender women.

Terminology

Across Australia, the terminology used to label this behaviour varies from narrow terms for criminal acts such as 'rape' and 'indecent assault' to broader definitions that better reflect the experiences of victim/survivors. Some states and territories have a preference either for the term 'sexual assault' or for 'sexual violence'. In this chapter we use 'sexual assault' and 'sexual violence' interchangeably. We use 'child sexual abuse' to describe adult women's experience of sexual assault through childhood and adolescence.

Victim/survivor

The term 'victim/survivor' is used in sexual assault services in Australia for children and adults who have experienced sexual assault. This term recognises that someone has been subjected to and survived the crime of sexual assault. 'Victim/survivor' also reflects the moment-to-moment, day-to-day feelings of those affected by sexual violence. Some victims of sexual assault add 'thriver' to 'victim/survivor' to highlight the fact that they experience times of joy, pleasure and satisfaction like everyone else. Victim/survivors may or may not identify with this term.

If you need to talk to someone straight away

Some readers may find some of the material in this chapter distressing or disturbing. If you would like more information or to talk to someone directly about sexual assault, child sexual abuse, sexual harassment or intimate partner sexual violence, please call the National Helpline on 1800 RESPECT (1800 737 732). The National Helpline also provides information and support to women experiencing family violence.

What is sexual assault?

Sexual assault is any sexual or sexualised behaviour that makes a person feel uncomfortable, apprehensive, intimidated, threatened or frightened. It is sexual behaviour that someone has not agreed to, where another person uses physical or emotional force, or the threat of physical or emotional force against them. It encompasses experiences such as child sexual abuse; sexual violence from intimate partners; sexual harassment; and unwanted explicit and offensive communication by word, graphic image or social media. Many forms of sexual assault are criminal offences. Sexual violence is never the fault of the victim/survivor.

Sexual assault may include behaviour such as:

- rape – forced vaginal, anal or oral sex
- unwanted physical contact – touching, pinching, embracing, rubbing, groping, flicking, kissing, fondling
- sexual harassment – dirty jokes, rude or explicit comments, invasive questions about sex or sexual activity
- stalking – repeatedly following or watching someone
- voyeurism – watching someone doing intimate things without permission
- sex-related insults – for example, 'slut', 'dyke', 'homo', 'slag'
- pressuring for dates or demands for sex – invitations that turn into threats, or not taking no for an answer
- indecent exposure – exposing or flashing genitals
- forcing someone to watch or participate in pornography – explicit photos, videos or movies of sexual acts

- offensive written or graphic material – dirty jokes, letters, phone messages, pictures
- drug and/or alcohol-facilitated sexual assault – having sex with someone who is severely affected by drugs or alcohol, spiking drinks with alcohol or drugs
- information and communication-facilitated sexual assault – using the internet or other technology to distribute explicit and offensive images or messages; or to coerce, expose, mislead or deceive someone into acts of a sexual nature

Some of these forms of sexual assault are often repeated and can be ongoing over a number of years and escalate in severity over time. A woman might experience sexual violence by a person well known to her, an acquaintance or a stranger; by a caregiver or professional; or by men acting alone or in groups. She may experience a number of assaults from a range of perpetrators.

What is sexual harassment?

Sexual harassment is any unwanted, unwelcome and uninvited sexual behaviour – dirty jokes, rude or explicit comments, invasive questions about sex or sexual activity, for example – (usually) in public contexts such as the workplace, school, sports or recreation facilities, that makes a person feel offended, uncomfortable, humiliated or intimidated. Sexual harassment is often trivialised and its serious effects on women's lives minimised.

Sexual harassment includes leering, pinching, patting, repeated comments, subtle or crude suggestions of a sexual nature, pressure for dates and sex, display or distribution of explicit and offensive graphic material, and stalking. It is not social interaction, flirtation or friendship; it is not mutual or consensual. Women usually experience sexual harassment from men, but may also be victimised by other women. Sexual harassment may be accompanied by other forms of bullying behaviour.

What is child sexual abuse?

A child or young person is sexually assaulted when any person who has more power uses their authority to involve them in sexual activity for the gratification of that person in authority. A sibling or older child may be in a more powerful position in relation to a younger or more dependent child. Child sexual abuse is a violation of a child's right to safety and protection from harm, and a betrayal of family and community trust.

Why we have included sexual assault in this book

Sexual violence and abuse are all too common experiences for many in our community – women and girls predominantly, boys and to a lesser degree men. This chapter deals with what is known about sexual assault in the lives of women and its possible effects on their health.

It is important that we present factual material here about sexual assault because the reality of the prevalence, nature and impacts of sexual violence challenges the many inaccurate and misleading ideas in the community about sexual abuse and sexual violence. For example, many people believe that sexual assault is rare, and that victims should be able to prevent it or make it stop. The reality is that sexual assault is common and can have significant and harmful effects. Sexual violence is never the responsibility of a victim/survivor: people who commit sexual assault are solely responsible for their violence.

Victim/survivors may find it difficult to recognise and name their experience as sexual violence. They may know that what happened was humiliating and frightening but not realise their responses are entirely understandable and valid. Or they may think they won't be believed or are not entitled to or worthy of support because they don't have any obvious or serious injuries. They may believe that everyone, especially women, has unwanted and frightening sexual experiences.

Much is now known about the impact sexual assault has on victim/survivors. Many of these consequences can directly affect women's health – emotional, psychological, mental, physical, spiritual, gynaecological and reproductive. Any traumatic experience may have systemic and recognisable effects on the human mind, body and spirit, but each victim/survivor will also have particular individual reactions and responses to violence perpetrated against them by another person. Every victim/survivor should therefore be provided from the outset with the opportunity to speak for herself about the impacts on her own life, and to be as in control as possible of what happens to her body, including her health care.

If you have experienced sexual assault at any time during your life and are in need of health care, it may be useful to take a copy of this chapter with you to assist your healthcare provider to better understand your experience and its impact on your wellbeing and health needs.

Children always have less power than adults: the closer the relationship between the child and the adult, the greater the dependency and therefore the greater the power the adult has over the child.

Children lack the necessary information and maturity to make an informed decision about sexual activities with an older person. They do not have adult knowledge of sex and sexual relationships, or the social meaning of sexuality and its potential consequences.

Child sexual abuse involves a wide range of sexual activity. It may include fondling of the child's genitals, or getting the child to fondle the perpetrator's genitals; masturbation with the child as either observer or participant; oral sex; vaginal or anal penetration by a penis, finger or any other object; fondling of breasts; voyeurism or exhibitionism. It can also include exposing the child to pornography or using the child for the purposes of pornography or prostitution, including the use of social media and other technological means of communication.

What is intimate partner sexual violence?

Women may experience intimate partner sexual violence in any intimate relationship from their teens through to their senior years. This includes in dating and brief encounters, longer term and lifelong spousal partnerships, heterosexual and lesbian relationships, cohabiting and separate living circumstances, and in current and past relationships.

The harm of intimate partner sexual violence may be compounded because sexual assault is a stark betrayal of individual and community values and ideals about trust and loving relationships. Sexual activity is never a requirement or obligation in intimate relationships. Free agreement, or consent, can never be presumed and can be withdrawn at any time.

Intimate partner sexual assault is often accompanied by other violent and controlling behaviour, including sexual harassment that denies a woman the freedom and opportunity to choose not to participate in sex. Sexual violence is almost always a reality or threat in family and domestic violence. It is often hard to recognise intimate partner sexual violence. Misinformation and misconceptions about sexual violence mean that in general the closer the relationship between victim and perpetrator, the less likely the assault is seen as rape, and the more likely a victim will be blamed and the harm of the violence minimised. See chapter 30 for more on intimate partner and family violence.

Sexual assault and the law

The aim and focus of this chapter is to help you understand the possible connections between sexual assault and your health and wellbeing. Victims of sexual assault are entitled to report their experience to the police if they want to, but this is never compulsory. It is not within the scope of this chapter to address the legal options in each state and territory.

If you would like to know more about the law and sexual assault in your state or territory you can check out the Australian Centre for the Study of Sexual Assault website at www.aifs.gov.au/acssa, contact a sexual assault centre or call your local police.

Sexual assault is a serious personal and social issue

The consequences of sexual violence primarily affect individual victim/survivors, but may also have detrimental effects on the family and friends of victims. Women make up half the adult population and the extent of violence against women, overwhelmingly perpetrated by some men, makes sexual violence a serious social problem. There are also negative social, cultural and economic consequences for our society as a whole if any woman feels reluctant or unable to participate fully in the life of her community because she feels apprehensive and affected by the experience or threat of sexual violence.

In every community there are many commonly held misconceptions about sexual assault that in general blame victims, excuse men who perpetrate sexual violence, trivialise sexual assault and minimise its impacts. These messages are harmful to everyone: women in general, victim/survivors in particular and the entire community. Unhelpful beliefs about sexual assault work to invalidate women's experience of sexual violence. They silence victims and confuse and mislead. Sexualised and often sexist portrayals of women in advertising and other media, including pornography, add to a social environment that reinforces attitudes supporting violence against women.

A violation of human rights

Sexual assault is a violation of the human right of sexual autonomy. Among other things, sexual autonomy means everyone has the right to freely choose *not* to participate in sexual activity at any time. It also means that no one ever has the right to pressure, coerce or force another person into any type of sexual activity. Everyone has the right to decline sex, say no, or abstain without fearing that something bad will happen to them, someone else or something they value.

If you have had sexual experiences that felt like sexual violence but you are not sure whether that label fits, you could ask yourself, 'Did I want to have that sex with that person? Did I feel like I freely and voluntarily agreed or was I intimidated or uncomfortable? At the time did I feel as though I could comfortably decline? Was I worried that something bad would happen to me? Was I frightened that they would do something bad to someone else? Was I sober enough or old enough to really understand what that person wanted of me?'

How common is sexual assault?

Australian and international research over the last 40 years shows that rates of sexual assault and other forms of violence against women are extremely high. For example:

- Up to one in three women will experience some form of sexual assault before the age of 16.
- Up to one in five Australian women will experience sexual violence in adulthood.
- Many young women experience sexual violence in early sexual relationships.
- Many women experience sexual harassment at work and in other social settings.
- One in two women experience physical and/or sexual violence from an intimate partner at some time during their life.

Overwhelmingly, sexual assault is perpetrated by men (98 per cent of sexual assaults), and the majority of victims are women and children. (This does *not* mean, of course, that 98 per cent of men commit sexual violence.) Although there is a misconception that sexual assault is usually committed by strangers, in fact most perpetrators know the victim in some way: as an intimate partner, acquaintance, friend or family member, or through family, social or work contact. Universally understood social expectations such as trust and a sense of fair play are attached to all of these relationships. Betrayal of this fundamental social and personal trust is a significant factor contributing to the harm of sexual assault. It may also add to confusion and difficulty in recognising such an experience as sexual violence.

Community misconceptions about sexual assault

There are many commonly held misleading ideas in our society that confuse and silence people – victim/survivors, friends and family, healthcare professionals – about sexual violence. Such misconceptions sometimes interfere with women receiving appropriate support when they talk about experiences of sexual assault.

Unfortunately, these harmful and biased ideas are very entrenched in our community, to a greater or lesser extent among women and men, regardless of social standing and education, and across most cultures. They generally define sexual assault very narrowly as rape by a stranger; attribute blame to women for causing sexual violence; and excuse perpetrators of responsibility for their actions. They also imply that women exaggerate or lie about sexual assault or make it up.

Misconceptions that support sexual violence suggest that somehow women provoke men or give them permission to commit sexual violence by wearing particular clothing, flirting, being in certain places, being unaccompanied, or being drunk or drug-affected. These misconceptions also suggest that women have the responsibility to protect themselves against would-be perpetrators, as if men who use sexual violence and abuse are predictable, recognisable and therefore avoidable. On the contrary, men who use sexual violence are usually very 'ordinary'-looking people. They act purposefully and strategically against women and children who know and trust them.

All of these prejudicial messages might make it difficult for a woman to recognise that she has experienced sexual assault, recently or in the past. They might make her reluctant to talk about her experience or to seek assistance and support because she feels ashamed or embarrassed. They might also discourage her from recognising that sexual assault can affect her health.

Impacts of sexual violence on women's health

Research over many years has shown some clear connections between sexual assault and women's health and wellbeing. The severity of these health consequences may be compounded by disbelieving and blaming responses at first disclosure, and the amount of time that often elapses between the sexual assault experience and receiving appropriate support, including relevant health care.

The consequences for women of child sexual abuse may be quite wide-ranging, long-term and complex. All aspects of human health –

emotional, psychological, physical, sexual, social and spiritual – are maturing through our childhood and adolescence. Violence such as sexual assault committed against a child has the potential to profoundly disrupt a child's world and the patterns and pathways of their unfolding life.

It is understandable that the experience of sexual violence may traumatise a woman and profoundly violate every aspect of her being. It can affect her emotional and physical health, her sense of self, her relationship with her body, and her sense of safety everywhere, including in intimate relationships and in healthcare settings.

Post-traumatic stress responses

Sexual assault is among the experiences that are known to cause post-traumatic stress responses. When an experience is so frightening as to feel life-threatening, it elicits powerful physical and psychological reactions over which we have little or no control. These are recognised as adaptive responses and the body's way of coping with the threat at the time. Post-traumatic stress is recognised as a cluster of reactions that continue well beyond the time when day-to-day stress reactions would have passed. Post-traumatic reactions can be intrusive and problematic and may seriously disrupt functioning in everyday life.

The cluster of post-traumatic stress reactions includes hyper-arousal, re-experiencing and avoidance. Hyper-arousal mirrors a state of being permanently alert to further threat. A victim/survivor may feel a continuous heightened sense of anxiety and danger that can interfere with everyday life, including sleep, and prevent relaxation. A constant sense of threat may also provoke watchfulness and protection over family members, especially children.

Re-experiencing may be triggered by any conscious or unconscious connection with the experience of sexual assault. It includes flashbacks, intrusive thoughts and nightmares in which a victim/survivor feels as though she is reliving the sexual abuse or sexual assault. Flashbacks may be momentary or of longer duration and are re-traumatising because victim/survivors re-experience the terror and disempowerment that accompany sexual violence. Fear of re-experiencing trauma might promote hyper-arousal and avoidance.

Avoidance actions might be deliberate or less conscious, and include strategies to prevent or contain further danger or feelings associated with trauma experience. Victim/survivors of sexual assault talk about isolating themselves from social or other triggering situations; avoiding stressful circumstances; shutting down emotionally; disconnecting and disso-ciating; and using alcohol and drugs, prescribed and illegal, to subdue feelings of fear, stress and anxiety. Dissociation is initially a protective process that separates a person for a period of time from associations with the experience of the trauma of sexual assault. It can sometimes persist and be less useful if it disrupts recovery and everyday functioning.

Alterations to thinking and mood have recently been recognised as associated with post-traumatic stress responses. These may include disruption to memories related to the traumatic experience; strong, persistent negative thinking about self and others; overwhelming feelings of, for example, guilt, shame, horror, anger. Victim/survivors may also feel alienated or estranged from others and uninterested in significant activities.

Talking about the experience of sexual assault to someone else

Some things that can prevent or lessen further harm to a victim/survivor include believing them and taking them seriously when they do talk about sexual assault, validating their feelings and reactions, and helping them to explore the options available for informal and professional support and assistance. It is very important that victim/survivors themselves make any decisions relating to their care and support, including the decision to talk about their experience, who they talk to and when; what happens after they tell someone; and that they feel they are in control of what happens to their bodies.

Victim/survivors may choose to talk to their healthcare providers about a history of sexual violence, past, recent or current, but no pressure should ever be placed on victim/survivors to disclose their experience to anyone. The quality and relevance of health care should not depend on disclosure; a victim/survivor should expect that medical and nursing staff will provide sensitive and respectful health care to everyone. This may include gentle and tentative questions about sexual violence as part of taking medical history, but again it is important that victim/survivors choose the time and people with whom they share their story.

The table below shows the health impacts known to be connected with women's experience of sexual assault, and reported by victim/survivors. The list is comprehensive but not definitive. Individual victims might experience some or many of these health issues. Any or all of these health problems can also occur with no connection to a history of sexual assault.

Possible impacts of sexual assault on women's health

Emotional health	Mental health
• Difficulties with trust • Sense of loss of control • Generalised anxiety • Emotional numbness • Guilt, shame, self-blame, confusion • Sadness and grief • Anger and rage • Out-of-body experiences • Discomfort with intimacy and touch • Nightmares and sleep disturbance • Constant sense of danger and lack of safety • Hypervigilance • Generalised fear of men	• Traumatic and post-traumatic stress responses • Depression • Anxiety • Self-harm • Eating disorders • Dissociation • Compulsive behaviours • Panic attacks • Flashbacks • Substance dependency, including tobacco and alcohol, illicit and prescribed drugs • Mental health disorders
Reproductive and physical health	**Social, cultural, spiritual and economic health**
• Chronic pelvic and other pain • Gastrointestinal disorders • Abnormal Pap test results • Pain with intercourse • Gynaecological disorders • Urinary tract infections • Increased rates of human papilloma virus and cervical cancer • Unwanted and early pregnancy • Terminations • Sexually transmitted infections	• Wariness and avoidance of social activities • Disruption to cultural identity and connections • Disillusionment with spiritual beliefs and supports • Disruption to school attendance and achievement • Interrupted work participation • Career disruption • Unemployment or difficulties in the workplace • Financial difficulties, debt • Homelessness, unstable housing • Disruption to family identity and connections
Psychological health	**Use of health services**
• Eroded sense of self-worth • Disrupted sense of self-efficacy • The feeling of going crazy • Suicidal thoughts • Suicide attempts	• Difficulties trusting healthcare providers • Reluctance or delay in accessing Pap screening • Late presentation for antenatal care and other care • Discomfort and fear of internal examinations • Avoidance of dental health care • Wariness of male medical practitioners

Support and assistance for victim/survivors

Victim/survivors are in the best position to say what sort of assistance they need at any time. However, there are some important guiding principles that friends, family and healthcare providers can take into account. Other service providers who may be supporting a victim/survivor in matters relating to sexual violence, such as police, lawyers, teachers, community workers and clergy, should also follow these principles.

Principles of effective support include belief and taking the matter seriously; letting the victim speak for herself; reassuring her that her responses to the trauma of sexual violence are normal; validating her feelings and individual reactions to the experience; exploring with her what she would like to happen now; and genuinely respecting her decisions. Victim/survivors report that a sense of emotional and physical safety is fundamental to support around disclosure and recovery. It is important for those supporting victims of sexual assault and abuse, including healthcare providers, to learn about what safety means to each individual and how to assist her in creating a sense of safety.

Among the decisions a victim/survivor might make are whether or not to seek professional support, including counselling, or report the assault or abuse to police. Victims of sexual abuse and sexual violence have the right to both these courses of action, but it is essential that the decision be theirs. Some Australian states and territories have time limits on reporting to police, and variations in eligibility for accessing government-funded free counselling and support. (For more information about the support options in your state or territory, see the Resources section at the end of this book.)

It is possible that when a friend or family member talks about past or recent sexual assault or sexual abuse, those listening might feel distressed and worried. Healthcare practitioners and other professionals might also feel disturbed and concerned. Sometimes people supporting a victim/survivor feel as though they have to do something special, or they are frightened that they will do or say the wrong thing and make the victim/survivor feel worse. Sometimes support people feel anxious and panicked about what has happened to the victim/survivor and want to do the 'right' thing immediately. There is no timetable: the best support is allowing a victim/survivor to set the pace and tone of the conversation and the course of events to follow. The important thing is that she has survived the experience. Her recovery will be assisted most by attention to and respect for her point of view.

Sexual assault and sexual abuse are such harmful experiences because they violate a person's sense of control over their own bodily integrity, physical, psychological and emotional: someone else has used force of some kind to dictate what they experience. It is therefore very important that those who are assisting and supporting victim/survivors behave in every way as unlike a perpetrator of sexual violence as possible. They need to resist the temptation to tell the victim what she should be feeling or doing, never assume they have greater knowledge or insight about sexual violence and what needs to happen, coerce or force a victim to take any particular course of action, undermine her sense of self-control by taking decisions out of her hands, minimise the consequences of sexual violence, be impatient by encouraging her to get over it; or be judgemental about her decisions.

The importance of belief

In a world that often blames victim/survivors for the sexual violence perpetrated against them and doubts their account of the experience, it is vital that every conversation with and action by people supporting a victim demonstrates belief. Conversations that question a victim's behaviour or reactions might register as blame and doubt. On the other hand, reassuring her that how she is feeling is normal, validating her reactions, attending to what she needs, talking through her options and respecting her choices will implicitly show that the supporting person believes the victim has experienced sexual assault and takes the matter seriously.

Self-care for support people

It is often distressing for family and friends who are supporting a victim/survivor of sexual abuse or sexual violence, and this distress might be ongoing and possibly long-term. There might be times when a support person doubts their own feelings and abilities. It is therefore often helpful for those supporting a victim/survivor to seek some assistance for themselves. Most Australian sexual assault services offer some level of telephone or face-to-face support for friends and family, and consultation and debriefing for community workers and healthcare providers.

Recovery from sexual assault

Recovery is a process that begins at the time sexual violence is experienced. All the instinctive reactions a victim/survivor has, as well as the more deliberate decisions she makes to survive sexual assault, can be understood and should be recognised as milestones on a journey of recovery.

Some people might interpret recovery to mean getting over the experience of sexual assault and getting back to 'normal', but it won't be possible for a victim/survivor of sexual violence to go back to being exactly the way they were before the sexual assault. Indeed, many victim/survivors of child sexual assault may not even have the luxury of knowing what they were like before.

Rather, what happens through recovery is a kind of reworking and an emergence of a new self. The self that emerges is one that incorporates three aspects: the pre-sexual assault self, the self who survived the experience of sexual violence, and a self with a new understanding of themselves and the world. This process is called post-traumatic growth.

There are times when victim/survivors feel that their experience of sexual violence or abuse overshadows all other aspects of their lives – relationships, work, family, leisure. During these crises, surviving seems to consume most of a victim/survivor's time and energy.

Establishing a sense of safety and control is vital in the process of ongoing recovery, but safety may be challenged or disrupted by post-traumatic stress symptoms. Regular and uncontrollable flashbacks, for example, may reiterate a sense of threat and danger. Victims of sexual assault may be assisted at this time by coping strategies that help them establish a sense of safety. Accessing counselling and support is one option for victim/survivors, along with a variety of self-help resources.

For recovery from sexual assault to develop, it is important for a victim/survivor to reconnect with her human rights, to know her options, and feel she has regained a sense of control over her own body. The more a victim/survivor is assisted to understand her rights and options and feel in control, the more likely she is to exercise those fundamentals and experience a sense of empowerment and self-determination.

Counselling and support groups

Many victim/survivors find that healing and recovery from the trauma of past or recent sexual violence is assisted by talking with people who understand what they have experienced. Victim/survivors report that talking to counsellors or to other victim/survivors in facilitated support groups helps them gain perspective and insight, and break through the silence and social isolation that surrounds sexual assault.

30

Family violence

Helena Maher

Love is very good for our health. Stable, trusting, caring relationships, and a life shared with family, friends and lovers have been shown to have profound benefits for our health and wellbeing. They are good for our stress levels, our blood pressure, our resilience and our happiness. Through the regard and respect of others, we feel our sense of self, confidence, autonomy and empathy nurtured and affirmed as a member of a just and fair society.

For many women, the experience of family and romance is none of these things. 'Family violence', 'intimate partner violence' or 'domestic violence' are terms used by professionals to mean women trapped in relationships with men who profess to love them but whose behaviour is focused on threats, isolation, punishment and control. While the vast majority of violence that women experience is from men, intimate partner violence can also occur in same-sex relationships.

Many women come into their adult life having already experienced or witnessed violence from members of their family or others in positions of trust in their community. In addition to the physical and emotional harm done to women's health, these experiences also increase women's vulnerability to violence and abuse in their adult relationships.

Family violence is a common experience for women, but it is also preventable. Prevention begins with individuals and the wider society acknowledging the extent of violence against women, refusing to blame women for men's actions and insisting that our police, courts and other institutions uphold women's and children's rights while holding men accountable.

This chapter is about violence experienced by women from men they know through intimate or family relationships, the serious impacts on women's health and the steps to take to get help, whether the violence is happening to you or someone you love.

Family violence is a crime

Until quite recently family violence was hidden or ignored because it was seen as private. Mostly, the law left alone men who were violent to their wives and it was socially acceptable for a man to feel entitled to control 'his woman'. The law is now clear that women do not lose their rights because they marry or are in a relationship, and that family violence is a crime.

At the legal and political level, Australian laws and government policies emphasise women's equality and the criminal nature of violence against women and children. All states and territories have laws aimed at protecting women and children from family violence, and governments fund specialist services to provide resources and support.

Most people agree that forcing someone to have sex, slapping someone, throwing or smashing objects with the aim of frightening them, yelling abuse and constant criticisms are forms of violence. The reality is that it may be a friend, colleague, or member of the local church or football team who behaves like this towards their partner or children. Exposure to violence in childhood, weak support for women's equality and support for traditional gender roles all contribute to a sense among some men that they are entitled to use violence to control women.

What does family violence entail?

More than just physical attacks, women in controlling relationships are subject to an insidious pattern of threats, intimidation and abuse that is just as harmful. Women talk about a wide range of deliberate behaviours focused on undermining their self-confidence: criticisms, put-downs, public humiliations and manipulative mind games. There is also a pattern of controlling a woman's everyday life: limiting access to money, friends or the clothes she wears; isolation from family and friends; demanding to know where she is or what she is doing; and accusations of being unfaithful. One of the hardest things for women to talk about is when the abuse they have experienced includes being raped.

How does family violence affect women's health?

Research has clearly established a link between our relationships and our health. A 2004 VicHealth study found that intimate partner violence was responsible for more ill health and premature death in Victorian women under the age of 45 than any other known risk factor. The impact is clearly seen in the rates of anxiety, depression, suicide, alcohol and substance abuse. Women with a history of intimate partner violence are more likely to smoke; have an abnormal Pap test; have contracted a sexually transmitted infection; have alcohol or drug problems; be diagnosed with a mental illness, chronic lung condition, heart disease, hypertension (high blood pressure), stroke or bowel problems; and suffer chronic pain and fatigue.

The impacts on health may vary according to the different stages of life:

- Exposure to violence as a child increases the risk of mental health problems, behavioural difficulties and developmental delays.

- Young women are at increased risk of having an unplanned pregnancy, an abortion or a miscarriage.

- Many women are assaulted when they are pregnant, increasing the risk of complications affecting both pregnancy and the baby's health.

- In midlife, women who have lived with a violent partner are more likely to experience depression and anxiety and to report diminished psychological wellbeing.

- Older women who have experienced violence from a current or past partner rate their health as poorer and use health services more frequently than other women, even after they are no longer exposed to the violence.

Why do men commit family violence?

Men's violence towards women is about the deliberate use of threats and violence to control or punish their partner, and is often supported by a sense of entitlement and enjoyment of the feeling of power that comes with domination. Men's attitudes about gender equality are a major predictor of their use of violence; violence is more prevalent where men hold to traditional beliefs about how women should behave, where men believe that physical violence is the normal way to resolve conflict and where these beliefs are shared by their peers. In relationships and families where men have control over all the major decisions, violence is used to uphold and reinforce this lack of equality. Growing up around men who are violent, abusive and disrespectful to women increases the likelihood of men using violence as an adult.

In contrast, in relationships, families, communities, institutions and societies where decision-making power is more equally distributed between women and men and gender roles are less rigid, there is less violence against women. In this way, community attitudes play a significant role in either supporting or preventing men's violence towards women.

The broader social context of family violence

In community surveys, one in three women reports experiencing physical violence at some point in their life since the age of 15. Ten per cent of women report that their current partner has been violent; 36 per cent report violence in a past relationship. Almost one in four children has witnessed violence against their mother or stepmother. Many people are shocked to learn how common family violence in our society is and how serious its effects are on the lives of women and their children.

Family violence is just one example of men's violence against women and children in our society. Sexual harassment – such as staring, leering, touching, requests for sexual favours, offensive jokes and intrusive questions – is common in workplaces, in schools and at sport and entertainment events. Sexting, stalking and bullying, or threatening to 'out' people or infect them with an STD are other forms of emotional and psychological abuse. Less familiar but just as damaging to women's physical and mental health are culturally specific practices such as female genital mutilation or cutting, so-called honour killing and forced marriage. In legal brothels in Australia women have been trafficked into prostitution. Many women and children have come to Australia as refugees, having escaped from countries where rape has been used as a weapon in war.

In 1993, the United Nations developed the following definition of violence against women to capture the range of violent behaviours to which women are vulnerable, and to support the elimination of gender-based violence from society:

> Any act of gender-based violence that results in, or is likely to result in, physical, sexual or psychological harm or suffering to women, including threats of such acts, coercion or arbitrary deprivation of liberty, whether occurring in public or private life.

The harm done to women's physical, sexual and mental health is at the core of this definition, and is supported by findings from a growing body of research that makes plain the toll on women's sense of wellbeing, relationships and quality of life.

You never would pick me as someone who has survived an abusive relationship. On the outside, we seemed like the happiest couple – afterwards people always said, 'But you two had so much fun.' And we did, but also there was all this horrible stuff: threats and manipulation, telling me off in front of friends, cutting me off from family. Sometimes I look back and wonder, 'What was I thinking?' But I wasn't – I was numb. Then one night he raped me, and that was it. I ran.

It took me years and lots of searching and lots of courage but eventually I found a counsellor who helped me face what happened, what led me into it and what got me out. I went to the police and I told my friends and family. Mostly I just sat with myself and felt the shame, the bitterness, the betrayal and the confusion. Going to the police was good, even though nothing came of it – there was no evidence, just my word against his. Even so, it made me feel I had the whole of society on my side now, and that who he really was was exposed. Telling people helped me see it wasn't my fault, and to feel that I was loved and cared for, that I didn't deserve that. The work those services do, domestic violence services, is incredible. Life-saving. Life-changing.

The challenges of leaving a violent relationship

All women who leave a relationship where their partner is violent experience significant difficulties.

The most likely murderer of an Australian woman is her past or current partner. Men practising coercive control are often terrifying in private and charming in public, and if you are in this position, you may find it extremely difficult to contact services without the knowledge or attendance of your partner. You must weigh up the danger you face if you ask for help from services that may fail in their duty to protect and support you. While services can make all the difference, social stigma and fear of judgement from professionals can also work to isolate women. In a society that plays down the prevalence, seriousness and harm associated with men's violence to women, women are easily trapped.

Escaping a violent relationship

It is important to understand how threats and abuse affect your ability to act and your own inner strengths, which will support you to escape violence.

The dynamics of abuse make you feel helpless by disconnecting you from society, family and friends and by making you feel that the violence is warranted. The fear of retaliation, community tolerance of violence, a lack of information or services, a lack of protection from police or the courts, language barriers, an insecure or low income, the loss of family or community: any and all of these factors can force women into crisis before they take the risk of seeking help.

There are many ways to counter these feelings:

- Violence is isolating, so neighbours, teachers, workmates and other contacts in your community can be essential sources of information about where you can go for help.

- Violence undermines your ability to trust. More and more though, as people recognise how serious and prevalent violence is in women's lives, it is easier to find professionals you can take the risk of opening up to.

- Violence is traumatising: the experience of being trapped or the feeling of being terrified can profoundly distort your sense of what is healthy and acceptable. Counselling can be an important part of reclaiming a joyful, loving life with affirming and fulfilling relationships.

- Your safety is vital; if you need immediate protection you can ring 000 for the police or the National Sexual Assault, Domestic Family Violence Counselling Service on 1800 737 732 to find your closest crisis support service. Domestic violence services can help you with free and safe accommodation, dealing with the courts or the police and linking you with other supports such as legal advice.

- Involving police is important but it's not the only option. Support groups run by services offer forums for sharing experiences, making friends and working through issues like parenting or getting control of your money after family violence.

Supporting someone you love

In the stories of women who have escaped from violent partners, it is clear that friends, family and community members play a vital role by listening and believing, and taking what they hear seriously without trying to tell women what to do.

If you know someone who is living with a violent partner, here are some practical ways that you can help:

- Violence is life-threatening, so it is important to honour her judgement about what course of action is safe for her at that point in time, and respect her choices. The process of getting free from violence can be slow and complicated as she struggles to reclaim her sense of self and reassert her independence. Be patient and provide practical support over the long term to help fortify her courage and endurance.

- Navigating legal avenues and the family violence system can be fraught with difficulties. It is not unusual for women to be let down by police, child protection, the courts and other professionals. Support her to persist with finding helpful expert professionals.

- Offer her social support – it can make all the difference. Research shows that abused women with a network of family members, friends and colleagues, or a community they belong to, have better mental and physical health than abused women with lower social support, irrespective of the severity or frequency of the abuse.

- Become involved in an organisation that fights for women's rights. Activism can be therapeutic. Women, as individuals and as part of feminist campaigns and organisations, have been essential in leading improvements for a fairer, safer, more just society for women and girls around the world.

- If you are a man, make your voice heard. Men have an important role in supporting the work of feminists to achieve equality for women and in challenging male friends, family members and colleagues who abuse their partner or children or excuse or trivialise men's violence towards women.

Be part of the change

Violence from men whom women know and trust causes serious harm to health and wellbeing. The burden of this violence on women's lives can be prevented through greater understanding from friends, family, colleagues and community members. Through refusing to trivialise violence against women, by understanding the pattern of behaviours that characterise men's violence, by responding with belief and empathy to women's experiences, and by being aware of the professional services that are available, we can make a major difference to the lives, health and wellbeing of all women and girls.

MIDLIFE

Introduction

Maureen Johnson

Like all life stages, the point at which midlife begins and ends is not neces-sarily clear. Generally, though, it is defined as between the ages of 40 and 60 (some put it as early as 35) and can be regarded as the bridge between adulthood and old age. For most women it is a time of change – physical and hormonal – as well as an important psychological developmental phase. It is also a time to prepare for 'successful ageing'.

As a woman, it can be hard to avoid the influence of societal attitudes during midlife. Cultural attitudes to fertility, childbearing and the roles women play vary markedly between cultural groups. In many cultures, increasing age signifies wisdom, status and power in the family and the community. By contrast, in Western society, where youth and beauty are held in high esteem, ageing can make women feel invisible and under-valued. Yet many of us arrive at midlife more confident and able, armed with a wealth of experience, knowledge and skills. Some women will reach the peak of their careers in their 50s; for example, studies in human resources show that on average, women take on their most senior role at the age of 53.

During midlife, most women experience more personal change or 'life events' than at any other time of life. These changes can be challeng-ing and difficult, and include poor health, marriage breakdown or divorce, or caring for ageing or sick parents or a sick partner. But changes at this time can also be positive, bringing new freedoms and opportunities, such as when children leave home, the opportunity to work less and the avail-ability of more time for socialising, holidays and other leisure activities. Becoming a grandparent can also bring great joy and new opportunities to enjoy families, without the immediate burden of responsibility that mothers often feel.

In many ways our midlife is a balancing act between the many chal-lenges we are presented with and the potential opportunities midlife brings. Of course our experiences of midlife are individual and influenced by a plethora of social issues, such as income, education, language, culture and our place in society.

Changes to the work environment for women over past decades have been enormous. Generally workplace changes have been in favour of women, but still experiences will vary. Some will find that midlife increases their opportunity to pursue long-held aspirations and plans, some find they are being replaced by younger employees, some have to come to grips with the 'glass ceiling', and others may have an opportunity to reduce their working hours or retire and enjoy family and new interests.

Physical changes to appearance have a significant impact on women in midlife. Midlife women start to lose their youthful appearance, and can find it more difficult to avoid gaining weight. As mentioned earlier, appearance is highly valued in our society, especially for women, so of course we worry about our bodies, and feel shame or embarrassment if we don't measure up to cultural standards. It can affect our confidence, our relationships and our ability to enjoy sex and sensuality. Societies that are youth-oriented, and in which stereotypes of ageing women are largely negative, do not provide a supportive environment for midlife women. While some women accept signs of ageing gracefully, others attempt to halt its appearance with Botox or collagen injections, plastic surgery and by other means.

A major event coinciding with, and often defining, midlife is menopause. There are physical and psychological effects attributed to the decline in oestrogen that occurs at this time, but social and cultural attitudes and beliefs also affect the way we experience menopause. For most women, menopause not only signifies a loss of fertility but also the onset of ageing, which, as we already mentioned, is associated in our society with decline and demise.

Sex is central to every life stage, though it is invariably affected by our physical and mental health. Our enjoyment of sex is also affected by our body image and how easily we accept the inevitable physical changes of ageing. We are generally very capable of being sensual and sexual beings throughout our lives and can continue to explore and enjoy sex with our long-term partners, if we have them, or with new partners if we don't. Enjoying and participating in sex may not always be as easy as when we were younger or when our relationships were new, but generally women in midlife and beyond are very capable of active and enjoyable sex lives. Sex and ageing is discussed in the final section of the book, in chapter 43.

Midlife demographics

Women are more educated, more qualified and more likely to be in paid employment throughout their midlife than ever before. Compared to previous generations, particularly in industrialised nations and particularly in white, Anglo-Saxon communities, we have more independent income and more money to follow some of our midlife dreams. Having said that, in midlife and beyond, the systemic discrimination against women can come into sharp focus for many of us. Women are also still more likely than men to be in part-time work and continue to earn less. There is more divorce or separation now than ever before, which means women, more so than men, are looking towards a future of living alone and often with a level of economic hardship. Separated women are also more likely to be in the rental market or in substandard housing. Women are more likely to have worked fewer hours across their careers due to interruptions to give birth and care for small babies, which may have affected their ability to progress in their careers or to earn enough for retirement.

How this book can help

This is our midlife. In the medical literature it is often defined as and limited to menopause or empty-nest syndrome, but it is more than that. The challenges we face go deeper than hot flushes and night sweats, and the impacts of our increasing confidence, self-acceptance and liberation can have far more significance than throwing out the tampon box. This is a time of transition. It is also a time where we need to pay more attention to our health, the way we eat and exercise, our mental health, our friendships and our social connections as we march towards life as independent and vital older women.

Not surprisingly, staying healthy, eating well, exercise and managing menopause were some of the themes that came up in our discussions with women in their late 30s, 40s and 50s. Chapter 31 focuses on eating well and maintaining health at this very busy time of life. Chapter 34 helps us to understand complementary therapies, which can include anything from acupuncture to Chinese medicine. Complementary therapies in the Western world are loosely defined as any therapy that does not fit within the realm of conventional medicine. The field is very broad and constantly changing and often, depending on the therapy, lacking in good research evidence. There are many reasons why the research is scant. Advocates argue that funding for research is skewed to Western medicines. Others say that Western research models and theories are contrary to alternative understandings of and approaches to health. Some therapies have been well researched and shown to have various levels of benefit – some have been shown to be very effective, some are effective in limited circumstances, some don't seem to make any difference at all and others need to be understood further. Overall, the research and medical community continue to improve their understanding of complementary therapies and how they can be used alongside conventional Western treatments.

To further complicate our understanding of complementary therapies, women in midlife are often perceived by commercial providers as being the most financially able and the most likely to buy complementary health products, which are often very expensive. Consequently, advertising campaigns carefully and effectively target this group of women with a range of these products. This is only an issue because while some products are effective, others are benign at best and dangerous at worst. The key is to be an informed consumer.

In chapter 32 we look at common medical conditions that may emerge during midlife. At this time we are most likely to experience the early effects of poor lifestyle habits, such as inadequate diet, alcohol or recreational drug consumption or lack of exercise, as well as our unique genetic tendency to develop particular diseases, such as lung disease, cardiovascular disease, type 2 diabetes and other immune-inflammatory disorders. We won't necessarily be aware of the signs and symptoms, and we won't necessarily understand their significance. Unfortunately, what we know about common diseases, their symptoms and treatments, tends to come from research done on men. It turns out that women have their own unique responses to a range of diseases and their treatments, which can make us very vulnerable with regard to early detection and appropriate action. More men develop heart disease, for example, but more women who have heart attacks will die. Heart disease symptoms can appear later in women and the 'known' symptoms for heart disease and heart failure, such as chest pain, are not necessarily as common in women as in men. Chapter 32 encourages us to be very proactive with our health and our health care, and to understand the range of symptoms that may be particular to us.

In chapters 35 and 36 we take a more detailed look at issues such as cancer prevention and screening. Prolapse and continence problems, which can start to emerge in the later stages of our midlife years, usually related to earlier pregnancies and births, are discussed in chapter 39.

Menopause is of course one of the most significant physical developments in our late 40s and early 50s. While many women sail through, others find it a very difficult time. In recent years hormone replacement therapy has become increasingly controversial. Women often find that they need to untangle truth from opinion and the evidence from fear-mongering to make decisions that are appropriate for them and for their health. Unfortunately, many women continue to suffer debilitating symptoms due to misinformation and fear. In chapter 33 you will be well informed about menopause, what it is and the various ways symptoms can be managed.

In chapter 41 we discuss the role of women as carers. For some women at this time, caring for elderly or sick parents, a disabled adult child or a partner is central to their day-to-day life. Being a carer can be overwhelming, isolating and relentless but it can also bring great pleasure and satisfaction if managed well and with good support. In this chapter you will read about ways to manage your role as a carer as well as caring for yourself.

The transition

Given that change is so common in midlife, it is not surprising that for some women, it can be a time of reflection, a time in which we wonder what is to come next. The midlife 'crisis' or transition is a phenomenon we tend to associate with men and to trivialise, reducing it to a red sports car or an affair with a younger woman. Women's midlife, on the other hand, is commonly reduced to menopause – a biological midlife event that is not generally associated with any psychological development beyond hormonal mood swings. But women may also experience a psychological shift at this time, not necessarily associated with menopause at all. While the male midlife crisis is often described as ego-driven or a search for affirmation, women during their midlife are more likely to move outside of themselves, to explore and experience life. Some commentators prefer to call it a midlife challenge, describing women's tendency to think in terms of growth and personal development. While men may be inclined to buy a sports car, women are perhaps more likely to trek across deserts, enrol in a university course or learn a new language.

Getting older

The journey towards our older years can be quite frightening, especially given the value our community places on youth. We also tend to look at old age through a stereotypical lens, which can obscure our view. Older women are very often presented in the media as dependent and as burdens on society, which undermines the true value of what women bring to the community, the economy and the family. Growing older doesn't have to be feared. It is a journey on which we can become more independent, more self-assured, less concerned about the opinions of others and more able to pursue creativity, ideas and learning.

Maintaining our health, a strong sense of wellbeing and purpose is crucial during midlife so we can continue our journey with vigour.

31

Food and nutrition for midlife

Jenny Taylor

In midlife we become more aware of the health problems that become more common as we age, such as type 2 diabetes, heart disease, cancer, hypertension (high blood pressure) and constipation. Healthy eating can help prevent or delay these conditions. Healthy eating means getting the right balance of nutrients, as well as balancing calories taken in with those burnt up by activity.

As we get older we need fewer calories, but our need for other nutrients remains unchanged. Quality becomes more important than quantity. In other words, we need to make what we eat count. There is little room for less nutritious, 'empty-calorie' high-fat or high-sugar foods, as most of us are not burning off as many calories as we used to.

Eating well

Use these guidelines to help ensure an adequate diet:

- Eat a wide range of foods covering all food groups. This way you are less likely to get too much or too little of anything.

- Eat at least three meals per day. It's difficult to cram the nutrients you need in a day into just one or two meals. Research shows that people who eat breakfast are less likely to be overweight.

- Enjoy all foods, but we recommend eating some in only small amounts. These are the foods with a large proportion of fat or sugar, such as fried foods, cream, biscuits, cakes and pastry. It can help to think of these as 'sometimes' foods rather than everyday foods. These foods contain higher amounts of unhealthy (saturated) fats, or are high in calories but poor in nutrients.

- Drink plenty of fluids for hydration and to prevent constipation, but limit highly sweetened drinks. Sweet drinks such as soft drinks, fruit juices and commercial iced teas contain far more sugar than most people realise, with up to nine teaspoons of sugar per 375 millilitres (one can).

- If you drink alcohol, limit it to two standard drinks per day. A standard drink is 375 millilitres of mid-strength beer, 100 millilitres of wine or 30 millilitres of spirits. Alcohol is also a rich source of calories, with nearly twice as many calories as sugar, so beware if you are watching your weight.

Recommended food intake

The list below of recommended foods for each day can look daunting, but if you eat regular meals containing carbohydrates, protein, vegetables or salad and you eat dairy foods each day, you are likely to be meeting your nutrient needs. These foods are recommended each day:

- **Meat and alternatives** – choose from lean meat, chicken, fish, eggs or vegetarian alternatives such as tofu, legumes (dried beans and lentils), nuts and seeds. Include them in one to two meals daily. These foods are a good source of proteins for repair and healing, as well as the minerals iron and zinc.

- **Dairy foods** – drink low-fat milk, eat yoghurt or cheese. If using other milks such as almond, rice or soy milk, check you have chosen a brand with added calcium. Aim for three serves daily, where a serve equals a cup (250 millilitres) of milk or yoghurt or a slice of cheese. These are good sources of protein and calcium.

- **Vegetables and fruit** – eat plenty of vegetables and fruit for vitamins and fibre. Their varying colours reflect different antioxidants and other nutrients that help maintain health, so include a variety of colourful fruit and vegetables. Five serves of vegetables and two of fruit are recommended each day (for examples of serve sizes, see the table on pages 88–9). Eating vegetables or salad with lunch and dinner helps you meet your vegetable quota and also helps with weight control, as they are filling but low in calories.

- **Whole grains** – eat wholegrain breads and cereals for fuel, fibre and B-group vitamins. Less processed foods such as whole grains tend to be richer in nutrients, beneficial for bowel regularity and more filling due to their fibre content, so you are less likely to eat too much of them.

- **Healthy fats** – eat 'heart-healthy' oils in small amounts, including olive oil or seed oils such as canola, sunflower, safflower, peanut and soy. Limit saturated fats such as animal fat, butter, cream, palm and coconut oil.

As we age, we are more likely to be diagnosed with or have risk factors for common health problems such as type 2 diabetes, heart disease or hypertension (high blood pressure). Fortunately, the diet for prevention and treatment of these conditions is similar to the healthy-eating recommendations for general health.

Do I need vitamin or mineral supplements?

If you eat regular meals with adequate food variety, you are likely to be meeting your nutritional needs without needing to take nutritional supplements. There are some exceptions, however:

- Vitamin D is recommended if you have low levels of this vitamin, and calcium supplements are advised if you don't eat much dairy food (see the 'Bone health' section below).
- A vitamin B12 supplement may be recommended if you are on medications that reduce stomach acid, such as Nexium. Stomach acid is needed to absorb vitamin B12, an important vitamin for nerve and brain function. Talk to your GP if you take this sort of medication.
- Iron supplements are unlikely to be needed by healthy women after menopause, as the need for iron to manufacture red blood cells decreases once periods cease. Most women can meet their iron needs with a varied diet.
- Multivitamin supplements can be beneficial if you do not eat a balanced diet but generally are not necessary for those who eat regular, varied meals. Seek advice from a doctor if you are taking high doses of vitamins or minerals, as these can affect the absorption of other vitamins and minerals.

Weight management and body image

Many women experience weight gain and shape changes in midlife and these can affect body image and self-esteem. Often more fat is deposited on the abdomen and trunk, causing 'middle-aged spread' or a 'spare tyre'. Whether these body changes are related more to ageing than menopause is not clear. As we age we have less muscle and our metabolic rate slows down, so we need fewer calories. At the same time, hormone changes can affect where the fat is stored.

Exercise

Exercise is particularly helpful for combating these changes. Sustained exercise that elevates your heart rate without puffing you out, such as brisk walking, is ideal, or you may prefer dancing, swimming or other sports.

Thirty minutes of exercise daily can help prevent weight gain and maintain general health, but you may need to increase this to 45–60 minutes if you need to lose weight. A pedometer (step counter) available from pharmacies and sports shops can help you achieve this. Aim for at least 10,000 steps per day, starting with 2000 more than you generally do and gradually increasing as your fitness improves. Walking in natural light can also help lift your mood, reducing stress and depression.

Healthy eating

Regular meals help maintain our energy levels and reduce the temptation to snack on unhealthy foods. Make sure you feel satisfied with what you eat. Eat a sustaining breakfast, and lunches and dinners that include protein, carbohydrate and vegetables or salad. Don't let yourself become overly hungry or you may have less control over the types and amounts of food you eat. If you need to, eat a healthy snack between meals.

Tune in to your body's hunger and fullness signals. You may not need the quantity of food you ate when you were younger. Many people eat from habit, with meal sizes larger than they may need. Even small imbalances in food eaten versus calories expended can cause weight gain.

Be aware of why you are eating. Is it to satisfy hunger or for another reason, such as boredom or stress? Recognise your 'non-hungry' eating and work out what you can do instead.

See chapters 13 and 14 for more information on managing your weight, and ideas for meals and snacks.

Bone health

Our bones become less dense as we age, especially after menopause, due to the drop in oestrogen. This increases the risk of osteoporosis, a condition where bones become fragile and easily broken. One in three women over the age of 60 will have a bone fracture at some stage due to osteoporosis.

As well as ageing, many factors are involved in bone strength, including genetics, diet, exercise, vitamin D levels and smoking. We can't do anything about some of these risk factors but getting enough calcium, vitamin D and weight-bearing exercise such walking, dancing or sports such as tennis can help maintain bone strength.

You can have your bone density and your risk of osteoporosis checked using a type of X-ray called dual-energy X-ray absorptiometry (DEXA; see chapter 32). This test may be recommended if you are over 70 or have certain other risk factors for osteoporosis. If low bone density is diagnosed, your doctor may prescribe vitamin D and calcium supplements as well as medication to help maintain bone strength if needed.

Calcium

Calcium is the main mineral in bones. On average, 60 per cent of our calcium comes from calcium-rich foods such as dairy foods. The remainder comes from smaller amounts in a range of foods. Calcium is added to most brands of soy milk, and some brands of rice milk, oat milk and almond milk, to the same level as that in cow's milk.

There is some debate as to how much calcium we need, as many factors affect how much calcium we actually absorb from our food, but for women over 50 eating an average Western diet, 1300 milligrams per day is recommended. This can be achieved by eating at least three serves per day of dairy or other foods from the list below. If you are regularly unable to achieve the recommended intake, we recommend a calcium supplement of 500–600 milligrams per day.

Each item on the list below will deliver one serve (or 300 milligrams) of calcium:

- hard cheese, 30 grams (1 thick slice)
- yoghurt, 200 millilitres (1 tub)
- milk, regular, reduced-fat or skim, 250 millilitres (1 glass)
- calcium-fortified soy, rice or almond milk, 250 millilitres (1 glass)
- ricotta cheese, 120 grams (½ cup)
- tinned salmon or sardines *if* bones are eaten, 100 grams (½ cup)
- firm tofu, 100 grams
- almonds, 100 grams (1 cup)
- tahini (sesame paste), 100 grams (½ cup)

Vitamin D

We need vitamin D for our body to absorb and use calcium. It may also play a wider role in contributing to our immune system and heart health.

Your GP can check your vitamin D level with a blood test, and will suggest supplements if necessary. Vitamin D deficiency is common in the

Australian population: 30–50 per cent of women have low levels. People with low vitamin D levels are not only more prone to brittle bones, but their balance is also not as good, which increases the risk of falls.

Only 5–10 per cent of vitamin D comes from food such as fatty fish, liver, eggs, margarine and some milks. Most is made in our skin when it is exposed to sunlight. Spending most of your time indoors, having darker skin or wearing concealing clothing increases the risk of a lower level of vitamin D.

Excessive sunlight exposure is not recommended due to the risk of skin cancer. The following amount of sun exposure is suggested for moderately fair-skinned people to help maintain adequate vitamin D levels while limiting the risk of skin cancer (bear in mind that the UVB rays that help make vitamin D don't pass through glass):

- in summer, six to seven minutes with arms uncovered at mid-morning or mid-afternoon
- in winter, seven minutes at noon in the northern states of Australia, or up to 30 minutes at noon in the southern states

People with dark skin may need three to six times more exposure, as their skin pigment reduces UV light absorption.

Menopause

The drop in oestrogen levels at menopause can cause symptoms such as hot flushes, vaginal dryness and mood changes in some women. There is debate about the effects certain foods may have on these symptoms.

Alcohol and caffeine may trigger hot flushes in some women, but a healthy diet, regular meals and regular exercise can help balance mood. The jury is out on whether the omega-3 fatty acids from oily fish can help improve mood and depression.

Phytoestrogens (plant oestrogens)

It is unclear whether plant oestrogens (phytoestrogens) can replace some of the oestrogen lost at menopause and help reduce menopause symptoms. Evidence from trials has been conflicting, so it is not certain whether they work any better than a placebo (inactive medication).

Phytoestrogens are present in whole grains, legumes (dried beans and lentils), seeds, fruits and vegetables. Soybeans and flaxseed (linseed) are particularly rich in them. Other substances in these foods may protect against heart disease, osteoporosis and cancer; they are therefore more likely to be beneficial than taking phytoestrogen supplements, which are best taken only with professional advice.

If you want to try getting phytoestrogens from food, 40–50 milligrams of phytoestrogens per day is a good level to aim for, which is the amount found in a traditional Asian diet. The average Western diet provides about 5 milligrams per day. The phytoestrogen level of plants varies according to the growing conditions, so the following list is just a guide. Each of the foods in the list contains approximately 45 milligrams of phytoestrogens:

- 100–150 grams (½–1 cup) soybeans, tofu or tempeh
- 35 grams soy flour
- 0.5–1 litre soy milk
- 45 grams flaxseed (linseed)
- 4–5 slices soy and linseed bread

Large amounts of phytoestrogens are not recommended for women with oestrogen-positive breast cancer or other oestrogen-dependent cancers, as they may stimulate growth of cancer cells.

Heart health

Heart disease is the biggest killer of women, but many people are not aware of this. The drop in oestrogen that occurs at menopause increases the risk of heart disease, so this is the time to get your blood fats and blood pressure checked.

Cut your risk of heart disease by doing the following:

- treating hypertension (high blood pressure)
- treating high cholesterol
- being physically active every day
- eating nutritious foods
- not smoking

Cholesterol and triglycerides are fatty substances made by the body; they have several necessary functions, but higher than normal levels can increase the risk of heart disease. High levels can be related to genetics, being overweight or diet. Our cholesterol levels can change as we grow older, with our LDL ('bad') cholesterol levels increasing and our HDL ('good') cholesterol levels decreasing.

In some people with high blood fats, dietary change and weight management can bring the levels down to normal. In others this will not be enough, and cholesterol-lowering medication will also be needed.

Cholesterol levels in the blood are affected by the types and amounts of fats and oils eaten, as well as other substances in food. Cholesterol in foods has less effect than types of fat eaten.

To help control your level of blood fats, limit the following:

- saturated fats from animal fats, butter, palm oil and coconut oil
- takeaways or creamy pasta dishes to once a week
- snack foods such as potato crisps to once a week
- cakes and pastries to once a week unless you have time to make your own with healthier oils; note that palm oil and coconut oil are often listed as 'vegetable oil' in baked goods but are saturated fats, in contrast to most vegetable oils
- fatty meats and full-cream dairy foods
- cholesterol-containing foods such as egg yolks, liver, kidney and brains; people respond differently to these foods, so if you have high cholesterol the degree of restriction depends on how you respond – most people can eat two to six eggs a week
- large amounts of refined carbohydrate (sugar) such as in highly sweetened drinks

It is beneficial to include the following in your diet:

- lean meat, vegetables and whole grains
- fish twice a week for healthy omega-3 fish oils; oily fish such as tuna, herring, sardines, salmon and mackerel are especially rich in these oils
- unsalted nuts and seeds, which contain healthy oils
- legumes such as dried beans, lentils, baked beans and kidney beans, which contain substances that can help reduce cholesterol
- oils such as canola, sunflower, soybean, olive and peanut oils; if labelled 'light', this refers to light flavour rather than lower calorie content – 'cold pressed', 'virgin' and 'extra virgin' refer to the level of processing, which affects flavour but does not have a big effect on nutrition
- margarines made from oils such as canola, sunflower, safflower or olive oil; cholesterol-lowering margarines to which plant sterols have been added that help reduce blood cholesterol levels are also available but

are no substitute for medication in most people. To gain maximum benefit you need to eat 1–1½ tablespoons a day, so beware of the added calories if you are not already eating spreads. There may be no benefit in eating these margarines if you don't have a problem with cholesterol.

High blood pressure

Blood pressure tends to increase as we age and is a risk factor for strokes and heart disease.

Watching our weight, limiting alcohol intake to a maximum of one standard drink per day, getting at least 30 minutes of exercise a day and limiting dietary salt will help keep blood pressure in check. Potassium, found in fruit and vegetables, and calcium from low-fat dairy foods, may also help reduce blood pressure.

Salt

The evidence that reducing salt can reduce blood pressure is stronger than ever. On average, we all eat around 9 grams of salt per day, when we only need 1–2 grams. As most salt comes from the foods we buy rather than salt added at the table, however, it's not always easy to know where to start when trying to limit salt intake. Most unprocessed foods are low in salt but it is added to many processed foods, especially sauces, savoury snack foods and takeaway foods. Even breads, most breakfast cereals and sweet biscuits contain appreciable amounts of salt.

Here are some tips for reducing your salt intake:

- Eat plenty of fresh foods such as vegetables and fruit, as these are naturally low in salt.
- Keep healthy snacks on hand, such as fresh fruit, unsalted nuts and low-fat yoghurt.
- Limit salty snack foods such as chips.
- Check food labels for salt to compare similar products and choose the lower salt options.
- Choose low-salt foods (less than 120 milligrams per 100 grams) where possible and avoid high-salt foods (greater than 500 milligrams per 100 grams).
- Use flavourings such as lemon juice, garlic, vinegar, herbs and spices when cooking. This will enable you to use less or no salt.

- Limit stock cubes and soy sauce where possible or choose low-salt varieties.
- Keep takeaways and fast foods to an occasional treat.
- Avoid adding salt to foods at the table.

Type 2 diabetes and impaired glucose tolerance

Type 2 diabetes is a condition in which there is too much glucose in the blood. Glucose is a type of sugar that comes from the carbohydrates we eat and is the body's main fuel source. Diabetes happens when insulin, the hormone that controls the metabolism of glucose, is not being produced in sufficient amounts or the body's cells don't respond to it properly. Genetic tendency, ageing, being overweight, poor diet and inactivity are all risk factors. In pre-diabetes, sometimes called 'impaired glucose tolerance' or 'impaired fasting glucose', the blood glucose is higher than normal but not as high as in diabetes.

Weight control, an active lifestyle and healthy eating can help prevent or delay the onset of diabetes, as well as treat it once it is present. The diet is the same as that recommended for general health – good food variety, limiting saturated fats and sweet foods, and eating regular meals with low-GI carbohydrates (see chapter 13) such as wholegrain breads and cereals to help prevent big swings in blood glucose levels.

If you have been diagnosed with type 2 diabetes or pre-diabetes and need further information, contact the diabetes organisation in your state.

Bowel problems

Constipation

Bowel problems such as constipation become more common as we age.

Increasing your intake of dietary fibre (the non-digestible parts of plants) helps increase bulk, making it easier for the muscles to move faeces along the bowel. Good sources of fibre include wholegrain bread, high-fibre cereals, vegetables, fruit, dried fruit, nuts and legumes.

Fibre can also be taken as supplements derived from plants such as Metamucil, Fybogel or Benefiber. Prunes and prune juice contain a substance that stimulates the bowel, and pears and pear juice can help keep bowel actions soft.

Low fluid intake is a common cause of constipation, so drink plenty of fluid to help keep bowel motions soft. Aim for around 2 litres or 6–8 glasses of water per day, more in hot weather.

Sometimes you may need to take laxatives. There are several different types that work by different methods. If you need to, ask your pharmacist or doctor for the type that is appropriate for you.

Irritable bowel syndrome (IBS)

IBS is a common condition that can cause varying symptoms including abdominal pain, bloating, flatulence, diarrhoea or constipation. It is not fully understood and the appearance of the bowel is normal when investigated. Research suggests that the nerves of the gut may become hypersensitive, resulting in pain or abnormal bowel contractions.

Often the cause is unclear, but triggers can include certain foods and stress. IBS is more common in women than men, so there may be a hormonal component. IBS can also occur after a bout of gastroenteritis.

The often-unknown causes can make treatment difficult, as can the fact that symptoms come and go. Generally, treatment focuses on dietary and stress-reduction strategies. It may also involve medication.

The following dietary strategies may help, but as many cases of IBS are not caused by diet, there is no point excluding foods if there is no improvement:

- Eat regular meals and snacks.
- Avoid large, fatty or spicy meals.
- Limit foods that irritate the gut, such as spices, caffeine and alcohol.
- Avoid 'windy' foods such as onions, legumes and cabbage.
- Try increasing fibre if constipation is a problem.
- If loose bowels or wind are a problem, try reducing highly fibrous foods.
- Keep a food and symptom diary to identify any trigger foods. Lactose, the sugar found in milk; yoghurt and unripened cheeses; or fructose, the sugar in fruit and some vegetables, can cause symptoms in some people, and different people can tolerate different amounts before symptoms occur.

Weak pelvic floor muscles can also be a cause of wind and the urge to evacuate the bowels. It may be necessary to seek specialised help from a physiotherapist to strengthen these muscles and from a dietician for the best foods to eat.

32

Common chronic medical conditions

Ines Rio

Having a chronic medical condition is common and rising; many Australians – and nearly all Australians aged 65 and over – have at least one medical condition that affects them over a long period of time. 'Chronic' is the word doctors use to describe a condition that lasts for a long time, often for someone's whole life.

Overall, more Australians are getting chronic diseases due to a range of factors, including our ageing population; early detection and improved treatments for diseases that previously caused death; and lifestyle factors such as obesity, physical inactivity, smoking and poor diet.

For some people it is even more complex as they may have more than one chronic health condition. In addition, acute (i.e. more short-term) medical problems and chronic conditions often affect each other. For example, if you have asthma, getting a cold may trigger your asthma or make it more difficult to control. Similarly, if your diabetes is poorly controlled you may be more likely to get vaginal thrush.

What are chronic medical conditions?

Common chronic medical conditions include:

- cardiovascular disease (16 per cent of the population)
- osteoarthritis (15 per cent)
- osteoporosis (4 per cent)
- diabetes (5 per cent)
- asthma (10 per cent)
- thyroid disease (5 per cent)
- long-term mental or behavioural conditions (11 per cent)
- cancer (2 per cent)

This chapter will look at six of the most common of these chronic conditions: cardiovascular disease, osteoarthritis, osteoporosis, diabetes, asthma and thyroid disease.

Mental health conditions are covered in chapters 10, 22 and 44.

Unfortunately, it is not possible to cover all chronic conditions in a book such as this, but we hope that if you have a chronic condition not covered here, you may still find parts of this chapter, such as 'Living well with a chronic illness', useful.

The information in this chapter is of a general nature only and should not be used as a substitute for medical advice or to alter medical therapy. Everyone's situation is different, so if you have a chronic condition you need to consult regularly with your GP and other qualified healthcare professionals to meet your own individual medical needs.

Living with a chronic medical condition

Having a chronic medical condition doesn't define who you are or prevent you from enjoying and participating in life, but it does make some aspects of your life more challenging. If you are affected by a chronic medical condition, its treatment requires a long-term holistic approach, often involving many healthcare providers and others (such as family, friends and support services). It is important that you:

- understand your condition and how best to manage it
- are closely monitored by your GP
- remember that you can do a number of things in your everyday life to help you manage your condition
- undertake preventative activities to lessen the progression of your disease and its complications, and to maximise your daily functioning and quality of life
- consider the interaction between your health conditions and other aspects of your life, such as physical activity, work, travel, driving, pregnancy, medicines, and drug and alcohol use

Managing your condition

Your GP is your first port of call to help you manage and understand your chronic condition. They may refer you to a range of other doctors and allied health professionals, and point you in the direction of support and quality information. Always bear in mind that not all information on the web is accurate.

It is important to reflect on your condition and work with your GP and others to understand it, how it affects you and how best to manage it so you can live well. You need to be at the centre of any decisions and management plan – only you know what your condition feels like and how it really affects you.

Each of the conditions discussed in this chapter has at least one peak organisation with a website that provides quality information (often also in languages other than English) including how to access support services and groups. These peak organisations are listed in the Resources section at the end of this book.

Cardiovascular disease (CVD)

Cardiovascular disease is any disease that involves the heart or blood vessels (arteries, veins and capillaries). It causes angina, heart attacks, strokes and kidney and leg circulation problems.

CVD is the biggest cause of deaths in Australia – heart disease and stroke together account for the deaths of one in three Australians. In midlife, CVD affects more men than women, although it is equally common in both sexes by the time people reach their 70s. Overall, it is the number-one killer in both sexes, so women need to address their risk factors as much as men.

The most common causes of cardiovascular disease are athero-sclerosis ('hardening' of the arteries) and/or hypertension (high blood pressure).

Atherosclerosis ('hardening' of the arteries)

Atherosclerosis is a build-up of fatty deposits (called plaques) in the lining of the walls of the arteries. These plaques can thicken, and calcium can be deposited in them, making them harder. Plaques can narrow the arteries to the point where they decrease the flow of blood through them. Sometimes a blood clot can form at these plaques, suddenly stopping the flow, or a piece of the plaque can flick off. Both of these can result in not enough blood, and therefore not enough oxygen, getting to where it is needed and therefore causing problems. If this happens in the heart, it causes angina or a heart attack; if it occurs in the brain, it causes a tran-sient ischaemic attack or stroke; and if it happens in the legs, it causes circulation problems.

Although cardiovascular disease usually affects older adults, early evidence of atherosclerosis begins in early life. This means it is very important to prevent atherosclerosis by having a healthy lifestyle from childhood if possible.

Coronary heart disease

To keep pumping, the heart needs a constant supply of oxygen-carrying blood. This is provided by coronary arteries that encircle the heart. As long as these arteries are healthy, they can keep the heart supplied with oxygen – even when it is pumping harder than normal, such as during exercise or sex. But if these arteries are diseased and become narrowed with atherosclerosis and/or clots, they do not carry enough blood to the heart muscle, and the heart will start to malfunction. This may lead to symptoms such as angina, or if some of the heart muscle dies, a heart attack.

Angina

Angina is caused when the blood flow to the heart is inadequate to provide the oxygen the heart needs, resulting in pain, 'heaviness', 'tightness' or 'pressure' in the chest. It is usually felt in the centre of the chest, but may spread to the neck, jaw or arms and sometimes the shoulders, back or abdomen. It can range in severity from a mild ache to severe pain. Some people don't feel any pain and may only get some of the other symptoms of angina, which can include sweating, shortness of breath and nausea. This is thought to be more common in women than men.

Typically, the pain comes when the heart requires more oxygen, such as during physical exertion, times of emotional distress or after a heavy meal, and stops quickly when the exertion ceases. It can also occur at rest, however.

Treatment for angina

There is a range of investigations and very effective treatment options for angina. The investigations aim to see where and how bad the coronary artery blockages are and how they affect the heart. This may include a 'stress' test – an ECG (a test of the electricity of the heart) taken while on an exercise machine or while the heart is stressed in another way (e.g., with medicine); special heart ultrasounds; or a special X-ray known as an angiogram.

Treatment always includes addressing risk factors through lifestyle changes: weight loss, improved diet and exercise, giving up smoking and getting the best possible control of high blood pressure, diabetes and high cholesterol.

A range of very effective treatments can be used to relieve pain and discomfort and reduce the risk of progression to more serious conditions such as a heart attack. These include medicines, the most common of which are nitrates such as nitroglycerine, which relax and widen blood vessels, allowing more blood to reach the heart muscle. Doctors may also prescribe other drugs to help reduce overall cardiovascular risk, such as beta-blockers, calcium-channel blockers, ACE (angiotensin-converting enzyme) inhibitors and antiplatelet or blood-thinning medicine.

If angina cannot be managed well using medicine and lifestyle measures alone, doctors may recommend a surgical procedure such as angioplasty or coronary artery stents to widen the arteries, or coronary bypass surgery.

When to see a doctor for angina

If you have angina, you should see your doctor or go to hospital straight away if:

- it is the first time you have experienced the condition
- the chest pain comes on during rest
- you are on medicine for angina, but the angina is more severe or more frequent than usual
- the chest pain doesn't go away quickly with normal angina medicine
- the angina doesn't quickly get better with rest

Heart attack

A heart attack happens when the blood flow to the heart is so insufficient that some of the heart muscle dies. Heart attacks can happen out of the blue or they can occur in people who have had angina. Symptoms of a heart attack vary from person to person.

While angina-like pain that does not go away with rest is the most common symptom, some people do not have pain and may get other symptoms such as intense nausea, dizziness, cold sweats, palpitations and shortness of breath. These types of symptoms are thought to be more common in women than men, which is why some women don't realise they are having a heart attack. Sometimes, there are no symptoms at all and the heart attack is only diagnosed much later when an ECG (a test of the electrical signals in the heart) or other tests reveal damage caused to the heart by a previous, 'silent' heart attack.

Treatment for heart attack

The quicker someone having a heart attack receives treatment, the less their heart muscle will be damaged, the more likely they will be to survive, and the greater their chance of a good result. If you've had a suspected heart attack, you will be given blood tests and an ECG to diagnose the heart attack, and sometimes other tests to assess the location and extent of the damage.

Treatment may include thrombolysis (clot-dissolving medicines); angioplasty, a balloon inserted into the artery to widen it (often followed by a tube, or stent, that remains in place to keep the artery open); or coronary artery bypass surgery, where blood flow is redirected around a narrowed artery to improve flow to the heart.

Almost all people will also be required to take ongoing medicines similar to those for angina to reduce the risk of further attacks, and of course address any other risk factors.

Seek immediate help for a heart attack

All heart attacks are a medical emergency because of the damage they can do to the heart. The death of heart muscle can lead to heart failure or an abnormal heart rhythm that may result in a cardiac arrest, where a person can suddenly collapse and may die.

If you suspect that you or someone else has had a heart attack, it is crucial to seek immediate emergency medical help by calling 000.

Stroke

A stroke happens when the blood flow to the brain is so insufficient that some of the brain dies. It is like a heart attack of the brain. It may also be associated with bleeding into the brain. They are most often not associated with pain, although they can be associated with headache.

Facial weakness, arm weakness and difficulty speaking are the most common signs of stroke, but they are not the only ones. Other signs of stroke include:

- paralysis, weakness or numbness of the face, arm or leg on either or both sides of the body
- difficulty speaking or understanding
- difficulty eating or swallowing

- dizziness, loss of balance, difficulty walking or an unexplained fall
- loss of vision, sudden blurred or decreased vision
- headache – usually severe, with an abrupt onset or changes in the usual pattern of headaches
- collapse or loss of consciousness

These symptoms can occur alone or in combination and can last from a few seconds to a very long time.

A transient ischaemic attack (TIA) happens when there is a temporary interruption to the blood supply to the brain that causes the same symptoms as a stroke, but these go away completely within 24 hours. It is like angina of the brain.

Strokes and TIAs both require immediate medical treatment to reduce the likelihood of permanent brain damage. The longer a stroke remains untreated, the greater the chance of permanent brain damage.

Treatment for stroke

The quicker someone having a stroke receives treatment, the less their brain will be damaged, the more likely they will be to survive, and the greater their chance for a good result with fewer long-term problems.

If you arrive at the hospital quickly and the stroke is due to a blood clot, you may be treated with a drug that breaks down blood clots. This drug is only useful for certain types of stroke, and needs to be given within a certain time of the beginning of a stroke.

Seek immediate help for a stroke or TIA

All strokes and TIAs are always a medical emergency – even if the symptoms don't cause pain or go away quickly.

If you suspect that you or someone else has had a stroke or TIA, it is crucial to seek immediate emergency medical help by calling 000.

CVD risk factors and prevention

There is no single cause for CVD, but there are risk factors that increase the chance of developing it. Risk factors that can't be changed include increasing age, being male and having a family history of CVD. Aboriginal and Torres Strait Islander people are also at increased risk of CVD.

The good news is that many important risk factors for CVD can be changed, including:

- smoking
- diet
- high total blood cholesterol and triglycerides (high blood lipids)
- high blood pressure
- diabetes
- being physically inactive
- being overweight
- drinking too much alcohol
- depression and a lack of social support

For most people, the best way to prevent CVD is to live a healthy life by maintaining a healthy weight, exercising regularly, eating a balanced diet, not smoking and ensuring their doctor is aware of all their risk factors, including any family history of heart disease. Other preventative measures depend on any other risk factors. For example, if you smoke you should see your doctor about help to give up, if you have high blood pressure you need to keep it well controlled, if you have high cholesterol this needs to be reduced, and if you have diabetes you need to make sure your blood sugar levels are under control.

If you already have CVD or are at high risk of getting it, your GP will need to monitor you carefully, and may also consider prescribing other medicine such as aspirin (to prevent blood clots) and statins (to lower blood cholesterol). Your GP is also likely to suggest you have the annual influenza vaccine, as getting the flu may put more stress on your heart and blood vessels.

High blood lipids (cholesterol and triglycerides)

Lipids are a group of naturally occurring and necessary fatty substances in the body. They have a variety of functions, including storing energy, signalling between organs and acting as structural components of cells. Although humans can both make and break down most lipids, there are some we cannot make and must obtain from our diet. These are called essential lipids and include omega-3 and omega-6 fatty acids.

There is good evidence to suggest that consuming some fats, such as the omega-3 fatty acids found in fish, has many positive health benefits, including on infant brain development, and decreases the risk of some cancers, CVD, and various mental illnesses such as depression and dementia. In contrast, there is good evidence that consuming other fats, such as trans fats (which occur in partially hydrogenated vegetable oils, mostly in processed foods), has negative health benefits as they both raise 'bad' (LDL) cholesterol and lower 'good' (HDL) cholesterol.

High LDL cholesterol and/or high triglycerides are common and are risk factors for CVD because they contribute to the atherosclerotic plaques that cause it.

Cholesterol is a type of lipid produced naturally by the liver. While our bodies need cholesterol to continue building healthy cells, having too much cholesterol can increase the risk of CVD. Some people make a lot of cholesterol, and this often runs in families. In addition, we get cholesterol from some foods, especially foods high in saturated fats such as animal fats.

Total blood cholesterol

The total blood cholesterol level includes two types of blood cholesterol:

- low-density lipoprotein (LDL), also known as 'bad' cholesterol because it can add to the build-up of plaque in the arteries and increase the risk of CVD

- high-density lipoprotein (HDL), also known as 'good' cholesterol because it helps protect against CVD

Most of the total cholesterol in blood is made up of LDL cholesterol, with only a small part made up of HDL cholesterol. It is best to aim for a low LDL cholesterol level and a high HDL cholesterol level.

Triglycerides

Triglycerides are another lipid normally found in the body and are used to store unused calories. You may have high triglycerides if your diet is high in sugars and other high-carbohydrate foods or high in alcohol; if you have poorly controlled diabetes, kidney or liver problems; or if you have a family history of high triglycerides.

Getting your blood lipids checked

- All adults should have their cholesterol and triglycerides checked every five years from the age of 45.

- If you are an Aboriginal or Torres Strait Islander this should start at the age of 35.

- If you are at increased risk of CVD or high lipids, your GP should check your lipids more often.

If you have high cholesterol or triglycerides, you need to work with your GP to understand this, address it and have it monitored. This should include:

- identifying and addressing other risk factors for CVD, such as diabetes, smoking, hypertension (high blood pressure), obesity and physical inactivity
- developing and maintaining a healthy diet, healthy weight and good level of physical activity
- prescription medicine if necessary

Diet

A healthy diet low in fat, high in fibre including whole grains and plenty of fresh fruit and vegetables, and low in trans saturated fats, decreases the risk of CVD. It is also thought that oily fish high in omega-3 fatty acids (see p. 490) may be beneficial. This diet acts to decrease the risk of being overweight and developing hypertension (high blood pressure) and diabetes, all risk factors for CVD.

High blood pressure

Blood pressure is the pressure of the blood on the arteries (the blood vessels that carry oxygen and nutrients to the body) as it is pumped around the body by the heart. Blood pressure depends on two main things: the amount of blood pumped by the heart, and how easily the blood can flow through the arteries (therefore the compliance of the arteries).

Our blood pressure normally goes up and down throughout the day, depending on the time of day and what we are doing. In high blood pressure, however, blood pressure is consistently high.

Family history, eating patterns, alcohol intake, weight and level of physical activity all have a strong influence on blood pressure. In some people, medicines, including the oral contraceptive pill, can also raise blood pressure.

High blood pressure can cause problems by:

- overloading and ultimately weakening the heart and coronary arteries because of the constant work for the heart, causing 'heart failure', a serious condition with symptoms such as tiredness, shortness of breath and swelling of the feet and ankles
- contributing to atherosclerosis

High blood pressure can also affect the arteries, and therefore blood flow, to other parts of the body, such as the eyes, kidneys and legs.

Getting your blood pressure checked

- All adults should have their blood pressure checked every two years between the ages of 18 and 50 and every year over the age of 50.
- If you are at higher risk of CVD or high blood pressure, your GP should check your blood pressure more often. This includes if you are an Aboriginal or Torres Strait Islander, have diabetes, kidney disease or high cholesterol, are overweight, have been assessed as having an increased risk of CVD, or have a family history of early CVD.

If you have high blood pressure, you need to work with your GP to understand this, address it and have it monitored. This should include:

- identifying and addressing other risk factors for CVD
- identifying and addressing any contributors to high blood pressure such as alcohol intake, medicine or kidney problems
- developing and maintaining a healthy diet, healthy weight and good level of physical activity and decreasing alcohol
- prescription medicine, if necessary

Physical inactivity

Regular physical activity is an important part of looking after our health and reducing our risk of coronary heart disease. From a CVD point of view, regular physical activity improves long-term health by reducing the risk of heart attack, helping you manage your weight and lowering blood cholesterol levels and blood pressure. If you have diabetes, it will help you control your blood glucose levels. Exercise guidelines for heart health are expressed in various ways, but all aim to encourage regular physical activity for life; for example, to have 150 minutes of moderately intense physical activity over a week, walk an extra 16–20 kilometres per week, or engage in moderate to vigorous exercise for more than 30 minutes on all or most days of the week.

If you have had a heart attack, regular physical activity will also help you recover more quickly.

Depression

Studies have shown that some people who have depression or are socially isolated are at greater risk of developing CVD. Depression can be treated with medication and/or talking therapies. If you think you have depression, talking to your GP is the best first step. See also chapter 40.

Family history, gender and age

Our family history of disease, which reflects our genes, can increase our tendency to develop many health problems, including CVD, high blood pressure, high blood cholesterol and diabetes. Having a family history does not mean that you will develop these problems, but if you do have a family history of CVD, it is important to reduce or remove your other risk factors and let your GP know.

Among midlife people, men are at greater risk of CVD than pre-menopausal women. Once past menopause, however, a woman's risk is similar to a man's. It is thought that this is due to hormonal differences among women and men – oestrogen may have protective effects. The production of oestrogen decreases after menopause, which may explain why a woman's risk of CVD increases then. Women who have experienced early menopause are more likely to develop heart disease than women of the same age who have not yet gone through menopause.

Cardiovascular disease – the important facts

- Cardiovascular disease is the number-one cause of deaths in Australia.

- The most common causes of cardiovascular disease are atherosclerosis ('hardening' of the arteries) and/or hypertension (high blood pressure).

- You can decrease your risk of CVD by maintaining a healthy weight, exercising regularly, eating a balanced diet and not smoking.

- All adults should have their blood pressure checked every two years between the ages of 18 and 50 and every year over the age of 50.

- All adults should have their cholesterol and triglycerides checked every five years from the age of 45.

- If you are at higher risk of CVD you need closer monitoring and management by your GP.

Unfortunately, there is evidence that women have more unrecognised and undertreated CVD, including coronary artery disease, than men, leading to worse outcomes. It is unclear why this is so. Perhaps their symptoms are less 'typical', they address these health concerns less, or people in general as well as health professionals generally think of heart attacks, angina, strokes and high blood pressure as occurring in men.

Osteoarthritis

Arthritis is a major cause of disability and chronic or persistent pain in Australia, with 3.85 million Australians affected.

Although arthritis is often referred to as a single disease, it is an umbrella term for more than 100 medical conditions that affect the musculoskeletal system. Osteoarthritis makes up more than 90 per cent of cases of arthritis in Australia. Some of the other types of arthritis that cause long-term problems include rheumatoid arthritis, gout, pseudo-gout and ankylosing spondylitis; as well as arthritis that can be secondary to another problem such as psoriasis, systemic lupus erythematosus (SLE) and inflammatory bowel disease. Although this chapter deals only with osteoarthritis, it is important that if you have any type of persistent problem or pain in your joints you seek the help of your GP, other health professionals and supports in order to have it addressed, diagnosed and managed as well as possible.

What is osteoarthritis?

Osteoarthritis is a group of joint problems where there is a breakdown and loss of the cartilage in one or more joints, leading to joint pain, tenderness, stiffness, locking and sometimes swelling. Cartilage is the firm, rubbery tissue that cushions our bones at the joints and allows bones to glide over one another.

Symptoms of osteoarthritis

Although any joint in the body can be affected, osteoarthritis most commonly affects the hands, feet, spine and large weight-bearing joints, such as the hips and knees.

As the cartilage breaks down and wears away, the bones rub together, causing the symptoms of osteoarthritis. These include:

- pain and stiffness
- sometimes swelling of the joint, with an accumulation of excess fluid in or around it

- weakness of the muscles and ligaments around the affected joints, perhaps giving rise to a feeling of joint instability
- possible formation of extra bone around the joint
- sometimes a crackling noise (called 'crepitus') when the affected joint is moved or touched

Pain and stiffness are the most common and earliest symptoms. Pain is usually worsened by using the joint and putting weight or pressure on it, and relieved by rest. In more severe cases, pain may occur while resting or wake you up at night. Humid and cold weather may increase the pain.

Due to irritation of the nerves supplying the joint, pain can often be felt in an area other than the joint. This is called 'referred pain', and means that osteoarthritis in the hip will often be felt in the groin or the front of the thigh to the knee.

The stiffness is usually felt on waking up in the morning or following any period of inactivity, usually lasts for 30 minutes or less, and is improved by mild activity that 'warms up' the joint.

The problems and severity people experience if they have osteoarthritis are variable. Some people get only mild symptoms that do not progress, while others have symptoms that are severe and disabling, interfering with daily tasks such as walking, showering, driving a car and cooking.

Causes of osteoarthritis

There is a widely held belief that arthritis is simply a consequence of age, the pain of growing old. It is certainly more common as we age – one in three people aged over 60 has osteoarthritis and almost everyone has some symptoms by the age of 70 – but it is not necessarily a natural part of ageing. Some older people never get arthritis, or only experience minor symptoms. In fact, many people suffering from osteoarthritis are of working age. Before the age of 55, the rates of osteoarthritis are equal in women and men, but after the age of 55, it becomes more common in women.

Osteoarthritis often has no known cause, in which case it is referred to as primary osteoarthritis. This osteoarthritis tends to run in families. When the cause of the osteoarthritis is clearly known, the condition is referred to as secondary osteoarthritis.

Factors that can lead to or contribute to osteoarthritis include:

- being overweight, which increases the stress on the weight-bearing joints such as the hip, knee, ankle and foot joints; next to ageing, obesity is the most significant risk factor for osteoarthritis of the knees

- fractures or other injuries to joints or ligaments, which can lead to osteoarthritis later in life, especially if they didn't heal well
- too much mechanical stress on joints, such as may occur with overly repetitive high-level activities either in sport or certain occupations; exercise in general, in the absence of injury, is not thought to increase the risk of developing osteoarthritis (nor has cracking one's knuckles been found to play a role)
- a congenital joint problem (one you were born with) that makes it more vulnerable to mechanical wear
- infection of a joint
- loss of strength in the muscles supporting joints or problems in the nerves supplying joints, which can lead to sudden or repetitive unco-ordinated movements that overstress joints
- medical conditions such as bleeding disorders that cause bleeding in the joint (e.g. haemophilia); problems that block the blood supply to a joint; and other types of arthritis, such as chronic gout or rheumatoid arthritis
- hormone problems such as diabetes and growth hormone disorders, which are also associated with early cartilage wear

Diagnosis of osteoarthritis

In most cases, a doctor can establish a pretty clear diagnosis of osteo-arthritis by taking a medical history and examining the affected joints. The doctor may order an X-ray – which may show changes in the joints such as narrowing of the space between joints, increased bone formation around the joint and cysts in the bone – but often this is not necessary. Sometimes other tests such as blood tests or a fluid sample taken from the joint are needed, mainly to rule out other types of arthritis, such as rheumatoid arthritis, but no blood tests are helpful in diagnosing osteoarthritis.

X-rays may not correlate with the findings of the physical examination or with the problems you experience. Sometimes the findings on an X-ray look like arthritis but you do not have any symptoms, and sometimes the X-ray findings seem minor and you have quite a lot of symptoms.

Management of osteoarthritis

As yet there is no outright cure for osteoarthritis, but a variety of treat-ments can help control it and reduce its effects and progression.

Every person with osteoarthritis is different. While pain and stiffness may prevent one person from performing simple daily activities, others can maintain an active lifestyle that includes high-level sport.

The more proactive you are in managing your condition, the less joint pain, stiffness and disability you will experience, and the greater your quality of life.

Exercise and physical activity

Affected joints usually feel better with gentle use but worse with excessive or prolonged use. Staying active and getting regular exercise is very important if you have osteoarthritis, as it helps decrease pain, keep joints mobile, increase muscle strength, strengthen bones and ligaments, decrease joint deformities, and increase fitness and wellbeing in general. In fact, recent evidence has shown that exercise and physical activity is one of the most important parts of managing osteoarthritis.

Regular gentle exercises are usually best, such as walking, tai chi or hydrotherapy (i.e. water exercises – the warmth and buoyancy of the water makes movement much easier). For most people, graded exercise (i.e. gradually increasing the intensity and duration of a physical activity) is an important part of management.

Ask your doctor or physiotherapist to recommend an appropriate exercise routine.

Maintaining a healthy weight

If you are overweight and have OA, it is important to lose weight. This will decrease the stress on your joints, help improve your symptoms and decrease the deterioration of your joints.

Minimising stresses on joints

It is important to become aware of the activities and body positions that stress individual joints and aggravate the symptoms, so these can be addressed. This may mean modifying activities such as housework and pastimes, or talking to your workplace and doctor about adjusting your work area or changing your work tasks. Many different aids and equipment are available for both home and work that can help maintain function, and these can be arranged through an occupational therapist or doctor.

Physical therapy for osteoarthritis

Most people find that physical therapy – such as physiotherapy – improves muscle strength, the motion of stiff joints and balance. After a full assessment, a physiotherapist will design a very specific rehabilitation program that includes pain management, muscle retraining and functional training to maintain independence, while protecting the painful joints. Hydrotherapy is often the preferred method to begin exercising as the painful joints are supported and warmed by water. However, land-based strength training and postural exercises are then needed to regain full function. Daily walking for 30 minutes is the most accessible type of exercise and is very suitable for those with hip or knee arthritis. A brace or splint may be needed initially to support the painful joints, or to allow them to move only in correct alignment.

Make sure you only see a registered and experienced physiotherapist who understands how to work with sensitive joint areas.

Splints and braces

These can sometimes support weakened joints or rest a joint that is very inflamed and painful. Some prevent the joint from moving, others allow some movement. You should only use a splint if your doctor or therapist recommends one, as using a brace the wrong way can cause problems.

You should also:

- control any other contributing factors (such as gout or diabetes)
- try not to overuse a painful joint at work or during activities
- apply heat and cold
- eat a healthy, balanced diet (see chapter 31)
- get plenty of rest

Medicine for osteoarthritis

Pain relief (analgesics) and anti-inflammatories

Paracetamol is the first line of medication treatment for osteoarthritis as it helps relieve pain and has few side effects. For more severe symptoms, non-steroidal anti-inflammatories (NSAIDs) are often used as add-on therapy as they will help both the pain and inflammation. While they tend to be more effective, NSAIDs also have more side effects, the most common of which is irritation of the stomach. Several NSAIDs are also available for topical use (i.e. as a cream); these have fewer side effects and appear to have at least some effect.

While doctor-prescribed opioid analgesics such as morphine and fentanyl improve pain, due to the high possibility of side effects and addiction with routine use, they should be used only rarely and for short periods of time.

Other medicine

Oral steroids are not generally used in the treatment of osteoarthritis due to their modest benefit and high rate of side effects. Injections of steroids into affected joints may, however, lead to short-term pain relief lasting for a few weeks to a few months.

Surgery for osteoarthritis

Severe cases of osteoarthritis may require surgery to replace or repair damaged joints. Surgical options include:

- arthroscopic surgery to trim torn and damaged cartilage
- changing the alignment of a bone to relieve stress on the bone or joint (osteotomy)
- surgical fusion of bones (arthrodesis)
- total or partial replacement of the damaged joint with an artificial joint (knee, hip, shoulder, ankle and elbow replacements)

Complementary/alternative treatments for osteoarthritis

As is often the case with chronic conditions where a cure isn't possible, there are many complementary and alternative treatments available for osteoarthritis.

Supplements

Two of the most common supplements are glucosamine and chondroitin, which are also produced naturally in the body to make cartilage. Other alternative medicines that purport to decrease the pain associated with

---

Osteoarthritis – the important facts

- Osteoarthritis becomes more common as we age but is not confined to the elderly.
- The cause of osteoarthritis is usually not known.
- The most common symptom of osteoarthritis is pain in the affected joints after repetitive use.
- The goal of treatment in osteoarthritis is to improve and maintain as much joint function as possible by reducing joint pain and inflammation.
- If you have osteoarthritis, maintaining a healthy body weight and engaging in regular physical activity are crucial.

arthritis include vitamins A, C and E, ginger, turmeric, omega-3 fatty acids, S-adenosylmethionine and electrostimulation techniques (NEST).

There is currently little scientific evidence to support the benefits of these. If you would like to try them, a sensible approach would be to discuss them with your doctor and stop them after three to six months if you have not noticed an improvement.

Acupuncture

Acupuncture is a treatment based on Chinese medicine. How it works is not entirely clear. Some studies have found that acupuncture may provide short-term pain relief for people with osteoarthritis, but it does not seem to produce long-term benefits.

Osteoporosis

Osteoporosis is a common condition affecting about 4 per cent of Australians (about 1 million people). In osteoporosis, bones become thin, weak and fragile, leading to a higher risk of fractures than in normal bone, such that even a minor bump or accident can cause serious fractures. Osteoporosis occurs when bones lose minerals, such as calcium, more quickly than the body can replace them, leading to a loss of bone thickness (bone density or mass) as well as structural quality. This usually takes place over many years.

More than eight out of 10 people with osteoporosis are women and most are aged 55 and over. Women are at a greater risk of developing osteoporosis than men, mainly due to the rapid decline in oestrogen levels after menopause. Oestrogen is an important hormone for maintaining healthy bones, so when oestrogen levels decrease after menopause, bones lose calcium (and other minerals) at a much faster rate.

One in two Australian women and one in three Australian men over the age of 60 will have a fracture due to osteoporosis during their lifetime. The most common types are fractures of the vertebrae (spine), hip, pelvis, wrist and forearm. Some people with these fractures, particularly those of the spine, may initially complain of no more than back pain for a few days, or even have no symptoms. Not only can these fractures cause pain and limit mobility and function, but they can also set in motion a cascade of events that may cause more problems (such as undergoing surgery, or developing bed sores, infections and blood clots).

As we cannot see or feel our bones getting thinner, many people do not know they have osteoporosis until they have a fracture or their doctor orders a test to check their bone density (sometimes called a bone mass measurement), because they have risk factors for osteoporosis. Bone density can be measured a number of different ways but it is usually performed using a special type of X-ray scanning called dual-energy X-ray absorptiometry (DEXA).

Besides being a woman, other risk factors for developing osteoporosis or osteoporotic fractures include:

- age
- having had a low-impact fracture or vertebral fracture in the past
- a family history of osteoporosis and fractures
- certain health conditions including rheumatoid arthritis, some thyroid and other hormone problems, coeliac disease and other chronic gut conditions, liver and kidney disease, and multiple myeloma (a type of blood cancer)
- some medicines such as long-term use of steroids and some breast cancer medicines
- early menopause
- a history of anorexia nervosa or another reason for periods stopping for more than six consecutive months under the age of 45 (excluding pregnancy, menopause or hysterectomy)
- smoking
- high alcohol intake
- inadequate calcium intake or vitamin D deficiency
- an inactive lifestyle over many years
- being significantly underweight
- recurrent falls

Prevention of osteoporosis

Some of the risk factors listed above we can do nothing about, such as being a female, family history, age, early menopause and a number of medical conditions. Several risk factors for osteoporosis can be addressed, however, such as smoking, excessive alcohol consumption, lack of physical activity, poor calcium intake, vitamin D deficiency and being significantly underweight. We call these modifiable risk factors.

If you have any of these risk factors, it is important to address them in order to decrease your risk of osteoporosis.

If you have had a low-impact fracture (that is, you fractured a bone without much trauma), you have lost height or started developing spinal curvature or back pain (which may indicate vertebral fracture), or you have some of the risk factors listed above and you think you may have osteoporosis, it is important to talk to your GP. They may then organise a bone density test to establish whether you have osteoporosis or not.

Routine checks for osteoporosis

Every woman from the age of 45 onwards should see her GP every year to have her risk factors for osteoporosis assessed and get advice on prevention. If you are over 45 and have had a low-impact fracture or vertebral fracture, or have other risk factors, you should discuss with your doctor whether you should have a bone density test.

Management of osteoporosis

If you have osteoporosis, you must then manage your condition at a number of levels, including:

- addressing modifiable risk factors
- managing the osteoporosis itself
- managing fractures

Addressing modifiable risk factors

Even if you have been diagnosed with osteoporosis, it is crucial to address the modifiable risk factors to decrease the progression of the condition and assist in strengthening bones. Depending on what these risk factors are, you may need to work with a number of health professionals, including your GP, pharmacist, physiotherapist and dietician.

See chapter 5 for more on maintaining bone health.

Ensuring adequate calcium and vitamin D

Ensuring adequate calcium and vitamin D intake is an important part of maintaining and improving bone health.

There is debate and controversy among doctors, dieticians and scientists about how much calcium and vitamin D we need and where we should get it from. The National Health and Medical Research Council's (NHMRC's) recommended daily intake (RDI) of calcium aims to enhance bone health and prevent deficiency in the general population. These RDIs vary with age.

Recommended daily intake of calcium

Life stage and age (years)	Recommended daily calcium intake
Childhood: 9–11	1000 milligrams
Adolescence: 12–18	1300 milligrams
Adulthood	1000 milligrams
Pregnancy	1000 milligrams
Midlife to old age: women over 50 and men over 70	1300 milligrams

Obtaining this recommended level of calcium is important for overall bone health. Blood tests for calcium are not useful for checking if you consume sufficient calcium and there is no evidence that any calcium intake higher than these recommended levels is of additional benefit.

If possible, it is preferable to obtain this calcium from your diet. People who, for whatever reason, cannot obtain enough calcium through their diet, may require a supplement, but it is not advisable to substitute a supplement for a poor diet. If a supplement is used the dose should be no greater than 500–600 milligrams per day (regardless of the type of supplement used).

Vitamin D is also needed for bone strength, as it ensures that the calcium consumed is properly taken up by the bones. Vitamin D levels can be determined with a blood test. Although there is no consensus among doctors as to what normal blood vitamin D levels are, there is general agreement that very low levels are insufficient.

We make most of our vitamin D in our skin after exposure to the UVB radiation in sunlight. We can also obtain some vitamin D from food, but with a Western diet this is generally only a small percentage of what is required. Regular, safe sun exposure is therefore recommended to maintain your vitamin D levels. The amount of sun exposure depends on the season, where you live in Australia and your skin type. It is important to balance the need for some sun exposure for vitamin D against the risk of skin damage and possible skin cancer from too much exposure. If you do not get adequate sun exposure, a supplement is recommended to maintain vitamin D levels (see also chapter 31).

People with osteoporosis or other risk factors for low vitamin D should have a blood test to check their vitamin D levels. Low vitamin D levels can be easily corrected by taking vitamin D supplements.

Managing the osteoporosis itself
Medicines

If you are diagnosed with osteoporosis or have a high risk of fracture, your GP will prescribe a medicine to strengthen your bones and help prevent fractures. Prescribed medicines play an essential role in the management of osteoporosis and may be used to both encourage bone formation and reduce bone loss. It is usually required for many years, for just as the bone loss may have taken place over many years, it takes time to rebuild bone strength.

A range of medicines for osteoporosis is available, and they are grouped into different 'classes' depending on their active ingredient. Some of the more common ones are:

- bisphosphonates, which reduce the reabsorption of minerals from the bones and can be taken as tablets – alendronate (Fosamax), risedronate (Actonel) – or as a once-yearly intravenous infusion – zoledronic acid (Aclasta)

- denosumab, which works in a different way from bisphosphonates but has the same effect of slowing the rate at which bone is broken down; it is usually given as a six-monthly injection (Prolia)

- strontium ranelate, which is absorbed into the bone in a similar way to calcium, and both increases bone formation and reduces bone loss, resulting in denser and stronger bones over time; it is usually taken daily as a powder dissolved in water (Protos)

- selective oestrogen-receptor modulators (SERMs), which act like the hormone oestrogen in the bones, helping to reduce bone loss; they are usually given as daily tablets – raloxifene (Evista)

- hormone replacement therapy (HRT), the active ingredient of which is the hormone oestrogen, although some HRT treatments (combined HRT) also contain progesterone. HRT helps slow bone loss and appears to be of greatest benefit to women under 60 who are at risk of fracture (and are unable to take other osteoporosis medicine). It is particularly useful for women who have undergone early menopause (before the age of 45). Over the age of 60, the risk of heart disease, stroke, blood clots and breast cancer increases and HRT is thought to increase these risks even further, so other osteoporosis medicines are generally recommended for women over 60.

- teriparatide, which increases bone formation and is currently restricted to people who have tried other treatments but continue to have very low bone density and further fractures. It must be prescribed by a specialist. After the course of treatment is finished another osteoporosis medicine is used so the new bone produced by using teriparatide is maintained and improved. It is usually given as a daily self-administered injection for 18 months (Forteo).

When advising you on the most appropriate medicine for you, your GP or specialist will consider many factors, including your age; the results of your bone density test/s; your fractures (if you have had any); what you have tried before and how effective this has been; the side effects of the medicines; your risk factors for problems; and other medical conditions and medicines you are taking, how they are administered and your preferences. In many cases, but not all, these medicines are subsided by the Pharmaceutical Benefits Scheme (PBS).

It is important to be aware of the potential side effects and adverse effects of any medicine you take and to take it only as directed to ensure you receive the most benefit and to reduce the risk of side effects. Talk to your doctor if you have any queries or concerns about your medicine.

Physical activity
The best exercises for bone health are dynamic, variable, moderate to high-impact exercises, using activities that are different from day-to-day ones. The most important muscles to target in bone health exercises are the thigh, the calf, and back muscles. Walking is often recommended, but it is not effective for bone health if it is not varied – for example, by walking faster, wearing a backpack, or up and down hills. Examples of good exercise for bones are dancing, line dancing, dance aerobics, tai chi, and gym work with hand or ankle weights. Less effective activities are cycling and swimming, during which the bones are not being strained. Once there is a diagnosis of osteoporosis, physical activity remains a priority for life in order to maintain good strength, balance and posture.

For those who are at risk of falls, the emphasis of activity changes to balance exercises and teaching strategies to prevent falls (such as wearing a hip protector). Strength training for lower limb muscles is still important, but at an appropriate level of intensity, as in tai chi. These physiotherapy programs will also emphasise pain management, postural re-education, joint flexibility and functional activity training.

Complementary medicine
Some people with osteoporosis decide to try complementary medicine in addition to the medicine prescribed by their doctor. These include

nutritional supplements, herbs and acupuncture, but there is currently little evidence that they are effective.

If you are considering complementary treatments, make sure you let your GP and any other health professional caring for you know, so that any interactions between them and your regular osteoporosis treatment can be minimised.

Managing fractures

If you have a fracture, it is important to have it diagnosed as soon as possible and address it in the best way possible. Some fractures will be more minor and just require pain relief and mobilisation, whereas others will be more serious and require hospitalisation, surgical procedures and the help of a number of allied health professionals, such as physiotherapists and occupational therapists, for rehabilitation.

Preventing falls

Avoidance of falls is an integral part of prevention of osteoporotic fractures.

You may be at increased risk of falls if you are older or have:

- a history of falls
- decreased muscle tone, strength and fitness as a result of physical inactivity

---

Osteoporosis – the important facts

- In osteoporosis, bones become thin, weak and fragile, leading to a higher risk of fractures than in normal bone.

- Many people do not know they have osteoporosis until they have a fracture or their doctor orders a test to check their bone density.

- There are a number of modifiable risk factors for osteoporosis that if addressed can decrease your risk of developing it.

- Every woman from the age of 45 onwards should see her GP every year to have her risk factors for osteoporosis assessed and get advice on prevention.

- There are many effective medicines available to strengthen bones and help prevent fractures when osteoporosis is diagnosed.

- If you have osteoporosis it is important to avoid falls.

- problems with balance and walking due to arthritis, stroke or Parkinson's disease
- poor vision
- cardiovascular problems resulting in light-headedness or loss of consciousness
- cognitive problems such as dementia
- medicine that results in sedation, light-headedness or poor coordination
- alcohol or other substance intake that results in confusion, sedation, light-headedness or poor coordination
- incontinence (which means you need to get to the toilet very quickly)
- extrinsic factors such as poor lighting, stairs, uneven floor surfaces, poorly fitting footwear and lack of equipment or aids

Diabetes

For our bodies to work properly, we need to convert glucose (a form of sugar) from our food into energy. Our pancreas, a large gland behind the stomach, produces the hormone insulin, which is required for most of our cells to take in glucose from blood so that it can then be converted into energy. Normally, our bodies release insulin in response to our blood glucose levels, and so maintain our blood sugar levels within a normal range.

Diabetes is usually a chronic (long-term) disease where the pancreas doesn't produce enough insulin, and/or there is a problem with how the body's cells respond to this insulin. So when someone with diabetes eats glucose or foods that break down to glucose, their cells can't take it up adequately and convert it into energy so it instead stays in the blood. This is why blood glucose levels are higher in people with diabetes than they should be.

There are three main types of diabetes:

- type 1 diabetes, which results from the body's failure to produce any insulin, and requires regular insulin injections or an insulin pump
- type 2 diabetes, which results mainly from cells being relatively resistant to the insulin produced
- gestational diabetes, which occurs when pregnant women without a previous diagnosis of diabetes develop type 2 diabetes during pregnancy (see chapter 17)

Type 1 diabetes

About 5–15 per cent of all diabetes is type 1 (also called insulin-dependent diabetes). Its onset can occur at any age but it usually starts in children and people under the age of 30 (which is why it used to be called juvenile diabetes). It occurs due to the loss of the insulin-producing cells in the pancreas, leading to insufficient insulin for the body's needs.

Without insulin, the body burns its own fats as a substitute. Unless treated with daily injections of insulin, people with type 1 diabetes accumulate dangerous chemical substances in their blood from the burning of fat, making their blood too acidic for the body to function. This is known as ketoacidosis and is life-threatening.

To stay alive, people with type 1 diabetes depend on up to four injections of insulin every day, or an insulin pump. There are different types of insulin and various regimes. They must test their blood glucose levels several times daily.

The exact cause of type 1 diabetes is not yet known, but we do know it has a strong family link and it is thought to be triggered in susceptible people at a vulnerable time in their life by specific viral infections.

We also know that it has nothing to do with lifestyle – most people affected are otherwise healthy and of a healthy weight when onset occurs – although maintaining a healthy lifestyle is very important in helping to manage type 1 diabetes.

At this stage nothing can be done to prevent or cure type 1 diabetes.

Type 2 diabetes

Type 2 diabetes (or non-insulin-dependent diabetes) is the most common type of diabetes, affecting 85–95 per cent of all people with diabetes and around 8 per cent of Australians aged 25 or older. While it usually affects older adults, younger people, even children, are now getting type 2 diabetes. Its incidence is increasing rapidly, and by 2030 it is estimated that it will almost double. This increase is linked to lifestyle factors (see below).

In type 2 diabetes, the pancreas makes some insulin but it is not produced in the amount the body needs, or the body's cells don't respond properly to the insulin produced. Most people with type 2 diabetes have both of these problems.

There is no single cause of type 2 diabetes; it results from a combination of lifestyle factors and genetics. The risk of type 2 diabetes increases with:

- a family history of diabetes
- age – first onset is most common after the age of 40, although the age of onset can be earlier
- being overweight, especially with the classic apple-shaped body where extra weight is carried around the waist; most, but not all, people with type 2 diabetes are overweight
- insufficient physical activity
- poor diet
- certain cultural backgrounds, such as Aboriginal and Torres Strait Islander, Pacific Islander, subcontinental Indian or Chinese
- giving birth to a child over 4.5 kilograms or having gestational diabetes when pregnant
- polycystic ovarian syndrome (PCOS; see chapter 24)
- taking antipsychotic medicine
- having abnormal blood glucose in the past, but not diabetes (called glucose intolerance).

It is estimated that more than half of type 2 diabetes cases can be prevented, and the rest better managed with having fewer complications, by a healthy lifestyle (see 'Management of diabetes' below).

Symptoms of diabetes

The symptoms of diabetes are caused by high blood glucose (hyperglycaemia), complications from having high blood sugar for a long time, and low blood glucose (hypoglycaemia). Some people have no symptoms at all.

Symptoms of high blood glucose

The high blood sugar levels that occur in diabetes can produce the classic symptoms of frequent urination (polyuria), increased thirst (polydypsia) and increased hunger (polyphagia). It can also produce other problems, including tiredness, poor healing of cuts, skin infections and rashes, blurred vision, weight loss, mood swings, headaches, dizziness and leg cramps. These symptoms may develop rapidly over weeks or months (especially with type 1 diabetes) or slowly over months to years (especially with type 2 diabetes).

Occasionally, symptoms associated with diabetes can be so extreme that it can become life-threatening and is a medical emergency. Symptoms may include altered consciousness, nausea, vomiting, abdominal pain and dehydration. This is particularly the case with type 1 diabetes, but can also occur with type 2 diabetes. Seek immediate medical advice by calling 000 if these symptoms occur.

Complications from having high blood sugar for a long time
Untreated diabetes can result in a number of long-term health problems, while managing diabetes well decreases the likelihood of these occurring. These problems typically develop after 10–20 years, but may be the first symptoms in people with undiagnosed type 2 diabetes.

Diabetes increases the risk of problems due to damage to blood vessels and nerves. These include:

- kidney damage (nephropathy)
- eye damage (retinopathy)
- nerve damage to the feet and other parts of the body (neuropathy)
- heart disease (e.g. angina or heart attack), stroke and circulation problems in the legs
- sexual difficulties, such as diabetes-related nerve damage causing vaginal dryness or loss of sensation or pain in the genital area; reduced testosterone due to chronic high blood sugar levels, contributing to decreased libido and low blood sugar (hypoglycaemia) after the physical activity of sex
- problems with circulation, nerve damage, foot ulcers or infections (especially in the legs)

Symptoms of low blood glucose (hypoglycaemia)
Symptoms of blood sugar levels getting too low include:

- unclear thinking
- irritation or aggression
- loss or change in consciousness
- weakness
- blurred vision
- headache
- shaking
- sweating
- pounding heart
- hunger

The most common causes of low blood sugar in people with diabetes are:

- taking insulin or diabetes medicine at the wrong time
- taking too much insulin or diabetes medicine by mistake
- not eating enough during meals or snacks after taking insulin or diabetes medicine
- missing or delaying meals
- exercising more or at a different time than usual
- drinking alcohol

Avoiding hypoglycaemia

Severe hypoglycaemia is a medical emergency that may cause seizures, loss of consciousness and death. Learn to recognise the early warning signs of hypoglycaemia and treat yourself quickly.

No symptoms at all

Many people do not have any symptoms at all when they develop type 2 diabetes, while other problems such as tiredness, lack of energy, blurred vision, headaches, dizziness, leg cramps, slower healing of sores or more frequent infections may be subtle and easily dismissed as a part of 'getting older'.

Unfortunately, often by the time type 2 diabetes is diagnosed, the complications of diabetes (see above) may already be present.

Management of diabetes

Diabetes is a chronic disease that cannot be cured except in very specific situations, but the complications of diabetes are far less common and less severe (and may never develop at all) in people who have well-managed blood sugar levels.

Although the specifics of treatment depend on the type of diabetes and individual issues, management concentrates on:

- keeping blood sugar levels as close to normal as possible, without causing hypoglycaemia (low blood sugar) by adopting a healthy eating pattern, exercising regularly, taking medicines and monitoring blood glucose levels

- addressing other risk factors and health problems that may contribute to diabetes itself or to the complications of diabetes, such as smoking, high cholesterol, obesity, high blood pressure and lack of regular exercise

- monitoring for control and complications, which means working with your GP to understand the range of complications, their symptoms and how they can be minimised, and having regular medical checks to monitor your blood sugar control and detect complications early. Your GP is also likely to suggest you have the annual influenza vaccine as the flu may affect your diabetes control.

The management of diabetes often requires a multidisciplinary approach, with your GP organising and coordinating your care to achieve the best outcomes. It is crucial that you develop a plan in conjunction with your GP and have regular checks, so you can best manage your diabetes together.

Eating well

Choosing healthy foods will help manage your blood glucose levels and your body weight. Healthy eating for people with diabetes is similar to recommendations for everyone, so there is no need to prepare separate meals or buy special foods.

The principles of eating if you have diabetes are to:

- eat regular meals spread evenly throughout the day
- eat food low in fat, particularly saturated fat
- eat food that has a low glycaemic index and is high in complex carbohydrates, such as wholegrain breads and cereals, beans, lentils and vegetables
- match the amount of food you eat with the amount of energy you use each day and avoid overeating

People with type 1 diabetes have to be particularly careful in planning their food intake, insulin and activity to best manage their blood glucose levels.

Keeping physically active

Along with healthy eating, regular physical activity can help manage blood glucose levels, reduce blood lipids (cholesterol and triglycerides) and maintain a healthy weight.

Being physically active plays an important part in diabetes management. For someone with diabetes, exercise helps:

- insulin to work better, which will improve diabetes management
- control weight
- control other risk factors for complications by lowering blood pressure and reducing the risk of heart disease
- improve sleep and reduce stress

As diabetes needs to be managed for life, it is recommended that you choose physical activities that are enjoyable and achievable. Walking is easy, cheap, and you can vary the speed and distance you walk as your fitness improves. Diabetes Australia recommends using a pedometer (a step counter) and increasing gradually to a level decided between you and your physiotherapist or doctor. This is commonly 10,000 steps per

---

Diabetes – the important facts

- People with diabetes have high blood glucose levels caused by a problem with the amount of and/or the effectiveness of the hormone insulin they produce.
- The three main types of diabetes are type 1 ('juvenile' or insulin-dependent), type 2 (non-insulin-dependent) and gestational diabetes (in pregnancy).
- All people with type 1 diabetes require insulin to stay alive.
- Type 2 diabetes is common and increasing due to lifestyle factors such as obesity, physical inactivity and poor food choices.
- It is thought that about half of type 2 diabetes cases could be prevented with a healthier lifestyle.
- Type 2 diabetes is often diagnosed late due to non-specific symptoms.
- Regular check-ups are needed to diagnose type 2 diabetes early.
- There is no cure for diabetes, but the symptoms and complications can be decreased and managed through good control, maintaining a healthy lifestyle and with regular check-ups.
- Diabetic emergencies can result from blood sugars that are too high for too long or sugars that are too low.

day. Incidental exercise – being active as much as you can during the day – makes your target step count achievable. Climb stairs, rather than use the lift, park the car further away from the shops, get off the tram or bus a stop earlier and walk the rest of the way home, move about while you are waiting in a queue, and go to the park or beach rather than watch a movie.

Precautions:

- Be aware of your own blood glucose response to physical activity. You may need to make adjustments to your medication or eating plan as your exercise intensity increases over time.

- Do not undertake strenuous physical activity if you are feeling unwell or ketones are present in your blood or urine.

- Take care of your feet – wear good-quality, well-fitting footwear.

Medicines for diabetes

Insulin is always required for type 1 diabetes. Type 2 diabetes can often initially be managed with healthy eating and regular physical activity, but over time most people with type 2 diabetes will need tablets and many will also need insulin. It is important to note that this is just the natural progression of the disease, and taking tablets or insulin as soon as they are required can result in fewer complications in the long term.

Asthma

Asthma is a disease of the small airways that carry air into and out of the lungs. In asthma these air passages become intermittently swollen and inflamed, resulting in narrowing and therefore making it harder for air to get through. This results in wheezing, coughing and difficulty breathing.

Asthma is common. More than 2 million Australians have asthma: about one in 10 adults and one in six children, although many children improve as they get older. These rates are high compared to the rest of the world. Although the rate of asthma in Australian children has declined over the past decade, it has remained the same in adults. It is not clear why this is so.

Asthma is more common among Aboriginal and Torres Strait Islanders than other Australians. More boys than girls have asthma, but after about the age of 15 it is more common among women than men.

Although asthma cannot be cured, it is a treatable health condition. With the right treatment, nearly all people with asthma will be able to join in sport and lead normal, active lives.

Symptoms of asthma

The most common symptoms of asthma are:

- coughing
- a tight feeling in the chest
- wheezing – whistling noise when breathing
- breathing problems (shortness of breath, struggling to breathe)

Acute asthma attacks often last for two to three days, but some people have chronic or lingering symptoms between attacks. This is an indication that the asthma needs better management.

Causes of asthma

The cause of asthma is usually not known, although we know there is a genetic component, as it often runs in families. There is also a strong link between asthma and allergy: around 80 per cent of people with asthma also have eczema, hay fever or allergies.

Many different things can start or trigger an asthma attack and these can be different for different people. The most common triggers are:

- respiratory infections such as colds and flu caused by a virus
- allergens such as dust mites, pollens, pets and moulds
- cigarette smoke (either active or passive); despite this, people with asthma smoke at least as much as people without asthma and around 8 per cent of kids with asthma live with someone who smokes inside the house
- exercise, although asthma triggered by exercise may be helped by medicine and/or warm-up exercises and once properly controlled, need not restrict activity; in fact people with asthma are encouraged to take part in exercise to improve their lung capacity
- weather – cold air, a sudden change in temperature, thunderstorms
- work-related triggers, such as wood dust and chemicals
- some medicines

It is helpful for you to know what triggers your asthma, so you can help avoid those triggers where possible. It is also important to know, however, that asthma can be unpredictable.

Treatment for asthma

With good management nearly all people with asthma can lead normal, active lives. The key steps are to:

- Understand your asthma.
- Avoid your asthma triggers.
- See your doctor for regular check-ups and work together to get the treatment you need to best manage your asthma.
- Follow your personal written asthma action plan (see below), developed with your doctor.
- Always make sure you have your reliever medicine with you.
- Make sure you are using your inhaler (puffer) correctly.
- Use your medicines as prescribed, even when you feel well.
- Live a healthy lifestyle – give up smoking if you smoke and exercise regularly.

Asthma action plans

It is essential that everyone with asthma has a personalised asthma action plan developed in conjunction with their doctor. The plan should include your medicine, how to prevent, recognise and manage asthma attacks and an asthma first aid plan in the event of severe symptoms. The plan should be kept in a place where you can find it easily.

If you have a child who has asthma, or are a carer for someone with asthma, it is also important that you and they know about their asthma, medicine and asthma action plan, and that other carers also know they have asthma and what to do during an asthma attack.

Asthma emergencies

Quick action may help prevent an asthma attack from becoming an asthma emergency.

Asthma emergency danger signs:

- Your symptoms get worse very quickly.
- You have severe shortness of breath, you can't speak comfortably or your lips look blue.
- You get little or no relief from your reliever inhaler.
  Call an ambulance immediately: dial 000.
  Say this is an *asthma emergency.*

Medicine for asthma

There are different groups of medicine used for asthma: relievers, steroids, preventers and controllers. What you need will depend on you and your asthma. This includes your triggers, if you know what they are, how often you get attacks, how bad they are, how easy or hard they are to control, and if you have any problems between attacks.

It is essential to work through these things with your doctor so your asthma management is the best it can be, and that you know how to take your asthma medicine.

Relievers

These work quickly (within a few minutes) to relax the muscles around the air passages, decreasing the narrowing of the breathing tubes and making it easier for air to get through, and therefore to breathe. They are almost always inhaled and include Ventolin, Bricanyl and Respolin. Inhalers can be tricky to use, so get your doctor to demonstrate and then practise while you are with them. They are sometimes used with devices to maximise their delivery to the lungs (for example, 'spacers').

Asthma can be unpredictable; you need to ensure you always have a reliever that is not past its use-by date and is easily accessible to you at all times.

If you need to use a reliever more often than every two to four hours or your use of it is increasing, you should seek medical attention.

Prednisolone

This is a type of steroid that reduces the swelling in the lining of the air passages and helps make the breathing tubes react more to relievers. It is usually given as a tablet, or a syrup for children. It takes about six to eight hours to work and is often only required during an acute attack. If you need it for longer term control, speak to your doctor about how to minimise possible side effects, including on your bone health.

Preventers

These help prevent attacks from happening and are usually inhaled. Not everyone needs preventer medicine, but if you do, you need to take them every day, not just when you have symptoms. They include Flixotide, Pulmicort and Singulair (a tablet). If you need a preventer, you must see your doctor regularly to ensure your medicine is working and you are on the correct dose.

Controllers

These are used when your asthma cannot be controlled using preventers alone. They help in a similar way to relievers but last or work for longer. Examples include Serevent and Formoterol. These should always be used in addition to preventers and as a result are often combined into one inhaler with a preventer. Seretide, for example, is a combination of Flixotide (a preventer) and Serevent (a controller), while Symbicort is a combination of Pulmicort (a preventer) and Formoterol (a controller).

A healthy lifestyle and asthma

Both active (smoking yourself) and passive (being exposed to others') cigarette smoke exposure is a well-known trigger for asthma. It can also cause other lung problems such as emphysema, which will compound any asthma symptoms.

If you smoke, it's important to give up. You should also avoid a smoky environment. If you are having trouble giving up smoking, see your doctor, as there is very effective treatment to help you quit.

Although asthma can be triggered by exercise, once properly controlled, regular exercise has been found to be beneficial for asthma as it improves lung function.

If your asthma is triggered by exercise, warm-up exercises and medicine before exercise may help.

Asthma – the important facts

- With the right treatment, nearly all people with asthma will be able to join in sport and lead normal, active lives.

- It is essential that everyone with asthma has a personalised asthma action plan developed in conjunction with their doctor.

- Asthma can be unpredictable; ensure you always have a reliever accessible.

- Both active and passive cigarette smoke exposure is a well-known trigger for asthma.

Thyroid disease

The thyroid

The thyroid is a small butterfly-shaped gland located in the lower part of the front of your neck. Its function is to secrete hormones.

The main hormones released by the thyroid are triiodothyronine (known as T3) and thyroxine (known as T4). These hormones are released into your blood and travel to nearly every cell in your body. Here, T3 and T4 attach to receptors and act to regulate your basal metabolic rate (the amount of energy you use when you are at rest); protein, fat and carbohydrate metabolism; bone growth; brain and nervous system development; and the effects of other hormones, vitamins and catecholamines (such as adrenaline). Thyroid hormones are therefore essential to the proper development and function of the human body, and affect a wide range of the body's metabolic and critical functions, such as temperature, energy level and heart rate.

The thyroid hormones produced by the thyroid gland are regulated by thyroid stimulating hormone (TSH), which is made by the brain's pituitary gland. In turn, TSH is regulated by both thyrotropin-releasing hormone, which is released by the hypothalamus in the brain (the hypothalamus receives and analyses lots of signals on how your body is functioning) and the thyroid hormones T3 and T4. When T3 and T4 are low, the production of TSH is increased, and, conversely, when T3 and T4 are high, TSH production is decreased. In addition, some pregnancy hormones stimulate production of thyroid hormones. The normal range of TSH varies with age, whether you are pregnant or not, and the way a laboratory measures it. There is still debate as to what constitutes a normal level of TSH, particularly in older people and in pregnancy.

Thyroid problems are common: more than 5 per cent of Australian adults are thought to be affected by them. Most thyroid problems are at least five times more common in women than men, with about one in eight women developing a thyroid disorder during her lifetime.

Symptoms of thyroid disease

Thyroid diseases encapsulate a range of diseases that cause a range of different symptoms and problems.

The symptoms of thyroid disease in adults can be due to:

- too little thyroid hormone
- too much thyroid hormone
- enlargement of the thyroid
- lumps in the thyroid

Too little thyroid hormone

This is called hypothyroidism. It occurs when the thyroid gland is under-active and there is not enough thyroid hormone for your body's needs. One of the most common causes of hypothyroidism is the autoimmune disease called Hashimoto's disease, in which antibodies gradually target the thyroid and destroy its ability to produce thyroid hormone. It affects about 1 to 2 per cent of the population, and is 10 times more common in women than in men, and more common in older women. Other causes include the surgical removal of the thyroid, radioactive iodine treatment for an overactive thyroid, some medications, iodine deficiency and congenital hypothyroidism.

Symptoms of hypothyroidism usually go along with a slowdown in metabolism, and include tiredness, weight gain, feeling cold, constipation, depression, forgetfulness, dry skin, heavy periods, hair loss and problems with low fertility. Hypothyroidism can also cause high cholesterol, heart problems and damage to nerves. Babies born to women with untreated thyroid disease may also have a higher risk of birth defects.

Subclinical hypothyroidism

Subclinical hypothyroidism describes the finding of a raised TSH but a normal level of thyroid hormones. In this case, as the level of thyroid hormone is normal, people don't usually have any symptoms and this finding is picked up after routine blood testing or checking if a goitre (an enlargement of the thyroid) or nodule (lump) is causing any problems.

Subclinical hypothyroidism is more common than hypothyroidism and more common as we age, and is found in about 8 per cent of women and 3 per cent of men. We don't yet know what, if any, the significance of it is and can't predict how it will progress in any one person. Sometimes with time it progresses to hypothyroidism and sometimes it settles back to normal.

There is still debate as to whether it can result in problems and if it should be treated, especially in pregnant women, those considering pregnancy, older people or those with heart problems. Therefore, if your blood tests show subclinical hypothyroidism, your GP is likely to talk to you about ensuring adequate iodine intake; the symptoms of hypothyroidism to be aware of; to organise follow-up tests every year or so (the optimum frequency of this has not been determined and depends on your doctor's clinical assessment); and they may discuss the pros and cons of the use of thyroid hormone replacement medicine.

Too much thyroid hormone

This is called hyperthyroidism. It is when the thyroid gland becomes over-active and produces too much thyroid hormone for your body's needs. The most common cause of hyperthyroidism is the autoimmune condition known as Graves' disease, where antibodies target the gland and cause it to speed up hormone production. Graves' disease is most common between 20 and 50 years of age. It affects about 1 per cent of the population and is 10 times more common in women than men. Hyperthyroidism can also be caused by a nodule or nodules releasing thyroid hormone (either with or without a goitre), or inflammation of the thyroid. Inflammation of the thyroid can be due to many things, including bacterial or viral illness; it can also occur after having a baby.

This post-partum thyroiditis occurs during the first year after giving birth, causing stored thyroid hormone to leak out of the inflamed thyroid gland and raising thyroid hormone levels in the blood. It affects about 5 per cent of women who have had a baby, and usually causes mild hyperthyroidism, which lasts between 1 and 2 months. Many of these women then develop hypothyroidism, lasting between 6 and 12 months before the thyroid regains normal function, although in some cases this hypothyroidism is permanent. It often recurs with future pregnancies.

Symptoms of hyperthyroidism usually go along with a speed up in metabolism and include irritability, nervousness, palpitations, anxiety, tremor, feeling hot, sweating, diarrhoea, muscle weakness, weight loss and sleep disturbances. It can also cause osteoporosis and heart problems, and cause vision and eye problems if it is due to Graves' disease.

Enlargement of the thyroid

An enlargement of the thyroid is called a goitre. A goitre can be a generally enlarged smooth thyroid or have nodules in it.

A goitre is the most common thyroid disease and affects women about 4 times more often than men, with about 3 per cent of women having one at any point in time. It is most common before menopause and its occur-rence declines with age.

The enlargement can be due to autoimmune problems (e.g. Hashi-moto's or Graves' disease), nutritional deficiencies in iodine (see below) or for an unknown reason. A goitre can cause an overactive or underactive thyroid, or not cause any problems in thyroid levels.

If you or your doctor notices a goitre, he or she will generally order a blood test to check your thyroid activity and to see if you have any antibodies against the thyroid. The doctor may also order an ultrasound to check the goitre and see if it has nodules in it.

Management will depend on the results of these tests, the size of the goitre and whether it is causing any problems by pressing on surrounding tissues.

Lumps in the thyroid

These are known as thyroid nodules and become more common as we age, with about 6 per cent of women and 1 per cent of men over 60 years having a noticeable thyroid nodule or nodules.

They may be associated with a goitre or the remainder of the gland being normal in size. Sometimes they are picked up via an ultrasound that has been performed to check a goitre, or you or your doctor may have noticed a lump in your neck, or you may have had symptoms of an overactive thyroid. If a nodule is noted, your doctor will usually organise a blood test and an ultrasound to further investigate.

Thyroid nodules can be solid or cystic (i.e. filled with fluid), single or multiple. They can be benign or cancerous and can be associated with normal or overactive thyroid activity.

Although thyroid nodules are common, thyroid cancers are rare and only a small number of thyroid nodules are cancerous, but sometimes a biopsy (where a needle is put into the nodule and cells are removed so they can be examined under a microscope) is needed to rule out cancer.

Causes of thyroid disease

Iodine deficiency is the most common cause of thyroid hormone problems. However, in Australia, most thyroid hormone problems, such as hypo-thyroidism or hyperthyroidism, are due to autoimmune thyroid disease.

Autoimmune disease means the body's natural ability to tell the difference between its own cells (which it should not attack) and bacteria, viruses or pathogens (which it should attack) becomes disrupted. This causes your immune system to wrongly mount an attack on parts of your own body by producing antibodies. In the case of autoimmune thyroid disease, these antibodies can either make the thyroid underactive or overactive, or sometimes both at different times.

The causes for autoimmune thyroid problems are largely unknown, but they can be associated with other autoimmune problems, or a family history of autoimmune or thyroid problems. However, we do know that, like other autoimmune antibodies, some people have antibodies against their thyroid but no thyroid problems at all.

Diagnosis of thyroid disease

The symptoms of both too much and too little thyroid hormone are highly variable between individuals. Only some of many possible symptoms may be present, and these symptoms are usually non-specific and occur with many other health conditions. They may vary in severity over time, and can develop slowly. So they can easily be missed by both sufferers and their doctors, and thyroid disease is therefore frequently diagnosed late or underdiagnosed. An estimated half of those with thyroid problems have never had their thyroid hormone problems diagnosed or, therefore, treated.

Generally, however, once a possible thyroid problem is considered, the diagnosis is relatively simple. A blood test to check thyroid function is often the first step. If it shows problems, a range of tests will usually be ordered to check for a range of thyroid antibodies. An ultrasound of the thyroid may also be ordered if a goitre or lump is noted, and a biopsy may be ordered if a nodule is found.

Management of thyroid disease

Most thyroid problems are lifelong conditions that, once diagnosed, can be well managed with the correct treatment, education and long-term medical attention, as well as by monitoring symptoms and with regular blood tests.

If there is too little thyroid hormone, the treatment is hormone replacement medicine (e.g. thyroxine). Hypothyroidism may become more or less severe over time, and the dose of thyroxine may need to change if it does so. But if you take your medicine every day and work with your doctor to get and keep your dose right, you should be able to keep your hypothyroidism and its symptoms well controlled throughout your life.

If there is too much thyroid hormone, the treatment depends on the cause and includes antithyroid medicine, radioactive iodine ablation (where radioactive iodine administered into the blood is taken up by the thyroid gland, where it destroys some thyroid tissue) and surgery.

Thyroid and iodine

To make thyroid hormones, the thyroid gland requires iodine, which we get from our diet and which can only be stored in small amounts in the thyroid. Iodine is therefore essential in a person's diet. Adults generally need approximately 150 micrograms of iodine per day (about ½ a teaspoon of iodised salt); pregnant and breastfeeding women need approximately 250 micrograms of iodine a day.

A long-term deficiency of iodine leads to the decreased production of thyroid hormones, and can cause the disease known as goitre as the thyroid gland enlarges in order to try to increase its function (see below).

People in some countries have very low levels of iodine in their diets as there is little in their soil, little in the foods they eat and no supplementation in those foods. Such countries tend to be in the remote and mountainous areas of South-East Asia, Latin America and Central Africa. In these areas, goitre is very common: it can be seen in as much as 80 per cent of the population. Unfortunately, in addition, mental retardation in children due to severe iodine deficiency in the pregnant mother is not uncommon. Iodine deficiency is the leading worldwide cause of preventable mental retardation.

Iodine deficiency has been largely confined to the developing world for several generations. However, a reduction in the use of iodised salt, and changes in the Australian dairy industry in the 1980s – when the use of iodine-based cleaners for the cleaning of milk vats ceased – has led in recent years to many Australians being mildly iodine deficient. For this reason, since late 2009 all commercially manufactured bread in Australia (excluding organic bread) has been fortified with iodine. This means that most Australians now get enough iodine in their diet.

Thyroid and pregnancy

During pregnancy, the thyroid needs to produce more hormones to keep up with the woman's increased body metabolism and to make enough thyroid hormone for both the fetus and the mother. During pregnancy, the thyroid normally enlarges slightly (a physiological goitre) in response to this, but usually not enough to be noticed.

Thyroid hormones play a critical role in both the development of a healthy baby – they are essential for the normal development of the baby's brain and nervous system – and in maintaining the health of the mother: pregnant women with undiagnosed or inadequately treated hypothyroidism have an increased risk of miscarriage, preterm delivery and developmental problems in their children.

You therefore need more iodine in your diet if you are considering pregnancy, are pregnant, or breastfeeding: about 250 micrograms a day, with a general recommendation that a pregnancy supplement with at least 150 micrograms of iodine per day is used (unless you have had thyroid problems before).

If you are pregnant and have thyroid problems, you can easily have a healthy baby and pregnancy by seeing your GP to talk to them about them, having regular blood tests to check your thyroid function (which may be required more often than usual in pregnancy), learning about pregnancy's effect on the thyroid and taking the required medications (which may need to change in type or amount during the pregnancy). It is preferable this is done before you get pregnant, or as early as possible in pregnancy, so any problems can be sorted out from the beginning.

Thyroid problems that first develop in pregnancy or in the post-partum period can be difficult to diagnose because so many of their symptoms (e.g. fatigue, difficulty sleeping, constipation, anxiety) are common to both a normal pregnancy, the post-partum period and thyroid problems; and because thyroid function tests are sometimes difficult to interpret in pregnancy.

If you have symptoms you think may be due to thyroid hormone imbalance, you have noticed goitre or have had problems with your thyroid in the past, please see your GP to discuss whether you should have a thyroid blood test.

Thyroid disease – the important facts

- Thyroid problems are frequently underdiagnosed or diagnosed late.
- If you have symptoms you think may be due to thyroid hormone imbalance or problems please see your GP to discuss whether you should have a thyroid blood test.
- Most thyroid problems are lifelong conditions.
- Once diagnosed, thyroid problems can be well managed with the correct treatment, education, long-term monitoring and medical attention.
- Thyroid problems in pregnancy need particular attention in order to maintain the health of the mother and ensure the proper development of the baby.
- Adults need approximately 150 micrograms of iodine in their diet per day; the general recommendation for women who are considering pregnancy, are pregnant or breastfeeding is to have a daily pregnancy supplement that contains at least 150 micrograms of iodine.

Living well with a chronic illness

We all want a healthy, rich and fulfilling life. Having a chronic medical condition doesn't change these aspirations, but it can mean more work to achieve and maintain maximal health in order to fully enjoy and participate in life.

With all medical conditions, it is important to understand the condition and the effects it has on you, and be an active participant in deciding on your goals and undertaking management towards those goals. This is especially true and important for people with chronic medical conditions.

Having a chronic health condition does make some aspects of your life more challenging. It lasts for a long time, often involves many health professionals and healthcare sectors, affects many facets of your life, and may affect those around you such as family and friends. All of these factors combine to make it especially important to understand as much as you can about your condition, to be an active participant in decisions and management, to be kept at the centre of quality care, and that there be excellent communication between you and your healthcare providers and between those providers.

It often takes some time for a chronic illness to declare itself. It may take more time for a doctor to diagnose that the sore joints are osteoarthritis, the sore back a symptom of osteoporosis or the lethargy a symptom of diabetes. The lead-up to diagnosis and afterwards can be busy and difficult: there are often many doctors' appointments and tests, visits to allied health professionals, different medicines and sometimes even operations. Not knowing what will happen over time, not knowing what the day-to-day level of problems will be and how they will affect your life, including work, relationships, family, leisure and finances, often leads to uncertainty, emotional turmoil and confusion.

It does take time and effort to adjust to having and managing a chronic condition. Over time, people often have different and fluctuating experiences with their health condition and its effects, the healthcare system and their emotional reactions and adjustment.

There is no single right response to learning how to best manage and live with your chronic health condition, but there are some principles that may help you. These include:

- working to find the right team of health professionals
- making the most of your appointments
- learning about your condition

- making sure health professionals and others understand what is happening
- setting goals and developing a healthcare plan
- being an active participant in your plan
- actively seeking support
- understanding your medicine
- keeping a record of important information
- developing and maintaining a healthy lifestyle
- managing pain
- coming to terms with your health condition

Working to find the right team of health professionals

- Find health professionals you can talk to, who listen to you and you trust.
- Have a regular GP – they get to know you and your situation over time and act as your central and regular point of contact, health care and monitoring, bringing together advice and information from various healthcare professionals and working with you to ensure a coordinated, quality approach to the management of your healthcare needs. They also work with you in other areas of your health care, including screening and other preventative health activities.
- Don't be afraid to ask for a second opinion or to question the role, frequency and function of the health professionals you see.

Making the most of your appointments

- Have someone you trust come to appointments with you. There is often so much information that it is good to have someone else there to take everything in. Remember to let them know that this is confidential information and they are not to speak to others about it without your permission.
- Think about and write down what you want to raise and ask before your appointments. This way you are more likely to give your GP and other health professionals the full picture of what is happening for you and get answers to the many issues that arise over time.
- Ask for an interpreter if you need one. Professional interpreters are used to translating medical terminology, which relatives aren't. It also

takes the responsibility away from friends or relatives, so they can just concentrate on your issues. Let your health professional know well before your appointment that you require an interpreter.

(See also chapter 3.)

Learning about your condition

- There is no such thing as a silly question. Ask questions, clarify and summarise what the health professionals and doctors have said. Ask for written information, diagrams or videos or about the cost of medicines, tests, procedures or consultations.
- Look up information on quality websites, visit a library, consider joining a support group or an online forum.
- Understand what to do if you have problems. Understand which symptoms it is really important to act on quickly and how to act.
- Understand the things you can do to lessen the risks of worsening your condition and increase the chance of alleviating it (preventative health).

(See also chapter 3.)

Making sure health professionals and others understand what is happening

- Talk to your health professionals about what you are experiencing, such as pain, difficulties or inability to do things, sleep problems, problems with medicine or their management and what is working and what is not.
- Show your doctor and other health professionals how you are doing the exercises you've been given, and where the pain is. It is surprising how often both patients and health professionals can misinterpret information.
- Consider and tell your health professionals the effect of your health conditions on all aspects of your life, including your emotions and fears, your mental wellbeing and adjustment, relationships, work, activity, leisure, hobbies, travel, driving, pregnancy, medicines and finances.
- Talk to your health professionals about your aspirations and what you want to achieve, including any plans to get pregnant.

- Tell doctors about the medicines you are using and how you are taking them. Let them know about any other over-the-counter or complementary medicine or drugs you are taking.

- It's important you tell your doctor if you smoke or use drugs or alcohol, as this may alter your management plan.

Setting goals and developing a healthcare plan

It is your body and your life, and ultimately you are the most important person in deciding on your health goals and how to achieve them – that is, your healthcare plan. In doing this, you should:

- Understand what the problems and options are, including their risks, benefits and costs, and actively share in making decisions with your health providers.

- Consider good advice.

- Communicate what you want to achieve, be realistic about what is achievable and its timeframe, and understand what you need to do to achieve the best life you can.

- Remember that some things may be especially challenging, require really tight control or alter your management approach. These include travel or an impending operation or procedure. Work with your GP and other healthcare professionals to define and set your goals and the plan of action to achieve them.

- Have a written healthcare plan, developed in partnership with your GP, and share this with all your other healthcare providers. See the sample healthcare plan at the end of this chapter for the kinds of things you might include.

- Clarify the roles and responsibilities of your various health professionals. Understand why you are seeing them and which to contact for what.

Being an active participant in your plan

You are the most important part of achieving the best possible health and life for you. After you leave a health professional's room, it is you who needs to implement the best management of your condition, such as taking the medicine, doing the exercises, monitoring your condition and making changes to your life. You should:

- Understand your role and responsibilities in the healthcare plan.
- Understand your role in organising tests and follow-up.
- Follow your healthcare plan.
- Watch for and manage the early warning signs and symptoms related to your condition.

Actively seeking support

- Actively seek knowledge, skills and support.
- Involve family, friends and colleagues as appropriate.
- Ask for help and support, but don't feel you have to disclose information if you don't wish to.

Understanding your medicine

Medicine can be very confusing. There are often different names and dosages for the same medicine; some medicine is taken with food, some on an empty stomach, and for some it doesn't matter; some need to be refrigerated; some can only be used for a maximum number of days; some start working in hours, some need to be used for months before you know if they are having an effect; some need regular tests for their levels, some need tests to check they haven't caused you problems, and some need no tests; some your doctor only wants you to take for a short time, some for a long time; some interact with other medicine, complementary medicine and even foods.

To help ensure your medicine works for you, you should:

- Understand what each medicine is for, how to take it, how long to take it and what the effects and side effects might be. Review the consumer medicine information (CMI) provided with your medicine to learn about the benefits and any possible side effects.
- Understand if any monitoring is required and if so how this will be organised, how you will be notified of the results and what action you need to take according to the results.
- Know when to stop your medicine, change your dosage or call your doctor.
- Talk to your doctor if you have any queries or concerns about your medicine.
- Keep a list of your current prescription and over-the-counter medicines and allergies with you.

- Tell your doctor about any complementary medicines you take.

- Tell your doctor about any allergies or sensitivities.

- If you have a serious allergy, make sure your family and friends also know about it, and consider wearing a medical alert bracelet.

Keeping a record of important information

- Keep a record of your medical information, including test results, medicines, allergies, diagnosis and healthcare providers. This may be in the form of a healthcare plan developed in conjunction with your GP. See the sample healthcare plan at the end of this chapter.

- Ask for copies of test results, surgical reports and discharge summaries and letters from hospitals.

The federal government has developed a personally controlled health record system – the eHealth record. This eHealth record allows you to access your own medical record and allows other healthcare providers to access and add information to this record. Ask your GP or visit the Australian Government's eHealth website, www.ehealth.gov.au.

Developing and maintaining a healthy lifestyle

A healthy lifestyle (considering diet, activity, weight, sleep, mental health, smoking, alcohol and drugs) is an important part of managing all chronic health conditions. It can reduce risk factors, improve management and lessen the progression of the disease and its complications.

In addition, a healthy lifestyle and undertaking preventative health activities give some protection against getting acute health conditions that can negatively impact your chronic health condition, lessens the chance of developing other chronic health conditions, and keeps your body and mind in the best shape to deal with your health conditions.

You should:

- Make choices and take action to develop and maintain a healthy lifestyle.

- Know the modifiable risk factors and recommended lifestyle for your chronic condition.

- Address these lifestyle factors so you can better manage your condition.

- Stay properly immunised, have whatever screening is appropriate (see chapter 2) and address the preventative health aspects that are relevant for you and your health condition.

Managing pain

Pain management is a crucial part of managing chronic health conditions that involve pain. Pain is an individual experience that only you can fully understand. In chronic pain, the intensity and duration of pain can be unrelated to the amount of damage to the body. See chapter 25 for more on managing chronic pain.

Develop a holistic pain-management plan that puts you in control and, over time, with the help and support of others, learn to manage the pain. You should try to:

- Have a support team, possibly consisting of your GP, other health professionals, friends, family, pain support groups and chronic pain clinics.
- Understand your pain – what it signifies and how it affects you.
- Understand what triggers, worsens and helps your pain.
- Understand your pain medicine, its effects and when and how to use it.
- Understand and use non-medicine strategies that work for your pain (such as rest, activity, hot and cold packs or stretching).
- Understand and use the power of your mind in managing pain.
- Establish goals and strategies to manage your pain.

Coming to terms with your health condition

To live well with a chronic condition you really do need to come to terms with it. It does not define you, nor does it mean that you need to accept that you will always have it, but you need to deal with it in the best way possible in order to minimise its negative effects, manage its impact on your body, emotions and relationships, and live well.

Some ways to achieve this are to:

- Understand how your health condition affects your body, mind and emotions, and the flow-on effects of this on the way you feel, think and act.
- Work through this to feelings, thoughts and actions that are positive for your health and the way you function and live your life.
- Take an active part in healthcare decisions and management.
- Rest – a chronic health condition can be tiring and drain your energy. Learn how to pace yourself, read the signs and communicate this to others. Understand what helps your stamina.

- Be clear with yourself, family and others about what you can and can't do. This can be especially difficult if you don't look sick or if you once did something you can no longer manage.

- Remember that the effect on your life often fluctuates. Just because you can't manage something today doesn't mean you won't be able to in the future.

- Remember what you can do, and try not to let what you can't do consume you. Work on what you can change and accept what you can't change. Don't lose time and effort in worry and regret.

- Actively seek support and work with your healthcare providers, family and friends.

- Learn and maintain good ways of dealing with difficulty (see chapter 2).

- Learn when to ask for help or seek support and professional help if you need to (see chapter 2).

> **Caring for someone with a chronic condition**
> Chapter 41 provides a detailed discussion of caring for someone with a chronic condition.

A sample healthcare plan

Date: May 2014

Name: Mary Isabelle Rosta

Address: 7 Healthy Lane, Heartwell

Date of birth: 16/12/1951

Home number: 1111

Mobile number: 111

Language/interpreter required: English/No

Medicare number: 1234

Private health insurance details: 2345

Partner's contact details: Nick Riley, mobile: 0413

Healthcare providers and contact details:

GP: Matthew Van Mark	1111
Diabetes Educator: Elinor Busso	2222
Dietician: Sarsha Kevins	3333

Podiatrist: Tom Henry   4444
Ophthalmologist: Gemma Dean   5555
Dentist: Lina Robb   6666

Allergies: Penicillin – bad rash

Medicine:
Insulin: NovoMix 30: 10–14 units twice a day by injection under the skin on my abdomen
Paracetamol: two tablets, only sometimes

Smoker: Never

Alcohol: 1–2 drinks most nights

Complementary medicine: fish oil tablets every day

Other medicine or drugs: None

About me: I'm a 62-year-old (mostly) happily married woman with two adult children living out of home and three grandchildren. I was born in Malta but came here when I was five years old. I worked as an administrative assistant but stopped two years ago. I have lots of friends and my husband works three days a week doing gardening. We have paid off our house and get by okay. We take our caravan to Queensland for two months every year. I enjoy cooking, book club and gentle yoga.

About my health: I was found to have diabetes five years ago after my doctor did a blood test because I was so tired and was getting vaginal thrush a lot. I started on tablets and tried to lose weight. The tablets weren't controlling my blood sugars well enough so I started on insulin four months ago. I had trouble doing it at first but am now confident in taking my blood sugars, using the insulin and changing the dose a little according to my blood sugars, if I'm sick and how I'm eating. The doctor also found my cholesterol was up a little. I am having trouble getting my weight down. I have never smoked but do drink a little. I don't take any medicine except for Panadol sometimes and what my doctor gives me.

My healthcare plan

Problem	Goal	Action	Who can help
Diabetes: sugar levels	• Improve sugar control: aim for HbA1C < 6 • No hypoglycaemic episodes • Hope to one day get off insulin to tablets again	Check blood sugars three times a day	Me
		Insulin amount changed as required as the diabetes educator taught me	• Me • Phone diabetes educator if problem
		Always have my diabetic lollies on me	• Me • Tell doctor if I get any hypoglycaemic episodes
		Think about my food and insulin matching	• Me • Diabetes educator
		Blood tests for HbA1C	GP – every three months
		See diabetes educator every two months and doctor every three months	Me to organise
Diabetes: complications	To get no problems with feet, eyes, kidneys, heart, brain and legs	Eye check with ophthalmologist once a year	Me to organise
		Foot check with podiatrist once a year	Me to organise
		Check feet every week, maintain nails as instructed, wear well-fitting footwear, tell doctor at first sign of problem	Me
Being overweight and not doing enough physical activity	Decrease weight to 80 kg in three months	• Keep to my eating plan • Weigh myself once a month	Me Dietician to review every six months – me to organise
	Do some exercise every day	Walk for 45 minutes every day	Me

Problem	Goal	Action	Who can help
High lipids (cholesterol and triglycerides)	Reduce lipids so I don't need tablets	<ul><li>Lose weight</li><li>Keep to eating plan</li><li>Be more active</li><li>Control sugars</li></ul>	GP – blood test every six months
Stay healthy	Keep active and doing what I enjoy, and keep my relationships strong	Check-up with my GP (blood pressure, weight, blood and urine tests)	GP – every three months
		Flu vaccination	GP – every year
		Mammogram	BreastScreen – every two years – me to organise
		Pap test	GP – every two years
		Faecal occult blood test (bowel cancer test)	GP – every two years
		Floss teeth every day	Me
		Yearly dental check	Dentist – me to organise
		Yoga twice a week	Me
		Book group once a week	Me
		Eat healthily, no alcohol for three days a week and only two glasses on other days	Me
		Holiday in Queensland every year	My husband and me

33

Menopause

Martha Hickey, Jennifer Marino

Menopause is a natural event for women. All women who live into their 50s will experience menopause, sometimes called 'the change of life', 'the climacteric', or simply 'the change'. Menopause is defined by the final menstrual period – which marks the permanent cessation of menstruation. In the lead-up to menopause the ovaries function less efficiently, resulting in changes in the levels of oestrogen and other hormones, until eventually your periods stop. You are said to be 'postmenopausal' after you have had no period for 12 months in a row. Menopause may occur naturally or as the result of medication or surgical procedures. Menopause marks the end of a woman's ability to conceive.

When does menopause happen?

The average age at menopause is 51, but it may occur at an earlier or later age, and the reasons for this are not well understood. When menopause happens before the age of 40 it is called 'premature', and when it happens before the age of 45 it is called 'early'; these are both discussed in more detail later in this chapter. For some women menopause may occur at roughly the same age as it did for their mothers and sisters. On average, smokers undergo menopause around two years earlier than other women, and women who have had a hysterectomy may have an earlier menopause. No clear relationships have been found between age at menopause and ethnic background, age at first period, use of oral contraceptives, or use of fertility medications.

Why does menopause happen?

Two hormones made by the ovaries – oestrogen and progesterone – control the activity of the ovaries and the environment inside the uterus (womb). During our childbearing years, these hormones act together to cause the release of a mature egg for fertilisation (ovulation) and the preparation of the uterine lining (endometrium) to accept a fertilised egg.

If no egg arrives, the hormone levels drop and the uterine lining is shed, as a menstrual period. As we age, our ovarian reserve – the number of eggs in the ovaries capable of being fertilised – begins to fall, and hormonal activity becomes more erratic and less synchronised. Eventually, the levels of hormones drop below those needed to stimulate ovulation or the growth and shedding of the endometrium, so menstruation ends permanently.

How do I know if I am experiencing menopause?

The most common symptoms women experience in the menopausal transition are changes in menstrual patterns, vaginal dryness, hot flushes and night sweats. In Western cultures, hot flushes and night sweats are the main symptoms of menopause. For some Asian women, body and joint aches and pains are the most troublesome symptoms. For women who experience these symptoms close to the average age of menopause (over 45) there is usually no reason to perform any special tests. For younger women (under 45), hormone tests may be helpful to confirm the diagnosis and to exclude other possible causes of their symptoms. Since hormonal levels commonly fluctuate on a daily basis, the blood tests may need to be repeated in order to confirm the diagnosis.

For more on symptoms, see below.

The stages of menopause

Perimenopause

For some years before the final menstrual period, body changes may occur due to changes in ovarian hormone levels. This time is known as peri-menopause (meaning 'around menopause'), or the menopause transition. During the menopause transition, oestrogen levels vary between high and low. Hot flushes, changes in the frequency and heaviness of menstrual periods, vaginal dryness, mood changes and sleeping problems are common during this time. Some women are still able to conceive during the meno-pause transition, so you should continue to use contraception until at least 12 months after your final period if you don't wish to become pregnant. Hormone replacement therapy (HRT) has no contraceptive effect.

Natural menopause

Natural menopause is the spontaneous, permanent termination of men-struation, not caused by any medical treatment or surgery. It is confirmed by 12 consecutive months without menstrual periods.

Postmenopause

The time that follows menopause is called postmenopause. This can make up a third of our lives, or more.

Changes around menopause

Changes in menstrual periods

Changes in menstrual flow and frequency are common during the menopause transition. A few women simply stop menstruating, but most women experience four to eight years of menstrual cycle changes before the last period. Periods may become irregular, and often cycles become shorter than 28 days. Bleeding may last fewer days or more days, and flow may become heavier or lighter, especially during late menopause, but this varies from woman to woman. These changes arise because ovarian hormone production varies and ovulation is less frequent. In late menopause, women often follow a missed period with a normal menstrual cycle. These changes can be annoying and inconvenient, but they are normal.

You should consult your doctor if you have any of the following changes, which may be abnormal:

- heavier menstrual bleeding
- periods lasting more than seven days, or two or more days longer than usual
- intervals shorter than 21 days between the start of one period and the start of the next
- spotting or bleeding between periods
- vaginal bleeding after intercourse

Eventually periods stop completely. Any woman who has vaginal bleeding after menopause should see her doctor to rule out serious problems (including cancer).

Changes in the body

Physical changes associated with menopause usually begin in our 40s, although some women experience them as early as their 30s. Some symptoms of menopause can also indicate problems such as thyroid disorders or depression, so it is important to discuss symptoms with your doctor. A major change of perimenopause is the loss of fertility. The declining number and quality of eggs, as well as age-related changes to the uterus, make it gradually more difficult for a woman to fall pregnant after her late 30s. The risks of miscarriage are also increased. During midlife, the risk of health problems for the mother, such as high blood pressure and gestational diabetes, also rises. Although women are less fertile during peri-menopause, they can still fall pregnant. If you do not want to conceive, you need to use appropriate contraception (see chapter 16).

Bone strength builds up through teenage life and our bones are strong-est between the ages of 20 and 30 (this is called peak bone mass). With menopause, the rate of bone loss increases for a time, with about a 15 per cent loss in the first five years, then slowing to 1.5 per cent a year. By the age of 65, one in four women has had a broken bone related to osteoporosis (meaning 'porous or weak bones'). By the age of 80, without intervention, many women have dropped to 70 per cent of their peak bone mass. The risk of osteoporosis is higher for women whose peak bone mass is lower, or who lose bone more quickly than normal. Family history, smoking, lack of weight-bearing exercise, more than two alcoholic drinks a day, use of certain medications (such as steroids), being underweight (with a BMI of less than 18.5; see chapter 14) and low dietary calcium or vitamin D all increase the rate of bone loss and the risk of osteoporosis and fractures.

Cardiovascular disease (CVD) is the leading cause of death in women. If you experience early menopause you may be at increased risk of CVD, and should discuss with your doctor how to maintain a healthy heart and blood vessels. (See chapter 32 for more on CVD.)

Menopausal symptoms

Hot flushes and night sweats

The most common menopause symptoms are hot flushes and night sweats, which affect around 80 per cent of women. Hot flushes can range from a warming sensation that lasts a few seconds to a sudden feeling of intense heat spreading over the upper body and face, with heavy perspira-tion and sometimes reddening of the skin, accompanied by nausea, racing or pounding heartbeat, or heavy breathing, lasting one to five or even as long as 15 minutes. Some women have chills instead of or after a hot flush. Night sweats are hot flushes with heavy perspiration that may wake you from sleep.

The mechanism of hot flushes and night sweats is not well understood, but it is thought that they arise as a consequence of changes to the hypo-thalamus, the part of the brain that acts as our temperature control centre. Ordinarily, above a certain temperature, the hypothalamus initiates sweating and other behaviours to lose heat, and below a certain temperature, it stimulates shivering and chills to gain heat. During menopause, these two threshold temperatures grow closer together, so you may react more extremely to warm and cool temperatures that previously did not bother you and so sweat and shiver more easily.

The pattern of hot flushes is usually consistent for each woman. Some women have flushes for only a few months, while others have them for many years. Flushes may be triggered by certain food or situations, and may be associated with feelings of embarrassment or anxiety.

Insomnia

In addition to the problems with sleep brought on by hot flushes and night sweats, insomnia is a common difficulty of menopause. Most adults require six to nine hours of sleep, and most people find that they experience less restful sleep as they age. The exact number of hours is not as important as whether you feel alert during your waking hours. Excessive daytime sleepiness should be investigated by your doctor, as there are many treatable causes of poor sleep other than menopause.

Mood changes

Mood changes affect many women during menopause. These may include tearfulness, mood swings, lack of energy, anxiety, panic attacks, or feeling blue, low, downhearted or depressed. Women who have a history of depression are more likely to experience depression at menopause. The link between depression and menopause is not well understood, but may relate to the frequency and severity of hot flushes, ongoing sleep disturbance or other life changes that are common at this time. Some women are distressed because they feel out of control of their bodies during this time of change. Others may be experiencing challenges typical of the midlife, such as ending or starting romantic relationships, the 'empty nest' (adult children leaving the home), the 'refilled nest' (adult children returning home), financial or career changes, or concerns about ageing parents. Just getting older can be a tricky proposition in a society that values youth.

Memory changes

Changes in memory and concentration are often a source of complaint, but there is no good evidence that menopause has any permanent negative effect on memory or thinking. These problems may instead be caused by sleep problems and stress.

Genital symptoms

Symptoms affecting the vulva (the outer part of the female genitals), vagina and bladder may arise from the menopausal change in hormones, or may be caused by other treatable problems such as sexually transmitted infections (STIs), skin conditions, thrush and allergies. The decrease in oestrogen can cause the tissues of the vulva and vagina to become thin, dry and inelastic, and may also cause a decrease in lubricating secretions during sexual activity. Changes in the bladder may lead to urinary frequency. In some women, this condition may worsen, resulting in inflammation. Inflamed tissues are more susceptible to injury during both everyday and sexual activity, and to infection. You should discuss any new or changed vaginal discharge, odour, irritation, burning, itch or pain with your doctor. (See chapter 26 for more on genital irritations and infections.)

Sex drive (libido) changes

Some women find that they experience changes in sexual desire during menopause. While some women find a new freedom from worry about unwanted pregnancy, others may find they are not as interested in sexual activity as they once were. Symptoms of menopause, such as mood changes, sleep disruption and genital discomfort, may negatively affect some women's desire for and enjoyment of sexual activity. Reduced ovarian production of oestrogen and testosterone may also affect sex drive. In addition, the life changes unrelated to menopause mentioned earlier may have varying effects on sexual desire during and after menopause. Sex drive changes become a problem only if you or your partner is troubled by them. Some couples are comfortable with a change in their sexual activity as they age.

Incontinence

Up to 50 per cent of women have difficulty with urinary incontinence (accidental leakage of urine) during midlife. Stress incontinence – loss of urine caused by weak pelvic floor muscles – results in leakage after coughing, sneezing, laughing or lifting objects. Lack of oestrogen can cause the thinning of the lining of the urethra (the tube that empties urine from the bladder), and ageing can weaken the surrounding pelvic muscles. Consequently, stress incontinence becomes more common during the menopause transition and postmenopause. Overactive bladder symptoms, caused by irritated or hyperactive bladder muscles, include frequent sudden urges to urinate, with occasional leakage. Mixed urinary incontinence is the combination of stress incontinence and over-active bladder. There are different treatments for incontinence and these may require specialised urinary tests (urodynamics) and either medical or surgical therapies. Physiotherapy can sometimes also be helpful (see chapter 18).

Prolapse

Prolapse, a condition where the supporting muscles of the vagina, bladder and bowel become weakened, is also more common with age. Prolapse is more common in women who have had children, especially those who have had difficult vaginal deliveries, as well as those who are overweight and those with a chronic cough (often smokers). Exercises and physio-therapy may help, but prolapse sometimes needs surgical treatment. For those who do not wish to have surgery, prolapse can also be treated using a vaginal pessary to support the uterus. This can be done as an out-patient procedure. (See chapter 39 for more on prolapse.)

Managing menopause symptoms

Lifestyle changes

Some lifestyle changes can address several menopause symptoms at once. Stress reduction (see the box below) helps improve sleep, mood and sexual desire, and may improve heart health.

Stress reduction

- Use meditation and relaxation techniques (www.themeditation podcast.com provides free meditation podcasts).
- Have a chat with friends.
- Make time for play, daily exercise and nutritious meals.
- Practise one-minute mindfulness: name five things you can hear, see, smell, touch right now (see www.marc.ucla.edu for informa-tion on mindfulness).
- Choose and watch a cloud or an ant – a detail of the world around you – for five minutes.
- Stand up and stretch – roll your shoulders up and around in a circular motion.

Sleep

Good 'sleep hygiene' is central to improving mood, memory and concentration. Sticking to a regular sleep schedule, with a consistent bedtime and rising time, is a good start. Keep your bedroom quiet, dark and cool, and reserve it for sleep and sexual activity. If you cannot fall asleep within around half an hour, get up, leave the room and engage in soothing, relaxing activity somewhere else, returning to bed when you become drowsy, so you do not form an association between your bedroom and anxious sleeplessness or restless activity. Avoid heavy meals in the evening, and keep alcohol, nicotine and caffeine to a minimum during the day. Earplugs and an eye mask may be helpful, although some people find them uncomfortable.

If you have problems with night sweats, dress in light cotton nightclothes and use sheets and garments that absorb moisture from the skin. Use layered bedding instead of heavy doonas, to allow you to adjust your temperature easily at night, and consider using a small fan to keep air moving at night. A frozen cold pack under the pillow will ensure you can always turn it over for a fresh, cool side on which to rest your head.

Exercise

Daily exercise may help with sleep, mood and concentration, and has a direct positive impact on heart and bone health. You should try to accumulate at least 30–60 minutes of moderate-intensity aerobic exercise (exercise that affects your heart rate and breathing) most days. You are exercising with moderate intensity if you still have the breath to carry on a conversation, but not to sing. Any form of movement is an opportunity to improve your health. Both formal exercise and increased activity in daily life contribute to good health. This could be as simple as gardening or getting off the bus a stop early and walking. If you have not been active for a long time, build up slowly to the recommended amount.

Recognising your hot flush triggers

You can help reduce the number and perhaps the severity of hot flushes by identifying and avoiding personal hot flush triggers. These might include spicy food, hot food or drinks, use of a hair dryer, having a bath, cigarettes, caffeine and alcohol. Avoid gaining weight, as this may make hot flushes worse. Cooling gels containing menthol may provide relief and refreshment, as may washing your hands in cold water or putting a cold compress on the back of your neck.

Non-prescription remedies for hot flushes

Non-prescription natural remedies can help some women. Soy foods, foods rich in phytoestrogens (see chapter 31) and isoflavone (phyto-estrogen) supplements have not been consistently shown to reduce hot flushes. The herb black cohosh may have a mild effect but studies have been inconsistent. These compounds may have oestrogen-like effects, so discuss with your doctor whether they are safe for you. Other botanicals promoted for this purpose – including evening primrose oil, dong quai, ginseng, licorice and sage – have not been shown to be effective in clinical trials.

Prescription medication for hot flushes

There are now a number of prescription medications that are effective for hot flushes and night sweats, some of which may also improve mood and sleep. These include a low-dose antidepressant such as venlafaxine, desvenlafaxine, escitalopram, citalopram or paroxetine, or other drugs including clonidine and gabapentin. Clonidine is generally used to treat high blood pressure, but can be used to reduce menopause-related hot flushes after breast cancer. Gabapentin is used to treat epilepsy and chronic pain, and can also be effective in reducing hot flushes. Non-hormonal treatments for hot flushes appear to be effective in one to two weeks. If there is no improvement over this period, talk to your doctor about modifying treatment approaches. Let your doctor know if you are also taking tamoxifen, as this may interact with some of these non-hormonal treatments.

Psychological treatments for hot flushes

Psychological treatments such as cognitive behaviour therapy may be effective in reducing the impact or troublesomeness of hot flushes and night sweats.

Hormone replacement therapy (HRT)

Many of the symptoms of menopause are thought to occur because of the change and eventual fall in ovarian production of oestrogen. Hormone replacement therapy (HRT) works by supplying oestrogen to relieve menopausal symptoms. Some HRT formulations, called combined HRT, also include a second hormone, progesterone. Oestrogen taken without progesterone ('unopposed oestrogen') can increase the risk of cancer of the lining of the uterus (endometrial cancer), so women who have not had a hysterectomy need combined HRT to protect against this type of cancer. Women who have had a hysterectomy can use oestrogen alone.

Oestrogens can be taken by mouth, in a patch, gel or cream applied to the skin, or in a gel or cream inserted into the vagina. Progesterone can be taken by mouth, by a patch, gel or cream applied to the skin, or by means of an IUS contraceptive device (Mirena; see chapter 16). Tibolone is a synthetic hormone taken by mouth that acts like both oestrogen and progesterone.

How do I decide whether or not to take HRT?

HRT is the most effective treatment currently available for troublesome hot flushes and night sweats. Clinical trials comparing HRT to a placebo (inactive medication) found that the severity of hot flushes decreased by nearly 90 per cent and frequency by around 18 flushes a week. Large trials have also shown that HRT decreases the risk of bone fracture, improves vaginal dryness, and may improve sleep, muscle aches and pains, and quality of life. Oral combined HRT increases the risk of blood clots in the legs and lungs, stroke and gallbladder disease. Women might also experience an induced premenstrual disorder when taking HRT, but usually your doctor will be able to find a type and/or dose of HRT that does not induce premenstrual-type symptoms. HRT should be avoided in women who already have heart disease, but it is not clear whether any formulation of HRT increases or decreases the risk of heart disease in healthy women. HRT does not help treat urinary incontinence.

Combined HRT is also associated with a slightly higher than average risk of developing and dying from breast cancer. This risk is increased with longer use of combined HRT. We do not know whether tibolone or unopposed oestrogen change a woman's risk of breast cancer. As mentioned above, unopposed oestrogen can increase the risk of endometrial cancer.

In addition to these negative events that affect only a few users, all formulations of HRT have side effects, including breast tenderness, nausea and vaginal bleeding. Although most side effects disappear after a few months, vaginal bleeding can also be a sign of other health problems, including endometrial cancer, so any bleeding should be evaluated by your doctor.

As HRT is a prescription medication, you will need to discuss your decision to use it with your doctor. You should feel free to ask your doctor any questions and raise any concerns you may have before you make a decision about using HRT. You should tell them if you have any personal history of breast cancer, uterine cancer, ovarian cancer, abnormal mammograms, blood clots or clotting disorders, high blood pressure, heart disease, stroke, liver problems or migraine. The risks of heart disease, blood clots, high blood pressure and stroke are higher among women who smoke, so taking HRT may not be safe if you smoke.

Early menopause

Women whose periods stop completely and permanently before the age of 40 are said to have premature menopause. This condition may arise because of surgery or treatment that removes or damages the ovaries at any age (called 'induced menopause'), or it may arise because of 'primary ovarian insufficiency' (POI). Women with POI have ovaries that are less responsive than normal to follicle stimulating hormone (FSH), resulting in irregular and infrequent periods, and elevated FSH levels in the blood. Women with POI do sometimes ovulate, so pregnancy is possible, and thus contraception is needed to avoid pregnancy. Women with POI may have menopausal symptoms even before menopause, and POI may go on for many years before menopause.

The symptoms of early menopause are the same as those of menopause at the usual time of life. When the cause of early menopause is surgery, the immediate drop in hormones can produce more noticeable and more disruptive symptoms. Menopause at a younger age increases vulnerability to bone loss and heart disease, because the protection of natural ovarian hormones is lost. It may induce intense, complex emotional responses, particularly in the context of being treated for cancer or another serious illness. You may also still experience a premenstrual disorder (see chapter 6 for more on this) even if you no longer menstruate. Early menopause is particularly difficult for women who have not yet started or completed their families. There may be still options for parenting, and these can be discussed with a fertility specialist.

Cancer chemotherapy and radiation therapy are both intended to injure or kill cancer cells and prevent tumours from growing, but both can also damage healthy tissue, including the ovaries. If you require cancer treatment, you should consider your plans for a family and discuss with your healthcare providers the available options for fertility preservation before treatment begins. In addition to causing menopausal symptoms (including vaginal dryness), some chemotherapy and pelvic radiation treatments can irritate and inflame the vagina and vulva. With some types of radiotherapy, some women need physiotherapy to prevent permanent shrinkage of the vagina.

Experiencing menopause

Movie stereotypes often wrongly portray menopausal women as crazy or hysterical. This is an unhelpful and inaccurate view of menopause. Realistically, most women have a positive attitude to menopause, and many see it as an opportunity to refocus on themselves.

Whether menopause has occurred naturally as part of a woman's life cycle or has occurred early as the result of medication or surgical procedures, there is evidence that a woman's attitudes towards and knowledge of menopause affects her experience.

It appears that women with more negative expectations of menopause may experience more troublesome symptoms. Age at menopause may also affect a woman's experience: women going through menopause closer to the average age may be less alarmed by their symptoms and, perhaps, more informed about what to expect than women going through menopause at a younger age.

Understanding what symptoms to expect, realising that most women are able to deal with their symptoms without treatment, and having a more positive outlook on menopause will all be helpful in managing this life stage.

34

Complementary and natural therapies and medicines

Vicki Kotsirilos

Recent studies demonstrate that up to 70 per cent of people are using some form of complementary medicine or therapy on a regular basis. The majority of people using these therapies are women over the age of 60, from many different backgrounds. In Australia, studies demonstrate that people are spending more out of their own pockets on complementary medicines than on pharmaceuticals.

What is complementary medicine?

The term complementary medicine is generally used to describe natural or non-drug medicines or therapies that are not part of mainstream medical care, but can be used alongside mainstream care. Many of our current pharmaceuticals are derived from herbs. For example, aspirin (salicylic acid) was chemically synthesised in 1860 from the herb white willow bark, which is rich in salicylates and was traditionally considered a useful painkiller.

In this chapter complementary medicine will be used broadly to describe these therapies. As the evidence accumulates over time for some complementary medicines, they will become integrated more into mainstream care. For example, some complementary medicines such as meditation, fish oils and vitamin D are already prescribed regularly by GPs, and many GPs offer acupuncture with a Medicare rebate.

For the majority of complementary medicines, however, there is a lack of scientific evidence of their usefulness, although some demonstrate better evidence than others. Complementary medicines that have useful supporting scientific evidence include acupuncture for pain; some herbs such as St John's wort for depression; and nutrients such as vitamin B6, vitamin D, magnesium, calcium and fish oils. Other complementary medicines significantly lack scientific evidence – such as homeopathy, kinesiology and reflexology; some have been shown not to work; and others may cause side effects and be harmful. Please check what these risks are with your doctor and other healthcare providers if you choose to trial complementary medicines. Some of the major complementary or natural therapies are outlined in the following list.

Alternative (or philosophical) medical systems

- Naturopathy
- Traditional Chinese medicine
- Traditional Indian medicine – Ayurveda
- Homeopathy
- Anthroposophic medicine

Mind–body medicine

- Meditation, relaxation therapies, breathwork, biofeedback
- Psychological therapies – cognitive therapies, psychotherapies, hypnosis, visualisation
- Support groups
- Spiritual healing, prayer, reiki, therapeutic touch, distant healing
- Creative therapies – art therapy, music therapy, dance therapy

Biologically based or medicinally based therapies

- Herbs: Western herbal medicine, Chinese herbal medicine, Ayurveda (Indian) herbal medicine, herbal extracts
- Dietary and nutritional changes
- Dietary supplements such as vitamins, minerals, amino acids, food supplements, natural supplements or extracts, dietary products
- Aromatherapy, Bach flower essences

Manipulative or manual-based therapies

- Therapeutic touch: massage, manipulation, chiropractic, osteopathy, acupressure
- Mind–body movements: Feldenkrais, Alexander technique, Pilates, yoga, tai chi, qi gong
- Reflexology, kinesiology

Energy or bioenergetic-based therapies

- Acupuncture
- Electromagnetic fields
- TENS (trans-electrical nerve stimulation)

Note: this list does not incorporate all complementary medicines and therapies, and some may belong to more than one classification.

What is integrative medicine?

Most doctors now prefer the term integrative medicine to complementary medicine as it describes the blending of complementary medicines with demonstrated scientific evidence into their medical practice; focuses on the whole person; and makes use of all appropriate therapeutic approaches, qualified healthcare professionals and disciplines when and if needed. Many people find integrative medicine appealing because it implies that their doctor, with their consent and decision-making input, will choose whichever treatment – be it orthodox or complementary medicine – is appropriate and suitable to their needs. Some doctors integrate more complementary medicines into their clinical practice than others.

Finding reliable information about complementary medicines

It is often difficult to know which complementary medicines are clinically useful for a particular condition and which are safe. Some people believe that because something is natural, it will be safe. While natural therapies and complementary medicines overall have been proven to be safer than surgery, pharmaceuticals or drugs, there are still issues of concern with them.

When using complementary medicines you should:

- Consider whether using them means you are delaying useful orthodox treatments or the treatments your doctor recommends, which may be detrimental for you and your condition.
- Be aware there may be risks if they do not work.
- Be aware that they may have side effects, known or unknown. Like all medicine and therapy, if it can be helpful, it has potential side effects.
- Ensure that you identify those that are safe and useful for your condition.

- Consider the costs associated with buying them or seeing a complementary medicine practitioner.
- Consider whether the complementary medicine practitioner is well qualified and informs you well.
- Be aware of all options for your health problem, including complementary medicines and orthodox medicine, and weigh the pros and cons.
- Check whether they interact with your pharmaceutical medicine(s).
- Check whether they are inappropriate for your health condition; for example, if you suffer from liver or kidney disease.
- Make sure you will benefit from them, and find out how long they will take to work.

It is a good idea to discuss your treatment options with your GP or specialist and allow them to monitor your response to the treatment. More and more doctors are now interested in this area and are learning more about complementary medicines, particularly the scientific evidence behind them and any safety concerns associated with their use. Most doctors understand and accept that many of their patients use complementary medicines. Mostly their concerns relate to those complementary medicines lacking scientific evidence or for which there can be safety concerns associated with their use or interactions with other therapies. GPs can also be concerned that in pursuing complementary medicines you may delay beneficial treatment.

Many people use the internet to find information about complementary medicines, which can be quite confusing. The volume of information and the different, changing research in this area can be overwhelming. When sourcing information about complementary medicines, you should seek reliable evidence from trusted sources. The Resources section at the end of this book offers some reliable web links and books you can trust to provide the real evidence.

Finding qualified complementary medicine or integrated medicine practitioners

Word-of-mouth is often the best source of recommendation for a good practitioner. A doctor who practises integrated medicine may advise you on the best treatment for you, be it a conventional treatment, a complementary treatment or a combination. If you decide to trial a complementary medicine in place of or alongside mainstream care, ensure that you and your doctor are satisfied with this approach, are fully aware of potential known risks, and are aware that other risks may be unknown. As mentioned, your doctor should monitor your response to the treatment and record your treatment outcome.

There are now a number of peak organisations that represent health practitioners with expertise in complementary medicines who are regulated by the federal government's Australian Health Practitioner Regulation Agency (AHPRA, www.ahpra.gov.au). These health practitioners include doctors, nurses, midwives, dentists, physiotherapists, podiatrists, psychologists, osteopaths, chiropractors and Chinese medicine practitioners among others (see the AHPRA website for the full list of practitioners and links to the peak organisations). This ensures some safety, as AHPRA regulates practitioners who are adequately qualified and can deregister or apply restrictions of practice to practitioners about whom concerns have been raised. Not all complementary and alternative practitioners are regulated by AHPRA, and even unregistered practitioners can continue to practise in the community, which can be dangerous.

Medical practitioners who practise integrative medicine and combine complementary medicines may be members of several organisations. Try the following websites to find a suitable medical practitioner with an interest in women's health:

- Australasian College of Nutritional and Environmental Medicine: www.acnem.org
- Australasian Integrative Medicine Association: www.aima.net.au
- Australian Medical Acupuncture College: www.amac.org.au

Naturopaths and herbalists are not registered with AHPRA. They are self-regulated through the Australian Register of Naturopaths and Herbalists (ARONAH, www.aronah.org), which sets minimum standards of practice for naturopaths and herbalists to ensure a level of safety.

Treating conditions with complementary medicine

Natural therapies for menstrual problems

Period-related conditions that may be relieved with complementary medicine include:

- premenstrual syndrome (PMS; see chapter 6)
- premenstrual dysphoric disorder (PMDD; see chapter 6)

- dysmenorrhoea, painful periods and menstrual cramps (see chapter 25)
- breast pain or swelling before periods (mastalgia; see chapter 37)

You can help some of the troubling problems associated with your cycles by improving your lifestyle. Research suggests that a healthy diet, avoiding salt in your cooking and food, reducing caffeine intake, restoring your sleep cycle, regular daily exercise and reducing stress may help improve your quality of life and significantly reduce the severity of PMS symptoms, including moodiness and painful periods.

Your attitude to your menstrual cycle

Your early experience with menstruation, and the attitude of your mother, friends, sisters, and others towards menstruation, may influence your experience and attitude towards your period. This is often an area that is overlooked.

Think about your early experience of menstruation. Was it positive? Was it negative? How do you view your period now? How does your partner view your period? Do you welcome them or despise them? This is important. Studies suggest that women who have supportive partners, friends, family, teachers and employers deal with symptoms of menstruation better.

If you experienced difficulties in the past, such as verbal, sexual and physical assault, which you feel may be having a negative effect on your body and menstrual cycle, speak with your doctor, who can refer you to a suitable counsellor or psychologist. They may be able to help you understand your feelings, and how they affect your body and the symptoms you may be experiencing with menstruation.

Many ancient cultures celebrate the onset of periods as a time of fertility. In some cultures, women are encouraged to rest when they are menstruating. In Western society we commonly view our periods as negative and a nuisance, often coming at the wrong time, and are fearful they will interfere with some event such as going camping or on a holiday. It's important we assess our thoughts about our periods and try to view them positively – our body is doing what nature intends for us and periods signify fertility. Perhaps you need to consider doing less and resting while menstruating and reducing your overall stress load.

Diet

A growing body of evidence suggests that diets rich in omega-3 fatty acids, calcium and vitamin D, and low in animal fats, salt and caffeine may reduce the risk of troublesome PMS symptoms. This includes a diet high in vegetables (five serves per day), fruit (two serves per day), nuts, seeds, fish (up to three serves per week) and other sources of omega-3 foods such as flaxseed (linseed) or chia seeds, low-fat dairy food, protein foods such as lean meat, legumes and eggs, and a variety of whole grains such as brown rice, traditional rolled oats, buckwheat flour, wholegrain organic breads, wholemeal pasta, couscous, millet or amaranth. Lean meat (red meat or free-range organic chicken) is an important source of iron and protein, especially for women with heavy periods. Avoid foods rich in saturated fats such as butter, cream, bacon and chips; limit salt and caffeine. Drink more water and calming herbal teas such as chamomile. Increase your intake of calcium-rich foods such as nuts, low-fat dairy products, fish with edible bones such as salmon and sardines, tofu, broccoli and bok choy.

Sleep

Studies have found that sleep disturbance is common in women who suffer severe PMS. Poor sleep can also contribute to mood disturbance, hormone irregularities and disturbed menstrual cycles. Shift workers are more likely to report menstrual problems. You can improve your sleep by trying the following:

- Exercise daily – exposure to sunlight can help produce the natural hormone melatonin, which induces sleep when released at night (see below).
- Avoid stimulants such as coffee and tea later in the day; avoid taking drugs such as caffeine, 'speed' and amphetamines.
- Avoid drinking fluids late at night to reduce your need to go to the toilet during the night.
- Avoid a heavy meal or spicy foods before bed, especially if you are prone to reflux.
- Develop a regular routine for bedtime.
- Go to bed the same time every day.
- Avoid bright lights before bed. Dim lights help the release of the sleep hormone melatonin.
- Relax before bed; have a warm bath with candles or a shower.

- Read a relaxing book before sleep as it may help.
- Use bedtime for sleep and sex; avoid arguments in bed with your partner or taking a laptop to bed.
- If you have stress or worries that are keeping you awake, speak to a friend or ask your GP for a referral to a counsellor to help deal with the worries and stop these negative thoughts keeping you awake.
- Use a diary to record your thoughts.
- Reduce your stress – try yoga and meditation.
- Drink calming teas – valerian, passionflower and chamomile teas may help induce sleep.
- Take melatonin supplements, which may help in some cases. Melatonin is a hormone and requires a prescription from your GP. It should only be used in the short term and under medical supervision. It is often used for jetlag. Homeopathic melatonin is available over the counter but has not been clinically trialled for efficacy.
- If you continue to have trouble sleeping, see your GP.

Sunshine and vitamin D

Sunshine may play a role in regulating hormones and sleep patterns by affecting the daily release of melatonin, a hormone produced in the pituitary gland in the brain from the chemical melanin, which is produced in the skin with sun exposure.

Sun exposure is also an important source of vitamin D. Ninety per cent of the vitamin D we get comes from skin exposure to sunlight, and less than 10 per cent from food sources such as fortified milk, eggs and some fish. Early research suggests that vitamin D may help normalise menstrual cycles (for example, in polycystic ovarian syndrome) and may help relieve muscular pains and mood disorders such as depression.

Exercise

Studies have found that women who exercise regularly are less likely to suffer menstrual pain, cramps and mood disturbance. We are not certain how exercise is helpful for PMS but studies demonstrate that exercise can release 'happy' hormones such as serotonin and endorphins, which may explain the benefit. Exercise daily for at least 30 minutes a day, outdoors if possible, for relaxation, sunshine and fresh air.

Yoga has been used for thousands of years as a mind–body approach to a number of health issues, including regulating the menstrual cycle, easing menstrual pain and helping hormonal imbalances.

Mindfulness meditation, stress reduction and relaxation therapies

Studies demonstrate if you are stressed, you are more likely to suffer severe symptoms of PMS and experience poorer quality of life. Regular relaxation is effective for reducing severe PMS, especially pain and emotional problems. Learn to practise deep-breathing relaxation or meditation. Local yoga centres often teach meditation, or ask your GP for a referral to a psychologist to help you learn relaxation strategies.

A small study found that weekly massages over five weeks improved the level of pain and mood disorders and reduced the fluid retention experienced by women during their menstrual cycle.

Recording your menstrual symptoms

Self-monitoring and recording your symptoms in a diary or on a calendar can help you understand your cycle and body better. A study found this helped women feel more comfortable with their symptoms, and reduced the severity of some of their premenstrual symptoms such as depression and moodiness. There are now many free apps that help you chart your symptoms in a calendar. You can learn more about your cycle and even estimate when you are most fertile using this method, although it is not entirely accurate.

Counselling

A number of studies have found that counselling or cognitive behaviour therapy that addresses negative thinking about periods and encourages positive thinking and behaviour patterns may help women feel more in control of their bodies, and help reduce the symptoms of PMS. When you feel good about yourself, you are more likely to eat better, exercise more, rest and look after yourself. Counselling can also help you explore any stress you suffer and deal with mood problems such as depression or anxiety. This also helps you deal with mood changes that may occur during your cycle. Counselling can also help women address recurring or persistent pelvic pain.

Physical therapies

Research suggests some physical therapies such as heat packs, TENS (trans-electrical nerve stimulation), acupuncture and acupressure are helpful for reducing menstrual pain and cramps. Physiotherapy may also be helpful for lower back pain associated with PMS.

Nutritional supplements

Many women take supplements such as vitamins, minerals and amino acids to help with the symptoms of PMS, but not all supplements have been shown to help. The table below lists supplements for which studies have demonstrated some scientific evidence of benefits, although more research is required with all of them. Check with your doctor to ensure there are no risks with you trying these supplements, some of which may interact with medication.

Nutritional supplements for PMS

Supplement	How it may help	Dosage and how to take it	Warnings and possible side effects
Vitamins B6 and B1	May reduce pain, cramps and mood disturbance	Vitamin B6: *do not exceed 50 mg a day*; vitamin B1: 100 mg a day Best if taken as a multi-B vitamin	Avoid high doses of vitamin B6 (more than 50 mg per day) and prolonged use, as this can cause nerve toxicity such as tingling, burning and shooting pains
Vitamin E (natural alpha-tocopherol)	May help reduce pain and menstrual blood flow	200 international units (IU) a day Commence two days before period is due and continue for first three days of period	This information is based on two small studies and more research is required May cause gut upset. Avoid high doses over 400 IU a day
Vitamin D	May help regulate menstrual cycle, relieve muscle pains, improve moods	1000 IU or more a day Check with your doctor, who will advise a suitable dosage for your needs	Vitamin D toxicity is rare but may occur with very high doses. This results in raised blood calcium levels, leading to feeling unwell, loss of appetite, thirst, constipation or diarrhoea, abdominal pain and muscle weakness, fatigue and confusion
Magnesium	May relieve menstrual cramps; improve premenstrual mood changes, especially irritability and anxiety; and help with muscle relaxation, muscle cramps and sleep	300 mg once or twice a day (best taken at night with calcium)	Reduce the dosage if you experience diarrhoea or loose stools May cause palpitations Avoid if you have kidney problems May lower blood pressure and cause heart arrhythmia, drowsiness and weakness in high doses

Supplement	How it may help	Dosage and how to take it	Warnings and possible side effects
Calcium	May reduce menstrual cramps, fluid retention, mood disorders and food cravings	1200 mg a day	May cause constipation or flatulence Avoid if you have kidney disease or high blood calcium levels May interact with blood pressure and heart tablets
Zinc	May reduce menstrual pain, cramping and depression, and provide immune enhancement	30 mg once to three times a day	This is based on small studies May cause nausea, gastrointestinal upset, a metallic taste in the mouth Avoid long-term use
Fish oils (omega-3 fatty acids)	May relieve menstrual pain, cramping, depression	1 g taken once to three times a day	May cause nausea and gastrointestinal upset In high doses, may 'thin' period blood (this may be useful if you have dark, thick menses) Avoid if allergic to seafood

Herbal remedies

The use of herbs for medicinal purposes dates back many thousands of years and is recorded in many cultures. The father of Western medicine, Hippocrates, prescribed many herbs such as St John's wort (*Hypericum perforatum*) and chaste tree (*Vitex agnus-castus*). Chaste-tree leaf was a favourite herb of Hippocrates, prepared as an extract soaked in wine for women to drink to relieve menstrual problems. Hippocrates recommended chewing the leaves of the white willow bark for pain relief during childbirth. White willow bark (*Salix alba*) is rich in the salicylates from which aspirin was derived. Fennel (*Foeniculum vulgare*) is a native of the Mediterranean region and was recommended for lactation problems. These herbs are now part of Western herbal medicine. There are many herbs also used traditionally in other cultures, such as in traditional Chinese medicine and Ayurvedic (Indian) medicine.

Today, science supports the use of St John's wort in the treatment of depression. St John's wort can interact with other medication such as the oral contraceptive pill and should never be taken with other anti-depressants, as this can cause a lethal reaction.

Several small studies suggest the berries of the chaste tree may help PMS and mood disorders associated with menstruation. A concentrated extract of fennel was shown to help reduce pain in women with menstrual cramps. Two trials of white willow bark found 'moderate evidence' that it reduces lower back pain and the need for medication when compared with a dummy tablet (placebo). Two small studies found that red clover (*Trifolium pratense*) may help reduce premenstrual breast pain due to their high phytoestrogen content. The research for this herb is weak and more studies are warranted to verify results.

Many herbalists also use a range of herbs such as dong quai (*Angelica sinensis*), cramp bark (*Viburnum opulus*), black cohosh (*Actaea racemosa*, formerly called *Cimicifuga racemosa*) and wild yam (*Dioscorea villosa*) for PMS and menstrual problems, but there is little evidence from research currently available that they work.

The table below lists the best researched herbs for the treatment of PMS, and the possible risks associated with taking them. Check with your doctor to ensure they are safe for you and will not interact with any medication you may be taking.

Herbal remedies for PMS

Herb	How it may help	Dosage and how to take it	Warnings and possible side effects
Chaste tree or chasteberry (*Vitex agnus-castus*)	May relieve PMS symptoms: irritability, mood changes, anger, headache, breast fullness and discomfort, abdominal bloating May help regulate menstrual cycle in PCOS	20 mg extract, one capsule a day	Generally safe but may cause gut disturbance or rash Avoid during pregnancy
St John's wort (*Hypericum perforatum*)	May relieve depression, mood disorders, premenstrual disturbed mood	300 mg twice to three times a day	Avoid taking with oral contraceptives, anticonvulsants and other antidepressants Check with your doctor if St John's wort interacts with your medication. Avoid during pregnancy. May cause dry mouth, gastrointestinal discomfort or skin rash

Herb	How it may help	Dosage and how to take it	Warnings and possible side effects
Evening primrose oil (*Oenothera biennis*)	May help reduce breast discomfort	1–3 g a day	Avoid if you suffer seizures or epilepsy
Red clover (*Trifolium pratense*)	May relieve premenstrual breast pain	40–80 mg a day	Avoid if taking blood thinners or if you have suffered oestrogen-sensitive tumours such as breast or uterine cancer
Traditional Chinese medicine	May help with PMS, hormonal disturbance	Must be prescribed by a trained Chinese herbalist	Check with a Chinese health practitioner

Natural therapies for menopausal problems

Menopause can affect us physically and emotionally and may cause a range of symptoms (see chapter 33). The most effective treatment for menopause is hormone replacement therapy (HRT), but many women are keen to trial lifestyle changes, complementary medicines and natural approaches before resorting to HRT. Things that may make menopausal symptoms worse include reduced physical activity, smoking, increased body weight and stress.

Many women find it a relief to have finished with menstruation, but some find it difficult to deal with the symptoms of menopause. In many cultures menopausal symptoms are not as common as in the West; this is the case, for example, for Greek peasant women and Mayan women in Mexico. It has been suggested that the diets of these women are rich in phytoestrogens derived from foods such as legumes and vegetables, which can help reduce the symptoms of menopause.

Studies suggest menopausal symptoms may be influenced by a range of factors, such as climate, diet, lifestyle, reproductive history, the mother's experience of menopause (how a mother expresses her experience and her attitude to menopause may influence her daughter's perspective and attitude to menopause), supports, religious beliefs, career, and attitudes regarding the end of reproductive life and ageing.

Reducing core body temperature

Higher body temperatures may precipitate hot flushes and may contribute to poorer quality sleep. Hot weather conditions such as summer may trigger more hot flushes. Staying cool in warmer weather, lowering the air temperature within the house, going swimming, and avoiding spicy and hot foods or drinks may be useful.

Relaxation and support groups

Nervous tension and stress are known triggers for hot flushes. One study found that counselling, slow, deep diaphragmatic breathing and relaxation therapies can help reduce the onset of a hot flush and the number of hot flushes, and improve quality of life.

Physical activity

Studies suggest that exercise can improve menopausal symptoms such as hot flushes, sleep disturbance, depression and moodiness by increasing natural levels of the opioid hormone endorphin. Data show that women who exercise regularly are less likely to experience menopausal symptoms. Exercise daily; walk at a modestly vigorous level at least 30 minutes a day, for example. Regular weight-bearing exercise such as walking is essential to prevent osteoporosis.

Yoga and meditation

A number of studies have shown that yoga and meditation can help reduce hot flushes and night sweats and improve memory, moods, attention and concentration. More rigorous studies are required, however, to assess the effectiveness of specific yoga and breathing techniques in the management of menopausal symptoms.

Nutrition and diet

During menopause, it is essential to consume a healthy, well-balanced diet high in vegetables and fruit, and increase your intake of calcium-rich foods for the prevention of osteoporosis and cardiovascular disease. Vitamin D supplements may be necessary, as studies suggest that vitamin D in combination with a high intake of dietary calcium reduces the incidence of fractures and falls. Recent research suggests that calcium supplements may increase the risk of heart disease in older women, but this does not occur with higher intake of dietary calcium. Increase your intake of calcium-rich foods such as nuts, seeds, low-fat dairy products, tofu, broccoli, bok choy, and fish with edible bones such as salmon and sardines.

Phytoestrogens, also known as plant oestrogens, are oestrogen-like compounds found in some plants that exert mild oestrogenic effects in menopausal women, helping to alleviate menopausal symptoms.

In general, an Asian diet has higher levels of phytoestrogens than a Western diet, which may help explain the lower incidence of menopausal symptoms and lower rates of cardiovascular diseases and some cancers among Asian women. Japanese women, for example, consume many products rich in phytoestrogens, such as miso, soybeans, flaxseed, soy grits, tofu, soy yoghurt, soy milk, soybean sprouts, sesame seeds (tahini), multigrain bread, hummus, garlic, mung bean sprouts, alfalfa sprouts, dried apricots, pistachio nuts, dried dates, sunflower seeds, chestnuts, dried prunes, fennel, yams.

Soy extracts

Soy supplements may play a role in the management of menopause and cholesterol, although soy in the diet is more important. The findings from studies are mixed. In some studies, 100 milligrams a day of soy protein extracts reduced cholesterol levels and menopausal symptoms such as hot flushes in postmenopausal women, while in other studies they showed no benefit.

Herbal remedies

Herbal medicines have traditionally been used to manage the symptoms of menopause. The best studied herbs for menopausal symptoms include black cohosh (*Actaea racemosa*, formerly called *Cimicifuga racemosa*), St John's wort (*Hypericum perforatum*) for depression associated with menopause, and red clover (*Trifolium pratense*). Clinical trials for dong quai (*Angelica sinensis*), ginseng (*Panax ginseng*), wild yam (*Dioscorea villosa*) and evening primrose oil (*Oenothera biennis*) have not shown any beneficial effect on menopausal symptoms.

Red clover

Red clover is a member of the legume family and contains high levels of phytoestrogens. Studies have shown mixed benefits for menopausal symptoms, and when there was a benefit, it was small compared with a placebo tablet. You should avoid using it if you have oestrogen-related health problems such as breast and endometrial cancers.

Black cohosh

Black cohosh was traditionally used in North American Indian medicine to treat menopausal symptoms. Numerous trials investigating the effect of black cohosh on hot flushes, urine urgency, vaginal dryness and mood swings have overall produced mixed findings. The fact that benefits have been observed in some studies but not others may be due to factors such as the dose and type of extract used, where the herb was sourced, and the level of active ingredients in the extract. The studies showing the best effects have used the isopropanolic extract of black cohosh root stock and ethanolic extract of black cohosh. Black cohosh does not have oestrogenic properties so it appears to be safe for use by women with oestrogen-sensitive breast cancer.

St John's wort

Several trials with combined herbal products containing black cohosh and St John's wort found they may alleviate hot flushes and improve moods in menopausal women. Another trial combining St John's wort with chaste tree found no benefit, however.

St John's wort can interact with other medications such as the oral contraceptive pill and can be lethal if taken with other antidepressants. Check with your doctor before taking St John's wort.

Hop extract

The hop plant (*Humulus lupulus*) contains high levels of phytoestrogens. Some studies have shown that hops can help reduce menopausal symptoms such as hot flushes and improve sleep.

Herbal remedies for menopausal symptoms

Herb	How it may help	Dosage and how to take it	Warnings and possible side effects
Red clover (*Trifolium pratense*)	May relieve menopausal symptoms: small reduction in hot flushes May help reduce bone density loss	40–80 mg a day	May cause headache, nausea, breast discomfort, heavy menstrual bleeding or vaginal spotting May increase the risk of bleeding Avoid if taking blood thinners
Black cohosh (*Actaea racemosa*)	May relieve menopausal symptoms	20–40 mg a day	Rarely, black cohosh may cause liver damage May cause gastrointestinal upset, headache, dizziness, weight gain, breast discomfort, vaginal spotting or bleeding

Herb	How it may help	Dosage and how to take it	Warnings and possible side effects
St John's wort (*Hypericum perforatum*)	May ease depression, mood disorders, menopausal depression.	300 mg twice to three times a day	Avoid taking with oral contraception, anticonvulsants and other antidepressants Check with your doctor if St John's wort interacts with your medication Avoid in pregnancy May cause dry mouth, gastrointestinal discomfort or rash
Soy extract	May relieve menopausal symptoms: reduction in hot flushes, breast pain and PMS	20–60 g soy protein (34–76 mg isoflavones) a day	May cause gastrointestinal upset Avoid if you suffer oestrogen-sensitive cancers such as breast or uterine cancer

Acupuncture and menopause

The use of acupuncture for the management of menopause is becoming more common, although most studies are of poor quality and to date have shown mixed findings. As the therapy is relatively safe, it is worth trialling for menopausal symptoms.

Natural therapies for vaginal problems

Treatment for atrophic vaginitis

Thinning and shrinking of vaginal tissue can cause soreness, pain, burning, irritation and infection, especially with sexual intercourse. (See chapter 25 for more details about atrophic vaginitis.) It occurs as a result of lowered oestrogen levels in menopause but may commence before menopause.

For relief of vaginal symptoms you may want to try some of the following treatments:

- almond or olive oil applied topically to vagina, especially for sexual intercourse
- vitamin E oil – prick a vitamin E capsule (200–500 IU) using a pin, squeeze out the contents and apply to the vulva and vagina most nights
- Sylk gel, derived from kiwifruit, for sexual intercourse

- vaginal dilators (see chapter 28) and/or finger penetration to help gently widen the vagina
- oestrogen cream – this needs a prescription from your GP

Treatment for vaginal infections

Vaginal infections, as opposed to sexually transmitted infections, usually occur from an overgrowth of some of the natural microorganisms in the vagina due to a reduction in *Lactobacillus* numbers in the vagina for some reason. They include bacterial infections such as gardnerella and parasitic infections such as trichomonas, which may cause bacterial vaginosis, or yeast infections (thrush) such as *Candida albicans* (most common) and *Candida glabrata*. In some women these infections do not cause symptoms.

There are many causes of vaginal irritation, malodour and vaginal discharge, such as vaginal atrophy due to menopause; skin conditions such as psoriasis, dermatitis, eczema and lichen sclerosus; STIs such as herpes simplex; and in rare cases cancer. Some vaginal discharges can be normal and fluctuate during the cycle with hormone changes. If you suffer persistent vaginal irritation or discharge, see your GP for an accurate diagnosis. If left untreated it may cause physical or psychological distress and interfere with your sex life. For more on genital infections, and their diagnosis and treatment, see chapter 26.

Candidiasis (thrush)

Candida is a type of yeast that lives naturally in the vagina. An overgrowth of candida can cause vaginal irritation, discomfort, a burning sensation and white discharge, and in some cases vulvar swelling and pain. Thirty per cent of women with candida have no symptoms and do not need treatment. Candidiasis may occur after a course of antibiotics, and from medications such as steroids and the oral contraceptive pill, or if you have a compromised immune system due to a condition such as AIDS or cancer. Candida infection may also occur in the mouth and gut. Recurrent candidiasis is defined as more than four to six episodes of symptomatic candida infections in one year. For the medical treatment of candida and other vaginal infections, see chapter 26.

Here are some natural ways to relieve vaginal infections and candidiasis:

- If possible, avoid medications that may cause yeast infections, such as antibiotics.
- Avoid tight clothing around the genital area, such as tight jeans and G-strings; wear loose cotton underwear, dresses and loose pants.

- Avoid rubbing and scratching the vaginal area as this can create an itch cycle.
- Reduce stress.
- Avoid sitting too much.
- Use non-drying soap substitutes and avoid washing the vagina regularly with soap and douches, bath salts and bubble baths.
- Avoid perfumed products, talcs or other powders in the genital area.
- Until the vaginal infection is cleared, avoid using tampons or wearing G-strings.
- Use condoms: they may help reduce recurrent vaginal infections.
- Use a sitz bath: sprinkle non-iodised salt (one teaspoon per litre) into a small amount of water in the bath and sit in it for 10–15 minutes every night until the discharge subsides; alternatively, swim at the beach for saltwater washes.
- Ask your doctor to check your blood vitamin D levels. Vitamin D deficiency may contribute to a poor immune system and has been linked to bacterial vaginosis. Vitamin D is mostly produced by the skin following direct sun exposure, but you may still need vitamin D supplements.
- Avoid sugar; honey; sweeteners; yeast; refined foods such as white breads; mushrooms; grapes; products containing vinegar; yellow, mature, processed and mouldy cheeses such as blue vein cheese or brie; fruits that show signs of mould and fermentation; and dried fruit. Avoid alcohol and bottled juices.
- Eat unflavoured yoghurt containing live probiotics (good live bacteria found in the gut such as *Lactobacillus* and *Bifidobacterium*); whole grains (brown rice, oats, barley, corn); flat pita bread without yeast; yeast-free wholegrain bread; white cheeses such as ricotta, feta and cottage cheese; legumes; garlic; protein foods such as fish, chicken, red meat, eggs, nuts and seeds; very fresh fruit (no more than two serves a day) and vegetables (five or more serves a day).
- Eat fermented foods such as sauerkraut, tempeh and miso; foods rich in the indigestible dietary fibre called inulin (found in globe artichokes); chicory root; dandelion; onions, garlic and leeks; bananas; unrefined rye and barley; soybeans; asparagus and other green vegetables; legumes; raw oats and berries. These foods are called prebiotics as they help promote the growth of probiotics by creating the right environment in the gut. There is a slight chance that probiotics might cause

irritation and infection, especially if your immune system is severely compromised with a condition such as AIDS or cancer.

Other treatments

An *occasional* vaginal douche using this recipe can help alleviate the symptoms of a vaginal infection. Use a well-washed squeezable plastic sauce bottle – you can purchase a new plastic bottle from a discount shop. To 200 millilitres of warm water add one teaspoon of probiotic powder or the contents of two capsules (to replace good microflora); and 20–30 millilitres (1–1½ tablespoons) of apple cider vinegar to improve the pH balance of the vagina. The probiotic powder may include bacteria such as *Lactobacillus acidophilus*, *Lactobacillus rhamnosus* and *Streptococcus thermophilus*.

For three or four consecutive days, lie on your bed with a thick folded towel under your buttocks, and lift your hips slightly. Insert the nozzle of the douche bottle into your vagina and gently squeeze a little into the vagina. Some liquid will spill out of your vagina. You can walk around after the douche or just roll over and sleep. The next day, wash and sterilise the nozzle of the bottle. Avoid reusing the douche if it has caused you any vaginal irritation. You can repeat the douche in a week's time if necessary.

If your male sexual partner is also suffering symptoms of penile infection (irritation is usually experienced at the tip of the penis, especially after sexual intercourse), he can try soaking his penis in a glass of this douche for about five to 10 minutes a day for up to four days.

You can also use diluted tea-tree oil (melaleuca oil) cream vaginally for seven nights for vaginal infections. Tea-tree oil has a mild antiseptic effect. Apply a small amount on your vagina the first night as a test dose, to ensure you are not allergic to the cream. Commence treatment with the tea-tree oil cream the following night if you do not react to the test dose.

You can make your own tea-tree oil remedy by blending five drops of tea-tree oil with one teaspoon of vegetable oil (such as olive oil). Soak a tampon in water first, then in the tea-tree oil blend, before inserting into the vagina. Leave overnight and repeat the following morning. Ensure you try the patch test with the tea-tree oil first, as described above.

If you suffer irritation of the vagina or vulva from sex, an infection or rash, for soothing effects try applying vitamin E oil (prick the top of a capsule containing 200–500 IU of vitamin E) or rosehip oil until the irritation settles. Give it about one week and if irritation persists, discontinue this treatment. Men can also try this to relieve irritation at the tip of their penis after sex.

You can try taking probiotic supplements such as one teaspoon of acidophilus powder or two capsules of acidophilus each morning before breakfast daily for two weeks, or until you have finished the bottle or packet. Repeat this step following a course of antibiotics. You could also take two garlic tablets after dinner for one week.

You may still need medical treatments, such vaginal antifungal creams for you and your partner, oral medication such as fluconazole (which is available over the counter in pharmacies), a course of nystatin tablets for the treatment of candidiasis, or antibiotics (vaginal and/or oral) for bacterial vaginosis. Speak with your doctor about these treatments.

35
Gynaecological cancers

Orla McNally

Cancer is a disease of the cells, which are the building blocks of all living things. Cells are constantly undergoing renewal or repair or death, depending on whether they need to be replaced, or have been injured or simply come to the end of their life. These processes are controlled mainly by genes, and all cancers arise as a result of problems with these genes. Most of the time the human body has the ability to fix these problems, but not always, and when this is the case cells can grow and multiply without control. This leads to a growth or swelling sometimes called a tumour.

While the focus of this chapter is on cancers of the female reproductive system, much of the information is very relevant to women with other, non-gynaecological cancers.

What causes cancer?

Although cancer is caused by problems in the genes, what causes these problems is not yet entirely clear. Many factors are likely to be involved, including lifestyle and dietary factors as well as substances in the environment. Smoking, obesity, asbestos and sun exposure are known risk factors for many cancers.

Tumours

Benign tumours

These tumours usually grow in a particular area, and do not move or spread outside a confined space. They often cause problems by putting pressure on normal organs in that area. Some benign tumours are pre-cancerous, which means they could turn into a cancer if not treated.

Malignant tumours

Cancer cells from these tumours have the ability to invade nearby tissues and/or leave the part of the body where they started and spread to other parts. The first tumour to appear where the cancer starts is called the primary tumour. When a cancer has spread, the new tumour is called a metastasis or a secondary tumour.

How tumours spread

In order for a tumour to grow, it must develop its own blood supply by creating new blood vessels. These new vessels allow the cancer cells not only to grow and multiply, but also to spread to other parts of the body. As well as travelling through blood vessels, the cells can travel in the lymphatic or lymph system, which under normal circumstances is responsible for cleansing the blood.

Stages and grades of cancer

The stage of a cancer is the degree to which the cancer has spread to other parts of the body. There are usually four stages, where stage 1 means the cancer is still confined to the place where it started (e.g. the ovary, uterus or cervix) and stage 4 means the cancer has spread quite far (e.g. as far from the genital area as the lungs).

The grade of a cancer indicates how well the cells resemble normal cells. Grade 1 cancers look very similar to the cells where they occur (such as the ovary, uterus or cervix), while grade 3 cancers look very unlike normal cells and as a result behave in a more aggressive way.

Recurrent cancer

A cancer is said to be recurrent when it grows again having been previously treated. This happens because some cancer cells can become resistant to treatment and remain dormant for a while before growing again. Even though the place where the cancer started has been removed, these cells can grow again either in the same area (called a local recurrence) or in another part of the body (a distal recurrence). It is often possible to treat recurrent gynaecological cancers, to manage symptoms or prolong life, but once a cancer recurs it is usually difficult to cure (i.e. make it go away forever).

What are gynaecological cancers

Gynaecological cancers are cancers that affect the components of the female reproductive system, including the ovaries, uterus (endometrium), cervix, fallopian tubes, vulva and vagina. The majority of cancers arise in

Symptoms of gynaecological cancers

Symptom	Frequency according to cancer type					
	Uterine	Ovarian	Fallopian tube	Cervical	Vulvar	Vaginal
Postmenopausal bleeding	Often	Sometimes	Sometimes	Often	Often	Often
Irregular periods	Often	Rarely	Rarely	Never	Never	Never
Bleeding between periods	Sometimes	Rarely	Rarely	Often	Sometimes	Often
Bleeding after sex	Sometimes	Rarely	Rarely	Often	Often	Often
Lump	Sometimes	Often	Often	Rarely	Often	Often
Abdominal swelling	Sometimes	Often	Often	Rarely	Never	Never
Vaginal discharge	Often	Rarely	Often	Rarely	Often	Often
Abnormal Pap test	Rarely	Rarely	Rarely	Often	Never	Never
Abnormal cervix	Rarely	Never	Never	Often	Never	Rarely
Itch	Never	Never	Never	Never	Sometimes	Sometimes
Pain	Sometimes	Sometimes	Sometimes	Sometimes	Sometimes	Sometimes
Pain with sex	Sometimes	Never	Never	Sometimes	Sometimes	Sometimes

these areas, but cancers arising in other areas such as the bowel or stomach can spread to the ovaries.

On average, 12 women in Australia each day will be diagnosed with a gynaecological cancer.

Gynaecological cancers may produce few symptoms until the cancer is quite advanced, as is sometimes the case with ovarian cancer, or may be detected as a result of a single episode of bleeding after menopause. See later in this chapter for more on the symptoms and treatment of the different gynaecological cancers.

Cancer health professionals

Usually the GP you first see with symptoms will arrange tests for you. He or she may then refer you directly to a gynaecological oncologist (a surgeon who specialises in the area of gynaecological cancers). If you come from a rural community, your GP may initially refer you to a local gynaecologist, who will arrange further tests. If cancer is suspected or confirmed, you should be referred to a gynaecological cancer centre, where a specialist or team of specialists will advise you about your treatment options. If you are not referred to such a centre or specialist, it is important to find out why you are not being given access to these services. Such a team will include:

- a gynaecological oncologist – a doctor who has completed specialised training in looking after women with cancers of the female reproductive system
- a medical oncologist – a doctor who specialises in cancer care and in particular in prescribing the right chemotherapy (anti-cancer drugs)
- a radiation oncologist – a doctor who specialises in cancer care and in particular in prescribing the right radiotherapy
- a pathologist – a doctor who specialises in diagnosing gynaecological cancers
- a radiologist – a doctor who specialises in reading X-rays and other imaging of women with gynaecological cancers
- specialist nurses – nurses who are experienced in looking after women with cancer and are there to support you through your journey
- a care coordinator – usually a specialist nurse who coordinates an individual's care and is available to answer any questions
- allied health professionals – including a dietician, psychologist, social worker, physiotherapist, occupational therapist and/or genetic counsellor

How your cancer might affect you

Prognosis is the word used to describe how your cancer is likely to affect you in the long term. It means the likelihood that you will be cured, or not die of your cancer. It is not possible ever to give 100 per cent assurance of a cure. Many factors influence the prognosis, including the grade and stage of the cancer (see above), and also other factors including the type of treatment possible and your other medical conditions. It is important to remember, however, that although statistics are very helpful when discussing diseases in general, they do not necessarily predict the behaviour of a cancer in an individual woman. A discussion with your specialist about your particular case will be much more accurate.

When you see your doctor or health professional, there are a number of questions you should ask:

- What type of cancer do I have?
- How extensive is my cancer? In other words, what is the stage and grade?
- What are my treatment options?
- What are the expected outcomes of each option, including the benefits and possible complications?
- What is the likely outcome of my treatment?
- What treatments do you think I should have and why?
- Are the latest treatments available at this hospital?
- Will I have to stay in hospital?
- How long will the treatment take?
- How much will it cost?
- Will it cause any pain?
- (If relevant) Will I be able to have children?
- How will it affect my sex life?
- How will you check if the cancer has responded to treatment?
- What about complementary treatments?

What you can do to help yourself

One of the difficulties for many women with a diagnosis of cancer is the feeling of a loss of control. Often they have been the main caregiver – the mother, the wife, the supportive daughter – and they now find themselves in a situation where everyone wants to help them, which can be very overwhelming. Women often ask what they can do to help with their treatment at this time. Here is a short list of things you can do, and that can all have a positive effect on a cancer journey:

- Look after yourself – you are number one for a while.
- Eat a sensible, balanced diet. There is no evidence that restriction of certain foods has any impact. Discuss the use of any vitamins and supplements with your doctor, as these may interfere with your treatment, especially if you are having chemotherapy.
- Do some exercise – there is increasing evidence that gentle and regular exercise during and after cancer treatment has a very positive effect not just on your sense of wellbeing, but also on recovery from treatment.
- Relax – reducing anxiety levels through relaxation is very helpful. The effect is similar to that of exercise.
- Find hope – a diagnosis of cancer, no matter how early or advanced, is a devastating life event, but learning about your cancer will usually be a source of hope rather than despair.

Participating in clinical trials

Advances in medicine have happened as a result of research. In cancer, this has involved testing treatments in the laboratory and then in humans. Testing or comparing treatments in humans is called a clinical trial. Many women with a gynaecological cancer will be offered entry into a clinical trial during their cancer journey, and will be supported by a specific research nurse and doctor should they consent to the trial.

Participating in any clinical trial has pros and cons. On the plus side, you might get a promising new treatment and might be the first to benefit from the new method. You are also helping others with the same disease now and in the future. On the minus side, the new treatment might not be any better than the normal treatment; there is a possibility of side effects or risks; and you might not be able to choose the treatment you receive. Ask your doctor about the pros and cons of participating in a particular clinical trial, as the possible risks and benefits will vary from trial to trial.

- Seek support – many cancers have specific support groups, and other groups such as Cancer Australia provide both general and if necessary specific support. Needless to say, your family and friends are likely to be a major support at this time. If they need support or advice, they can also contact a cancer organisation. See the Resources section at the end of this book for more information and contact details.

- Find out about your family history. A proportion of cancers arise as a result of a defective gene that passes from one generation to the next. You are likely to be asked about any cancers in your family, and the more information you can obtain about this yourself before you see the specialist, the better. Note that the majority of cancers appear to occur out of the blue.

Types of treatment

There are national and international guidelines for the treatment of all cancers, which have been developed as a result of research and experience over many decades. A number of factors will influence how cancer will be treated in each individual, including where the cancer started (such as the ovary, uterus or cervix), the stage and grade of the cancer (see above), and specific factors such as general health, other medical conditions and fertility requirements.

Gynaecological cancers are treated with surgery, radiotherapy, chemo-therapy or hormone therapy, but sometimes a combination of these treatments is necessary, either at the same time or one after the other.

Surgery

See the sections on individual cancers later in this chapter for more details on surgery options.

Radiotherapy

This treatment uses X-ray radiation to kill cells or injure them so they cannot multiply. The radiation may be given from the outside (external radiotherapy) in small doses each day over four to five weeks; or given inside (internal radiotherapy), such as directly to the cervix or top of the vagina over a few hours with a special applicator placed in the vagina. The side effects of radiotherapy include lethargy, loss of appetite, diar-rhoea, pubic hair loss, menopause, loss of fertility, shortening or narrowing of the vagina, cystitis (inflammation of the bladder) and skin changes. Most of these side effects disappear after the treatment has been completed, but some, such as menopause and loss of fertility, are irreversible. See chapter 24 for information on preserving fertility from cancer treatments.

Chemotherapy

Chemotherapy uses drugs to kill or interfere with the growth and multiplication of cancer cells. How chemotherapy is given depends on the type of cancer and the type of chemotherapy being used. Some chemotherapy can be taken orally, as a liquid, capsule or tablet, at home, and others might require an injection into a muscle, the spine or abdominal cavity. Chemotherapy for gynaecological cancers is usually given intravenously (into a vein) by a specialist nurse under the guidance of an oncologist. Most chemotherapy is given during a day admission, but occasionally a stay in hospital is required. Side effects include lowered production of blood cells, thrush, nausea and vomiting, mouth sores, loss of appetite, hair loss, menopause, effects on fertility, skin rashes, tingling nerves and joint pains. As with radiotherapy, many of these side effects are not permanent, but some are: hair grows back, but nerve damage may be permanent.

Hormone treatment

Many cancers contain proteins called hormone receptors, which influence the growth of cancers and can sometimes be blocked using other hormones such as progestogens (Provera) and tamoxifen. Side effects include breast tenderness, nausea, fluid retention, hot flushes and headaches.

Fertility, sexuality and body image and cancer

Many cancer treatments can affect body image, particularly with treatments such as chemotherapy causing hair loss and weight changes. Although the removal of any of the female organs is not always outwardly obvious compared to removal of a breast, for example, the effect on a woman's perception of herself can be profound. This can lead to lack of confidence, difficulty in relationships, and lack of interest in intimacy and sex. Treatment for cancer of the vulva does lead to changes in physical appearance, although to minimise this, a non-surgical treatment such as radiotherapy may be chosen, particularly if the cancer is near the clitoris.

Unless a gynaecological cancer is found early, treatment for cancers of the uterus, cervix, fallopian tube and ovary usually lead to loss of fertility. If this is a concern, you will be referred to a specialist in fertility to discuss fertility options that might be appropriate for you, such as leaving the ovaries in place for surrogacy using your eggs; ovarian suppression (turning the ovaries 'off' during chemotherapy); or freezing ovarian tissue, eggs or embryos until you are ready to use them. (See chapter 24 for information on preserving fertility in these circumstances.)

The gynaecological cancers

Uterine/endometrial cancer

This is the most common gynaecological cancer, with 1900 Australian women diagnosed every year. It accounts for 4 per cent of all cancers in Australian women. The incidence is rising, probably as a result of the rising obesity problem. Endometrial cancer usually occurs over the age of 50 but can occur in younger women, particularly those who develop a condition called hyperplasia, where the cells in the lining of the uterus multiply and can become abnormal if not treated.

Adenocarcinoma is the most common type of cell in this type of cancer, and usually has not spread outside of the uterus at the time of diagnosis. Other cell types – clear cell, serous and sarcoma – are known as high-risk types because there is a high chance they will already have spread at the time of diagnosis.

Stages of uterine/endometrial cancer

The stages of endometrial cancer are:

- stage 1, in which the cancer is confined to the uterus (lining and/or wall)
- stage 2, in which it has spread to the cervix
- stage 3, in which it has spread beyond the uterus and cervix to the ovaries, fallopian tubes, vagina or nearby lymph nodes
- stage 4, in which it has spread further, to the rectum or bladder, or outside the pelvis to the abdomen or lungs

Causes of uterine/endometrial cancer

It is not known exactly what causes endometrial cancer, but there are known risk factors:

- age
- late menopause
- hyperplasia
- a family history of bowel, breast, endometrial or ovarian cancer

- oestrogen replacement therapy (HRT) without progesterone
- tamoxifen (used for treating breast cancer)
- obesity
- high blood pressure
- diabetes
- never having had children
- previous pelvic irradiation
- ovarian tumours
- polycystic ovarian syndrome (PCOS; see chapter 24)

Prevention of uterine/endometrial cancer

Regular exercise, weight loss (maintaining or achieving a normal BMI; see chapter 14), a healthy balanced diet, pregnancy, the oral contraceptive pill and the Mirena IUS are known to reduce the risk of developing endometrial cancer.

Symptoms of uterine/endometrial cancer

Postmenopausal bleeding is a common symptom of endometrial cancer. Once periods have stopped for at least six months it is essential that any further bleeding is investigated, as one in 10 women with bleeding after menopause will have an endometrial cancer. This cancer may also cause abnormal vaginal discharge and, in young women, irregular bleeding. Other less common symptoms are period-like pain in the pelvis, pain passing urine and pain during sex. Occasionally a Pap test will pick up cancer cells from the lining of the uterus, but this test is mainly designed to pick up abnormal cells from the cervix.

Diagnosis of uterine/endometrial cancer

If you have any of the above symptoms your doctor will perform a physical examination. This will include a speculum examination to look at the cervix and vagina, and if possible passing a fine tube through the cervix to sample the lining of the uterus (this is call a pipelle or endometrial biopsy). If this is not possible as an outpatient, you will be admitted to hospital for the day and, under a short general anaesthetic, your cervix will be dilated so that a camera can be used to examine the endometrium and the lining scraped or curetted (a dilatation and curettage, or what doctors call a D&C). You will also have an ultrasound scan of the pelvis.

If you are found to have endometrial cancer, further tests to check the stage of your cancer will be arranged, including blood tests, a chest X-ray, an MRI or CT scan of the pelvis and abdomen, and possibly a PET scan. (See chapter 3 for explanations of these tests and scans.) At this stage you will be under the care of a specialist gynaecological cancer team.

Prognosis for uterine/endometrial cancer

Because endometrial cancer usually presents at an early stage, most women are cured. Even with advanced disease treatment is still possible, but the likelihood of long-term cure is lower.

Treatment for uterine/endometrial cancer

An individualised treatment plan will be formulated with your specialist. Uterine/endometrial cancer is usually treated with an operation to remove the uterus, fallopian tubes and ovaries. The lymph glands may also be removed to check for any signs of spread. Surgery may be done through a large incision in the abdomen or by keyhole (laparoscopic) surgery.

Everything that is removed at surgery is examined by the pathologist, and this determines whether any further treatment is required in the form of radiotherapy, chemotherapy or hormones (see earlier in this chapter).

Cervical cancer

In Australia, seven in every 100,000 women will be found to have a cervical cancer every year; that's 734 cases. This accounts for 1.7 per cent of all cancers for Australian women. There has been a significant fall in incidence since the national cervical screening program began in 1991.

The cervix has two types of cells: squamous cells, which are flat and occur mainly on the entrance to the cervix; and more raised glandular cells inside the cervical canal. Eighty per cent of cervical cancers are of the squamous type, and the rest are mainly adenocarcinomas originating in the glandular cells. If the cancer has invaded only a few millimetres it is called a micro-invasive cancer. Once it has invaded beyond a few millimetres it is called an invasive cancer, and is more likely to grow locally and spread through the fine capillary tubes of the lymphatic system.

Stages of cervical cancer

The stages of cervical cancer are:

- stage 1, in which it is confined to the cervix
- stage 2, in which it has spread beyond the cervix to the vagina and the supporting tissues of the cervix

- stage 3, in which it has spread to the rest of the pelvis
- stage 4, in which it has spread beyond the pelvis to areas such as the bladder, rectum and abdomen

Causes of cervical cancer

The human papillomaviruses (HPV; see chapters 8 and 26) are the main cause of cervical cancer. Other significant risk factors are smoking, not having regular Pap tests, age (being in our 40s and 50s), long-term use of the Pill (more than five years) and having many children. It can also occur in women who were exposed in their mother's womb to a drug called diethylstilboestrol (DES), which was used in the 1950s to prevent miscarriage.

Prevention of cervical cancer

The HPV vaccine will reduce the risk of cancer significantly in women who have it before they become sexually active. There is, however, evidence that the vaccine has an effect even if it is administered after sexual activity has started, by preventing infection with the HPV types covered by the vaccine, which are thought to be responsible for some cancers. Women who stop smoking significantly reduce their chance of abnormal changes on the cervix and consequently cancer. Australia's National Cervical Screening Program recommends regular Pap tests every two years from the age of 18 or two years after commencing sexual activity (whichever comes sooner) until the age of 70.

Symptoms of cervical cancer

Cervical cancer may cause bleeding between periods, bleeding after intercourse and bleeding after menopause. Sex may become painful, or there may be a persistent vaginal discharge. When the cancer is in the early stages, there may be no symptoms. When it is advanced there may be back pain, leg swelling and tiredness.

Diagnosis of cervical cancer

Examination of the cervix with a speculum at the time of a Pap test may reveal an obvious cancer, but sometimes magnification with a colposcope (see chapter 36) may be required. A biopsy (a small piece of tissue) will be removed to send to a laboratory to confirm the diagnosis. Sometimes this is done during an examination under anaesthesia. Other tests will be performed to establish the stage of the cancer, including blood tests, a chest X-ray, and CT, MRI or PET scans.

Prognosis for cervical cancer

Most women with early cancer of the cervix will be cured. Even with advanced disease, treatment can usually alleviate symptoms and prolong life, although it is less likely the cancer will be cured.

Treatment for cervical cancer

If the cancer is found early and you want to stay fertile, an operation that just removes the cervix (called a cone biopsy or trachelectomy) may be possible. The standard operation for early cancer is, however, a hysterectomy – which may be simple (without removing part of the ligaments that support the uterus) or radical (removing part of the ligaments) – as well as removal of the pelvic lymph nodes and possibly the fallopian tubes and ovaries.

If it is unlikely that surgery can adequately remove a cervical cancer, then the best treatment is radiotherapy (external and internal), to which a small amount of chemotherapy is added. This is called chemoradiation.

Ovarian cancer and fallopian tube cancer

The ovaries are made up of a covering called an epithelium and internal cells, which comprise the egg cells (called germ cells) and supporting cells that produce female hormones (called stromal cells). Most ovarian cancers arise from the epithelium and account for the 1300-plus women diagnosed each year in Australia. Ovarian cancer can occur at any age but most epithelial cancers occur in women over the age of 50. Germ cell tumours, which are much less common, usually occur in women who are in their 20s. Sadly, three out of four women with ovarian cancer die within five years, compared to one in four women with breast cancer.

Fallopian tube cancer arises in the fallopian tubes and is also epithelial in nature. It is less common than ovarian cancer but causes similar symptoms and is diagnosed and treated in the same way, so will be considered with ovarian cancer in this section.

Stages of ovarian/fallopian tube cancers

The stages of ovarian cancer are:

- stage 1, in which it is confined to the ovary
- stage 2, in which it is found in one or both ovaries and has spread to other areas in the pelvis such as the uterus, fallopian tubes, bladder or bowel

- stage 3, in which it is found in one or both ovaries and has spread outside the pelvis to the omentum (a fatty part of the peritoneum, the lining of the body cavity surrounding the organs in the abdomen), the intestines or lymph nodes in the pelvis or abdomen
- stage 4, in which it is found in one or both ovaries and has spread outside the abdomen (usually in the outer lining of the lung), or has spread to inside the liver

A similar staging system is used for fallopian tube cancer.

Causes of ovarian/fallopian tube cancer

In most cases the cause of ovarian cancer is not known but is likely to be due to a number of factors. It is known to occur more often in women who have not had any children or have had fertility treatment, and in women who are obese. Approximately 10–15 per cent of ovarian cancers arise as a result of a gene mutation (see 'Hereditary breast and ovarian cancer' below).

Prevention of ovarian/fallopian tube cancer

There are no screening tests for ovarian or fallopian tube cancers to date. Certain things seem to be protective, however, including having children, using the oral contraceptive pill and not being overweight. Some women are at increased risk of ovarian cancer because they have a strong family history of ovarian cancer or breast cancer (see 'Hereditary breast and ovarian cancer' below). If you have a strong family history, you may elect to have your ovaries and fallopian tubes removed at an appropriate time after discussion with a familial cancer specialist and a specialist gynaecologist. A Pap test doesn't detect ovarian or fallopian tube cancer. It's designed to detect cervical cancer. The best thing you can do is know your body and be aware of the symptoms (see below). If you're still concerned about a persistent symptom, you should always get a second opinion.

Symptoms of ovarian/fallopian tube cancer

The symptoms of ovarian cancer are often vague and can be similar to the symptoms of many other conditions that can be part of everyday life, particularly at the age (around menopause) when ovarian cancer most commonly occurs. The most common symptoms that may indicate ovarian cancer are:

- abdominal bloating/feeling full
- abdominal or back pain
- appetite loss or feeling full quickly

- changes in toilet habits, including needing to urinate often or urgently
- unexplained weight loss or weight gain
- indigestion or heartburn
- fatigue

If any of these symptoms are unusual for you, and they persist, it's important to see your doctor.

The Ovarian Cancer Australia website has an online symptom diary, a very useful app for women who are concerned about their symptoms (see www.ovariancancer.net.au/awareness/symptoms).

Diagnosis of ovarian/fallopian tube cancer

To make the diagnosis a doctor will carry out a full examination, including examination of the breasts and an internal examination. Blood tests, and in particular a blood test for a tumour marker called CA125, will be performed. An ultrasound of the pelvis, a CT scan and an MRI scan will be performed for further information. Usually the diagnosis of cancer cannot be made until surgery to remove the ovary or fallopian tube, but sometimes fluid called ascites is present in the abdomen and pelvis, which can be drained off and sent to be examined for cancer cells.

Prognosis for ovarian/fallopian tube cancer

Ovarian and fallopian tube cancers confined to the ovary or tube may be cured with surgery alone. Most of these cancers, however, are not early (stage 1), and so treatment involves surgery and chemotherapy. These do have a chance of cure in a small percentage of women, but in the majority the cancer will return after a period of remission and is unlikely to be cured.

Treatment for ovarian/fallopian tube cancer

Unless the cancer is thought to be confined to one ovary or tube, surgery usually involves a hysterectomy, along with removal of the tubes and ovaries, the pelvic lymph nodes and those around the aorta, and the omentum (see above). The aim of surgery is to remove as much of the visible cancer as possible. Sometimes this is only possible by removing part of the bowel. This might require a colostomy bag, which in most cases is temporary. For younger women who wish to preserve their fertility, if the cancer is early it might be possible to leave one ovary and the uterus in place.

Except when the cancer is confined to one ovary or tube, chemotherapy is recommended. This usually involves six cycles (treatments) of two chemotherapy drugs at three-week intervals. Sometimes chemotherapy is used first to 'shrink' the cancer if it has spread, in order to make surgery possible. This is called neo-adjuvant chemotherapy.

Radiotherapy is usually reserved for recurrent cancer in one or two areas.

Vulvar cancer

In Australia 280 women out of 100,000 will be affected by cancer of the vulva each year. It usually occurs between the ages of 55 and 75.

Cancer of the vulva is a skin cancer and so the cell types that occur are similar to those of skin cancers elsewhere in the body. The most common is squamous cell cancer, followed by melanoma, adenocarcinomas and, more rarely, verrucous cancers and sarcomas.

Causes of vulvar cancer

There are a number of precancer conditions of the vulvar skin that can lead to vulvar cancer, probably as a result of chronic itching and therefore trauma. These include vulvar intraepithelial neoplasia (VIN), which is usually associated with the HPV. Other chronic conditions such as lichen sclerosus and genital herpes may also be precancerous. (See chapter 26 for more on these conditions.) Smoking is a major contributing factor, and any condition that affects the immune system can also increase the risk.

Prevention of vulvar cancer

Treatment for any precancer conditions of the vulva mentioned above is important, as is keeping a regular check on the vulvar skin. Smoking is a significant risk factor so giving up is a major preventative step.

Symptoms of vulvar cancer

A vulvar cancer may not cause any symptoms, but itching, an ulcer or a lump may occur. Itching in an older woman should not be assumed to be thrush (candidiasis) without a full examination.

Diagnosis of vulvar cancer

The vulva is examined and a small biopsy taken to confirm the diagnosis. The groin is carefully examined too, to check for signs of spread. Further tests, including blood tests, a chest X-ray, and CT and MRI scans, are usually organised.

Prognosis for vulvar cancer

Most women with early cancer of the vulva will be cured. Even with advanced disease, treatment can usually alleviate symptoms and prolong life, although it is less likely the cancer will be cured.

Treatment for vulvar cancer

This is usually determined by the location of the cancer and its size. Unless the cancer involves the clitoris or is close to the anus, surgery is the preferred treatment, although it is physically and psychologically challenging because it is mutilating. Surgery may involve only a small excision, but may be radical, including removal of the lymph nodes in the groin. Occasionally plastic surgery may be required.

Radiotherapy to which a small amount of chemotherapy may be added (chemoradiation) may be used before surgery if the cancer is large or involves the clitoris or the anus.

Vaginal cancer

Cancer of the vagina is rare. About 90 Australian women are newly diagnosed with vaginal cancer each year. Vaginal cancer accounts for less than 0.5 per cent of all cancers in Australian women.

There are two main types of vaginal cancer: those that start in the vagina itself (primary vaginal cancer), and those that spread into the vagina from another part of the body (secondary vaginal cancer). Only primary vaginal cancer will be discussed here.

There are two main types of primary vaginal cancer, which are named after the cells from which they develop:

- Squamous cell carcinoma – this is the most common type of vaginal cancer, and means the cancer originated from the skin cells. It is usually found in the upper part of the vagina, and most commonly affects women between the ages of 50 and 70.

- Adenocarcinoma – this type of vaginal cancer begins in the glandular cells in the lining of the vagina. It usually affects women under the age of 20, but occasionally occurs in other age groups.

Other very rare types of vaginal cancer include melanoma, small cell carcinoma, sarcoma and lymphoma.

Stages of vaginal cancer

The stages of vaginal cancer are:

- stage 1, in which it is confined to the vagina

- stage 2, in which it has begun to spread through the wall of the vagina but has not spread further into the walls of the pelvis

- stage 3, in which it has spread to the pelvis and may also be in the lymph nodes close to the vagina

- stage 4, in which it has spread to the bladder or the bowel, or to other parts of the body such as the lungs

As mentioned earlier, if the cancer comes back after initial treatment, this is known as recurrent cancer. Vaginal cancer may come back in the vagina or in another part of the body.

Causes of vaginal cancer

As with cancers of the cervix and vulva, HPV can also cause precancerous changes in the vagina that can lead to cancer. In fact, any HPV-related precancerous or cancerous condition of the female genital tract increases the risk of a precancer or cancer in another part of the genital tract. Smoking is also a risk factor.

Symptoms of vaginal cancer

There may be no symptoms, as this type of cancer may be found early, at a routine examination such as a Pap test. Bleeding may occur spontaneously or be provoked by activity including sex. Pain in the pelvis or back area may occur at later stages.

Diagnosis of vaginal cancer

A full physical examination will be required, including an internal examination. Sometimes an examination under anaesthetic will be recommended to obtain further information and in particular to obtain a biopsy. Blood tests, a chest X-ray, and CT and MRI scans will be arranged to determine the stage of the cancer.

Prognosis for vaginal cancer

Most women with early cancer of the vagina will be cured. Even with advanced disease, treatment can usually alleviate symptoms and prolong life, although it is less likely the cancer will be cured.

Treatment for vaginal cancer

It is possible to remove small cancers with surgery without removing too much of the vagina so that sex is still possible. If the cancer is large, radiotherapy, to which a small amount of chemotherapy is added (chemoradiation), is the treatment of choice. This means the vagina will be affected but not removed.

Inherited cancers

A strong family history means having several close blood relatives (on your mother's or father's side of the family) who have had breast or ovarian cancer, bowel or uterine cancer, especially if this was diagnosed at an early age.

Hereditary breast and ovarian cancer

Some women are at increased risk of breast or ovarian cancer because a family member is known to have inherited a fault in a gene associated with these cancers.

If ovarian cancer is caused by inheriting a faulty gene, this is called hereditary cancer. There are several genes for which inherited faults may be involved in the development of breast or ovarian cancer. These are genes that normally prevent a woman developing breast or ovarian cancer.

Two genes associated with ovarian cancer are called BRCA1 and BRCA2 (breast cancer one and breast cancer two). If you have inherited a fault in one of these genes, you have a high chance of developing ovarian cancer or breast cancer, although it does not mean you are certain to develop either cancer. Between 10 and 15 per cent of all ovarian cancers may be explained by an inherited gene fault in BRCA1 or BRCA2.

If you are concerned about your potential genetic risk, visit www. ovariancancer.net.au/awareness/genetic-risks, which has information about genetic risks. The Cancer Australia website has a helpful online assessment tool (see canceraustralia.gov.au/clinical-best-practice/gynaecological-cancers/fra-boc/evaluate).

Hereditary uterine/endometrial cancer

Some women are at increased risk of endometrial cancer because a family member is known to have inherited a fault in a gene associated with this or other cancers, including bowel and prostate cancers and melanoma. This is known as Lynch syndrome, and endometrial cancer is often the first cancer to occur in women who have inherited one of the faulty genes.

Life after cancer

There have been many advances in the treatment of cancer and as a result many more women are living longer after a cancer diagnosis. Getting back to 'normal' after treatment can sometimes present challenges, and there are now a number of programs aimed at providing ongoing support, as well as advice about general health issues and any other issues that might be relevant as a result of treatment, such as menopause. These programs may be available at the hospital where you were treated or through organisations such as Ovarian Cancer Australia and BreaCan. See the Resources section at the back of the book for more information on these organisations.

36

Abnormal Pap tests: dysplasia

C. David H. Wrede

Dysplasia is a general pathological term used to describe abnormal growth of a set of cells in a particular organ. For the purposes of this chapter, it refers to abnormal changes to the superficial cells of the cervix, usually identified from a Pap test. Most abnormal Pap test results are not due to cancer but to other less worrying abnormalities that can be easily treated.

The cervix

The cervix forms the neck of the uterus and is located at the top of the vagina. The cervix is covered by two different types of cells, those on the outer part of the cervix and those in the cervical canal. The outer part of the cervix, closest to the vagina, is covered by flat skin-like cells (squamous cells) that lie in layers.

The inner part of the cervix or the canal that leads from the vagina into the uterus is known as the endocervical canal. The column-shaped cells that line the endocervical canal are called columnar or glandular cells. These cells form a single layer. The area where the flat squamous cells and the glandular cells meet is known as the transformation zone.

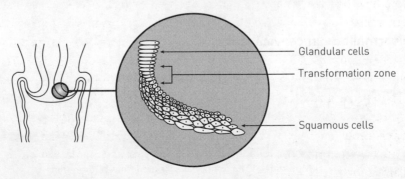

Glandular cells

Transformation zone

Squamous cells

Detail of lining of cervix

Normal changes to the cervix

The location of the transformation zone on the cervix can vary from woman to woman and according to age. After menopause, for example, the transformation zone is usually in the endocervical canal. In young women, when hormone levels are higher, this area may be on the outer part of the cervix; when this occurs it is called an ectropion. The transformation zone of the cervix is where many changes in the cells occur. Some changes are quite normal and occur most frequently at puberty and during pregnancy. These changes are known as metaplasia.

Inflammation on the cervix, also known as cervicitis, is common and may not have a specific cause, but sometimes it is due to an infection, and can cause such changes to the cells. These changes may be a normal response to the usual organisms and acidity in the vagina, in which case they do not require treatment, but a specific infection by a recognised disease-causing organism (such as chlamydia) will require a course of antibiotics.

Abnormal cell changes

Abnormal changes in the cells of the cervix also occur at the transformation zone, and these types of changes are called dysplasia. There are two kinds of changes: cervical intraepithelial neoplasia (CIN), when the abnormality is in the squamous cells; and less frequently adenocarcinoma in situ (ACIS), when it is in glandular cells. Dysplasia or abnormal growth in the surface cells of the cervix is graded from mild to severe (see the table below).

Dysplasia, either CIN or ACIS, is not cancer, but if not monitored or treated can lead to cancer. Treatment for these abnormalities is simple, safe and nearly always successful.

Abnormalities in cervical cells

Type	Severity	Description
Low-grade abnormality – CIN 1	Mild	The abnormal cells are only in the bottom third or less of the surface layer. In less than 10% of cases these can progress to high-grade changes. Frequent Pap tests will be necessary to pick up those that do get worse.
High-grade abnormality – CIN 2	Moderate	The abnormal cells are in the bottom third or two-thirds of the surface layer.

Type	Severity	Description
High-grade abnormality – CIN 3	Severe	The abnormal cells occupy the full thickness of the surface layer.
ACIS	n/a	A less common form of abnormality in the glandular cells.

Pap tests

A Pap test is an important cancer-screening test because it can find pre-cancerous changes in the cervix. Sometimes these cell changes may lead to cancer if they are not monitored or treated. This process usually takes many years.

During a conventional Pap test, cells are collected from the cervix with a spatula and/or brush and are fixed to a glass slide and sent to a laboratory for testing. If you receive an abnormal result from your test, you will be recommended to visit your doctor for follow-up. If your abnormal test requires an opinion from a specialist gynaecologist, the first appointment will include an examination called a colposcopy (see below). During this examination the doctor may need to take a biopsy.

Pap test follow-up

Following the examination the doctor will discuss the findings with you and the possibilities of treatment or follow-up. You should receive a letter about two to three weeks after your appointment telling you if you will need treatment, if you just need a review with the gynaecologist in six to 12 months, or if you simply need to return to your doctor for another Pap test in one or two years' time.

Your Pap test result

The result on your Pap test may have been reported in one of the following ways:

- negative/within normal limits
- possible low-grade intraepithelial lesion – changes in cells that may represent a low-grade abnormality but are not clear enough to justify a definite diagnosis
- low-grade intraepithelial lesion – minor changes consistent with human papilloma virus (HPV) infection

- possible high-grade intraepithelial lesion – changes in cells that mean a high-grade abnormality is suspected but are not clear enough to justify a definite diagnosis; with this result you would be referred for a colposcopy

- high-grade intraepithelial lesion – changes in cells that mean a high-grade abnormality is present; with this result you would be referred for a colposcopy

- atypical endocervical (glandular) cells of undetermined significance – changes in cells that are unusual in appearance and whose exact nature is uncertain; referral for colposcopy would still be recommended

- possible high-grade glandular lesion – changes in cells that mean a high-grade glandular abnormality is suspected but are not clear enough to justify a definite diagnosis; again, a referral for a colposcopy would be recommended

- adenocarcinoma in situ – changes in cells that indicate a less common high-grade abnormality inside the canal of the cervix; referral for early colposcopy would be recommended in this case

    Very rarely Pap tests may report:

- squamous cell carcinoma (SCC) – the presence of cancer in the squamous cells of the cervix; with this result you would be referred to a specialist gynaecological oncologist

- adenocarcinoma – a less common cancer affecting the glandular cells of the cervix rather than squamous cells; again, you would be referred to a specialist gynaecological oncologist

Only a *very small minority* of abnormal tests suggest there is an invasive cancer present. For more on cervical cancer, see chapter 35.

What causes abnormal cells to develop?

Most types of dysplastic abnormalities of the cervix and nearly all cervical cancers are linked to the human papilloma virus (HPV; see chapters 9 and 26). More than 100 different types of HPV have been identified. The virus causes changes in the cells that are divided into two groups:

1. those considered low-risk, usually causing low-grade abnormalities to develop, most of which will go away naturally within two years as the immune system responds locally to the infection and attacks cells containing the virus

2. those considered high-risk (14 recognised types), which can cause high-grade abnormalities (CIN2/3) to develop and if left untreated can progress over a period of 10 years or more to cancer of the cervix; they therefore need to be treated

The human papillomavirus (HPV) and abnormal cervical changes

Viruses are microscopic organisms that survive by spreading from one part of the body to another. Symptoms vary depending on the type of virus and the organ infected, but many infections cause no overt symptoms. There are more than 100 types of HPV affecting various parts of the body. Of these, about 40 types affect the genital area, including the cervix.

The types of HPV that infect the genital area are spread primarily through genital contact. More than 80 per cent of women and men who are sexually active will be exposed to the HPV virus during their lifetimes. In Australia the most common HPV types that cause genital infection are types 6 and 11 (associated with warts and low-grade changes), and types 16 and 18 (associated with high-grade changes).

Most HPV infections have *no* signs or symptoms. This means that most infected people are unaware they are infected and yet can transmit the virus to someone else during sex. This will often happen to people in their late teens and early 20s. More than 95 per cent of infections are cleared naturally by the immune system, while in the 5 per cent that persist it can be months or even years before abnormalities occur. Condoms offer only about 70 per cent protection from HPV infection.

Most people who have the virus will never develop warts or cell changes. The vast majority of women with HPV do not develop cervical cancer. Women will only find out they have had an HPV infection if they develop warts or if their Pap test reports an abnormality (less than 5 per cent of all tests taken).

Smoking is an important risk factor because it can lower immunity, and allow infection to persist and abnormalities to develop. Other things that may affect immunity include active Hepatitis B and C, HIV infection, recent glandular fever and immunosuppressive drugs taken for diseases such as rheumatoid arthritis or after organ or bone marrow transplants.

Monitoring and treatment of abnormal cells

If you have had an abnormal Pap test, there are various options available to you.

Colposcopy

After a positive or abnormal Pap test result and referral to a specialist, further examination and tests will be carried out before decisions can be made about the best treatment, if any, for your condition. The main examination is a procedure called colposcopy. The procedure is quite safe for pregnant women and will not harm the baby.

Colposcopy is an examination of the cervix that allows the specialist to locate cell changes and assess the extent of the changes. This examination is uncomfortable, but should not be painful, and should last only five to 10 minutes. Colposcopes are sometimes connected to a TV monitor so you can see what is happening, if you are interested.

A colposcope is a magnifying instrument, like binoculars, with a bright light, on a stand. You will be asked to undress from the waist down and will be provided with a gown to wear or covering for your lower half. At the start of the examination your legs will be placed in leg supports. These can be adjusted to suit you, so if you are not comfortable, ask for them to be adjusted before the examination begins.

A speculum is inserted into the vagina (exactly as for a Pap test) to hold the walls of your vagina slightly apart so that the specialist can see the cervix using the colposcope, which remains outside the body.

The examination usually starts with a repeat Pap test. The first smear is taken from the outside of the cervix using a spatula. The second is taken from the canal of the cervix using a thin brush.

After taking the Pap test, the specialist will dab the cervix with very mild acetic acid solution to help identify any abnormal cells. Most women do not find this painful although it may sting a little. Using the colposcope it is possible for the specialist to see the area and pattern of abnormality. It is important for them to check if the abnormal area is only on the outside or if it goes into the canal of the cervix. A brown dye (iodine) may then be used to outline the changes.

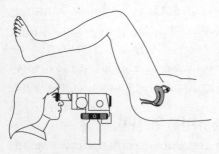

The colposcope

Biopsy

In order to confirm a diagnosis, during the colposcopy the specialist may take a tiny sample of cervical tissue. This is called a targeted biopsy. The biopsy will be sent to a pathology laboratory for further testing. Many women experience

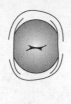

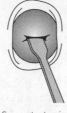

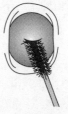

View of cervix through | Smear test using | Smear test using
a colposcope | a spatula | a brush

Taking a Pap test

no pain with this procedure, while others report some stinging or mild period-type cramping. It is very important that the abnormality be correctly diagnosed before any treatment decisions are made.

After the examination the specialist will be better informed to discuss the findings of the Pap test with you. It may be helpful to have someone with you so that you feel confident to ask questions and to help you to remember details of the discussion. The specialist may have a fairly good idea from the examination of the degree of abnormality present, but will need to await confirmation from the biopsy before making any decisions about treatment.

In most clinics, you will receive a letter outlining the results of the tests and a recommendation for the future management or treatment of your condition about two or three weeks after your visit. A copy will also be sent to your doctor. In some units you might also be able to telephone a dysplasia nurse to discuss the results if you do not receive or understand them.

The biopsy may show any of the results outlined below.

Low-grade abnormality

This indicates a CIN1 or wart virus (HPV) change. You will be advised to return to your GP for a Pap test in 12 months. This is because we know that these changes will disappear in over 80 per cent of women over a two-year period – in other words your own immune system will most likely get rid of the virus.

If these low-grade changes have been present for some time (more than three to four years), you may be advised to have another colposcopy in six to 12 months, or to have the cells removed. It is very important that you continue to have your Pap tests according to your doctor's recommendations because in the remaining 15-20 per cent of women, the low-grade changes persist and in a minority high-grade dysplasia may develop.

High-grade abnormality

This indicates CIN2 and CIN3, in which case you will need treatment. Your specialist will advise you on what this should be and when it can occur. If you are pregnant treatment can usually and safely be deferred. Your specialist will probably ask to see you later in your pregnancy and 12 weeks after the birth. Treatment will involve destroying the abnormal cells with a laser ablation of the cervical lesion or removing them with a LLETZ or LEEP procedure, or more rarely with a cone biopsy. All of these treatments are described below.

ACIS or precancerous glandular changes

If your biopsy or Pap test indicates these changes, you will need a cone biopsy (see below) or similar excisional treatment to treat the condition.

The abnormal area cannot be seen

If the abnormal area and transformation zone extend into the endocervical canal with the upper limit out of sight (technically called an unsatisfactory colposcopy), the specialist may advise you to have a cone biopsy (see below).

Minor cell changes

If the biopsy shows minor cell changes such as inflammation, infection or normal healing changes (metaplasia), that are not dysplasia (and therefore not precancerous) the recommendation will be to return to your GP in 12 months for a Pap test. This check-up is very important to ensure that the minor changes detected are improving or have returned to normal.

Treatment for abnormal changes to the cervix

The anaesthetic

Your specialist will discuss whether your procedure will be performed under local anaesthetic (while you are awake) or general anaesthetic (while you are asleep). Laser and LLETZ (also known as LEEP) treatments may be performed under local or general anaesthetic. Cone biopsy requires a general anaesthetic. If you have a particular preference for your anaesthetic, you should notify the doctor at your colposcopy.

Local anaesthetic

If you have a local anaesthetic, you can drink and eat normally before the procedure. Check with your specialist, but it can be helpful to take paracetamol or a non-steroidal anti-inflammatory drug (e.g. ibuprofen) half an hour before coming to the hospital for your treatment.

Local anaesthetic requires you to stay in hospital for two to three hours, after which you should be well enough to drive yourself home.

General anaesthetic

If you have a general anaesthetic it is best to take the day off work. You must not eat or drink any fluids (including water) for six hours beforehand. It is also not advisable to smoke for 48 hours beforehand. Immediately following your treatment you can expect to be in hospital for two to three hours. You will need to arrange for someone to take you home.

Types of treatment

Laser ablation treatment

The laser we use in dysplasia treatment is a very strong thin beam of infrared light that can be focused on pinpoint areas of the surface of the cervix. The heat from the beam destroys abnormal cells by burning and vaporising them.

Because the laser burns the cells, there will be a small amount of smoke, which will be removed from the vagina using a smoke evacuator. Everyone in the room will wear protective glasses and surgical masks. You will also be asked to wear a pair of the protective glasses during the procedure.

The laser leaves a raw area, which usually heals very well in about three weeks with minimal scarring. This is usually not painful, although you may experience a period-type cramp following the procedure. You should be able to return to work within 24 hours.

Wire loop excision (LLETZ or LEEP)

Large loop excision of the transformation zone (LLETZ, also called loop electro-surgical excision procedure or LEEP) removes a similar amount of

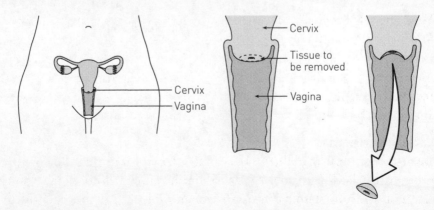

Wire loop excision

tissue to the laser. A wire loop with a very high-frequency electrical current is used to remove rather than destroy the abnormal cells. Afterwards the piece of tissue removed (loop biopsy) is sent to a pathology laboratory for examination, to confirm the diagnosis and to check if the abnormal cells have been completely removed.

Cone biopsy

A cone biopsy is a minor operation to remove a cone-shaped piece of tissue from the cervix. This can be performed using standard surgical techniques (scalpel) or electro-surgery.

A cone biopsy may be recommended when:

- Abnormal cells extend into the endocervical canal and therefore cannot all be seen during the colposcopy. In older women who are near or through menopause there is a greater chance of needing a cone biopsy because the transformation zone is usually in the canal.

- The Pap test results repeatedly show abnormal cells but the colposcopy appears normal. The abnormal cells may be coming from higher within the endocervical canal than can be seen.

- The Pap test or biopsy has shown abnormal glandular cells.

- The specialist is concerned that the abnormal cells may have formed an early cancer.

As well as helping to make an accurate diagnosis, the cone biopsy is usually an effective treatment in itself. The tissue removed during the cone biopsy will be examined to confirm the diagnosis and to check if

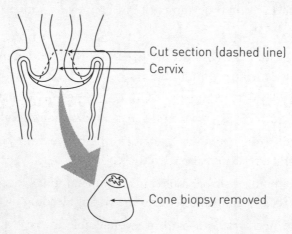

Cone biopsy

the abnormal cells have been completely removed. In a minority of cases, further treatment may be recommended.

On the day that you are admitted you will have a chance to talk with the specialist about the operation. It may help to make a list beforehand of any questions you want to ask.

The operation is performed on the day you are admitted to hospital under general anaesthetic. When the anaesthetic has worn off you may experience some period-type pain or cramping.

After a cone biopsy, it is best to take a couple of days off work and get help from family or friends so you can rest. For the following week you will need to avoid too much physical activity, particularly any lifting.

You can expect some bleeding and pinkish discharge. If it becomes heavier than a period you should contact your local doctor or emergency department. You should not have sexual intercourse for four weeks.

Following a cone biopsy, women who get pregnant will need special check-ups between 12 and 28 weeks, as having a cone biopsy increases the risk of premature delivery from a usual rate of 5–7 per cent to 10–15 per cent.

Radical diathermy

Radical electro-diathermy uses an electric current to produce heat that destroys the cells. It can cause more tissue damage, pain and scarring, and consequently is rarely used in Australian hospitals these days.

What to expect following treatment

- You may have a vaginal discharge. It may be pink, blood-tinged or dark brown. You may have spotting or bleeding for one to two weeks after treatment. About a week after the treatment it is quite normal to pass a small blood clot which might look like a piece of tissue. This is usually followed by a small amount of bleeding.

- You may have mild to moderate discomfort similar to period pain. You may take pain-relieving medication such as paracetamol to relieve this.

- You should avoid strenuous exercise for three to four weeks; light training can be restarted after two weeks.

- You should not have sexual intercourse or use tampons for four weeks. This helps with healing and reduces the risk of bleeding or infection.

- You should not soak in a bath; it is preferable to have a shower or sponge bath for the first two weeks at least.

If any of the following happen you should go to your local doctor or emergency department:

- vaginal bleeding heavier than a period or soaking a maxi pad in one hour (go to the emergency department rather than waiting to see your GP)
- a fever above 38 degrees Celsius
- offensive and smelly vaginal discharge
- severe abdominal pain that is not relieved by paracetamol

The first follow-up appointment is usually six months after the procedure. It is very important to attend to determine if the treatment has been successful.

Frequently asked questions

How can I prevent cancer of the cervix?

The best way to prevent cervical cancer is to have a regular Pap test (every two years between the ages of 18 and 70). An abnormal Pap test result or any unusual symptoms will lead to further investigations. Vaccination against four types of genital HPVs is available free for all children and is licensed for women up to the age of 45 (see below). If you are a smoker you are two to three times more likely to have an abnormal test, so we strongly recommended that you give up smoking.

Is there a cure for HPV?

There is no medical cure for HPV infection, but in the vast majority of women the infection goes away without intervention due to the local immune reaction. Any treatments are directed at the changes in the cervical skin caused by HPV infection, such as obvious warts or dysplasia.

What is the connection between HPV infection and cervical cancer?

All genital types of HPV can cause mild Pap test abnormalities that do not usually have serious consequences. Approximately 14 of the 40 identified genital HPV types (so called high-risk types) can lead, in a minority of cases, to cervical cancer. Research has shown that for most women, genital HPV infection will become undetectable within two years. Regular Pap tests and careful medical follow-up and treatment are the best way to ensure that abnormal cell changes do not develop into cervical cancer.

Is my partner affected by HPV?

Generally, the virus will not affect a male partner but he may carry it on his skin. Woman-to-woman transmission can occur through either direct genital contact or the shared use of sex aids.

Could the HPV vaccine help me?

Of the two vaccines currently available, the one commonly used in Australia (Gardasil) protects against infection by four genital HPV types. It does not treat pre-existing infection. The vaccine requires three injections over six months and works by causing the body to produce its own protection (antibodies) against four HPV types: 6, 11, 16 and 18. Two of these types, 16 and 18, cause 70 per cent of cervical cancers in women. The other two types, 6 and 11, cause approximately 90 per cent of genital warts. It is important to note that the vaccine only helps to protect against 70 per cent of cervical cancers, so you must still have regular Pap tests to detect any abnormal cell changes due to other HPV types.

The HPV vaccines were originally designed to protect people who have not yet come into contact with genital HPV. The vaccine commonly used in Australia is approved for use in females aged 9–45 and school-aged boys. It is funded under the Immunise Australia Program for girls and boys aged 12 or 13. As natural infection with the virus does not provide immunity that prevents new infection, there is potential benefit for women to have the vaccination even after known previous HPV infection or test abnormalities. Unfortunately, there is no Medicare rebate for receiving the vaccine after school age.

For further information contact your GP or women's healthcare provider.

I'm feeling scared – is this typical?

Knowing you have abnormal cells and that you need tests and possible treatment can be stressful or frightening. It can make you feel very vulnerable. It is particularly difficult because you probably didn't know anything was wrong before your Pap test result. You may feel that things seem to be out of your control. These feelings are quite normal.

Because the abnormal cells are hidden in a sexual area and are linked with the possibility of precancer, it can be very frightening. Try to remember that having abnormal cells does not mean you have suddenly become seriously ill or have cancer. Talking about your fears and concerns with your partner, family or friends can help you overcome some of these feelings. It is quite usual to feel a little anxious until you have had all the tests and know what treatment, if any, is required.

The vast majority of abnormal Pap test results do not mean you have cancer. Pap tests are designed to detect precancerous changes so that cancer can be prevented.

What if I'm pregnant when the abnormal test result is found?

If you are pregnant and you have an abnormal Pap test result, a colposcopy examination can be performed without any harm to the pregnancy. The abnormal area will be checked at regular intervals throughout the pregnancy. If the dysplasia is still present after you have had your baby, it is recommended that you have treatment then.

Will the treatment affect my fertility?

In general the treatments do not affect your ability to become pregnant. Cone biopsies and larger LLETZ/LEEPs for dysplasia might weaken the cervix and increase the risk of premature delivery. It is therefore important to inform your obstetrician about any treatments you have had in the past.

Does smoking cause dysplasia?

Many studies have indicated that smoking increases the risk of dysplasia by a factor of up to three. For help with giving up, call the Quitline on 137 848.

What check-ups will I need after treatment?

You will probably see your specialist six months after your treatment for a follow-up Pap test (after laser) and colposcopy (after LLETZ/LEEP or cone biopsy). At each appointment you will be advised when to see your specialist again. When your specialist is certain that the abnormalities have been successfully treated they will return you to your GP for care. In most cases you will be asked to see your GP one year after treatment for a Pap test and a test for HPV. This will be repeated two years after treatment.

If your Pap test and HPV tests are negative after two years, you can safely return to the routine screening of a Pap test every two years. If your Pap tests are normal but you test positive for HPV, Pap tests will be repeated annually until the infection is gone. In almost all cases, the immune system will keep the virus under control or get rid of it completely. It is very rare for HPV to lead to cervical cancer.

What are the chances of recurrence?

Up to five per cent of women will have further problems with recurrent dysplasia. You will need regular cervical screening according to the guidelines of the National Cervical Screening Program and what your doctor recommends.

Is dysplasia hereditary?

Dysplasia and cervical cancer are not hereditary, but your immune system and the way your body responds to infections are influenced by your genes.

Is there anything I can do to help my dysplasia?

The main aim is to maintain your immune system at the best possible level. If you are a smoker it is best for you to give up.

Complementary therapists may talk about the benefits of beta-carotene, folate and vitamins C and E in the treatment of dysplasia. While there is no harm in trying them, there is no scientific evidence to prove they will be helpful.

You should always tell your doctor if you are taking any alternative medicines, including any herbs, vitamins or other complementary remedies.

What if it's cancer?

It is very unlikely that you will be found to have true invasive cancer after a colposcopy or even after treatment. For the few women for whom this is the case, the cancer will usually have been detected at a very early stage and the chance of being cured will therefore be high.

Future developments

Australia's National Cervical Screening Program is currently under review, and new recommendations will be published by the federal government after consultation and review by national experts. Information about this review can be found at: www.cancerscreening.gov.au/internet/screening/publishing.nsf/Content/ncsp-renewal.

It is possible that the test used for screening, the frequency of testing and the age of commencement may all be changed as a result of this review. Any changes would be preceded by extensive public information releases and advertisements.

37

Breast health

Bruce Mann

Breast changes are common as we grow older and change. Breast development commences during fetal development, and is the same in boys and girls. At puberty, the next stage of breast development occurs. The ducts and glandular tissue develop, resulting in the adult breast that is a mixture of glandular tissue (breast parenchyma) and fatty (adipose) tissue. During pregnancy, another stage of development occurs under the influence of the hormonal changes, with a dramatic increase in the glandular tissue and development of the lobules where milk is made. Once the baby is weaned, the breast undergoes another series of changes as it goes back to the 'resting' state. After menopause, the level of circulating female hormones is greatly diminished, and the breasts undergo further change, with much of the breast glandular tissue disappearing.

In tandem with the cyclical hormonal changes between menarche (the start of your periods) and menopause, there will often be noticeable changes in the breasts, often with variable pain, tenderness and lumpiness. These may be uncomfortable – extremely so in some cases – and at times you or your GP may be concerned about the possibility of a serious problem in the breast.

Breast density relates to the ratio of parenchyma to adipose tissue, and varies from woman to woman. In general, young women have higher breast density than older women, but it is also influenced by genetic and other factors. It has been shown that women with higher breast density are at increased risk of developing breast cancer, and also that a small breast cancer is more difficult to detect by mammography in a woman with denser breast tissue.

Lumps and lumpiness

Breast lumps or lumpiness are a common reason for a woman to seek medical attention. Sometimes these lumps or lumpiness are painful, but the usual concern is that the lump or change might represent cancer. There are a large number of causes of breast lumps. The most common is simply a prominent area of breast tissue in a lumpy breast. These lumps might seem prominent at one point, but later might seem to have disappeared.

Common causes of a discrete lump (a lump with defined edges as opposed to the lumpiness described above) include fibroadenomas (a common, harmless lump made of fibrous tissue surrounding normal breast ducts that most often occurs in young women), cysts, fat necrosis (a lump that can form after trauma due to some of the fatty tissue in the breast losing its blood supply), abscesses and cancer. While cancer is the most feared cause of a breast lump, it is certainly not the most common.

When a lump is found, or there is lumpiness that needs further investigation, an ultrasound is often the most valuable investigation. Ultrasound uses soundwaves to image the breast tissue, and may be able to show that there is a discrete abnormality within the breast, or that what is being felt is most likely to be simply prominent breast tissue. If there is a discrete lump, the ultrasound can distinguish between cysts (fluid-filled lumps) and solid lumps, which are generally more of a concern.

A discrete solid lump in a woman younger than 40 is most often a fibroadenoma, although further imaging and some form of needle biopsy is usually necessary to confirm the diagnosis. A fibroadenoma does not need to be removed.

Breast pain (mastalgia)

Breast pain is experienced by most women at some time during their life. It is usually cyclical, most often bothersome before a period, and may need no investigation or treatment. There are times, however, when the pain is severe enough for a woman to seek medical attention. A doctor's standard approach to the problem of breast pain is to look for and exclude serious underlying problems and then address the pain. Cancer is rarely painful, but there are cases where pain is the first symptom of what turns out to be cancer. It is important to emphasise that this is rare, but excluding cancer is an important first step.

The most common cause of pain is related to hormonal effects on the breast. This pain occurs during the reproductive years, and is most common during the 20s and 30s. Investigation typically reveals no under-lying problems. If there is associated lumpiness, or a specific lump, then investigation may show some form of benign breast condition such as 'fibrocystic change', which may or may not be related to the pain. Factors that may be associated with it include the contraceptive pill – changes in the Pill may bring on pain, and similarly a change in the kind of Pill used may be effective management of the pain; smoking, which seems to sensitise breast tissue to pain; and caffeine. Treatments commonly used for benign breast pain include evening primrose oil and vitamin B6. The evidence for the effectiveness of these treatments is not strong, but many women believe they are very helpful. Some women request surgery to remove a specific area that seems to be causing the pain; in most cases this should not be done, as it may not fix the pain, and the site of surgery often causes pain for a long time.

Other causes of pain include chest wall pain, which is frequently mistaken for breast pain. This pain is most often just beside the breast-bone (sternum), and often responds to treatment with anti-inflammatory medications. Infections of the breast tissue (mastitis) are also painful. Mastitis is most common during breastfeeding, and is particularly a problem in the first few weeks of feeding a first baby. This usually starts with cracked nipples, and leads to a tender and red area in the breast. Mastitis generally responds to continued feeding or expression of milk, and to antibiotics, although sometimes it progresses to a more serious infection, including formation of an abscess. The other group of women who experience infections tend to be smokers in their 30s to 50s. These infections occur close to the nipple and do not result in the severe pain and fevers of infections related to breastfeeding, but can be difficult to treat and often recur if the woman continues smoking.

Breast cancer

Breast cancer is more common in older women: 6 per cent of all breast cancers occurring in women under 40; 17 per cent between 40 and 50; 24 per cent between 50 and 60; 26 per cent between 60 and 70; and 27 per cent over 70. Put another way, women at 20 have an approximately 0.1 per cent chance of developing breast cancer in the next 10 years, whereas women at 30, 40, 50, 60 and 70 have about a 0.8 per cent, 1.5 per cent, 2.5 per cent, 3.5 per cent and 2.5 per cent chance respectively of developing breast cancer over the next 10 years.

In most cases of breast cancer, there is no obvious precipitating reason. In 5–10 per cent of cases, a woman who develops breast cancer has inherited a mutation in one of a number of breast cancer susceptibility genes (such as BRCA1 and BRCA2; see chapter 35) that means that she had a very high chance of developing breast cancer and requires specialist risk management. In a further 20 per cent of cases, there is a family history, but this is usually not very strong and may simply be due to bad luck or shared environmental factors. For more see 'The genetics of breast cancer', later in this chapter.

A number of lifestyle and environmental factors are associated with an increased risk of developing breast cancer. Having a child early in life appears to be protective, and prolonged breastfeeding is also associated with a reduced risk of breast cancer. Women who have no children, and those who delay their first pregnancy until their mid-30s, thus do have a higher risk of the disease. Being overweight or obese is also associated with increased risk, especially if the weight is gained after the age of 18. Alcohol intake is associated with increased breast cancer risk. Low vitamin D levels have also been associated with increased risk of breast cancer and a poorer outcome if cancer develops; whether this is a direct effect of the vitamin D (and therefore treatable with supplementation) or an indirect reflection of lifestyle and other dietary factors is unknown. Exercise has recently been shown to be beneficial after a breast cancer diagnosis. Specific associations between aspects of diet and breast cancer risk have not been identified, and in particular there is no evidence that breast cancer risk can be altered through specific dietary supplementation or modification.

Postmenopausal combined oestrogen/progesterone hormone replacement therapy (HRT) has been associated with an increased risk of breast cancer. Use of HRT for up to five years has not been shown to have a detectable impact on breast cancer risk but use for longer than that is associated with an increased risk, and the duration of use is directly related to the level of increased risk. Women who have used postmenopausal HRT for 10 years have a risk of breast cancer about 30 per cent greater than women who have never used HRT. This means that 4 per cent of 65-year-old women who have used HRT since the age of 55 have a risk of developing breast cancer in the next 10 years, as opposed to a risk of about 3 per cent for women who have not used it. A lot of work is being done to identify the component of HRT that is responsible for this increased risk. It appears that it is due to the progesterone rather than the oestrogen, so that women who have had a hysterectomy (and therefore do not need the progesterone to protect against endometrial cancer) have a much lower risk of developing breast cancer from HRT.

Screening for breast cancer – mammograms

A national mammographic screening program was introduced in Australia in 1993 to improve the outcome of breast cancer through early detection. A successful pilot project was conducted in Melbourne and developed into the program that is now conducted by BreastScreen Australia. The aim of the program is to maximise the detection of small and early breast cancers. The target age range for this program is 50–69, as this is the group that has been shown to have the greatest benefit from mammographic screening in randomised clinical trials. Women between 40 and 50 and those over 70 are eligible to attend, but they are not actively recruited, as the evidence for benefit in these age ranges is not conclusive.

There has been some controversy over the value of routine mammographic screening. Five large randomised studies in the 1970s and 1980s addressed the question of whether mammographic screening in healthy women without any symptoms led to a reduction in breast cancer mortality. The overall results of these studies suggest that it does, by about 15 per cent. More recent analysis has suggested that the impact is lower than this, and that the dramatic improvements in the outcome of breast cancer seen in recent decades are more the result of improved treatment rather than earlier diagnosis. Most experts believe that it is the combination of early diagnosis and improved treatment that has led to the significant reduction in the chance that women in Australia will die from breast cancer.

An area of concern to many is that some abnormalities detected in a screening program would never have caused a problem during the natural term of the woman's life. This is impossible to measure directly, as it would require deliberately withholding treatment after diagnosis of something that is potentially dangerous. It is accepted, however, that a number of cases of early precancer (known as low-grade ductal carcinoma in situ) are likely to be 'over-diagnosis'. The problem is that no one can be certain if any particular case of cancer needs treatment or not. An important aim of research is to ensure that the diagnosis of these conditions does not lead to unnecessary over-treatment with surgery, medications or radiotherapy.

The genetics of breast cancer

As mentioned above, about 5–10 per cent of all cases of breast cancer occur in women with a genetic predisposition. These women have a strong family history, with multiple relatives on the same side of the family developing breast and/or ovarian cancer at a young age. It is important to note that these mutations can be passed through the father's side of the family as well as the mother's, and so breast or ovarian cancer in aunts and grandparents on the father's side may be significant for a woman's breast cancer risk.

Cancer Australia has developed a very helpful classification system based on family history. Less than 1 per cent of the population can be classified as very high risk, possibly due to an identifiable inherited mutation, and should undergo specific risk management under the care of a specialist. A larger group is classified as moderate risk, and may consider having yearly screening mammograms instead of the standard timeframe of every two years. Most women are classified a 'population risk', and need no more than to be 'breast aware'; that is, to be alert to any persistent changes in the breast and have these assessed and appropriately investigated, and have a surveillance mammogram every two years over the age of 50.

Treatment for breast cancer

Cancer treatment is specifically tailored in every case to the nature and severity of the particular cancer, and the needs and views of the individual woman. Until the late nineteenth century, breast cancer treatment was very unsatisfactory. The only treatment option was surgery, and removal of the breast cancer was usually followed by a recurrence in the breast, meaning that the treatment often did not help the unfortunate patient.

In the early twentieth century, an effective surgical treatment was introduced: the radical mastectomy, where the breast, the overlying skin and underlying muscle were removed, as well as the lymph nodes from the axilla (armpit). This was effective at stopping the cancer from coming back on the chest wall, but was very disfiguring, and the cancer often came back elsewhere.

Throughout the twentieth century, surgical treatment for breast cancer became more refined, and the radical mastectomy was replaced by the simple mastectomy (leaving the muscle behind) and then mastectomy was replaced by breast conservation – simply removing the cancerous lump and a rim of normal tissue, then treating the remainder of the breast with radiotherapy. This is a standard treatment option available to most women diagnosed with breast cancer. Where mastectomy is still required or chosen by the woman, reconstructive techniques have been developed, using either an implant (prosthesis) or the woman's own tissue, most often from the lower abdomen. Reconstruction can sometimes be done during the same operation as the mastectomy (immediate reconstruction) or delayed to a later date (see chapters 27 and 38 for more).

A complication of the removal of the axillary lymph glands is lymphoedema, the accumulation of tissue fluid (lymph) in the arm or breast, which ranges from bothersome to painful and disabling. In the mid-1990s, the technique of lymphatic mapping and sentinel node biopsy was developed, which allows the surgeon to identify and remove the key lymph node that would be involved with breast cancer should it spread. This means that where the cancer has not spread to the lymph nodes, a very small operation removing a single node can be done, and the risk of lymphoedema is dramatically reduced. It also means that breast cancer surgery can generally be done as a day procedure.

The other crucial development in breast cancer management is the introduction of 'adjuvant' therapies. These are treatments given after breast cancer surgery to reduce the risk of cancer recurrence. Adjuvant radiotherapy is frequently given to either the breast or the chest wall after surgery to remove the cancer, to reduce the risk of recurrence in the breast or chest wall. Adjuvant chemotherapy or hormonal therapies are given to reduce the risk of the cancer recurring at a distant location, such as in the bone, liver or lungs. Depending on the situation, these adjuvant therapies can reduce the risk of recurrence by more than 50 per cent, and are responsible for much of the improved outlook for women faced with a breast cancer diagnosis.

Breast cancer is not a death sentence

The number of women diagnosed with breast cancer is more than six times greater than the number of women who die from it. In other words, more than 85 per cent of women diagnosed with breast cancer will not die from it – they will be cured. This is remarkably better than 40 years ago, when the number was around 65 per cent.

38
Plastic surgery in midlife

Dean Trotter

By midlife, some women will have suffered some form of cancer or trauma, and reconstructive plastic surgery can be an important step in their path to recovery. This is also the period where age begins to show on the face and body, and some women undertake cosmetic surgery to improve their appearance in these areas.

Plastic surgery after cancer

Cancer surgery may result in a loss of function or may change appearance, and plastic surgery may be considered to reshape, repair or rebuild tissues affected by cancer surgery. This surgery may be as simple as revising a bad scar, or as complex as transferring tissue (for example, skin grafts or tissue flaps) or using implants to reconstruct damaged or diseased structures, such as a breast.

Breast reconstruction surgery

Breast cancer becomes more common with increasing age, and reconstructive breast surgery following breast cancer can be very important in restoring self-image. Surgery may involve techniques such as augmentation or reduction for symmetry, or complete breast reconstruction with tissue flaps or silicone implants.

Breast reconstruction may be performed at the time of mastectomy (immediate reconstruction) or at a later time, once all the necessary treatment for the breast cancer has been completed (delayed reconstruction). Both techniques have very high rates of satisfaction and improvement in quality of life. The major benefit of immediate reconstruction is that more breast skin can be preserved and then used to reconstruct the breast; this means that the reconstructed breast is more like the original breast. If the reconstruction is delayed, a large amount of breast skin needs to be removed to ensure a good mastectomy scar. This breast skin then needs to be replaced during the reconstruction, which generally means more scarring on the chest.

See chapter 27 for more information on breast reconstructive plastic surgery.

Virginia is 56 years old. When she was 42 she underwent a left total mastectomy and axillary lymph node clearance. She also had post-operative chemotherapy and radiotherapy. At the time she had three children between the ages of eight and 14 and was working full-time. She was not offered reconstruction, but even if she had been, she said she would have been too busy to contemplate it, preferring just to have her cancer treated and get on with her life.

Since having the surgery she had heard that reconstruction was possible. She had a friend who had had it and said it had changed her life in a positive way. Virginia felt that it was something she would like to do once her children had moved out of home.

Virginia's GP referred her to a plastic and reconstructive surgeon. The surgeon discussed reconstructive options and showed her some pictures of other people who had had delayed breast reconstruction.

After some further thought, Virginia decided that she would like to undergo surgery. The surgery lasted four hours. The skin and fat from her abdomen were moved to her chest and shaped into a breast, pre-serving the abdominal muscles. The blood vessels supplying the tummy tissue were connected with microsurgery. The abdomen was sutured closed, giving Virginia a tummy tuck. Everything went smoothly post-operatively and she stayed in hospital for five days. Virginia took six weeks off work to recover from the operation. When she first went back to work she found she was tired by the end of the day, but this feeling soon disappeared and after three months she felt she was back to normal.

After six months Virginia had surgery to recreate a nipple on her recon-structed breast. She also had a breast lift on her other breast to place the nipple and areola in a better position and reshape the breast, providing a more symmetrical result. This surgery required only one night in hospital and took 90 minutes. Virginia took two weeks off work to recover from the surgery.

Virginia's final phase of reconstruction was a tattoo to colour her new nipple and simulate an areola on her new breast. This occurred about three months after her previous operation.

Virginia is very pleased she had the surgery; in fact, she now feels she would have liked to have had it earlier, had her circumstances allowed. She had given up wearing a breast prosthesis some time before and had changed her wardrobe to suit her new body. Her self-confidence has improved and she likes that she can wear any clothing she wishes. She also now feels she has beaten her cancer and can really look forward to enjoying her life.

Genital surgery

Genital surgery for cancer may be followed by referral to a plastic surgeon for reconstruction. Surgery in the genital region can be very distressing and uncomfortable. This is a complex area of the body, and surgery needs to remove the problem but also be mindful of trying to avoid creating new and ongoing problems. One of the more common situations arises when a woman is being treated for vulvar cancer. This may require cutting out parts of the vulva, vagina and skin around the anus, and sometimes the anus, urethra, bladder or rectum are involved too. Reconstruction is complex and varied, depending on the exact problem. A common reconstruction involves moving tissue from the groin crease or thigh (called a flap) to fill the defect created by the surgery to remove the tumour.

Jo was diagnosed at 62 with vulvar intraepithelial neoplasia. She had been advised that around half of her left vulva, the lower part of the vaginal wall and some skin between her vulva and anus needed to be removed (these tissues are all part of the perineum). She was referred to a plastic and reconstructive surgeon to determine what form of reconstruction was best. Jo was fit and well and took no medications. She had stopped smoking more than 20 years before. She was of average height and weight.

Jo's plastic surgeon advised her that she was a good candidate for what is called a 'lotus petal' flap. This is where a piece of tissue is moved from the upper thigh or groin crease and used to fix the defect created by removing a tumour. The tissue includes skin and fat, with the blood vessels to keep it alive. The tissue looks like the petal of a lotus flower, hence the name.

Jo underwent surgery under a general anaesthetic to remove the tumour. Jo was admitted to hospital on the same day and needed no special preparations other than not eating or drinking for six hours before the operation. Once she was anaesthetised, a urinary catheter was inserted to drain her bladder and then the tumour was removed. The lotus petal flap was then removed from her groin and moved into the area where the tumour had been. The flap reconstructed the lower vagina and vulva, and replaced the skin that had been removed between the anus and vagina. It was attached with dissolving sutures and a silicone draining tube was inserted into the thigh where the flap had been harvested. The whole procedure lasted less than two hours. Jo stayed in hospital for four nights.

She was not in much pain initially because the surgeons had injected local anaesthetic into her wounds while she was still under the general anaesthetic. The pain was worst on the first and second days but was well controlled with strong tablet painkillers. Jo found the biggest issue was that she couldn't sit down normally as she had to avoid all pressure on the flap. Once Jo went home she continued to avoid pressure on the flap, and spent her time watching TV, reading books and using her computer. The sutures started to dissolve after about three weeks, and by six weeks things were starting to get back to normal. Jo still had some discomfort and the flap was still a little swollen, but she could now walk normally and was able to resume swimming. Although her perineal anatomy was not the same as it had been before and she had some scarring, she was pleased that the tumour had been removed and she was able to get back to the things she used to do. It took some months for her to return to sexual activity with her partner, but she was eventually able to do so.

Skin cancer surgery

Skin cancer is very common in Australia. The importance of protecting ourselves from the sun has really only been appreciated for the last 20 years or so, which means that generations of Australians have been exposed to high levels of solar radiation. This is known to lead to skin cancer, and the risk is higher in those with fairer skin. Skin cancers develop more commonly on sun-exposed areas, especially the face, forearms and legs.

The three main types of skin cancer are basal cell carcinoma (BCC), squamous cell carcinoma (SCC) and melanoma. BCC is the most common type of skin cancer. It may look like a small ulcer, a scaly spot, a firm lump or a flesh-coloured mole. Usually there are no symptoms. BCCs do not spread through the bloodstream or lymphatic system, but will continue to grow in the spot where they developed until they are treated. Treatment may involve using a cream or surgery. The type of treatment offered depends on how big the BCC is and where it is. If it is large or in an area that is cosmetically sensitive or without loose skin (such as the nose), then a reconstruction may be required. This may involve skin grafts or rearranging the skin in the local area (a flap) to fill the defect created by removal of the tumour.

SCC is the next most common form of skin cancer. It can spread through the bloodstream or lymphatic system but fortunately this is not common, especially with smaller lesions. It often appears as a scaly spot or ulcer. Its treatment is similar to that of BCC.

Melanoma affects around one in nine Australians. Fortunately, although it is a potentially fatal disease, it is generally not fatal as most melanomas are diagnosed at an early stage. They usually appear as dark or black spots, bubbles, blisters or scabs. They may arise in an existing mole or develop in an area of previously normal-looking skin. The thickness of the melanoma is one of the most important factors in making a prognosis and determining what treatment is best. The tumour is usually cut out with an appropriate margin of normal skin, to try to reduce the chance of it recurring. Other tests may be advised, such as a lymph node biopsy or radiological investigations, such as a chest X-ray, MRI, CT or PET scan or ultrasound (see chapter 3 for more information on these tests and scans).

Skin cancer is common and can be appropriately treated by any suitably qualified doctor. If you require skin grafts and flaps or surgery in cosmetically sensitive areas such as anywhere on the face, you should consider a consultation with a plastic and reconstructive surgeon.

Cosmetic surgery

Cosmetic surgery may be considered by older women seeking to restore a more youthful appearance. This is commonly aimed at rejuvenating the face or the neck (face lift or neck lift). This type of surgery is usually entirely elective and always needs careful consideration; the motivation for the surgery needs to be defined and the goals clearly set.

Ageing is a normal, inevitable process, and surgery is unable to prevent it. As we age, our tissues lose elasticity and volume and tend to become saggy and empty. The speed of this process is influenced by a number of factors, including smoking, sun damage, weight changes, medications and genetics.

Surgery generally attempts to rejuvenate the affected part of the body by restoring tissues to their previous positions, and restoring volume where appropriate. There are many options available and the best choice for any individual should be decided over a number of consultations with a properly trained plastic and reconstructive surgeon.

Botox and fillers

Non-surgical methods are popular and include using injectable products, such as botulinum toxin (botox) and 'fillers' such as hyaluronic acid, hydroxyapatite and collagen. Botulinum toxin is used to temporarily paralyse muscles, weakening them and allowing the wrinkles that develop due to the action of those muscles to smooth out. It tends to work best around the eyes and mouth and on the forehead. The toxin is effective for around three months and then needs to be reinjected. It is quite a safe drug with minimal side effects. There is a small chance of bleeding or infection and an extremely rare chance of overdose. It is, however, expensive and if not regularly repeated the effects will wear off and the wrinkles treated by it will recur.

Fillers are often used in conjunction with botulinum toxin to smooth out wrinkles. Some wrinkles will disappear with the toxin alone, but others are deeper and if filled with a substance may become shallower and less noticeable. Various products are available, and new ones regularly come onto the market. Many are based on a substance that is produced naturally by the body: hyaluronic acid. Fillers made of this substance are gradually broken down by the body and rarely induce a bad reaction from the immune system. They are intended as a short- or medium-term solution and may help soften the appearance of wrinkles if used properly in some people. Other fillers are made from substances that are not normally produced by the body or cannot be broken down in the body. These include silicone and various types of plastics. Use of these needs to be carefully considered as they have a high rate of complications. Often the consequences are permanent and untreatable – sometimes they are devastating.

In general, if you are considering botulinum toxin or fillers, we strongly advise a consultation with a properly trained medical practitioner.

39

Prolapse and incontinence

Marcus Carey, Margaret Sherburn

Pelvic organ prolapse

Prolapse is a protrusion or 'dropping down' of the pelvic organs into the vagina or even outside the vaginal opening. Prolapse can affect the bladder (in which case it is referred to as a cystocele), uterus or rectum (rectocele). It occurs when the ligaments and muscles that support the pelvic organs become stretched, weakened or torn. It is a very common disorder that may be experienced by young, midlife and older women.

While ageing is a factor, other factors can cause prolapse, including loss of muscle tone, menopause, pregnancy and childbirth, obesity, family history, pelvic trauma, previous pelvic surgery, repeated heavy lifting,

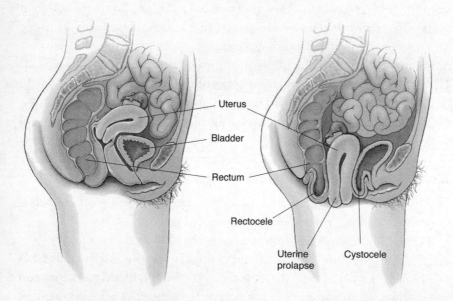

Uterus

Bladder

Rectum

Rectocele

Uterine prolapse

Cystocele

Normal support, no prolapse

Pelvic organ prolapse

chronic constipation, chronic coughing, smoking, and certain medical conditions that weaken the body's connective tissue. It may also occur in tandem with other pelvic floor disorders such as urinary incontinence.

Prolapse has four stages, for which the reference point is the vaginal opening. Stage 1 is the mildest form of prolapse, and means that the pelvic organs have prolapsed to a position that is at least 1 centimetre above the vaginal opening. Stage 2 means the prolapse is situated 1 centimetre above or below the vaginal opening. In stage 3, the prolapse protrudes more than 1 centimetre below the vaginal opening. The most severe form of prolapse is stage 4 and occurs when the entire vagina is outside the vaginal opening.

How common is prolapse?

Prolapse is very common. Fifty per cent of women who have had a baby will develop some degree of prolapse at some stage, but most women with prolapse experience only minor symptoms or even no symptoms at all. Just over 10 per cent of women with prolapse require surgery.

How do I know if I have prolapse?

Prolapse can cause a variety of symptoms. If you have prolapse you may become aware of a lump or bulge protruding from your vagina. You may also experience a sensation of fullness or heaviness in the vaginal area. Lower back pain and pelvic discomfort are also common symptoms. Prolapse of the bladder may cause difficulty with bladder-emptying and frequent bladder infections. Prolapse of the lower bowel into the vagina may cause constipation and difficulty passing a bowel motion. Prolapse can also cause problems with sexual intercourse, such as reduced sensation, a feeling of the vagina being too loose, discomfort and even pain. The majority of women with prolapse experience mild symptoms or even no symptoms.

Non-surgical treatments for prolapse

The two most common non-surgical treatments for prolapse are pelvic floor muscle training and the use of a vaginal pessary.

Pelvic floor muscle training (see chapter 18) is used to strengthen the group of muscles and ligaments that support the urethra (which takes urine from the bladder to the outside of the body), bladder, uterus and lower bowel. Regular exercise of the pelvic floor muscles is recommended throughout life to prevent or correct weakness. Exercising weak muscles regularly over a period of time can strengthen them and make them work again. Pelvic floor muscle training can be effective if you have a mild (stage 1 or 2) prolapse.

A vaginal pessary is a device that supports the vagina. It may be preferred over surgery by women who are planning to have further children; who have a medical condition that makes surgery more risky; or who simply do not like the idea of surgery at this stage. Vaginal pessaries are generally successful in relieving prolapse symptoms. They can be used for as long as you wish but a new pessary needs to be fitted every three to six months. The pessary sits inside the vagina and when it is in the correct position you should not be able to feel it. After the pessary has been inserted you can resume all of your normal day-to-day activities, including sexual activity.

Surgery for prolapse

Many different operations can be used for prolapse. The type of surgery recommended will depend on many factors, such as age, the severity of the prolapse, and having had a hysterectomy or previous failed prolapse surgery. Prolapse surgery can be performed along with surgery for urinary incontinence, and about 35 per cent of women who have prolapse surgery will need this. The most common operations used for prolapse are detailed below.

Vaginal repair using sutures (colporrhaphy)

Repairing a prolapse with sutures (stitches) is often referred to as a colporrhaphy. This type of surgery is usually recommended for a mild degree of prolapse (stage 1 and 2 prolapse; see above) in women who have not had previous prolapse surgery. A vaginal repair using this technique can be performed in combination with other procedures, such as surgery for urinary incontinence and hysterectomy.

Prolapse surgery can be performed with a regional (spinal) anaesthetic or general anaesthetic. Incisions are made inside the vagina and the tissue supporting the vagina repaired and strengthened with stitches. This may be at the front or back walls of the vagina or both, depending on the type of prolapse. Sutures provide reinforcement of the weakened vaginal tissue. An additional stitch (sacrospinous ligament fixation stitch) may be required at the top of the vagina for additional support. The incisions that were made in the vaginal walls at the start of surgery are closed with stitches that will dissolve after two weeks. At the end of the operation a catheter is inserted into the bladder to drain urine, and a gauze pack placed in the vagina to prevent bleeding. These remain in place overnight.

Hysterectomy

Some women with a moderate or severe prolapse of the uterus require a hysterectomy as part of their surgical treatment. Hysterectomy, if required, is usually performed through the vagina so that no abdominal incisions are required.

Sometimes the hysterectomy is performed with laparoscopy (keyhole surgery) or through an incision in the lower abdomen. Usually the ovaries are not removed during hysterectomy for prolapse unless there is a specific reason, such as a family history of ovarian cancer.

Prolapse surgery using a synthetic graft (mesh)

The use of a synthetic graft during prolapse surgery is sometimes recommended if for an advanced or recurrent prolapse. Advanced prolapse means the prolapsed vagina or uterus protrudes outside the vaginal opening (stage 3 or 4). Recurrent prolapse means prolapse has recurred after prior prolapse surgery. The aim of a synthetic graft (often referred to as mesh) is to improve the long-term success rate of the prolapse surgery. The failure rate for surgery using a synthetic graft is about 50 per cent lower than for the traditional technique of using sutures only (colporrhaphy). This type of surgery is best carried out by doctors who are very experienced in the use of synthetic grafts.

A synthetic graft is an inert material specifically designed to increase wound strength and is permanent. They have been extensively used in surgery, especially in hernia repairs. The synthetic graft provides a framework of support and has many holes within it to allow the body's own tissue to grow into the graft. It can also be placed underneath the vaginal skin during a colporrhaphy.

Sacrocolpopexy

Sacrocolpopexy is an operation that suspends the vagina or uterus using a synthetic graft that attaches to the front of the tailbone (sacrum). This provides good support for the top of the vagina or uterus. A repair inside the vagina may also be required at the same time. This operation can be performed in combination with other procedures. Studies from the Women's show that it has a success rate of more than 90 per cent.

Sacrocolpopexy is usually made available to women with a stage 3 or 4 prolapse or who have already had a hysterectomy. It may also be used to support a prolapsed uterus in younger women if they wish to retain their uterus. This surgery is very technical and is best performed by doctors who are experienced in it.

The operation is performed under general anaesthetic. It may require an incision in the abdomen or be performed by laparoscopy (keyhole surgery).

Colpocliesis

Colpocliesis is a very simple operation that supports the uterus and vagina by closing the middle segment of the vagina using sutures (stitches). This operation is usually reserved for elderly women who haven't been able to use a vaginal pessary successfully. It is relatively quick to perform, often taking only around 30 minutes, and for some women can be completed under a local anaesthetic with sedation instead of a general anaesthetic. It is not possible to have sexual intercourse ever again after a colpocliesis.

The surgery involves partial closure of the vagina in order to prevent prolapse of the uterus and other pelvic organs such as the bladder and the rectum. A portion of the front and back walls of the vagina are removed and sutured together using stitches, resulting in a partial closure of the central part of the vaginal cavity. Women generally make a rapid recovery following a colpocliesis operation and typically leave hospital the day after surgery.

Recovery after surgery for prolapse

Most women stay in hospital for three to five days following surgery, going home when they feel well and are able to pass urine. The suggested pain relief is paracetamol (such as Panadol) every four hours for two weeks if necessary. (It is best to avoid medications with codeine, such as Panadeine, to avoid constipation.) It is also important to maintain good bowel habits to avoid constipation or 'straining': try to drink approximately 1.5–2 litres of fluid each day, maintain a healthy diet and use Metamucil or a similar preparation (available at chemists), if required, to promote soft stools.

It is important to rest and allow the area to heal. Recommended recovery instructions and things to look out for are, for the first two weeks:

- restrict activity and rest as much as possible
- there will be a small amount of light pink blood loss from the vagina for up to two weeks

For two to four weeks:

- keep your activity light and easy
- avoid heavy lifting (nothing heavier than 4 kilograms) including shopping bags, washing baskets and children
- avoid playing sport, swimming and moderate-impact exercises such as jogging or jumping
- any stitches present will fall out once they dissolve in about ten days (and up to three weeks)

For the first six weeks:

- Do not have sexual intercourse

You may drive a car after two weeks; however, check with your car insurance provider first to see if insurance will cover you after such a procedure.

You will likely have a follow-up appointment six to eight weeks after your surgery.

Possible complications with prolapse surgery

There are general risks involved with having such an operation, including anaesthetic problems, bleeding and blood transfusion, infection within the pelvis or wound, and clots in the legs that can travel to the lungs (pulmonary embolism). Antibiotics are given during surgery and continued after the operation to reduce the risk of infection. Medication to thin the blood is given during surgery and during the hospital stay, to reduce the risk of developing blood clots. It is rare to experience serious bleeding or to need a blood transfusion. Generally there is improved sexual function after most prolapse surgery, but about 2 per cent of women may experience painful intercourse after surgery and may require further treatment.

Whenever a synthetic graft is used, there is a small risk of a small portion of the synthetic graft protruding into the vagina, usually referred to as a vaginal mesh exposure. This is usually treated with vaginal oestrogen preparations (vaginal oestrogen cream or pessaries used three times a week) if the vaginal skin is thin, or a small vaginal operation to remove the exposed section of synthetic graft (the entire graft will not need to be removed). Occasionally bladder problems can occur after surgery, such as difficulty with bladder-emptying, cystitis or urinary leakage. These problems usually settle down soon after, but if incontinence remains a problem a small operation or medication may be required. Pain may occur immediately after surgery but this generally disappears after a few days or weeks.

Prolapse can sometimes recur after surgery, either at the same site or at a different site from where the surgery was performed (in which case it is referred to as de novo prolapse). Some doctors (urogynaecologists) specialise in pelvic floor problems and have had additional training in treating prolapse, particularly recurrent prolapse and complex prolapse. Some of the more complex operations for prolapse, such as sacro-colpopexy and surgery using synthetic grafts, are frequently performed by urogynaecologists.

Female urinary incontinence

Urinary incontinence is the involuntary or accidental leakage of urine. It affects 30–50 per cent of women. Although the rates increase with age, incontinence among young women is also quite common. Pregnancy, childbirth and ageing are considered to be among the most common causes of urinary incontinence, but many other factors can cause it, such as some types of medication or a chronic cough.

Many women with bladder problems are reluctant to discuss them and may be too embarrassed to acknowledge they have a problem. Sometimes women are made to feel these conditions are 'normal', especially as they get older, and that, since these sorts of bladder problems are rarely life-threatening, they are not really a problem. The truth is, though, that incontinence can have a very significant impact on quality of life.

The good news is that the majority of women who seek help for bladder problems and receive appropriate assessment and treatment will experience significant improvement.

The types of urinary incontinence

Female urinary incontinence can be grouped into several distinct categories. The most common type of incontinence is stress incontinence, where urine leakage occurs with increases in abdominal pressure (physical stress) from activities such as coughing, sneezing and exercising. The next most common type of incontinence is urge incontinence. This is often referred to as an overactive bladder. Urge incontinence occurs when urine cannot be held long enough to reach the toilet in time. Urge incontinence is usually associated with a strong desire to pass urine. A combination of stress and urge incontinence is called mixed incontinence. Often a woman may first experience one kind of leaking and find that the other begins to occur later.

Diagnosing urinary incontinence

The first step towards diagnosis, is keeping a bladder diary, which is used to record fluid intake, frequency of urination, volume of urine voided and any episodes of urinary leakage. A bladder diary is useful in distinguishing between stress incontinence and an overactive bladder. It also gives useful information about fluid intake and urination habits.

Urodynamic testing evaluates the ability of the bladder to fill and empty, and provides a diagnosis of the underlying cause of the urinary incontinence. Urodynamic testing can be very helpful in sorting out which parts of the bladder and urethra are functioning correctly, and which parts are not. The results of urodynamic testing will often help the treating doctor determine the best treatment for the patient.

The type of urodynamic test undertaken will vary from hospital to hospital and depend on the person's health. The tests range from simple observations (how long it takes to empty the bladder, the volume of urine passed and whether the patient can stop the urine flow in midstream) to highly sophisticated testing that uses imaging equipment to take pictures of the bladder at work or pressure sensors that monitor the pressure inside the bladder. None of these tests should hurt. You may need to arrive for testing with a full bladder or having stopped some medications.

Non-surgical treatments for female urinary incontinence

Pelvic floor muscle training is used to strengthen the group of muscles and ligaments that support the urethra, bladder, uterus and lower bowel. The pelvic floor muscles also help control bladder function, allowing you to 'hold on' until an appropriate time and place. We recommend that all women exercise their pelvic floor muscles regularly throughout their life, to prevent or correct weakness. Exercising weak muscles regularly over a period of time can strengthen them and make them work effectively again. Around 75 per cent of women experience an improvement in stress incontinence with pelvic floor muscle training under the supervision of a physiotherapist or nurse with expertise in managing female incontinence. For women with overactive bladder symptoms such as urinary urgency, frequency and urge incontinence, pelvic floor muscle training in conjunction with bladder retraining is an effective management strategy. For information on how to do pelvic floor exercises, see chapter 18.

Women with urge incontinence (overactive bladder) often benefit from a range of medications that can relax the bladder muscle. These medications are generally effective in around 85 per cent of women and can be prescribed by a GP. Lifestyle changes such as reducing caffeine and alcohol intake, giving up smoking, losing weight and avoiding constipation can also improve bladder function.

Surgery for female urinary incontinence

Surgery is often considered for women with stress incontinence who fail to respond to conservative therapy (see later in this chapter), but is only rarely performed. Operations for stress incontinence include mid-urethral sling, colposuspension, rectus fascial sling and urethral bulking agents.

Mid-urethral sling operation

The most widely used operation for stress incontinence is the mid-urethral sling procedure, often referred to as the tension-free vaginal tape or TVT operation. This minimally invasive operation involves the placement of synthetic mesh tape to support the urethra and prevent stress incontinence.

This operation is sometimes performed in combination with other procedures such as surgery for prolapse. The two types of mid-urethral slings most commonly used are the retropubic (TVT) and trans-obturator (TOT) slings.

Women can comfortably have the operation with a local, regional or general anaesthetic. The surgeon makes a small incision in the vagina just below the urethra. For a retropubic sling, two tiny incisions will also be made just above the pubic bone. If a trans-obturator sling procedure is performed, the additional tiny incisions will be made in the groin on each side. The sling goes under the urethra to provide lift and support.

This operation takes approximately 20 minutes and most women return home within 24 hours. Pain relief tablets are usually enough to deal with any postoperative discomfort. It is important to rest after the operation and allow the area to heal. Generally restriction of physical activity is recommended for 25 days after surgery, and abstinence from sexual intercourse for six weeks.

Studies show that mid-urethral sling surgery is successful in treating stress incontinence in 80–90 per cent of cases. Women with both stress and urge incontinence can also expect a 50 per cent improvement in their urge incontinence symptoms.

Possible complications with incontinence surgery

There can be complications with any type of surgery but serious complications are uncommon with this operation. There is a small risk of damage to the bladder, urethra or blood vessels when the tape is inserted. After surgery about 5 per cent of women will have trouble going to the toilet and may need a catheter for a few days until they can establish normal bladder-emptying. In rare circumstances, if bladder-emptying doesn't settle, division or adjustment of the tape will be required. Approximately 5 per cent of women may experience a bladder infection after surgery and need antibiotic treatment. Bladder irritability after surgery can occur in a small number of cases and may require medication.

Anal incontinence

Anal incontinence is the accidental or involuntary loss or seepage of solid or liquid faeces. Injury to the anal sphincter muscle or the nerves to this muscle sustained during childbirth is the main cause of anal incontinence. This explains why anal incontinence is around eight times more common in midlife women than in men. Following childbirth, 4 per cent of women experience anal incontinence. Less common causes include prolapse of the rectum through the anus, inflammatory bowel disease (ulcerative colitis and Crohn's disease), fistula (leakage of faeces through the vagina), haemorrhoids, severe constipation and neurological conditions (such as spinal injury).

Female anal incontinence requires careful assessment to determine its precise cause. Specialists use investigations such as an ultrasound examination of the anal sphincter and anal pressure studies (anal manometry) to gather valuable information and determine a diagnosis and treatment approach. They may also study pelvic floor and anal sphincter nerve function using electromyography (EMG) in some cases.

Treatment for anal incontinence

Early detection and surgical repair is an important aspect in the management of anal sphincter damage resulting from childbirth. Women who sustain tearing of the lower birth canal or have an instrumental (forceps or vacuum) delivery are at increased risk of a sphincter injury. All women who have had an instrumental delivery or a delivery complicated by trauma to the lower birth canal should be carefully examined by the midwife or attending doctor for the presence of a sphincter injury. If a sphincter injury is identified, it should be surgically repaired by an experienced doctor under a regional or general anaesthetic. This should be followed up with assessment and treatment of any ongoing anal symptoms. Often delivery by elective caesarean for any future pregnancies is recommended for women who have had a significant anal sphincter injury.

Most women with anal incontinence can be managed by conservative treatment (see below). Surgical treatment is generally reserved for severe anal incontinence or if conservative treatments are ineffective.

Conservative treatment for anal incontinence

A variety of conservative treatments are used for anal incontinence. Pelvic floor muscle training (see chapter 18), dietary modification and the use of stool bulking supplements (such as psyllium husk) can be useful, simple measures in managing anal incontinence. Medication that reduces the motility of the large bowel and increases water absorption from the gut in order to ensure solid, formed bowel motions can reduce anal incontinence. These medications can have some side effects, such as constipation, nausea, abdominal bloating and colicky abdominal pain. Regular bowel enemas can be useful for some women to ensure that the rectum is kept relatively empty.

Surgery for anal incontinence

Surgery to repair a damaged anal sphincter is considered only for women who fail to respond to conservative treatment and only if a sphincter defect has been identified by ultrasound imaging of the sphincter muscle. These operations can include the use of an artificial bowel sphincter, perianal (around the anus) bulking agents and anal slings to support the anal muscles. Women whose anal incontinence is caused by pelvic floor nerve damage may be considered for sacral nerve neuromodulation (surgical insertion of a small device that stimulates the nerve controlling the anus). Surgery to divert the bowel (such as colostomy) is considered as a last resort for very severe cases of anal incontinence.

Conservative management of prolapse and incontinence

Pelvic floor muscle training is the mainstay of conservative management of prolapse and incontinence. It is recommended as first-line treatment for all women with stress, urge or mixed incontinence. Evidence of its effectiveness for the management of prolapse is growing as recent research endorses this training.

Managing risk factors

The list of risk factors for prolapse and incontinence includes several modifiable risks, such as low muscle tone, lifting, coughing, smoking, obesity and constipation, though some are inevitable (menopause, ageing). Physiotherapists or continence nurses work with women to manage these risk factors, using strategies such as:

- taking up some low-impact exercise to increase muscle tone and lose weight: walking, cycling, swimming (rather than high-impact exercise such as running, netball, some gym classes)
- increasing fruit and vegetable intake and possibly taking a fibre supplement for constipation
- lifting heavy items correctly or avoiding lifting entirely
- reducing the load on the pelvic floor by using ergonomic ways to lift, push, pull and pass a bowel motion without straining

What is actually meant by pelvic floor muscle training

Is it just doing the 'squeeze' exercise? No. The aim of pelvic floor muscle training is to build on the basic pelvic floor exercises (see chapter 18). To combat unwanted leakage, a base level of muscle strength is needed. The muscle then has to learn to contract quickly and on command to combat coughs and sneezes. It also has to combat the urge to go to the toilet for long enough to reach a toilet. Then the muscle must be trained

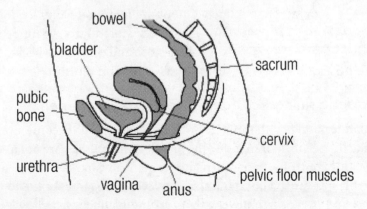

Pelvic floor muscles

to contract before a stressful activity such as lifting – a pre-contraction before effort. The anal sphincter can also be trained for both strength and speed to combat anal incontinence. All of these factors make up pelvic floor muscle training and require working with a physiotherapist or continence nurse.

Details about how to do a basic pelvic floor muscle exercise are in chapter 18.

Improving urine flow

Some women have difficulty getting urine to flow easily. This is called voiding difficulty and is combatted using the technique of double voiding. This involves semi-standing up after the flow has slowed or stopped, moving or jiggling the pelvis then sitting down again to finish emptying the bladder. It is important never to strain when trying to empty as this can put pressure downwards on the pelvic organs and over time create susceptibility to prolapse.

Improving bowel movement

Likewise, if a bowel motion is difficult to pass, usually due to constipation, sitting on the toilet in a position that enables best passage of the motion

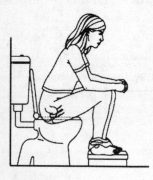

is the key to not straining and avoiding tissue damage. The technique is to sit forward with a straight back, feet flat on the floor, and let the abdomen relax for the whole time the bowel motion passes, gently pushing or bearing down with the diaphragm (bottom of the chest), and feeling that the abdomen and pelvic floor are relaxed during the motion. If this is unsuccessful, do not strain or stay on the toilet. Leave and only come back when the urge to pass a motion returns.

Toilet position

Bladder training for urgency and urge incontinence

In bladder urgency the muscles of the bladder wall become overactive. Unlike the pelvic floor muscles, the bladder wall muscles are not under our conscious control – they contract automatically, like our heart muscles. For this reason, bladder training involves using the brain to change habits and override the overactivity in the bladder wall muscles rather than doing muscular exercises. For some women this can be a slow and effortful process, while others, once they understand the techniques, can have a 'light bulb' moment and begin a new way of thinking and behaving immediately.

Bladder training involves using cognitive behaviour strategies to gain improved control over the sense of urgency. Most women with bladder problems are anxious about where the next toilet is, so go to the toilet just in case, resulting in many trips to the toilet day and night. Urinary frequency means going to the toilet more than seven times per day, and getting up to go to the toilet more than once per night (called nocturia). The bladder then 'learns' over time to give the signals to void when it has not filled anywhere near its capacity. Anxiety about leaking increases, trips to the toilet increase in frequency, and so a vicious cycle develops.

Bladder training could also be thought of as a bladder-stretching program. The techniques are:

- Stop and relax – do *not* rush to the toilet. If you run, the bladder has won.

- Breathe slowly and evenly.

- Apply perineal/vaginal pressure: sit on the arm of a chair or the edge of a desk, sit on a rolled-up towel or cross your legs.

- Curl your toes repeatedly or hold them firmly curled.

- Stretch your calf muscles and hold the stretch.

- If you are walking, slow your pace and emphasise heel-to-toe walking.

- Squeeze and lift your pelvic floor muscles and hold them tight.

- Distract yourself. Do *not* think about the toilet or about leaking. Distract yourself with a physical or mental task – such as counting

---

Normal bladder habits

You will know you have achieved success when your bladder habits are normal.

Normal bladder habits are:

- going to the toilet four to six times per day and not more than once after you have gone to bed

- drinking 1.5–2 litres of fluid a day (mostly water rather than fizzy drinks or tea or coffee)

- regularly voiding 200–400 millilitres of urine (each time) backwards from 100 by threes or sevens; thinking of three Australian towns starting with A, then with B, then C and so on; or doing a crossword puzzle – or making a phone call.

The value of conservative treatment

The good thing about conservative treatment for incontinence problems is that there are no known side effects or complications. Success is determined by many factors, but overall the success rate of conservative treatment varies from 75 to 85 per cent. The large number of risk factors and their complex interactions determine the final success rate for each woman, but the most important factors for success are adherence to the training program, the intensity of the exercises performed, and being supervised by a qualified physiotherapist or continence nurse.

A pelvic floor muscle training program before and after surgery for prolapse or incontinence has been shown to improve the success rate of the surgery and reduce the risk of recurrence after surgery. Strong pelvic floor muscles give durability to the surgery.

The most important thing is to just do it, and keep on doing it! Don't give up before the treatment has had a chance to work. Would you stop cleaning your teeth because you got sick of doing it? No. Make your pelvic floor or bladder training program like cleaning your teeth and do it for life.

40

Mental health in midlife

Fiona Judd

Midlife is a time of multiple biological, psychological and social changes and challenges for women, and every woman will have their own perspective on the meaning of ageing. These factors may have a profound effect on the mental health and wellbeing of women in midlife. While the majority of women do not experience significant mental health problems, anxiety and depression will affect as many as one in four midlife women.

The psychological stage of midlife

As we saw in chapter 4, personal development occurs in stages, which involve psychological tasks, variously described by different theorists. For example, Erik Erikson, a psychologist and psychoanalyst, has suggested that successful negotiation of each life stage results in development of psychosocial strength to help us through the remaining stages of our lives.

Midlife is the time to develop an appropriate balance between the stages of generativity and stagnation. Generativity involves a concern for future generations and contributing to positive changes that benefit other people. It is a period in which women raise children, and/or contribute to the world in a variety of other ways including occupational, social and volunteer activity. By contrast, stagnation is a period of self-absorption, caring for no one.

This developmental stage includes the time sometimes referred to as the 'midlife crisis', a time of questioning what or for whom we are doing all this for. Handled badly, this question can lead to panic at getting older and attempts to recapture youth. Handled well, it leads to a capacity for caring that serves us well through the rest of our lives.

Depression

Depression, or a depressive illness, is characterised by a sustained and persistent low mood – that is, low mood that lasts for weeks or longer – together with loss of enjoyment of things that usually bring pleasure. It often involves loss of interest in usual activities – including work, social activities and even spending time with loved ones – along with loss of motivation and finding things a chore. It often includes loss of appetite and weight loss, poor sleep, loss of energy, trouble concentrating and memory problems. In addition to feeling sad or depressed, it can involve feeling anxious, irritable and angry. These symptoms persist for periods of several weeks or longer and interfere with daily activities. Severe depression can cause problems doing even simple tasks. Sometimes depression leads to suicidal thoughts and plans. If you experience these thoughts, you should seek assistance immediately by calling Lifeline on 13 11 14.

Risk factors for depression

Depression is a common problem, experienced by 8–10 per cent of women. Several risk factors for depression have been identified, including: adverse life events, particularly 'loss' events such as the loss of a role (e.g. children leaving home, retirement from work, marital separation, death of a loved one); a genetic predisposition (i.e. a family member having depression); and a history of depression including postnatal depression. Physical health problems may be associated with depression, particularly neurological conditions such as stroke or Parkinson's disease, chronic painful conditions such as arthritis, and life-threatening illnesses such as cancer. Some prescribed medications (e.g. some medications for high blood pressure, some anti-inflammatory drugs and steroids) can also cause depression.

Many women who experience depression in midlife have had depression before, with the first onset often during their teens or 20s. These women will probably readily recognise what the problem is, but even if they have been depressed before, they may mistake their current symptoms for something else, or the depression may affect them differently this time, particularly if there are new or additional factors influencing its onset.

Many women experience mood changes along with the biological changes that occur at the time of the transition to menopause. Low or variable mood, crying, loss of confidence and sleep disturbance are common menopausal symptoms. Although these symptoms might also occur as part of a depressive illness, when they occur during the time of transition to menopause it does not necessarily imply depression. There is an important distinction between mood disturbance as part of menopausal changes, which is best treated as part of the overall management of menopausal symptoms with, for example, hormone replacement therapy, and mood disturbance that is part of a depressive illness, which will be best treated with psychological therapies and/or antidepressants.

Where to seek help for depression

Usually the best person is your doctor, who will be able to assess your symptoms and determine whether you are depressed or if there is another cause for the way you feel, how severe your depression is and what factors may be contributing to it, and advise you about appropriate treatments.

Treatment for depression

Treatment is guided by the factors causing the problem as well as the severity of the depression. For example, if you have recently started a new medication for a physical health problem and this has precipitated your depression, the solution may be to change this medication. If your depression is mild, psychological therapy will probably be the most appropriate treatment. If it is moderately severe, your doctor may recommend an antidepressant. If it is more severe, and if you are feeling suicidal, your doctor may suggest you see a psychiatrist and/or that you be admitted to hospital for treatment.

Self-education

If you have depression, a good place to start your treatment is to learn about the problem. Information and a variety of resources about depression and treatment for depression are available from beyondblue, the Black Dog Institute and SANE Australia (see the Resources section at the end of this book). These resources highlight how lifestyle factors, such as stress, poor work–life balance, and excessive use of alcohol, can contribute to depression, and the importance of addressing these issues. Improved work–life balance, regular exercise, healthy eating and regularly engaging in pleasurable activities are very effective means of avoiding and/or treating depression.

Psychological (talking) therapies

Psychological therapies for depression include cognitive behaviour therapy (CBT) and interpersonal therapy (IPT), both of which require a specialist therapist, so make sure your GP refers you to a clinical psychologist with the necessary expertise. CBT focuses on thoughts and behaviours and how these may influence mood, and can be particularly helpful at combating patterns of thinking that reinforce low mood and behaviours that lead to avoidance of potentially pleasurable activities. IPT focuses on loss and role change, so it can be particularly helpful for depression precipitated by these types of psychosocial issues.

Antidepressants

A variety of effective antidepressants is available, but they work in different ways and produce different side effects. Some can be safely taken with other medications, while others cannot. Your doctor will prescribe a particular antidepressant by taking into account whether you have had an antidepressant in the past with good or problematic effects, its possible side effects now and how it may react with any other medications you are taking. The most commonly used group of antidepressants is the serotonin selective reuptake inhibitors (SSRIs), which include Sertraline, Paroxetine, Fluoxetine and Citalopram. Generally, these medications can be taken safely with other drugs and most people experience few side effects.

Shirley was 46, married with three children. She had not had any mental health problems in the past, but over the past six months she had become teary and irritable, and had trouble sleeping. Her doctor referred her to a clinical psychologist for assessment and possible treatment for depression.

When interviewed by the psychologist Shirley indicated that these feelings were very uncharacteristic for her. She noted that she'd always been a happy person, very content with her life and comfortable with her lifestyle. She described her husband, David, an accountant, as very supportive, and indicated that she did not understand why he had started to annoy her and why they had started having frequent disagreements.

On further questioning, Shirley acknowledged that she was at times a 'bit of an uptight person', one who liked to be in control of things. She admitted she was having some difficulty adjusting to her children growing up and changing their focus from home to other interests and friends.

Shirley also talked of her sadness about the decision she and David had made to place her mother in a nursing home. As the eldest child in the family, the responsibility for this decision had fallen on her, and so too had the guilt, since the family had planned, after their father died, that Shirley's mother would always live with one of the children. Worsening dementia had meant that this was no longer possible.

Adding to these problems was Shirley's concerns about menopause. Her periods had been irregular and infrequent over the past 18 months and she was experiencing hot flushes. She described these as over-whelming and embarrassing, and especially troublesome at night. Shirley was also worried about her memory; she had noticed she was becoming forgetful, misplacing things, and, given her mother's problems with dementia, was fearful that she might be experiencing early symptoms herself. She noted she had put on weight, especially over the past six months, as she'd lost interest in her golf.

Shirley reported that, by contrast, David was excited about their children growing up, and was looking forward to travelling as they had always planned. He was thinking about downsizing his business, giving him more time for leisure, but if he did so, there would be no need for Shirley to continue working part-time with him as she'd done for the past 10 years. She saw this as an indicator of her being of 'no use to anyone'.

The psychologist told her that she did not think Shirley had a depressive illness, but that she was experiencing low mood and difficulty adjusting to change – in her role as a mother and as a carer for her mother, in a sense grieving for the loss of these roles – and coming to terms with the transition through midlife. The psychologist also noted that the severity of her hot flushes and changes to her periods indicated that she was in the menopause transition, and that hormonal changes might be affecting her mood and her memory.

In order to deal with these issues the psychologist suggested Shirley talk to her GP about the potential benefits (and risks) of hormone replace-ment therapy for her menopausal symptoms. She also said that she could assist Shirley with the role transitions using psychological therapy. Shirley agreed to try short-term therapy (around six sessions) using interpersonal therapy (IPT). Together Shirley and the therapist identified the main issues to be addressed as her role changed from needed, nurturing mother to mother of adult and independent children, and as a result of her mother's declining health and loss of independence. While they both acknowl-edged the broader issue of Shirley's own ageing, they did not choose it as a primary target for therapy at that time.

Anxiety

Anxiety symptoms, sometimes labelled stress, are common at times of change, or when we are under pressure, which means they are often experi-enced by women in midlife. Typical symptoms of stress include irritability, feeling keyed-up or on edge, muscle tension (sore neck, headaches), sleep disturbance and fatigue, and trouble concentrating. These symptoms are more severe and persistent in people with generalised anxiety disorder. (See box below.)

It can be difficult to distinguish between stress and an anxiety disorder, and if your symptoms are erroneously labelled as 'just a bit of stress', you may not seek effective treatment. When the symptoms are severe and persistent, and coupled with worry about various events or activities, they are likely to indicate an anxiety disorder. The best way to be clear about what the problem is, and how best to deal with it, is to talk to your doctor.

What can I do if I am stressed?

The most important thing if you experience symptoms of stress is to recognise them, and acknowledge that you need to do something about them. Sometimes it is easy to pinpoint the cause, although doing something about it may be less straightforward. Often there is not one cause or a simple cause, however, and you may need instead to manage the effects of the stress.

Relaxation is a useful technique for stress management. This may be formal relaxation therapy, which can include progressive muscle relaxation, imagery and visualisation, and meditation; mindfulness-based approaches; ensuring time out for regular exercise; or making regular time for a relaxing activity or hobby such as gardening. Your doctor or therapist can also teach you about structured problem-solving, activity scheduling and time management, and can refer you for problem-focused counselling, such as financial counselling.

Anxiety disorders

There are several different types of anxiety disorder. They share some features, such as feelings of tension, worry, fear or dread that are prolonged or excessive – that is, out of proportion to any current threat or problem – and interfering with day-to-day activities. The disorders are all characterised by three groups of symptoms: autonomic nervous system overactivity (shaking, sweating, racing heart), thoughts focused on a perceived threat, and actions and behaviours designed to avoid or deal with the perceived threat. Common perceived threats include having a serious physical illness (e.g. heart attack, stroke, brain tumour), something going wrong (e.g. someone having a car accident, fear of making a mistake), and something negative about the future of the world (e.g. severe drought, major calamity). The main anxiety disorders and their key features are listed below.

Panic disorders

Panic disorders are characterised by recurrent panic attacks – abrupt, unexpected and unpredictable attacks of fear and discomfort, reaching peak intensity within minutes.

Panic attacks

Panic attacks are sudden episodes of severe anxiety characterised by physical symptoms and fear of dreadful consequences. The physical symptoms include:

- palpitations, pounding heart or accelerated heart rate
- sweating
- trembling or shaking
- sensations of shortness of breath or being smothered
- feeling of choking
- chest pain or discomfort
- nausea or abdominal distress
- feeling dizzy, unsteady, light-headed or faint
- numbness or tingling sensations
- chills or hot flushes
- feelings of unreality (derealisation) or of being detached from oneself (depersonalisation)
- fear of dying
- fear of losing control
- fear of 'going crazy'

Phobic disorders

Phobic disorders are characterised by excessive and unreasonable fear that leads to avoidance of places or situations. There are three subtypes:

- **agoraphobia** – fear and avoidance of a variety of situations (e.g. crowds, public places, public transport, being home alone, going far from home) from which escape may not be possible, or where help might not be available if a panic attack occurs

- **social phobia** – fear and avoidance of scrutiny or being the focus of attention in case of acting in a humiliating or embarrassing way (e.g. shaking, blushing, stammering, having a panic attack)
- **specific phobia** – excessive and unreasonable fear and avoidance of a specific situation or object (e.g. spiders, heights, lifts, tunnels, thunderstorms)

Obsessive compulsive disorder (OCD)

OCD is characterised by obsessions and/or compulsions where obsessions are recurrent intrusive thoughts that cannot be ignored, resisted or reasoned away (e.g. worries about germs or contamination) and compulsions are excessive and inappropriate repetitive acts performed in a set way or according to certain rules (e.g. checking, counting, cleaning). Compulsions temporarily reduce the anxiety caused by obsessions.

Generalised anxiety disorder

Generalised anxiety disorder is characterised by persistent tension, anxiety and uncontrollable worry over everyday events and problems, together with a range of symptoms. The core symptom is tension, which has typical psychological and physical aspects, and recognised consequences. The psychological aspects include:

- nervousness
- feeling keyed-up or on edge
- inner restlessness
- difficulty concentrating or mind going blank
- irritability, feeling cranky, easily annoyed or angry
- hyper-vigilance, feeling constantly on alert and easily startled

  The physical aspects include:

- muscle tension, stiff neck, back pain, tension headache
- muscle spasms
- tremor, muscle jerks

  The consequences include:

- sleep disturbance (difficulty falling or staying asleep or restless unsatisfying sleep)
- fatigue, exhaustion

Post-traumatic stress disorder (PTSD)

PTSD is characterised by recurrent intrusive recollections of and re-experiencing (e.g. through mental images, nightmares, flashbacks) a traumatic event together with high levels of arousal and distress.

Risk factors for anxiety disorders

Anxiety disorders affect almost one in five women, generally begin in the teens or early 20s and are usually recurrent. It is much less common for an anxiety disorder to begin for the first time in midlife, so if you do develop anxiety at this time, it will probably be a recurrence of a problem you have experienced previously. However, stress may affect anybody at any age, and can certainly be a problem for the first time in midlife. Anxiety can also occur as a result of a medical problem such as thyroid disease, some prescribed medications such as some asthma medicines, some over-the-counter preparations such as cold and flu tablets, or excessive caffeine. Using alcohol to deal with stress can result in anxiety as the body adjusts to the absence of alcohol the next day.

Anxiety may also occur as part of a depressive disorder; in fact, even though the primary problem may be depression, it can cause severe anxiety symptoms from panic attacks to feelings of general anxiety (see above).

Treatment for anxiety disorders

Self-education

The first step in dealing with anxiety is to identify and change any lifestyle factors that are causing or exacerbating it. Common factors that can worsen anxiety include alcohol use, excessive caffeine intake, excessive work and inadequate sleep. Education about anxiety and the ways it can be treated is also important. Excellent information is available from beyondblue and SANE Australia (see the Resources section at the end of this book).

Psychological (talking) therapies

Anxiety disorders are usually best treated using psychological therapies, but if symptoms are more severe medications may also be used. If you have an anxiety disorder, the first step will usually be to learn some form of relaxation technique, and then practise it regularly. This might be relaxation training provided by a therapist, but may also include other forms of relaxation such as meditation, yoga or tai chi. The most common psychological therapy used to deal with specific anxiety symptoms is cognitive behaviour therapy (CBT; see above under 'Depression'). Different CBT techniques are applied depending on the disorder being treated.

Medications

The medications used for the treatment of anxiety disorders have changed over the past few years. Previously the benzodiazepines (e.g. diazepam, sold as Valium; oxazepam, sold as Serepax; and alprazolam, sold as Xanax) were widely prescribed, but this is no longer the case. While these drugs are effective in treating anxiety, they are associated with a range of serious side effects including excessive sedation with impairment of concentration, memory and judgement, as well as being highly addictive. The most commonly used medications now are the selective serotonin reuptake inhibitors (SSRIs). Although these medications may take several weeks to yield any benefits, they are effective for the treatment of anxiety and can be safely continued long term.

Anxiety or hot flushes?

Hot flushes are a core symptom of menopause, and so are experienced by many women at some time in midlife. They generally occur together with other menopausal symptoms, such as night sweats, sleep disturbance and vaginal dryness. These symptoms may occur together with, be mistaken for, or contribute to the development of anxiety symptoms. There are physical similarities between anxiety symptoms, particularly panic attacks (see above), and these common menopausal symptoms, including rising sensations of heat in the chest and head, flushing and sweating, and palpitations. It is important for a doctor to identify these symptoms correctly as either part of the menopause, and so best treated with hormone therapy, or part of an anxiety disorder, and so effectively treated by other means.

Schizophrenia and bipolar disorder

Schizophrenia and bipolar disorder (generally called psychoses) each affect around 1 per cent of the population. Both most commonly begin in early adult life, although onset in midlife does occur. If you have one of these disorders, you will probably have experienced more than one episode of illness and will have developed a management plan that maintains your mental wellbeing and prevents relapse.

A number of factors may increase vulnerability to relapse in midlife. First, the stresses of midlife, and its changes and losses, may trigger an episode of illness. Secondly, the side effects of medication, such as weight gain and reduced libido, may become more problematic in midlife, which prompts some women to attempt to change or reduce their medication. While it's important to minimise these problems (which are also common in midlife women in general), it is essential that any medication changes be made in consultation with the prescribing doctor and with careful monitoring by all concerned to avoid relapse.

A common concern for women with these disorders is whether hormone replacement therapy to treat menopausal symptoms will worsen their mental health condition. In fact, there is some evidence that oestrogen is protective against psychotic illness, so, if anything, hormone replacement therapy is likely to benefit rather than adversely affect any existing psychotic illness. A doctor should include evaluation and treatment of any menopausal symptoms in an overall mental health treatment plan.

Preparing for successful ageing

Healthy or successful ageing generally means adding quality of life to quantity of life. This encompasses freedom from chronic disease and the ability to function effectively, both physically and mentally, in old age. Earlier, we referred to Erikson's proposition that successful negotiation of each life stage results in development of psychosocial strength, which helps us through the rest of the stages of our lives. Older age is described as the time of ego integrity versus despair. Ego integrity – described by Erikson as coming to terms with your life, accepting your life as you have lived it and the development of wisdom – might also be considered successful ageing.

Research has identified factors that permit us to continue to function effectively, both physically and mentally, into older age. Importantly, the influence of some of these factors begins in midlife and it's possible to modify their effects. They include health behaviours such as not smoking, limited alcohol use, a healthy diet and regular physical activity, as well as minimising psychological stress and maximising social support. Focusing on wellbeing in midlife can not only enhance your current quality of life, but is also an investment in your future physical and mental wellbeing in older age.

41

Being a carer

Andrea Ball

At some point in our lives, most of us will be a carer or will need a carer. According to the Australian Bureau of Statistics' Survey of Disability, Ageing and Carers, in 2009, there were 2.6 million carers in Australia who provided unpaid care and support to family members and friends who were aged and frail, or who had a disability, chronic or life-threatening illness, mental illness, or drug or alcohol problem.

Caring is an important part of our experience as humans, and taking on a caring role is a significant life event that can be both very rewarding and very challenging. Being a carer can strengthen your relationship with the person you are caring for and may provide opportunities to grow and learn new skills. Many people who are carers and those who are receiving care describe their relationship as loving and supportive. But caring is also very demanding, affecting your ability to work, your finances, and your own physical and mental wellbeing.

If you are in a caring role of any kind, it is important that you receive the support you need. Looking after your own physical and mental health, taking time out from your caring role, finding support networks to assist you and getting financial assistance where it's available will all help you manage the demands of caring and balance caring with the other parts of your life.

The information in this chapter will provide practical ideas and a guide to the range of support services available to help lighten the load of caring and protect a carer's long-term health. Leaning on these services and the support of family and friends may help you feel happier and more satisfied as a carer and in all other areas of your life.

Who are carers?

Across all age groups, 13 per cent of women are involved in a caring role, compared with 11 per cent of men. The number of people in caring roles increases with age, and in the 45–54 age group, 23 per cent of women and 16 per cent of men are carers. The number of women in caring roles is highest in the 55–64 age group, where 25 per cent are carers.

The gender difference is greatest when you look at primary carers – people who provide the majority of unpaid care for another person. About one-third of carers are primary carers, and of these, 68 per cent are women.

Women often move in and out of caring roles at different times in their lives. Ninety-two per cent of primary carers for children with an illness or a disability are women, and women make up 70 per cent of children who care for their parents.

Anyone can be a carer. You may be the partner, parent, child, sister, friend, niece or neighbour of the person you care for. Every care situation is different. You may have gradually become a carer as your partner's or an older relative's health has deteriorated over time. Or your caring role may have started suddenly, after a health crisis like a heart attack or an accident.

Caring roles can range from a lifetime of caring for a child with a disability to providing 24-hour nursing care for a seriously ill partner, or helping someone live independently by helping out when needed with transport, shopping and banking. All carers give a lot of themselves and play a vital role in families and the community by helping the person they care for to remain as independent as possible and enjoy good quality of life.

Caring affects your health, finances and relationships

All this caring can come at a high cost to health and wellbeing. Carers often report poor physical, mental and emotional health as a result of their caring responsibilities. The more hours spent caring each week, the greater the impact on the carer's health and wellbeing. Carers are more likely to experience chronic health problems, anxiety and depression. Many carers are worn out and desperate for a good night's sleep.

Caring often has a big impact on finances, too. Half of all carers and 62 per cent of primary carers are on low incomes. This is because it's often not possible to keep up paid work while caring – this is especially true for women, who are more likely to be primary carers. There are also many extra costs involved in caring. Extra money may be needed for expenses such as medicines, transport, meals, power bills and respite care. The combination of a low income and these extra expenses can make it really tough to make ends meet.

Relationships often change when we take on a caring role. The situation that created the need for care can cause a major change in a relationship – especially if a partner or child has been diagnosed with a serious illness or has been in an accident. You may even find yourself caring for someone, such as a parent or parent-in-law, with whom you have always had a diffi- cult relationship: 22 per cent of people caring for more than 40 hours a week say they have a strained relationship with the person they are caring for. But caring can also strengthen relationships: 36 per cent of primary carers say that caring has brought them closer to the person they are caring for.

The person being cared for is struggling too

Caring for someone changes the power balance within a relation- ship. While you are taking on new responsibilities, the person you are caring for is adjusting to being more dependent on you. This can be a difficult adjustment for both of you.

As part of your caring role, try not to take over decision-making or other tasks the person you are caring for is still capable of. Aim to help them be as independent as possible, knowing that this may change over time. It is very important, for example, for many older people to have a sense of control over their finances. Even if they can no longer do their own banking, show them their bank statements and involve them in decisions about how they spend their money.

Carers often have complicated feelings

It's normal to have complicated feelings about your caring role, and your feelings will change at different times. Carers say they often feel over- whelmed, confused and shocked, especially in the early stages of caring or if they suddenly become a carer when someone they are close to is diag- nosed with a serious illness.

It is also very normal for carers to feel frustrated, angry, lonely and isolated. There may be times when you feel you don't want to be a carer and wish that other family members would step up and help more (see 'Support from other family members' later in this chapter for help with this issue). You may then feel guilty about resenting your caring role. You may grieve for the relationship you have lost with the person you now care for and for the loss of the life you used to know.

Any of these feelings can become overwhelming at times. You may find that your feelings spill over into other relationships and cause you to behave in ways that you don't like very much. Your feelings might make it difficult to think and make decisions.

Who can help carers work through their feelings?

Many carers find it helpful to talk to someone about how they are feeling; it's too much for most people to deal with by themselves. Joining a support group or talking to a counsellor are options that can help.

Support groups for carers

A support group offers you the chance to meet other carers who can relate to your situation and provide you with a safe place to let off some steam. You can share your experience of caring, receive emotional support and learn practical information about services that can help. A support group can also be a great way to feel less isolated and meet new friends. Support groups come in all shapes and sizes: some general groups are open to all types of care situations, while other groups focus on a specific illness or disability. To help you find a group with the right fit for you, contact your local Carers Association on 1800 242 636.

Counselling

Talking to a qualified professional who understands the problems carers deal with every day can help you sort through your feelings, make useful changes, develop coping skills and improve stress management. Talking to a counsellor is not a sign of weakness or that you are not coping. It is about looking after yourself better, which in turn will help you care better as well.

The National Carer Counselling Program (NCCP) can help by offering short-term counselling services. To contact the service, call your local Carers Association on 1800 242 636 and let them know you want to know more about counselling for carers. There is usually a small fee for the service and the amount you pay depends on your income and the type of counselling you need. You can talk to a counsellor over the phone, by email, Skype, or in person. Counsellors who speak languages other than English are available in some areas.

For more on managing stress and looking after your own health, see 'Support from other family members' and 'Looking after yourself' later in this chapter.

Abuse in care relationships

Abuse can happen in all types of relationships, including those where someone is caring for another person. Both the person receiving care and the carer can be at risk of abuse. Abuse can take many different forms: it may be physical, sexual, emotional or verbal. In caring situations, there is also the potential for financial abuse and neglect.

Carers who are under stress and having difficulty adjusting to their caring role may abuse the person they are caring for. Care recipients with dementia, mental illness and drug and alcohol problems may be aggressive or abusive towards their carer. There may be a previous history of abuse within the relationship (on either side) before the care situation began, and abuse may increase with the stress and difficulties of giving or receiving care.

It is important to seek help if you think abuse is happening, whether you are concerned about your own behaviour as a carer or the behaviour of the person receiving care.

Help with abuse in care relationships

- Call 1800 RESPECT (1800 737 732), Australia's national sexual assault, domestic and family violence counselling service. Telephone counselling is available 24/7. The website www.1800respect.org.au has helpful information and online counselling.
- Call your local Carers Association on 1800 242 636.
- Talk to your GP.
- If the situation is dangerous, call the police on 000.

For more on family violence, and the strategies and services to help, see chapter 30.

Carer support services

There are many support services designed to help make a carer's job easier and to help people stay at home for as long as possible. Caring is a very demanding job and no one expects you to do everything yourself – and neither should you. Some people feel reluctant to ask for help and feel they should be able to manage everything by themselves or just within the family, but this can take its toll on their own health and relationships. It's often useful to get help with the tasks you aren't so good at (cooking might not be your thing, for example) or that you find physically difficult (such as house maintenance and repairs, perhaps) so you can focus on the things you do well. Sometimes, it's just a good idea to have extra help with home nursing or practical home help, so you can have a break and a little bit of extra time for yourself.

Have a look through the different types of support services listed on the next pages and think about which could be helpful for you. Most of these organisations will want to assess whether their service is suitable for you, which could mean they will need to make a full assessment of the care situation. This can mean quite a few questions, paperwork and your time. It's often helpful if you can ask different family members to organise different areas of support to share the workload.

The Australian Government's My Aged Care service is a good place to start the search for any of the support services listed below, even if the person you are caring for isn't aged (call 1800 200 422 or visit www.myagedcare.gov.au and choose 'Find a service'). You can search for all types of services (such as housework, home maintenance, meals and more) for your town, suburb or postcode. The services listed may be provided by community, private, church-based or charitable organisations. Depending on the organisation providing the service, different charges will be involved, while some services are provided free of charge or at a low cost.

Some of the different types of services you might want to think about using are:

- **home care services** – which can help with practical tasks at home including cleaning, shopping, laundry and some personal care such as bathing and dressing. As well as looking on www.myagedcare. gov.au, you can find services by doing an internet search for 'home care services' and including your city, town or nearest regional centre.

- **home maintenance and modification services** – which can provide essential home repairs and make changes to a home such as installing safety ramps and support rails

- **home nursing services** – which provide a trained nurse to visit people at home and help with bathing and the toilet, giving medicines and injections, and changing dressings. These services may be provided by a community nurse or by private nursing agencies.

- **community health centres** – which offer a range of health services, including physiotherapy, podiatry, speech pathology, dietary advice and social work

- **food services** – which can deliver nutritious fresh or frozen meals. Different food services can provide different levels of support, from occasional meals when you need time out to a regular delivery service. Meals can be tailored to specific health, religious or cultural needs. Search for food services in your local area on www.myagedcare.gov.au or visit www.mealsonwheels.org.au, which delivers meals during the week for a small charge.

- **transport services** – which can help if neither you nor the person you care for have their own transport and can't use public transport. You can use these services to attend medical appointments, go shopping or enjoy social outings.

- **volunteers** – who make an extraordinary contribution to the community and to the life of carers, especially in rural areas. They may provide home visits, help with shopping or transport to appointments, and offer other personal and home services. To find volunteers who may be able to help out, do an internet search for 'volunteer home services' and include your city, town or nearest regional centre. Your GP, community health centre or local council may also be able to help you find volunteer services.

- **the Australian Government** – which provides a range of programs designed to help older people retain their independence at home and in the community. These include the Home and Community Care

---

Do you have an emergency care plan?

When you care for someone who depends on you, it makes good sense to have an emergency care plan: a list with contact details for people who have agreed to provide emergency care when needed, and with instructions for care, such as medicines that need to be given and support services you have in place.

You can download a template of an emergency care plan and fill in all the relevant details yourself. Visit www.health.gov.au/internet/main/publishing.nsf/Content/ageing-carers-carerkit.htm for the emergency care plan. You can also call 1800 200 422 to have a copy of the plan sent to you.

You should keep a copy of the completed plan in a safe place where it is easy to see and give a copy to each of your emergency carers. Update your plan every year, or whenever care details change.

(HACC) Program for people who need basic home help, and many other programs and packages that can provide more complex or higher levels of care. The person you are caring for will need to be assessed to work out eligibility and the best type of program for their needs. Call 1800 200 422 to find out more.

Support from other family members

In many families, even in large ones, the main responsibility for caring often falls on one family member. Sometimes other family members don't understand how much this person is doing.

Holding a family meeting can be a really helpful way to talk openly about any concerns and care issues, and to make decisions together. You may be able to ask other family members to help with specific tasks depending on their skills. People always like to be asked to do something because you've acknowledged they are good at it. If a family member is a great gardener, ask them if they would be able to help plant some flowers or herbs to cheer up the house or mow the lawn every two weeks. You could ask a family member who is handy to help out with repairs. A family member with computer skills could set up a spreadsheet to keep track of caring and medical expenses. Even young family members can help share the load by reading stories and playing board games with the person you are caring for. Many families find it helpful to draw up a roster of jobs that everyone has agreed to help with.

Do your best to keep meetings positive so that family members will be happy to come along and contribute. If you are having difficulty getting other family members to support you and cooperate, you can call your local Carers Association on 1800 242 636 for more ideas to help.

See later in this chapter for information about respite services that allow carers to take a break from their caring role.

As the daughter of Italian immigrants, Sophia's role as a carer began when she was just 12 years old and became her parents' interpreter at healthcare visits. Sophia describes how her role as a carer has grown as her parents have aged.

'As my parents aged and their health deteriorated, I became much more than just their interpreter. I became their taxi driver, shopping assistant, home help, financial assistant, counsellor and, most important of all, their case worker when dealing with the health system.

'In 2006, my father's health declined dramatically. He was in and out of

hospital, and with each admittance, his health worsened and his dementia increased. While he was in hospital, I would go in before work to see that he was okay and keep him calm, and would come back in the evening to make sure he ate and then stay with him till bedtime. Throughout this time, I was lucky to have a very understanding workplace. If I needed time off work, I could take it, and they made allowance for my performance and output because they knew the strain I was under. In his final months, my father needed constant care and so I quit work to help my mother care for him at home: she would take the day shift and I looked after him at night. I look back on this time and wonder how I survived it.

'After my father passed away, my primary carer role shifted to my mother. She had kept herself strong throughout my father's declining years, ignoring her own health to look after his, and this had taken its toll. My mother became completely dependent on me. She also became a falls risk, so I decided it was time to move in with her.

'For the most part, moving in with Mum has been a good thing, though it did take a while to adjust. I hadn't factored into the equation how much I would miss my independence, what little of it I did have, and how much I would grieve the loss of my own home I had lived in for 17 years. But luckily I have found my own space within her space.

'You may ask why I have done all of this for my parents. It's partly cultural: obligation to family is instilled in us, especially if you are female. But mostly, it's because of my deep love for both my parents and my wish not to see them suffer in their final years. As much as I have given to my parents I get back more. Difficult as it has sometimes been, I feel like they deserve this little piece of my life I have been able to give them.'

Juggling work and caring

Taking on a caring role can affect your ability to continue with paid work. Over half of women aged 30–64 who are primary carers are not in paid employment. For those women who are in paid work, the work is more likely to be part-time.

Many carers would like the opportunity to keep up their paid work. As well as providing income and helping build up superannuation, it can offer a great deal of satisfaction, is good for self-esteem and provides the chance to mix with other people. Paid work also provides a life outside caring.

It can be tricky to juggle paid work with caring, but having extra support at work and more flexible work arrangements can make the juggling act easier. Employees have certain rights, and it's important to know your rights to help you negotiate with your employer.

Your rights at work

Your legal rights as a carer are covered by various national and state or territory laws or in national modern awards, which set our minimum workplace conditions. Under these laws and awards, most employees can request flexible working arrangements and take both paid and unpaid leave to cover sickness and caring responsibilities.

If you want to negotiate working arrangements to help you in your caring role, it is best to start by researching your rights:

- Talk to your HR or personnel department at work.
- Talk to co-workers and find out if anyone else is juggling work with caring, and how the company has responded to any requests they have made for flexible work arrangements.
- Visit the Working Carers Gateway at www.workingcarers.org.au and read their Employee Guide.
- Contact Fair Work Australia on 13 13 94.

Negotiating with your employer

Once you know your rights, think carefully about what you would like to negotiate with your employer. You may want to start or finish work at different hours on certain days, work fewer days, do some of your work from home, work split shifts or job-share with another employee.

Think about how you can still get all your work done with the new work arrangement you are requesting. This may be by working through some lunch hours, asking co-workers to cover for you at certain times and doing some extra work at home. Working out these details will help you present your employer with a positive business case.

Once you have thought about the details, make an appointment with your employer to talk about your caring responsibilities and use these tips to help you negotiate:

- Explain your caring situation positively and tell your employer you want to be able to work *and* care. Don't apologise for caring.
- Tell your employer you have researched your legal rights as a working carer and that there is an increasing trend for employers to support staff who are working and caring.

- Present your employer with a solution rather than a problem – that way you are much more likely to get a positive result. For example, you could say something like: 'I've been thinking about how I can combine my work with caring for my mother in a way that won't inconvenience any customers. Because we are usually busiest after 10.30 am, I was wondering if I might be able to start work then instead of at 9 am. I usually catch up on emails and do other admin work before we get busy in the shop, so I thought I might be able to do that work from home at night instead.'
- Be prepared with solutions to likely objections from your employer.
- Remember that your skills and experience are valuable to your employer and that many workplaces are becoming increasingly aware of the benefits of family-friendly work policies.

You may like to give your employer a copy of the 'Carers and work' fact sheet, available in the 'Employers' section of www.workingcarers.org.au.

Your employer needs to approve or refuse your request in writing within 21 days. If your request is refused, your employer needs to give the reasons why. If you are not satisfied with your employer's response, you should contact the Fair Work Australia Ombudsman on 13 13 94 about the next steps to take or visit www.fairwork.gov.au.

Payments for carers

Many carers are entitled to government benefits and allowances that can help them cover some of the extra costs associated with caring, or help them continue caring if they are not able to stay in substantial paid work.

Some carers are hesitant to apply for assistance: they may not realise they are eligible or may feel like the application process is too complicated. Some people think they should be able to manage without government

---

The National Disability Insurance Scheme (NDIS)

The NDIS is a scheme that will completely change the way people with a permanent disability are cared for and supported in Australia. One of the key aims of the NDIS is to provide better support for families in their caring role.

The NDIS is being rolled out around Australia from 2013. Visit www.ndis.gov.au or call the helpline on 1800 800 110 to find out when changes will begin in your area.

assistance. The government has money set aside to specifically help carers and the people they care for, so it makes good sense to access these payments and ease some of the financial strain.

You or the person you are caring for may be eligible for a number of different payments and concessions, outlined below.

Carer Allowance

Carer Allowance is a supplementary payment for carers who are providing daily care of at least 20 hours a week. The allowance isn't affected by income or assets and it is not taxed. This means you can still work or study without the allowance being affected and it can be paid *in addition to* other benefits such as the Carer Payment, Age Pension or other Centrelink payments. Carer Allowance is made up of a small fortnightly payment and an annual supplement.

Carer Payment

Carer Payment can provide income support for people who are providing full-time care and are unable to take on substantial paid work because of this caring role. The payment is affected by your own income and assets, as well as the income and assets of your partner (if you have one) and of the person you are caring for.

Disability Support Pension

The Disability Support Pension is a payment for people who have an illness, injury or disability that affects their ability to work. Payments are also available for parents who are caring for a child with a disability.

Better Start for children with a disability

The Better Start initiative provides funds to allow access to early intervention services such as physiotherapy and speech therapy for children up to the age of seven (parents need to register by the time their child is six).

Children are eligible for the program if they have been diagnosed with any one of a range of disabilities listed on www.betterstart.net.au

To learn more or to register your child for Better Start, call your local Carers Association on 1800 242 636 or visit www.betterstart.net.au

Concessions

If you or the person you care for receives a Centrelink payment, you may also be eligible for a Pensioner Concession Card or a Health Care Card. These cards may entitle the holder to concessions on prescription medicines, transport, car registration, education costs, council rates, water rates, some telephone services and power bills.

If you receive Carer Payment or a Disability Support Pension, you may also be eligible for rent assistance.

More information on payments for carers

You can find out more about all these payments and concessions by visiting www.humanservices.gov.au or calling Centrelink on 13 27 17. If you do not speak English very well, you can contact the Centrelink Multilingual Service on 13 12 02.

The Department of Veterans' Affairs (DVA) provides some financial assistance to war veterans, war widows and widowers, their families and carers. You can call DVA on 13 32 54 to find out if you are eligible for DVA assistance.

If you are unclear about what allowance you are eligible for or have any problems completing application forms, your local Carers Association can provide you with assistance on 1800 242 636.

Make sure you keep copies of your applications and supporting documents in case there are any questions or problems regarding your application.

If Centrelink turns down your first application, you can appeal their decision and have the right to a second appeal if necessary. Sometimes you need to be persistent to get the allowances you are entitled to.

Carer and Companion Cards

The Carer Card gives you benefits and discounts on a range of products and services from government and participating businesses.

The Companion Card allows someone with a significant permanent disability to buy tickets to various events and on public transport so a carer can accompany them at no extra charge.

The Carer and Companion Card systems vary in each state and territory. Your local Carers Association can provide you with more information.

Looking after yourself

Taking good care of *you* is one of the most important things you can do as a carer. Looking after your own physical and emotional health will help you keep up with the demands of caring and, importantly, all the other parts of your life.

Healthy eating

Healthy eating will help your body keep functioning well and give you the strength and energy you need. Sometimes the demands of caring can make people too tired or busy to cook or too stressed to eat properly. Here are some useful ideas that have helped other carers:

- Try not to rush meals or eat them on the run. Taking time out to sit down and enjoy a relaxing meal is good for your social and emotional wellbeing.

- Keep a well-stocked pantry with plenty of long-life ingredients that make it easy to create quick meals. Good staples include: pasta, noodles, rice, lentils and couscous; canned chickpeas, kidney beans, cannellini beans, baked beans and lentils (choose low-salt varieties); canned tuna, salmon and sardines (choose low-salt varieties); frozen vegies; canned fruit in natural juice; and plenty of dried herbs, spices and low-salt sauces to spice up your meals.

- Have a few very simple dishes in your regular meal rotation so you know you will always have the ingredients on hand to put dinner together with minimum fuss. Easy, tasty and inexpensive options include: baked jacket potatoes with baked beans; scrambled eggs or an omelette with salad; pasta with a tomato and tuna sauce; or canned sardines on toast with salad. One-pot dishes such as soups, risotto, stews and curries are also easy to prepare and save on washing up.

- Make extra food when you have the time and energy and freeze the leftovers in meal-sized containers. Better still, ask another family member or good friend to cook a large casserole or soup you can freeze.

- See the information on food services earlier in this chapter. You don't need to commit to using a food service all the time. You can buy a selection of frozen, nutritious meals to have on hand when you are too tired to cook.

You will find more information on healthy eating in other chapters of this book:

- Chapter 5 includes useful information to help you get all the nutrients you need for good health, to stay at a healthy weight, and to help keep your bones healthy and reduce the risk of heart disease.

- Chapter 13 includes plenty of practical tips for preparing healthy meals for women of any age.

- Chapter 14 focuses on healthy eating habits (not diets) to help you reach or stay at a healthy weight.

Sleeping well

Many carers say that they sleep poorly and often feel tired. You may have problems falling asleep, staying asleep or with the quality of your sleep. Eating well, staying active and managing stress will all help you get into a better sleeping pattern, and sleeping better will then help you to manage stress better too.

Health professionals often talk about 'sleep hygiene', which really just means developing good sleeping habits, such as sticking to a regular sleep schedule, avoiding heavy meals and caffeine close to bedtime, and so on. You'll find some helpful ideas for better sleep in chapter 33. This chapter focuses on menopause but don't worry if you are years away from or years past menopause – women of any age will find these ideas helpful.

Staying active

Finding time for around 30–60 minutes of physical activity every day is important for overall health and for keeping up with the physical and emotional demands of caring.

We all know that being active has many physical benefits, but it is also good for our emotional and mental health: it encourages better sleep, helps reduce stress, anxiety and depression, and increases energy. These are all very important for anyone in a caring role.

It may not be easy to fit extra activity into your day, but it is one of the most valuable things you can do for yourself as a carer – so don't ignore it. Here are some ideas:

- Regular walking is an easy, fun and inexpensive way to get active. Snap on a pedometer, grab a friend (two- or four-legged), and aim to increase your steps each week.

- Following an exercise DVD or fitness program on a games console at home is a good option on days when you can't get out of the house.

- It doesn't matter if you're active for 30 minutes (or more) all at once or if you break up your activity into 10-minute sessions when you can fit them in throughout the day.

- All kinds of incidental activity add up, too: use the stairs instead of lifts, walk to the shops, get busy in the garden if you can get out of the house, turn up the music and get physical with the housework!

- Community centres often have well-priced classes in all types of activities, including tai chi, yoga and Zumba. These can be a good option if you enjoy exercising with other people and can be great use of your time when you have organised respite care.

Check with your doctor before starting a new exercise program if you haven't been active for a while, if you have any health problems or if you are taking any regular medicines.

You will find more information on physical activity in other chapters of this book:

- Chapter 5 includes lots of practical ideas to increase your daily exercise and about the role of exercise in preventing many common health problems.

- Chapter 14 focuses on being active for health and weight loss.

Managing stress

Caring is a demanding job and it is very common for carers to experience physical and emotional stress. The greater the demands of your caring role and the less supported you feel, the more likely you are to feel stress. High levels of ongoing stress can take their toll and increase your risk of other health problems.

The best way to start helping yourself is to recognise that you are experiencing symptoms of stress and then work out what you can do to deal with the stress.

The signs of stress

Do you recognise any of these signs that your stress levels are high?

- problems sleeping – problems getting to sleep or staying asleep, or restless, unsatisfying sleep
- feeling tired a lot of the time

- feeling negative or uninterested in people or activities you normally enjoy
- being forgetful and unable to make decisions
- overeating or losing your appetite
- feeling tense, on edge, angry or irritable
- feeling helpless or worthless
- a racing heart, sweating, headaches, digestive problems or muscle tension that have no other obvious cause

These are all signs that you need to slow down, look after yourself and talk to someone to get the support you need. Here are some practical ideas that have helped other carers:

- **Change what you can.** You may not be able to change the main demands of your caring role, but it's usually possible to make small changes that can help. Ask family members and friends to help out, enlist the help of an extra support service or consider some extra respite care.
- **Learn new skills to help you manage.** There will be many things you cannot change, so it is really helpful to learn skills that will help you to manage the demands of caring. Your doctor can refer you to someone who can teach you practical skills such as structured problem-solving, activity scheduling and time management, or can refer you for problem-focused counselling such as financial or conflict resolution counselling.
- **Talk to your family, friends, a counsellor or other support group members** about how you are feeling. People who are looking in from the outside can often make creative suggestions to help.
- **Practise relaxation.** You might want to try progressive muscle relaxation, imagery, visualisation or meditation. There are lots of good CDs that can guide you through these techniques (try your local library) or do an internet search for 'free relaxation podcasts'.
- **Take regular time out to recharge.** Everyone needs time out to do their own thing. Try your best to do something that is just for you every day – keep up your outside interests and hobbies or learn something new, spend time with positive friends outside your caring role, go to the movies, read a good book or take a long bath. See later in this chapter for information on respite care that will give you some time to yourself.

Female carers are especially at risk of anxiety and depression. If you are experiencing some of the signs of stress listed earlier, especially if they are overwhelming or continue for weeks at a time, it may suggest that you are experiencing anxiety or depression. These are real and treatable illnesses. Start by talking to your GP, who can help find the best treatment for you. Most women in this situation find that once their anxiety or depression is treated, they are better able to manage the demands of caring.

For more information about stress, anxiety and depression see chapters 40 and 44 in this book, or contact beyondblue (see the Resources section at the end of this book).

Looking after your own health

When people spend a lot of time caring for someone else's health, they have a tendency to neglect their own health. The physical and emotional demands of caring can affect your health: lifting the person you care for, for example, may strain your back or joints. The time you spend caring may also make it difficult to take time out to be active and to keep on top of regular health checks.

Chapter 2 includes information about healthy lifestyle choices, health checks, tests and vaccinations that are important for all women.

Getting the break you need – respite care

Respite means taking a break – for you and the person you care for. There are many different types of respite care available. Depending on what services are available in your area, it is often useful to use a combination of respite care to meet your needs.

Respite can include:

- in-home care from a support worker
- community-based respite, where the person you care for joins a day program at a community centre or in a community house
- residential respite care, where the person you care for has a short stay in a care facility such as an aged-care home
- family, friends or a volunteer providing care so you can take a break
- emergency respite care if you need to deal with sudden illness or emergencies

Respite may be for a few hours, overnight or for longer periods. Most types of respite care will involve some cost.

Many carers are initially reluctant to consider respite care, but it really is essential for their health and wellbeing, can help them care better and can also benefit the person they are caring for. When carers start using regular respite care they usually can't understand why it took them so long to get started. Think of respite as an important *part* of your caring role rather than something that interrupts your role.

Carers often say they get the most out of respite care when they plan carefully what they will do in their break. Otherwise, it's tempting to use up all your time pottering at home and catching up on jobs. Respite is the ideal time to take up a new activity or an exercise class, to catch up with friends or enjoy a bit of pampering.

Here are some starting points:

- To find out about respite options in your area, contact your Commonwealth Respite and Carelink Centre on 1800 052 222.
- For emergency respite care outside business hours, call 1800 059 059.
- For help planning respite care and for emotional support, contact your local Carers Association on 1800 242 636.

Residential aged care

If you are caring for an older family member or friend, there usually comes a time when you can no longer provide care at home and you need to start thinking about moving the person you care for into a residential aged-care facility.

There are many practical, emotional and financial issues to consider when this time comes, and the aged-care system can be a bit of a maze.

To find out more:

- You will find a really helpful series of fact sheets for carers and family considering residential care on www.survivingthemaze. org.au.
- There's also useful information on the Australian Government's My Aged Care website: www.myagedcare.gov.au.
- If you'd rather talk to someone to point you in the right direction, call either My Aged Care on 1800 200 422 or your local Carers Association on 1800 242 636.

Ella describes herself, first and foremost, as the mother of six beautiful children. She is also the full-time carer of her profoundly disabled 17-year-old son Samuel. Samuel was born with several medical conditions. When he was 11 months old he had surgery on his skull. The surgery was a success and he recovered quickly, but within a few months his health declined. He had headaches and vomiting and then started to stare into space. Eventually Samuel had an epileptic seizure, stopped breathing and had a stroke. Ella was told that her son was 'brain dead'.

Ella says, 'My life changed forever that day. We said our goodbyes and a few days later we turned off his life support and waited for him to die.' But to everyone's surprise, Samuel kept breathing. Samuel woke up but would never be the same again: he had severe brain damage, vision impairment and epilepsy, and would never be able to walk or talk. Ella says that's when her struggle with life began. She was pregnant with her fourth child and became very depressed and unable to sleep. She cried constantly and started drinking to numb her pain. She was eventually prescribed antidepressants and slowly began to feel better and more able to deal with things.

Within a few months, Samuel started vomiting and again stopped breathing. He was resuscitated many times and two weeks later, doctors sent him home to die. Ella says she had a lot of support at that time, but she pretended everything was okay so people would think she was coping. Ella became obsessed about caring for Samuel and so there was no room for anyone else to come in and help. She ended up in therapy and Samuel had to be put into care for a number of months. Ella says, 'I started to learn how to accept help and how to let people know when I wasn't coping. I had to learn to be open about my needs. It was, and still is, a long journey.'

Recently, Samuel was diagnosed with further serious health problems. Ella says, 'My little boy has amazed everyone and has made me the person I am today. He is a strong, lovable and most precious boy. Every day with him is a bonus. He has taught me and helped me so much and I hope in the future I can offer my support to other families.'

Planning for the future

Planning ahead can help give you and the person you are caring for peace of mind. This planning may include organising various legal documents that clearly set out the person's wishes while they are still able to make these decisions. What you need to do will depend on your relationship to the person you care for, and their abilities, views and age. It's always a good idea to talk about and make these plans while both you and the person you care for are still quite well and able to make important decisions.

Enduring power of attorney

An enduring power of attorney (EPOA) is a legal document that allows someone to choose a person they trust to make financial and legal decisions on their behalf when they can no longer make these decisions for themselves. These types of decisions may include banking, changing investments or selling a home. Someone can only appoint an EPOA for themselves, and they can only do this while they understand what they are doing.

It is a good idea to talk to the person you are caring for about appointing an EPOA while they are still well enough. This is a very personal decision and they may wish to appoint you or another family member or close friend.

We should all ideally appoint an EPOA for ourselves while we have the capacity, so it's something you should think about doing for yourself, too. It can save a lot of future anxiety.

Advance care planning

Advance care planning is all about making plans for medical care in advance. It is a good idea for everyone to think about advance care planning, including you as a carer and the person you are caring for. Planning keeps you and the person you care for involved in medical decisions now and in the future. If you or the person you care for become very unwell in the future and either of you is unable to speak or make decisions, the plan provides a way of communicating personal wishes about medical and end-of-life care to family, friends and healthcare professionals. This can help to avoid a lot of confusion.

Part of advance care planning involves writing a document called an advance care plan (which may also be called an advance health directive, an advance care directive or a living will). A plan might include information about whether or not the person wants to be resuscitated if their heart stops and whether they would want to be on life support. Once you and the person you care for have an advance care plan, it is important to let others know about it. A copy should be kept in their medical file and at home with other important documents.

Visit www.respectingpatientchoices.org.au to read more about advance care planning. Choose 'Advance Care Planning for everyone' for an easy step-by-step guide to preparing an advance care plan.

Wills

Everyone should have a will – a document that sets out your wishes for your property, money and belongings after you die. It's normal to feel uncomfortable about making a will or talking to the person you care for about their will, but if they don't make one, their wishes can't be carried out and this can cause a lot of anxiety in families. It's important for you and the person you care for to make a will while you still have the capacity. It can be a very simple document and the contacts below can help.

Help with future planning documents

For help appointing an enduring power of attorney, guardian or administrator, or preparing an advance care plan or will, contact:

- your community legal centre or legal aid (check your phone book)
- your solicitor
- the guardianship board or tribunal in your state or territory (in some states this is called the Office of the Public Advocate). Do an internet search for 'guardianship board' and include your state or territory, or check the phone book.

There's no doubt that caring is one of the most rewarding and challenging roles anyone can take on. Always remember that to go the distance in your caring role, you need to keep yourself healthy, take regular time out and make good use of the support networks that are there for you. When you put your own needs much higher up the list, you will find you can be a better carer – and you will feel healthier and happier yourself. All the best in your caring role.

LATER YEARS

Introduction

Maureen Johnson

Life expectancy at birth for women in Australia is 83 years, or 73 for Aboriginal and Torres Strait Islander women – a shameful but persistent disparity in our society. At the beginning of the twentieth century, women were lucky to survive menopause; nowadays menopause marks more of a midpoint in a woman's lifespan. So, at 65, the point at which our later years are thought to begin, there are potentially many more years to be lived and, for most women, there is no reason why those years can't be healthy, active and full. For most older women in Australia that is already the case; 60 per cent of women in Australia aged 56–69 are in good health with no disability, an increasing percentage are still in the workforce and most are living independently in their own homes, despite the dominant perception that they are in nursing homes and requiring high-level care.

The less optimistic perspective, though, is that there are many older women who are not necessarily in the very best of health. In 2004, nearly 100 per cent of people aged 65 and over reported one chronic health complaint. The social picture is also of concern: older women are more likely to be widowed, and while living alone is a sign of ongoing health and independence, some will tolerate less than adequate living conditions in order to stay in their home. Many women are socially isolated and more likely to be economically vulnerable than their male counterparts. This often reflects a lifetime of disparity, as women continue to be paid less and have more interruptions to their working life, due to pregnancy and family duties.

Based on this information, government projections are grim and in alignment with prevailing views: an ageing population, more disability and more demand on health and aged services. We must add to this the fact that many of us will enter our later years with health beliefs that are, to use a youthful phrase, 'so last century'. Many older people are less inclined to take an active interest in their health, believing that the need for exercise diminishes with their advancing years or that vigorous exercise is a risk and light or gentle exercise is pointless – and so their health deteriorates.

But here is the good news. As mentioned earlier, for many women this is increasingly not how it is, and for others it is certainly not how it has to be. For women in their 60s, 70s, 80s and older, 'the times they are a-changing'.

The truth about social networking sites

Lots of older people think that using Facebook or similar social networking sites must be bad for you. Many think it would take up too much of their time, while others just can't see the point. A small but promising study by the University of Arizona's Psychology Department, however, has shown that using Facebook may increase the cognitive function in people 65 and older by up to 25 per cent.

It is thought that the benefits may be due to increased social engagement and reduced isolation, due to the complexity of inter-actions Facebook offers or the myriad information it allows people to gather at any one time, or all of the above.

Social networking is a good way to keep cognitively active, but it is also a good way to stay in touch with family and old friends. Of course it won't be everyone's cup of tea, and it is very important to have good support and a teacher who can make sure you are keeping your profile secure and safe. It is also not the only way to be cognitively engaged – but it is good to know it has its benefits.

Health in older women

A doctor tells the story of a woman in her later years who thinks she may have continence problems. She tells him that generally she is okay, except when she is on the trampoline with her grandchildren. In many ways, this interaction epitomises the changing character of today's 'older' woman. A generation ago the pursuit of health and fitness featured less in the priorities of older women, and the powerful links between lifestyle and healthy ageing were not nearly as clear. Nowadays we are increas-ingly cognisant of the important role of physical activity, nutrition and social engagement in maintaining our ongoing health. Our later years, which have traditionally been painted in the sombre tones of autumn, are starting to take on a summer glow – with a sense that so much is still possible, that rapid physical and mental decline are not inevitable and that jumping on a trampoline with our grandchildren can be the rule rather than the exception.

We now know that physical activity can significantly improve our quality of life. For many women, who may have spent their adult years struggling with body image, it can be quite liberating to finally be exercising for all the right reasons: strength, mobility, self-esteem, increased self-confidence and social connectivity, and feeling good. Healthy ageing is not to be confused with the secret to eternal youth. All of us, no matter how hard we work to maintain our physical health, will still turn grey, our skin will still wrinkle and our breasts will still submit to the inevitable demands of gravity.

In many cultures these signs of ageing are respected and valued, and associated with wisdom, respect and knowledge. Unfortunately, in Western society, the same signs of ageing can be a cloak of invisibility, obsessed as we are with youth and beauty. It's no wonder that our changing body can make us very sad or frightened. Negative stereotyping can also feed our negative health beliefs. It can be disheartening if the purpose of physical activity is to stave off the signs of ageing, only to find that no matter how hard we try, their arrival is as inevitable as the physical and biological transformations of adolescence. But grey hair and wrinkles do not have to have an impact on our strength, vitality or overall health, and the more we are able to bounce on trampolines with our grandchildren or at least remain active and engaged citizens, the more we will shift misconceptions, reverse negative stereotyping and paint a picture of ageing that is positive and aspirational. Strong, vital, active ageing women are powerful and beautiful!

How this book can help

When we were developing this book we spoke with older women and asked them about the issues that would be important to them in a book about women's health. They talked about issues they felt were central to ageing, including mental health and dementia, nutrition, self-care, and sex and sexuality.

Early in this book, in chapters 2 and 3, we talk about the importance for all women of maintaining a strong relationship with their doctor. Health checks are critical as we enter our later years, and while some screening tests are considered less important as we age, others are increasingly so.

For some, the later years can bring an increased risk of osteoporosis, for example, which also means the risk of falls increases. Your GP will ensure that your risks are monitored to help you stay healthy.

Many women in their later years are living alone, often because their partner has died or because a relationship has ended. Some women will be in new relationships; some may begin relationships well into their later years. The issue of sex can be quite confronting, especially for those who haven't been in a sexual relationship for a long time. Women who are still in very long-term relationships can also find sex very difficult: long-term couples can become extremely ritualised in their lovemaking and sometimes it can become too familiar, losing some of the thrill of earlier years. In chapter 43 we talk about sex and debunk a few myths about what it means to us in our later years. Believe it or not, older women can have an increased risk of sexually transmitted infections. This is because there is no longer a risk of pregnancy and women and their sexual partners can become complacent about using condoms.

In chapter 44 we talk about mental health as we grow older. The good news is that there is evidence to show we are less inclined to worry and suffer from depression in our later years, although there are mental health issues that are very specific to this life stage. Loneliness, for example, can be a big issue as we approach our later years, particularly if physical or mental health conditions impede our ability to participate in activities outside the home. Our lives become increasingly bounded by the home as we age, and the home often represents our independence and ongoing health. Our home helps us maintain an attachment to the past and keeps our memories and the concept of family contained, even if the people have long gone. This means we may hang on tightly to our home even when it is no longer suitable to our needs, and even if this compromises our connection to the outside world.

In chapter 42, we discuss nutrition, an area that many women in their later years are inclined to neglect. As we age, our sense of taste can change and our appetite may not be quite so voracious. Some older adults can actually become quite malnourished. While as older women we do not need as many calories, we still need essential vitamins and nutrients, which are best delivered through food. The Women's dieticians offer ways for us to think about food and ideas for us to maintain a healthy diet, even in the most difficult of circumstances.

Life as an older woman

Our later years are, in many ways, the longest journey of all of our life stages. They are also a time when we are likely to face some of our most challenging and confronting health issues. Saying you should eat well, exercise and stay connected with your community, friends and family can make it seem very straightforward and easy, but of course it doesn't take into account the complexity or the context of your life, your history, your circumstances or your existing health. You may have days when it is too hard, but we hope there will also be days when you can consider some of the health advice in this section.

Other sections in this book may also be useful to you: if you are caring for a sick partner, parent, son or daughter, you will find chapter 41 on carers useful; there is also some good information in chapters 2 and 32 about general health checks to prevent the onset of common diseases such as heart disease and diabetes, for example.

Women in their later years are significant contributors to society: to family, home and the workplace, as well as in informal activities that support the economy and the community. Many women are still working into their 70s; many volunteer into their 80s. Some take on the full-time care of their grandchildren, while others continue to provide care for disabled adult children. As a society we are still learning to respect and to value our elders, and it is incumbent upon each of us, as we enter our later years, to live active, engaged and vital lives and to impress upon the elders of tomorrow that it's a good place to be.

42

Food and nutrition for older women

Jenny Taylor

Being well nourished improves mental and physical health and quality of life at all stages of our lifespan, but as we pass through midlife into older age our nutritional concerns may change. Our nutrient needs don't decrease, but our calorie needs and appetite may. This means we may need to take more care to ensure an adequate diet. As well as lack of appetite, worry about cholesterol, weight or blood sugars may cause older people to overly restrict their eating. Malnutrition is extremely common among elderly people: 38 per cent of those who live at home are at risk of malnutrition and the percentages are even higher for people in hospital or aged care. Malnutrition can mean lack of calories or a lack of nutrients, such as iron or vitamin B12, needed for the body to function at its best. Being malnourished increases the risk of falls and illness, and delays recovery.

Poor food intake

Reduced appetite is common as we age, and there are many reasons for it. Our senses of taste and smell may become less acute, making food less flavourful. Illness or medications can reduce our appetite and affect the taste of foods. We may not be doing enough physical activity to stimulate our appetite. Lack of saliva, poor dental health or trouble swallowing can also make eating an effort and so reduce intake. On top of these difficulties, changes in digestion may cause some nutrients to be poorly absorbed into the body.

Other factors include loss of interest in cooking and eating due to living and eating alone or illness, depression, bereavement, alcoholism, dementia or confusion. Poor nutritional knowledge or cooking skills may result in filling up on monotonous, nutrient-poor foods such as toast or biscuits. Low income may restrict food intake and variety, as can an inability to shop or cook due to poor mobility.

Over-restricting food quantity or variety due to concerns about weight, blood sugar or cholesterol may be inappropriate in the elderly. Concern for these conditions needs to be balanced against the need for good nutrition. A slightly higher body weight may be beneficial in older people. There is evidence that mildly overweight older people tend to live longer, perhaps because they are less frail. Losing weight at this stage of life risks losing muscle and bone strength, which increases the risk of falls and reduces the ability to cope with illnesses, and so may do more harm than good.

Signs of malnutrition

As the signs of malnutrition overlap with other conditions, they are not always easy to spot. Losing weight without trying is a red flag for malnutrition, but malnutrition can also occur without weight loss. Being overweight does not protect against malnutrition if you are not eating a good diet. It is still possible to carry excess fat but lack nutrients that are needed for the body to function at its best.

Malnutrition can contribute to memory loss and confusion, and to low immunity, increasing the risk of infections, poor wound healing and skin ulceration. It causes fatigue and muscle weakness, too, which increase the risk of falls.

Keeping your body in good nutritional shape

As we age, the amount of nutrients we need stays the same, but we don't need so many calories, we need quality, not quantity. This means there is little room for large amounts of low-nutrient foods such as biscuits or soft drink.

The best way to stay well nourished is to eat a good variety of foods from the major food groups each day. Choose nutrient-rich foods according to the following guide:

- Include iron- and protein-containing foods such as red meat, chicken, fish and eggs, or vegan alternatives such as dried beans or nut butter, in one or two meals a day. If chewing is a problem, choose soft foods such as minced meat or casseroles. You may also find soft foods easier to eat if your appetite is not good, as they require less effort to eat.
- Aim for three serves a day of dairy foods for calcium and protein. These can include milk, soy milk, cheese or yoghurt, custards and

dairy-based desserts such as rice pudding, which are easy to eat even if your appetite is not good.

- Have some vegetables or salad with lunch and dinner and a couple of serves of fruit during the day for vitamins and fibre. Stewed or canned fruit is a good alternative to fresh if chewing is a problem.

- Add a carbohydrate serve to each meal for energy (bread, dry biscuits, rice, pasta, potato or breakfast cereal).

Fluid intake is important. Inadequate fluid can lead to dehydration, constipation and feeling unwell. Nine cups (2.25 litres) of fluid a day are recommended. This can include tea, coffee, soups, milk-based drinks and juice, but not alcohol.

Vitamin D deficiency is a common problem among older people, affecting muscles and bones and increasing the risk of falls and fractures. As our vitamin D comes mostly from exposure to sunlight rather than food, we can be low in this vitamin even when eating a varied diet. Our skin becomes less able to make vitamin D as we age, thus increasing the risk of deficiency. Sitting in gentle sun for a few minutes each day or going for a morning or late-afternoon walk with bare arms will help maintain vitamin D levels without risking excess sun exposure. Your doctor can easily determine your vitamin D level with a blood test, and vitamin D can be taken as a supplement if needed.

Tips for improving appetite and food variety

If your appetite or food intake is not good, the following tips may help:

- Eat small, frequent meals and snacks. Large meals can be off-putting for people with poor appetites, and small amounts taken often can add up to a substantial amount of food. Good snacks include milk-based drinks, crackers and cheese, toast with peanut butter, toasted cheese sandwiches and yoghurt.

- Eat meals and snacks before filling up on low-nutrient foods or drinks such as coffee or biscuits.

- Tasty foods with extra seasoning may tempt jaded tastebuds. Try adding flavourings such as lemon juice, herbs and spices.

- Make drinks such as coffee or Milo more nourishing by basing them on milk.

- If your appetite is very poor, drinks may be easier to take than food, but avoid filling up on drinks that are insufficiently nourishing, such as soft drinks or fruit juice. Nourishing soups containing vegetables and meat, split peas or lentils are appropriate, as are milk drinks such as smoothies made with milk, fruit, yoghurt or ice-cream. Supplements such as Sustagen, Proform and Ensure are 'food drinks' containing all the nutrients and calories present in food, and can replace solid food. These are different from multivitamin tablets in that they also contain calories, protein, carbohydrate and fat, and not just vitamins and minerals.

- Physical activity such as a daily walk helps stimulate the appetite, as does eating in pleasant surroundings such as at a set table or in company when possible.

- Maintain good oral care and if you have dentures make sure they fit well.

- Use support systems to help maintain good nutrition and well-being. If necessary, take advantage of family, friends or community supports for help with shopping. Use a shopping list so you don't forget important foods. Meals on Wheels and frozen meals from the supermarket can take the pressure off if health problems make cooking difficult. Take advantage of opportunities for socialising such as local council-run activities for older people, which often include meals.

Bowel problems

Constipation is a common problem that not only causes discomfort, but also can reduce appetite. It can be helped by drinking plenty of fluid and increasing fibre intake from food such as fruit, vegetables, whole-meal bread and high-fibre breakfast cereals. Fibre supplements such as Metamucil, Benefiber or Fybogel are a good alternative if you are unable to eat sufficient fibre from food due to tooth or appetite problems. Other things that may help are pear juice, which contains a substance that helps keep bowel actions soft, and prunes and prune juice, which contain a substance that stimulates the bowel. If constipation continues to be a problem and you need laxatives, seek advice from your doctor or pharmacist on the best type for you.

In contrast, weak pelvic floor muscles or digestive problems can cause loose bowels or the need to use your bowels urgently. If this is the case, you may benefit by limiting coarse, fibrous foods such as grainy bread, muesli, fruit skins and dried beans, and instead choosing white or smooth wholemeal bread and soft or cooked fruit and vegetables.

Weight control

While it is beneficial in our older years not to be too thin, being over-weight can make joints and mobility worse as we age, and contribute to other health problems. Losing weight at any age is hard, but as we get older this is compounded by difficulty exercising and our lower calorie needs. A realistic goal might be to gain no further weight or perhaps to lose a few kilograms slowly.

As we still need to stay well nourished while watching our weight, the foods and drinks that can be spared are those that are rich in calories but not nutrients. Biscuits, chocolate and pastries provide a lot of calories for their size and can be eaten as treats rather than everyday foods. Also be miserly with butter, margarine and oil for cooking. Soft drinks, cordials and juices contain more sugar than many people realise: at around five teaspoons per glass, they can soon add up. Alcohol is also a rich fuel source that can contribute to weight problems.

If you are able, regular exercise such as walking or water exercises will help build muscle and burn calories.

43

Sexuality in older women

Susan Carr

A woman aged 65 today in Australia will live well into her 80s, according to the Australian Bureau of Statistics. While a lot of attention is given to sex and sexual problems during menopause, by the time a woman reaches 65, she is usually well past the worst symptoms of menopause and recognises and accepts physical changes due to her changed hormonal status but can still encounter difficulties with sex.

It is often forgotten that sexual attraction is triggered primarily by the emotional response to another person, and this does not decline with age. Although the physical mechanics of the sexual act may become slower or less comfortable with age, the emotional excitement can remain as intense as in youth. Many women in their 70s and 80s say, 'In my head I still feel 21, it's just my body that's changing.'

This aspect of sexuality is largely incomprehensible to a society focused on youth and physical perfection, and can make older people too embarrassed to admit, or discuss, their sexual feelings. What sustains older people in a sexual relationship is a shared sense of humour, and an ability to enjoy the 'lows' as well as the 'highs' of their sexual contacts.

At this age you may be single or married, in a heterosexual or same-sex relationship or widowed. You may be a mother, grandmother or possibly a great-grandmother, or you may be childless. It is a time when you can hope to have a fulfilling sexual relationship, if that's what you want. It is a time free of concerns about contraception, fertility or acute menopausal symptoms. Many women enjoy healthy sex lives well into their 80s and beyond. A Japanese study asked women and men in their 80s and 90s if they were interested in sex. Both women and men said they were ... but the women said they had difficulty finding partners.

Problems may arise with sexual activity and relationships at this stage, as in any other phase of life, and it is important not to ignore these problems.

Sex may even be an important issue in the terminal stages of diseases such as cancer, and the patient should be allowed to express these wishes. (There is more information on this later in the chapter.)

Sexual health

Many women are in new relationships at this age due to changing social circumstances. Women who are divorced or widowed are less inclined nowadays to fade away in society. The increased social and financial independence of many women, as well as their use of social media means they can socialise and meet people as never before. On the other hand, some women feel safer and more sheltered in their own familiar environment, and often partner with old and close family friends. It has often been said that the worst affliction of all is loneliness, and for many women good companionship and consensual sex at any age is life-enhancing.

It is easy to ignore or dismiss concerns about sexually transmitted infections (STIs), and the older age group is very guilty of being sexually reckless and abandoning condoms. Many older men say they are not used to using them, or may have partial erectile failure, which makes them difficult to use. Older women know they can't get pregnant, so they assume they don't need to worry about condoms. Age does not offer any protection, however, from STIs, so condom use with a new male partner is always advised. It is possible to become infected with HIV or HPV at any age, both of which can be prevented by condom use. One clinic visitor was even thrilled to have a diagnosis of trichomonas, saying, 'It makes me feel young again to have an STI.'

Another possibility at this age is developing gynaecological cancer. See chapter 35 for comprehensive information on this topic. Always see your doctor if you experience any bleeding or pain with sexual activity, which could indicate vaginal or cervical cancer. These symptoms would be unlikely at this age to indicate ovarian or endometrial cancer.

Sexual difficulties

A general population-based study in the United States showed that 37 per cent of men and 43 per cent of women will have a sexual problem at some point in their life. The group most likely to have a problem of this nature is postmenopausal women. There is now general recognition of the sexual problems faced by women in their 50s and beyond. The impact of menopause is lifelong, and the acute symptoms can last for up to 10 years. At any age the emotional impact of vaginal dryness can be enormous, and there are many problems a patch or tablet cannot fix. If you have a chronic or new illness, you may need to make some physical adjustments to the way you express your sexuality.

The most common sexual problems at this age are pain on penetration (dyspareunia) and loss of libido.

Dyspareunia (pain during sex)

It is common in postmenopausal women for the vagina to shrink and become dry, due to lack of oestrogen. This can cause discomfort on penetration, but the dryness can be corrected by using a good lubricant, or oestrogen cream or pessaries if advised by the doctor.

Another common cause of a dry vagina at any age is lack of arousal. As we get older it can take longer to become sexually aroused. Lack of sufficient foreplay before penetration will cause painful sex. This sometimes becomes so uncomfortable that a woman may end up avoiding sex altogether.

Sex need not always involve penetration. There are many pleasurable ways of being sexual with or without a partner, and experimentation can be fun. Stimulating your erogenous zones using either a vibrator, a partner or masturbation, may be exciting. Sex toys are not only for the young, and can be bought on the internet if going to a sex shop doesn't appeal.

Maria, aged 82, has been married for 51 years to Peter, aged 81. They have four children and six grandchildren. Maria is in good health; she had a breast cancer diagnosis and treatment six years ago and is now well. Peter had a minor heart attack 18 months ago, after which he became a little depressed.

Maria visited her doctor for a check-up. She was very vague at first, but it eventually transpired that she and Peter had always had a good sexual relationship, but sex had become less frequent over the years. Over the last year or so, sex had become painful, and Maria was worried there might be something wrong.

Maria had a full gynaecological screen, and apart from some vaginal atrophy (shrinkage), all was well. She said she always used lubricant cream before sex and when she was referred to the psychosexual clinic, it became clear the problem was not with Maria. Peter had increasing erectile dysfunction, which made any attempts at penetration painful. Peter was given medication and sex improved for them both.

Loss of libido

When we get older, our interest in sex may lessen for many reasons. This includes the hormonal changes of menopause, any illnesses causing pain, fatigue or loss of function, or simply overfamiliarity with a long-term partner. Any past loss or hurt we think we have dealt with, may return to our subconscious at unexpected times and have an impact on our daily life. The loss of health or a loved partner, loss of material goods and past losses such as abortions or miscarriages can affect a sexual relationship in later life. If this is the case for you, good psychological or psychosexual counselling can help you come to terms with the past and improve the present.

Often in a longstanding relationship, sex just becomes boring, over-familiar or irrelevant. If both partners have the same attitude to their sexual relationship, then there is no problem. If, however, one wants sex and the other does not, it can put enormous strain on the relationship. Communication is often the key: talking to one another about sex is vital.

Many people in this situation don't want to broach the topic for fear of hurting their partner, or of allowing past problems to resurface. If it is too difficult to bring up the topic, a visit to a sexual or relationship counsellor can help.

The important thing is to ask for help. You are entitled to a satisfying sex life at any age.

Layla was 68 with two children in their 30s who had left home, and was married to Archie, aged 69. They had been married for 40 years and Layla was retired, but her husband had his own business and was still working.

Layla said she had never felt the same since her menopause, and now vaginal dryness was making sex so uncomfortable that she was avoiding it. She also said she was having problems sleeping. Her GP prescribed sleeping pills and vaginal oestrogen cream, but Layla said that although the pills were helping her sleep, she still didn't feel like having sex. The doctor gave her vaginal oestrogen pessaries instead of cream.

A few months later Layla went to the surgery complaining of a sore shoulder, saying she had tripped over a chair at home. She had some bruises. The GP asked about her general health, and mentioned her loss of libido. She told him it was no better.

Two years later, she was hospitalised with a broken arm, and only then, after sensitive questioning, did she break down and admit her husband was an alcoholic who was occasionally violent. She left him, met an old schoolfriend, and her libido returned.

As Layla's case shows, a loss of sexual interest can be due to many complex factors, and it is important to look beyond surface issues for a solution.

Sex and terminal illness

This can be a very difficult area for people to discuss. The limited research involving people with a terminal disease such as cancer and their partners shows that some people would like to express their sexuality with their partner, particularly at the palliative phase (when recovery is no longer possible). This may just be holding and cuddling, but the physical and emotional barriers of palliative care may be a hindrance.

One of the main problems is privacy and a suitable bed, especially in a hospital setting. If the subject is sensitively broached with your doctor or care coordinator, there may be an opportunity for time as a couple, without family, friends or the clinical team. The couples who do wish sexual contact when one partner is dying, often as a last expression of life, find it very hard to express this to anyone, and may need some help or advice, even on the practical level. At a time of overwhelming emotions ranging from acceptance and grief to rage and denial, it is important to respect the wishes of the couple right up to the end.

Single women and sex

Women don't need a partner to enjoy good sexual stimulation, arousal and orgasm. This can be achieved with a good imagination and a comfortable knowledge of our body.

Sexual fantasies are cost-free and private, and can trigger strong feelings of arousal. Masturbation or self-stimulation techniques vary from woman to woman and usually women in their older years are very familiar with their own bodies. If not, there is time to learn, and there are a lot of self-help books about female anatomy and masturbation techniques.

Remember, self-stimulation is for pleasure and cannot harm you or anyone else. It works at any age, although it takes longer to climax as we age.

Talking to doctors about sex

Communicating about sex can be difficult at any age, both for women and their doctors. As the age gap between doctor and patient widens, however, it may become even harder. An 81-year-old lady in a new relationship is unlikely to be comfortable discussing lack of orgasm with a doctor or nurse who is the same age as her grandchild. Conversely, a younger doctor may find it almost impossible to imagine that the old lady in front of them is capable of or interested in having sex.

We are all entitled to help for sexual difficulties, and doctors or nurses will deal with any issues we raise in a professional and confidential manner. Never assume you are too old for sex, and never assume your doctor is too old or young to listen.

44

Mental health in older women

Christina Bryant

In Western societies we tend to think of old age as a time of decline – that we reach the prime of life sometime in early adulthood and can expect a steady decline in all aspects of our life thereafter. Certainly, we still live in a society that values youth much more highly than old age – we only need to walk through our local shopping centre and see beauty treatments being offered with the promise of 'reversing ageing'. Coupled with ageist views about older people, it is no wonder women say they feel invisible once they are past midlife, and under pressure not to look their age. Although it is true that some aspects of our psychological abilities do decline with age, the view that old age is a time of irrevocable decline is now quite outdated.

So what can we expect as we get older? This chapter covers the normal psychological changes that take place as we age, and talks about the risk factors for developing depression and anxiety. It also explains the difference between forgetting things and dementia, and the major causes of dementia. While people can experience loss and bereavement at any age, older people are more likely to experience a variety of losses, which we will discuss. Finally, we will say a few words about how to maintain mental health and enjoy a long and happy life.

Normal changes as we age

A number of changes take place as a normal part of ageing, and these are often divided into physical, cognitive (how we think and remember things), emotional (how we feel about things) and personality changes.

Physical changes

Over the past two centuries, life expectancy in the developed world has doubled from about 40 to well over 80, with women living approximately seven years longer than men. As we live longer, though, we become more vulnerable to chronic and degenerative diseases, many of which have a strong link to environmental or lifestyle factors. Today, heart disease and cancer account for more than half of all deaths in people aged over 40, yet it has been estimated that a significant proportion of cancers are related to factors we can do something about: around one-third are related to smoking, and a further third to diet. While there is much we can do to prevent chronic diseases, however, we cannot halt the biological process of ageing completely. As we get older, for example, our muscle strength declines and our bone density decreases, yet even some of these processes can be ameliorated by ensuring a good diet, maintaining a healthy weight, and engaging in regular moderate physical exercise.

Cognitive changes

It is well known that the speed at which we can process information slows down as we get older – and, in fact, this slowing down starts as early as our mid-20s. This means that we might find it harder to remember a telephone number very quickly, or it might take us longer to react to a red light. Older people also tend to be more easily distracted, and take longer to learn new skills, such as using new technologies. At the same time, though, we get better at seeing different sides of a story, and have large stores of personal experience to draw on when approaching issues and making decisions. This is what we could call wisdom.

Emotional changes

One of the stereotypes of ageing is that, as we get older, it is natural to feel miserable, or even depressed. In fact, most older people describe themselves as satisfied with their lives, and with time we tend to worry less. This is partly because we develop coping skills as we go through life, and partly because it seems that older people do not react as strongly to emotional stresses as younger people. On top of that, it seems that as we get older we pay more attention to positive experiences. Research has found, for example, that when older adults are asked to remember positive images (such as a smiling baby) and negative images (such as a duck in an oil spill), they remember far more of the positive than the negative images. This so-called positivity effect starts in midlife and seems to continue into advanced old age.

Changes in personality and social roles

Although personality is, by definition, a set of stable characteristics and ways of responding to situations, there is some evidence that as we get older we become more agreeable and less inclined to worry and be irritable – contrary to the stereotype of the 'grumpy old woman'. The majority of older people continue to carry out a wide range of roles as they age, and while the balance of these may change, they can provide much life satisfaction. Retirement, for example, may afford greater opportunities for involvement with grandchildren or hobbies. We have all heard newly retired people say they do not know how they ever found the time to go to work. Not surprisingly, it seems that being involved with other people and having a range of interests is good for our wellbeing.

In summary, old age is not all about decline. For an increasing number of people, it is a time characterised by a positive outlook, reasonable health, and time to do things they have always wanted to do. And while some things, such as remembering names, might get harder, think of all that accumulated life experience and wisdom we can now bring to bear on problems!

Mental health in older age

Older people do sometimes develop mental health problems and it is important to realise that it is *not* normal to feel sad or anxious, and it is not just part of being old. If you have persistent feelings of sadness or worry, or find yourself avoiding activities you used to enjoy, it is important to consider the possibility that you may have a depressive or anxiety disorder.

Depression

Most of us feel down from time to time or have periods when we find it hard to motivate ourselves, but this is very different from having depression. People are considered to be depressed if they have a range of symptoms that include a sad or depressed mood on most days, which they cannot shake off even if they do something they would normally enjoy. Additional symptoms of depression include a loss of interest in previous activities, loss of motivation, poor concentration and memory, difficulty making decisions, and fatigue and loss of energy. It may also involve feelings of guilt – people with depression sometimes worry about minor misdeeds from a long time ago, feel that they are a burden to others, or feel that things are hopeless. In older people, the physical symptoms of depression may be particularly prominent, including pain, dizziness, difficulty sleeping and loss of appetite.

When the feelings of hopelessness or being a burden become entrenched and severe, some people can begin to feel that life is not worth living or contemplate suicide. Between 2001 and 2010, 1796 Australians over the age of 65 suicided, and for men over the age of 85 the suicide rate was comparable with that for younger men. Depression is a strong risk factor for suicide. One study found that 75 per cent of older people who suicided had visited their GP in the four weeks before their death. It could be that older people will visit their doctor when depressed but, because they cannot find a way to talk about emotions, report physical complaints instead. Therefore, persistent low mood and negative thinking in an older person should be taken just as seriously as they are at any other time in the lifespan.

Is depression different in older people?

Studies have shown that many older people who are depressed do not describe themselves as feeling sad, and that their symptoms are weighted more towards the physical ones, such as pain, and changes in sleep and appetite. There is also some evidence that fewer older adults meet all the criteria for a diagnosis of depression, but are more likely than younger people to report some symptoms of depression. This means that, as an older person, even a few symptoms of depression might affect us disproportionately. If we feel unmotivated, lacking in energy and are not sleeping well, for example, we may not technically be depressed, but we could find it increasingly difficult to continue basic activities such as shopping and cooking, or may withdraw from social activities.

'Vascular depression' is a term used to describe a subtype of depression that usually emerges in later life. Its features include less depressed thinking but greater apathy and impairment in carrying out daily activities; a poorer response to treatment; and more prominent cognitive difficulties, especially in the area of thinking and planning. Unlike depression earlier in life, vascular depression is thought to have a much clearer physical cause, namely vascular disease. Vascular disease is any condition that affects the blood vessels, such as narrowing of the arteries or blockages in blood vessels. When the blood vessels in the brain are affected by vascular disease, cell death occurs, either as the result of a major acute (sudden) stroke, or a series of minor strokes. Getting older increases the risk of vascular disease, but smoking is the biggest (and most preventable) cause of vascular disease.

What causes depression?

Although old age is not a cause of depression in and of itself, it does increase the risk of developing certain other conditions associated with depression, such as vascular disease (see above). Poor physical health increases the risk of depression, and conditions such as Parkinson's disease and heart disease become more common as we age. According to some estimates, up to 35 per cent of older people in hospital are depressed, up to 40 per cent of those with heart disease are depressed, and about 25 per cent of those with Parkinson's disease are depressed.

The way these conditions are linked to depression is quite complex: on the one hand, the effect of their physical symptoms may restrict the ability to carry out normal activities, leading in turn to social isolation and other losses. This can then start a downward spiral in which the person with depression does less and less, and eventually becomes so depressed that they feel unable to attempt even small activities. Some research suggests, however, that depression and some physical conditions, especially heart disease and strokes, might both be caused by the same underlying physical process. One such process receiving quite a bit of attention is the inflammation of cells, which is caused by a complex reaction of the body to injury. These so-called inflammatory processes, which are known to play an important role in the development of heart disease, may also be involved in depression.

Some risk factors for depression in old age are the same as those for younger people. These include genetic factors – depression does tend to run in families – and experiencing losses and major life adjustments. In addition, women are at a higher risk of depression, except in late old age. The reasons for this are still subject to debate, some saying it is hormonal, and others emphasising the often complex and sometimes disadvantaged lives women lead. Women often have a heavier burden of caring for others than men, for example, are more likely than men to be widowed (because they live longer), and may experience the financial disadvantage that comes of having had fewer opportunities to work and amass retirement income.

Treatment for depression

Often the most helpful first step if you think you might be depressed is to talk to a GP, who can make sure you have no untreated physical conditions that could contribute to or mimic depression. Generally, the first stage of treatment for milder depression is to try to identify whether there is a specific cause or trigger that could be resolved. If your health is making it harder to carry out activities that you previously valued, for example, finding ways to return to these or modify them might be helpful. This might be a matter, say, of arranging for a neighbour to give you a lift to the shops, or if arthritis no longer permits you to work in your garden the way you used to, it might be possible for you to still tend a smaller flower-bed or direct your energies to other activities. While there is a practical element to this, making adjustments also requires mental and emotional changes, and having somebody to talk to about these matters can be helpful. Counsellors, pastoral and community workers and good friends may all be able to help in this situation.

If your depression is more severe or persistent, you should seek pro-fessional help. Your GP might refer you to a clinical psychologist, who can provide more intensive, structured treatment for depression, or they may prescribe an antidepressant medication. The available evidence suggests that older people respond just as well to antidepressants as younger people, but your doctor may need to consider the interaction of these medications with other medicines you may be taking for physical health conditions. Psychiatrists who specialise in the treatment of older people are best placed to advise on these potential drug interactions.

Anxiety

While feeling nervous about an upcoming challenge or worrying about an issue some of the time is quite normal, anxiety can become a problem when it is linked to unpleasant physical symptoms, such as heart palpita-tions or trembling, and causes people to avoid things they used to do in order to prevent themselves from feeling anxious. If your anxiety becomes so strong that it is out of proportion to the circumstances, it is likely that you have developed an anxiety disorder.

There are a number of different anxiety disorders, depending on the exact symptoms involved. Generalised anxiety disorder is characterised by persistent worry accompanied by physical tension and feeling keyed-up, whereas post-traumatic stress disorder (PTSD) occurs after people have been exposed to a life-threatening experience, and involves symptoms such as re-experiencing the trauma through flashbacks and nightmares, as well as feeling numb and avoiding reminders of the trauma.

For more on the types and symptoms of anxiety disorders, see chapter 40.

Is anxiety different in older people?

The symptoms of anxiety are more common in older age than symptoms of depression, and many older people experience some symptoms of anxiety without necessarily meeting the criteria for a recognised anxiety disorder. Often these problems go undetected and therefore remain untreated. There are a number of possible reasons for this. Older people may be reluctant to talk about their anxiety or worries, feeling they should be able to cope with these on their own. Another problem can be that it is easier for older people to avoid situations that make them anxious. A physical problem, such as a hearing or continence problem, that makes it hard to be in social situations could mask avoidance of these situations due to anxiety. This can be made worse by family members thinking this is a normal part of getting older.

What causes anxiety?

Anxiety, like depression, is caused by many factors. Some people have a personality that predisposes them to worry and become easily upset by events, and this seems to have a strong genetic basis. At any time of life, women are at a greater risk of developing anxiety than men. Sometimes anxiety symptoms are triggered by life experiences. People who are exposed to major traumatic events, such as wars, sexual assault or natural disasters, for example, are at risk of developing PTSD, while the diagnosis of a health problem in ourselves or a family member might trigger severe worry that develops into generalised anxiety disorder.

Physical health problems and the early stages of dementia can increase anxiety, and a careful assessment is needed to ensure that symptoms of anxiety are not missed. Older people are sometimes in caring roles, such as looking after a partner who has developed dementia and needs supervision and assistance. This can be very stressful, and it is well established that carers have high levels of anxiety.

One of the specific forms of anxiety older people can experience is fear of falling. This is thought to be the most common fear of older people, and although having a fall increases the risk of developing a fear of falling, the fear can also develop in people who have never had a fall. It is characterised by acute symptoms of anxiety provoked by the anticipation of walking.

Treatment for anxiety

Often the most helpful first step is to talk to a GP, who can address any physical conditions or medications that can cause anxiety. Sometimes relatively simple strategies, such as learning to relax or finding other ways of coping with stress, can be helpful. More specialised treatments can be provided by clinical psychologists. Doctors can also prescribe medications for anxiety in older people.

For more on treatment for anxiety, see chapter 40.

Dementia and delirium

Dementia is a leading cause of disability in older people, and increasing age is the strongest risk factor for the development of dementia. Dementia refers to a cluster of symptoms with certain characteristics that can have many causes. Alzheimer's disease is the most common cause of dementia, accounting for 50–60 per cent of cases. Among the many other causes of dementia, some may be reversible, so it is important to seek a medical opinion if changes in memory, thinking or personality are noticed either by someone themselves or a relative.

The characteristics of dementia

Dementia is an acquired condition (unlike an intellectual disability, such as Down syndrome, that someone has from birth), and represents a decline from previous functioning. Memory impairment is a core feature of all the common forms of dementia, but other areas are also affected, including personality and other aspects of cognition, such as the ability to recognise objects, and the ability to initiate and plan activities. Some types of dementia, particularly frontal lobe dementia, are associated with 'disinhibition' or a reduced ability to restrain behaviour. Someone who has always been polite and considerate, for example, may become aggressive or sexually inappropriate. These problems give rise to difficulties in carrying out activities of daily living and occupational roles. Finally, a key feature common to all dementias is that they are progressive – that is, the person will show irreversible decline over time.

The characteristics of delirium

Dementia should be distinguished from delirium, which is very common among older people, especially those with poor physical health or who are in hospital. Delirium is an acute disorder characterised by rapid onset, a fluctuating course, and disturbances in thinking and consciousness. It usually disappears when the underlying condition (e.g. a urinary tract infection) is treated. Someone suffering from delirium may feel muddled and experience a reduced awareness of time and where they are. Gaps in memory and hallucinations can also occur in the acute stages of the condition, and can be very distressing for family members to observe.

The causes of delirium usually involve a combination of vulnerability factors, such as an existing diagnosis of dementia, or vision and hearing impairments, together with an acute (short-term) illness, such as a urinary tract infection. Some medications have the potential to cause delirium, and surgery is another common cause. Although delirium is a short-term problem for most people, for about 30 per cent of patients it becomes a prolonged or recurrent condition. Treatment for delirium involves finding the underlying physical cause (e.g. an adverse reaction to medication) and addressing that.

Dementia versus age-related decline

Another important distinction to make is between dementia and normal age-related changes in memory. Many older people find that their memory for certain things, such as the names of people they have just met, sometimes lets them down. This normal age-related decline is often related to reduced attention and taking longer to process and later recall new information. If prompted, they will be able to recognise the name or fact they were trying to recall. In contrast, the loss of memory experienced with Alzheimer's disease, for example, is characterised by rapid forgetting: new information is lost almost as soon as it is heard, and is therefore not stored. This means that no amount of prompting will trigger retrieval of the memory, and this can lead to the repetitive questioning carers can find so trying.

Alzheimer's disease

Alzheimer's disease is the most common cause of dementia, and accounts for 50–60 per cent of all dementias. First described more than 100 years ago by the German psychiatrist Alois Alzheimer, it is characterised by slow onset, progressive decline and prominent memory problems. People with Alzheimer's find it very difficult to learn new material; they also exhibit changes in personality, which friends and family can find very disturbing and hard to understand. In the early stages of the disease, sufferers can have difficulty finding the right word, so that instead of saying 'cup', for example, they might say 'the thing you drink out of'. As the disease progresses, people with Alzheimer's get lost even in familiar places, are no longer able to manage dressing and bathing themselves, and their speech begins to lack meaning. In the later stages (usually within five to eight years of onset), they completely lose the ability to care for themselves and to speak. Perhaps most distressing to relatives is that they can no longer recognise their spouse and children, or sometimes mistake them for somebody else.

Other causes of dementia

Other common causes of dementia include cerebrovascular disease, which accounts for approximately 20 per cent of dementias. Cerebrovascular disease can cause either a major stroke or multiple small strokes, some-times called infarcts, and the resulting dementia is often characterised by prominent problems with motivation and depression. The onset of vascular dementia is often sudden (rather than insidious, as is the case with Alzheimer's), and the progression is through step-by-step decline, rather than the slow, steady decline more typical of Alzheimer's.

Lewy body disease is thought to be the cause of approximately 10 per cent of dementias, and is related to Parkinson's disease. People with Lewy body dementia have some of the physical symptoms of Parkinson's disease, such as stiffness and slow walking, as well as vivid visual hallucinations and fluctuating cognition. Lewy bodies are abnormal accumulations of protein that develop inside nerve cells.

Frontotemporal dementia tends to have an earlier age of onset than most other dementias, and disinhibited behaviour is often a prominent feature. A previously mild and gentle person, for example, might start to be sexually inappropriate or aggressive, causing much embarrassment to family members.

How is dementia diagnosed?

Sometimes people in the early stages of dementia are aware themselves of difficulties with their memory or thinking, but more often it is family members who become concerned and initiate the first appointment with a doctor. The first step in diagnosis is for the doctor to establish a good history of the problem. As one of the diagnostic criteria for dementia is a deterioration in mental state from its previous level, family members are important sources of information and should be involved early on if possible. Medical examination and blood tests are important to exclude any possible reversible causes of the impairment, such as medication.

The next step is to establish the extent and nature of the cognitive impairment, often by a neuropsychologist. This will involve tests to thoroughly assess many aspects of cognition, including memory, attention, mental flexibility, and the ability to plan and solve problems. This kind of assessment is often carried out in a multidisciplinary memory clinic. Often a CT scan or MRI will be performed to determine the extent of the changes in the brain.

Once a diagnosis has been made, it is now the usual practice to convey this information to both the sufferer and their family. It is very difficult to tell somebody they have a progressive disease for which there is no definitive medical treatment, but there are good reasons to do so. It helps people and their families to plan for the future; to make decisions as to whether driving, for example, is still safe; and, importantly, to determine whether medication may be beneficial.

Treatment for dementia

Most of the medications prescribed for people with dementia are choline-sterase inhibitors (e.g. donepezil, rivastigmine and galantamine). While they do not treat the underlying cause of the disease, they have been shown to slow deterioration in people with Alzheimer's disease, which may enable them to be cared for at home for longer than they otherwise would. Local Alzheimer's disease organisations provide the best starting point for information about a range of services that inform and support carers of people with all forms of dementia, as well as groups that help people live with their impairments.

In the early stages of dementia, the sufferer will still be able to enjoy a range of activities, and it is important to maintain social and leisure interests, including physical exercise as far as possible. There is some evidence that involvement in moderate regular physical exercise, such as walking, can slow cognitive decline.

Caring for someone with dementia is very demanding and carers are at heightened risk of depression and anxiety, so if you are a carer it is essential to monitor your own mental health, as well as that of the person you are caring for.

Is there anything we can do to prevent dementia?

To some extent this depends on the type of dementia. The most important risk factors for vascular dementia are potentially preventable, namely untreated high blood pressure and heart disease. With Alzheimer's disease, a number of non-preventable risk factors have been identified, including advancing age and having a specific genetic mutation affecting a protein called ApoE.

On the other hand, a range of preventable risk factors is now also emerging, and they overlap considerably with those related to healthy ageing in general. It has been estimated that the risk of Alzheimer's disease and some other forms of dementia could be substantially reduced by not smoking and increasing physical activity, which would also reduce the risk of diabetes, obesity, high blood pressure and heart disease. Another important factor is mental stimulation – not so much through specific memory-training exercises, but through being involved in a broad range of stimulating activities and learning new skills that use different parts of the brain.

Preparing for decline

One important reason for sharing the diagnosis of dementia with the affected person is so they can begin to make appropriate financial and legal arrangements. Early planning enables them to have a say in how their affairs are handled in the future. The two principal means of doing this are through appointing an enduring power of attorney (EPOA), and making a will (see chapter 41). A power of attorney is a legal document through which we can appoint someone else to act on our behalf with regard to medical, financial or lifestyle decisions when we are no longer in a position to make those choices ourselves.

It is a good idea for someone with dementia to appoint someone to act as their EPOA soon after they are diagnosed. In fact, it is probably a good idea for us all to do this, because we can only appoint an EPOA while we still have the capacity to do so. In this context, *capacity* (sometimes also called *competence*) has a specific meaning: a person has capacity if they understand the issues they are facing, the choices they could make, and the possible consequences of those choices. You should choose to appoint somebody who would make decisions on your behalf based on the values and wishes you would have expressed were you still able.

Once you lose capacity, you cannot make a will, so it is important to make one while you still can. With the help of a lawyer, this document ensures that your wishes with regard to property and assets will be carried out after your death. There is increasing interest in living wills or advance care plans (see chapter 41), legal documents that allow us to convey our decisions about end-of-life care ahead of time. They provide a way for us to communicate our wishes to family, friends and healthcare professionals, and to avoid confusion later on. These decisions might include questions such as whether you want to be resuscitated if your heart stops, whether you want to be on life support, and so on. Although most people believe that advance care plans are a good idea, very few people actually make them, perhaps because it is not always easy to know what treatment choices would actually be available and what we would want in a specific situation.

Grief and loss in later life

Although losses can occur at any time in life, they are almost inevitable in later life, and can take many forms. Grief is the emotional and physical experience we have when we have lost something or somebody. Bereavement is a specific type of loss, namely that of a person, and usually through death. Mourning is the process we go through in adapting to a loss. The losses we experience most intensely are probably those of loved ones, either through death or relationships coming to an end, but other losses can also have a profound effect on us emotionally and practically. Moving from a house we have lived in for many years, losing a job, losing physical abilities and sensory losses can all give rise to grief and necessitate a period of mourning. And because women live longer than men, they are more likely to be widowed and experience grief.

Grief is characterised by a range of feelings most of us can recognise, including deep sadness, often accompanied by crying, and yearning for what has been lost, together with intensely physical feelings of fatigue, aloneness, hollowness in the stomach and tightness in the chest (or you could say heart). At first there is often a feeling of disbelief, especially if the loss has been sudden, which can be followed by numbness or pre-occupation with the loss or the circumstances surrounding it. Gradually the intensity of these feelings reduces, and we can regain involvement in our life, even if it has altered forever.

Sometimes a loss is not just a cause of grief, but may prompt more positive feelings. When death has come at the end of a long illness, for example, family members may feel relief; and when a very controlling partner dies, feelings of liberation would not be out of place. All these feelings are part of normal grief, but people might find them more difficult to express because they feel they should not have these more positive reactions.

People often ask how long is it normal to feel grief, and when the process of mourning is complete. The process of mourning is very individual, depending on the type of loss, its circumstances, and the supports available to the grieving person. In the case of bereavement and relationship break-up, the first year is likely to be extremely difficult as repeated first anniversaries arise (birthday, wedding anniversary, the first Christmas, and so on). Often the poignancy of the feelings diminishes after about two years, but many people say we never completely get over a major loss, even though we may adapt to new circumstances and enjoy life again.

Losses and relationships ending either through death or separation and divorce can also be opportunities for growth and for learning new skills. A woman whose husband always took control of the finances, for example, may gain satisfaction from learning to take responsibility for this aspect of the household. After a period of adjustment, it may be possible to form new relationships or, alternatively, enjoy the freedom of living independently. Indeed, there is evidence that women who live alone have good emotional and physical health and satisfaction with life, provided they have a good network of supportive friends. And the good news is that most women are good at picking up the phone, organising to have a coffee and talking to each other.

Positive ageing

For thousands of years we humans have been interested in how to prolong our lifespan, and over the years people have come up with some quite unusual ideas about how to do so. Early in the twentieth century, for example, a Russian scientist called Elie Metchnikoff came up with the idea that sour milk would neutralise harmful bacteria and have a rejuvenating effect, which led to a brief but international craze for sour milk. Fortunately, nowadays we do not have to go to these lengths in order to live a healthy and happy life. The promotion of healthy or active ageing is now the priority of many governments across the world. Healthy ageing is a holistic concept comprising not just physical health, important though that is, but also cognitive health (an active mind with a well-preserved ability to think and remember), emotional health, and a high level of social engagement and participation.

How do we live an active, healthy life? For a start, it's never too early or too late to make positive lifestyle changes. Secondly, we now view mental and physical health as closely related, so that anything that is good for your heart is also good for your brain. Evidence is accumulating that adopting a healthy lifestyle in the middle years of life is the best way to embark on old age in good health. We all know that maintaining a balanced diet and healthy weight are important for physical health, together with eliminating smoking, keeping alcohol consumption within safe limits, and engaging in moderate levels of physical activity. Sometimes it can be hard to make those changes – and maintain them – but they are our best chance for good cardiovascular fitness and mobility, which, in turn, enable us to lead an active and interesting life. These provide the foundations for good emotional health, which we can define as not merely the absence of depression or anxiety, but positive wellbeing and a sense of satisfaction with life.

Also very important for our satisfaction with life are our relationships with other people, and this is where women may have some real advantages over men. Although older women are more likely to live on their own or be widowed than men, they are also good at making supportive relationships with others, which can compensate for living alone. In a variety of ways, women seem to be skilled at staying socially connected: they tend to initiate social contacts more than men, and use those relationships for support at times of stress and as a springboard for other activities, such as going for a walk or seeing a movie, all of which help support wellbeing.

Women also tend to be involved in a range of volunteering and caring roles, for example with grandchildren, and while these may at times be burdensome, they also help keep women connected to society and their extended family. We are also fortunate to live in an age where technologies can help us keep in touch with friends and family even when we are physically apart. Skype, smartphones and email all provide ways to share news and experiences at the press of a few buttons. Some older women feel daunted by these technological advances, but many local organisations offer classes in making use of these technologies.

Most people adjust well to the challenges that come with ageing, such as retirement, moving to a smaller house and having less physical stamina, and do not experience depression, anxiety or dementia. Some of the negative consequences of ageing have more to do with illnesses than with age itself, and there is much we can do to prevent these illnesses by actively adopting a lifestyle that is physically healthy, mentally stimulating and connected to other people.

Some people do develop depression or anxiety, however, and it is important that these conditions not be dismissed as an understandable part of getting old. On the contrary, they can interfere greatly with the enjoyment of life if not treated. The process of ageing well, however, goes beyond the efforts an individual can make themselves. We all need to work to change our society by challenging the stereotypes of ageing and ensuring that all women have access to the resources they need to build a safe, healthy and happy life.

Afterword

We at the Royal Women's Hospital developed *The Women's Health Book* because we wanted to do a number of things for women.

We wanted to provide you, the reader, with practical, comprehensive information written by women's health experts who work with women every day. This information can be used to improve your health and wellbeing, and the health and wellbeing of the people around you.

This book not only provides you with new information on health problems and staying healthy, but also with the knowledge and confidence you need to question the medical advice you are given until you understand fully what it means, in particular for you as a woman. It offers strategies and alternatives so you can take control of your health and most effectively use the health system when you need to. Talk with your doctor about how the advice he or she is giving affects you as a woman and what alternatives, if any, might suit you better.

We also want this book to give you an appreciation of how social issues impact our health, because the first step in eradicating social issues that affect health is identifying them. Our ability to maintain our health and take action when it is threatened is dependent on so much: our cultural background, our income, where we live and our access to good health care. Our relationships and the support we receive to care for children and take time for ourselves also impact our ability to be healthy and to act when our health is compromised.

In most families, women continue to be the primary carer and to put the needs of their family before their own. We put off going to the doctor or doing exercise because we have to do the shopping or take the kids to basketball. To enjoy a long, healthy life, we need to prioritise our own health and encourage other women to do the same. We definitely don't want to teach our children that a woman's health and wellbeing comes after everyone else's! As Dale Fisher, the former chief executive of the Women's and the woman behind the concept of this book, used to say, 'It's like the safety advice you are given when you fly: you need to put on your own oxygen mask before you can help others.'

I must admit, though, that we also developed this book because we wanted *you* to do things for us! Please start talking about women's health. Discuss issues such as mental health, endometriosis, pelvic pain and heavy menstrual bleeding so that we can demystify and destigmatise them. Talk to your teenagers, both daughters and sons, about sex and contraception. Educate those who don't understand that violence against women is a health as well as a criminal issue. Advocate for equal pay to improve financial stability for women. Share your knowledge of the inequities in medical research and our health system with friends and family. Be a vocal advocate for women's hospitals and for gender-specific research or care conducted anywhere. Write to your local hospital, or get involved with their community participation efforts, and hold them to account to consider sex and gender when they provide care. Without a concerted effort to achieve gender equity in health, future generations of women will continue to receive health care designed for men. And that's not good for women *or* men.

You can let us know what other health topics you would like to know more about by emailing us at womensbook@thewomens.org.au.

Finally, I want to say thank you on behalf of the Royal Women's Hospital Foundation. Some of the proceeds from this book will support the Royal Women's Hospital's comprehensive research program, which is improving the health and wellbeing of women and newborns everywhere.

Sarah L. White, PhD
Director, Royal Women's Hospital Foundation

Acknowledgements

A book like this is a very large and complex team effort. On behalf of the Royal Women's Hospital Foundation, I would like to acknowledge and sincerely thank the following people for their role in taking this book from idea to reality.

First, thanks to Ms Dale Fisher, the chief executive of the Women's from 2004 to 2013, who recognised the need for a book like this, and had the drive and vision to make it happen.

Thanks, too, to the members of the Editorial Group who guided the production of the book so expertly: Associate Professor Leslie Reti, Ms Dale Fisher, Professor Martha Hickey, Professor Fiona Judd, Professor Suzanne Garland, Dr Jennifer Marino, Associate Professor John McBain, Dr Ines Rio, Ms Maureen Johnson, Miss Orla McNally, Ms Tanya Maloney, Dr Sarah White and Dr Jan Davies. Associate Professor Leslie Reti, Chair of the Women's Health Book Editorial Group, must be singled out for providing leadership and wisdom throughout the entire process of developing content and working with writers and editors. Ms Maureen Johnson and Dr Ines Rio are due special thanks for responding to so many requests for more information. Dr Jan Davies, who managed the production of the book on behalf of the Women's, also deserves a special mention.

The writers of the content, the clinicians from the Royal Women's Hospital and other experts gave so generously of their time and shared their expertise to provide this resource for women. Many others, both clinicians and non-clinicians, read drafts of chapters and provided valuable comments to help make the book accessible to all.

Hundreds of women shared their views with us about what they thought should be in the book in surveys, consultation groups, individual meetings and a national online forum. I thank them for helping us and hope this book reflects their ideas.

Clare Forster at Curtis Brown introduced us to Random House Australia, and provided advice and guidance at key times.

The Random House Australia team was passionate about the book from the outset. Thanks are especially due to Ali Urquhart, publisher;

Brett Osmond, marketing and publicity director; and Nikki Christer, publishing director, for their enthusiastic support throughout the process.

Managing editors Brooke Clark and Anne Rogan, Random House editor Catherine Hill and copyeditor Nicola Young used their great skills to give the chapters one voice, and make complex health information simple and accessible. They were continually positive, encouraging and helpful.

Maureen Johnson and Marino Norio from the Women's Consumer Health Information team helped to source the illustrations in the book. To Beth Croce and Bill Reid for beautiful and sensitive medical illustrations, and Carmel Reilly for the non-medical illustrations, thank you.

There is always a dedicated administrative and project group behind the scenes and in the wings of every big endeavour. This group at the Women's includes: Tanya Maloney, a super maternity-leave cover executive sponsor, who provided support to keep the process on track; Karen Cusack, the Women's legal counsel, who provided expert advice; Tanya Carter, communications manager, and Dilys Luciani, volunteer coordinator, who helped with consumer consultations; Nathalie Kemp, marketing manager, who helped with marketing concepts; Melissa Hegedis from the Women's Foundation, for managing all that paperwork; and Lauren Calleja, Cathy Sandlant, Suzanne Henty and their colleagues in the Women's Finance Department, for answering many questions.

Sarah L. White PhD
Director, Royal Women's Hospital Foundation

Resources

The following organisations and websites provide information and support that are focused on women's needs and on the needs of specific groups of women. The listings will give you a starting point if you would like more information on a particular area covered by the book. All listings are alphabetical within chapters.

General women's health information and support services

Australian Women's Health Network (AWHN)
www.awhn.org.au
AWHN is the peak organisation for women's health in Australia and is the umbrella organisation for women's health services in each state and territory.

Visit www.awhn.org.au, choose 'Women's Health Services' and select your state or territory to find a listing and contact details for your local service.

Each organisation on the website supports women's health and well-being, offering services that may include health information, community programs, women's groups and counselling, as well as access and referrals to free and low-cost women's health services.

Better Health Channel
www.betterhealth.vic.gov.au
The Better Health Channel provides health and medical information that is quality-assured, reliable, up-to-date, easy to understand, regularly reviewed and locally relevant. It does not have any advertising or sponsorship and is fully funded by the state government of Victoria. It has an A-Z of conditions and provides typical treatment protocols in Australia.

health*insite*
www.healthinsite.gov.au
This is an internet gateway that links you to a wide range of up-to-date and reliable information on all areas of health and wellbeing for everyone in Australia – including information on women's health, parenting, living with a disability and ageing. You'll also find links to many health services in your state or territory.

Jean Hailes for Women's Health
www.jeanhailes.org.au
Jean Hailes for Women's Health is a national not-for-profit organisation providing a range of health services and information for women across Australia. There are separate Jean Hailes websites with easy-to-understand information on ageing well, bone health, menopause and early menopause, endometriosis, PCOS and general women's health.

Royal Australian and New Zealand College of Obstetricians and Gynaecologists
www.ranzcog.edu.au/womens-health/online-patient-information
The Royal Australian and New Zealand College of Obstetricians and Gynaecologists (RANZCOG) trains and accredits doctors in the specialties of obstetrics and gynaecology in Australia and New Zealand. They have a section on their website for patient information.

The Royal Women's Hospital
www.thewomens.org.au/health-information
The Royal Women's Hospital, Melbourne, was one of the first Australian hospitals to be given the World Health Organization designation of a Health Promoting Hospital and provides information on a wide range of women's health issues in English and other community languages. Women from anywhere in Australia can access this information online. The Women's also publishes downloadable fact sheets that are a useful reference tool. Health information areas include: breast health and feeding, fertility, incontinence and prolapse, menopause, mental health, pregnancy and birth, miscarriage and pregnancy loss, periods, sex and sexuality, unplanned pregnancy and abortion, staying well, sexual assault and violence against women, vulva and vagina health, and women's cancers.

Aboriginal and Torres Strait Islander women

National Aboriginal Community Controlled Health Organisation (NACCHO)
www.naccho.org.au
NACCHO is the national peak body representing Aboriginal Community Controlled Health Services (ACCHS) across the country. Choose 'About Us' from the Home page and then choose 'Affiliates' from the dropdown menu. This will give you a list of ACCHS in each state and territory, where you can find out more about local programs and services.

Deaf, hearing-impaired or speech-impaired women

National Relay Service
www.relayservice.gov.au
If you are deaf or hearing- or speech-impaired, you can call any health services through the National Relay Service using the internet, a telephone typewriter (TTY), Auslan or a regular phone (if you have a speech impairment).

TTY users call 1800 555 677 to reach a service that has a free 1800 number, or 133 677 to call any other number.

Speak and Listen users call 1800 555 727 to reach a service with a free 1800 number, or call 1300 555 727 to call any other number.

There are a number of other options available for making calls – there is more information about them on the Relay Service website.

Financial health

MoneySmart
www.moneysmart.gov.au
Looking after your finances is an important part of looking after your health. MoneySmart website is run by the Australian Securities and Investments Commission (ASIC) to help ordinary Australians make smart choices about their personal finances – including useful tips, plans and calculators to help at different life stages and when your finances are under stress. The site is for all Australians: young or old, rich or poor, investing or paying off debt, and includes specific information for women and Aboriginal and Torres Strait Islander people.

Health interpreters

Translating and Interpreting Service (TIS)
13 14 50
www.tisnational.gov.au
If English is not your first language, you can call TIS and tell them the number of another service that you want to call (such as a women's health service or your local hospital). TIS will then call the number and talk to the service and to you through an interpreter on the same line. This service is free.

If you need an interpreter to attend a doctor's appointment or you need health information translated into a language other than English, your healthcare professional can usually organise this for you at no cost. Interpreters need to be booked in advance, so you need to ask for one when you book your appointment.

Lesbian, bisexual and transgender women

National LGBTI Health Alliance
www.lgbthealth.org.au
The National LGBTI Health Alliance is the peak health body for organisations that provide health-related programs, services and research for LGBTI people. Choose 'visit our member organisations' from the home page to find member organisations in your state and territory that offer health information, support and counselling services.

Women from non-English-speaking backgrounds

Multicultural Women's Health Australia program
1800 656 421 (free call)
www.mcwh.com.au/mwha/mwha.php
This program is run by the Multicultural Centre for Women's Health, a national, community-based organisation that works to improve the health of immigrant and refugee women around Australia. Visit the website or call the free 1800 number to be put in touch with bilingual health educators or an interpreter, to find health information in your language, or to be referred to multicultural and women's health organisations in your state or territory.

My Language
www.mylanguage.gov.au
My Language is a joint partnership between the State & Territory Libraries. The website aims to provide a hub where public libraries and culturally and linguistically different (CALD) communities can actively share information resources and programs to support CALD communities. Translated information includes health, legal, education, settlement and libraries.

Women with a disability

Women With Disabilities Australia (WWDA)
www.wwda.org.au
WWDA is the peak organisation for women in Australia with all types of disabilities. The website includes an Information and Referral Directory (look under Service Directory on the Contents page) to help women with disabilities find information about services and organisations that can assist them.

1 Why women's health matters

Australian Human Rights Commission
www.humanrights.gov.au/our-work/sex-discrimination
The 'Our Work' section of the Australian Human Rights Commission website has guides describing sex discrimination and sexual harassment and how to recognise and address them. There is also information on pregnancy discrimination, and articles on legislative and advocacy work being undertaken to ensure economic security for women and balancing paid work and family responsibilities.

2 Staying healthy

All About Acne
www.acne.org.au
This website is an independent, up-to-date site providing practical, evidence-based information from health professionals. There is also information especially for teens and carers of teens.

Australian Hearing
www.hearing.com.au

This is an Australian government agency providing hearing services to help people manage their hearing impairment. They provide a full range of hearing services for children and young people up to the age of 26 and eligible adults.

Better Health Channel
www.betterhealth.vic.gov.au

The Better Health Channel provides health and medical information that is quality-assured, reliable, up-to-date, easy to understand, regularly reviewed and locally relevant. It does not have any advertising or sponsorship and is fully funded by the state government of Victoria. It has an A-Z of conditions and provides typical treatment protocols in Australia.

beyondblue
www.beyondblue.org.au

This organisation has resources for people who experience depression and anxiety, their partners, family and friends, and for health professionals who work in mental health. You can read their information online, download it or order printed copies.

Cancer Australia
www.canceraustralia.gov.au

This organisation has excellent information about different cancer types on its website. It also provides an Australian-wide directory of gynaecological oncology services.

Dementia Care Australia (DCA)
www.dementiacareaustralia.com

DCA is an independent information and education organisation specialising in supporting both people with dementia and their carers, whether they are family members, professional carers, employers or friends.

Diabetes Australia
www.diabetesaustralia.com.au

This organisation helps people affected by or at risk of diabetes. On their website you can access information on different types of diabetes, the diagnosis and treatment of diabetes, diabetes and pregnancy, diet and other relevant topics.

health*insite*
www.healthinsite.gov.au
For falls prevention, see this non-commercial, government-funded health information service that provides easy access to reliable, quality, evidence-based information from trusted sources. Go to their home page and enter 'falls' into the search bar.

Healthy Teeth
www.healthyteeth.org
This is a Canadian website providing information on oral care for people of all ages.

Heart Foundation
www.heartfoundation.org.au
This is a charity established to reduce premature death and suffering from heart, stroke and blood vessel disease. On their website you will find information including how to minimise the risk of cardiovascular disease, the warning signs of heart attack and how to get treatment.

Immunise Australia
1800 671 811
www.immunise.health.gov.au
This government program aims to increase national immunisation rates by funding free vaccination programs, administering the Australian Childhood Immunisation register and communicating information about immunisation to the general public and health professionals.

Kidney Health Australia
www.kidney.org.au
This is a not-for-profit organisation that aims to improve kidney health outcomes for people with kidney and urinary tract diseases, their families and carers. It funds medical research and provides health programs and services, including a network of education, care and support for patients, their families and carers.

myGov
www.australia.gov.au/topics/health-and-safety
This Australian government website has excellent health and safety information, as well as valuable information on alcohol and drugs, their use and misuse and minimising risk.
www.australia.gov.au/topics/health-and-safety/drug-and-alcohol-use

Oral Health Promotion Clearinghouse
www.adelaide.edu.au/oral-health-promotion
This is a national online resource that promotes effective strategies to improve the oral health of Australians.

Osteoporosis Australia
www.osteoporosis.org.au
Osteoporosis Australia has information on risk factors, diagnosis, treatment, and calcium, vitamin D and exercise.

Quitnow
13 7848
www.quitnow.gov.au
This Australian government website has information, links and resources to help you quit smoking.

Skin Cancer Foundation
www.skincancer.org
This is an international organisation devoted solely to education, prevention, early detection and prompt treatment of the world's most common cancer.

Vision Australia
1300 84 74 66
www.visionaustralia.org
Vision Australia is a national provider of blindness and low vision services. It is a not-for-profit organisation providing services and support for clients through centres in NSW, ACT, Queensland and Victoria. Clinics are also held in other locations and there are outreach services to the Northern Territory and Tasmania.

3 Getting the most out of your health consultation

The ABC Health and Wellbeing Consumer Guide
www.abc.net.au/health/consumerguides/stories/2006/06/19/1837215.
htm
'How to Choose a GP' is a useful guide to choosing the right doctor for you.

ADOLESCENTS
4 Adolescence and puberty

Better Health Channel
www.betterhealth.vic.gov.au
The Better Health Channel provides health and medical information that is quality-assured, reliable, up-to-date, easy to understand, regularly reviewed and locally relevant. It does not have any advertising or sponsorship and is fully funded by the state government of Victoria. It has some useful and clear information on teenage health:
www.betterhealth.vic.gov.au/bhcv2/bhcarticles.nsf/pages/Teenage_health

Center for Young Women's Health
www.youngwomenshealth.org
This is a website developed by Boston Children's Hospital in the USA but aimed at teenage girls from all around the world, with a variety of information addressing normal and abnormal development and other aspects of young women's health.

likeitis
www.likeitis.org.au
This is an Australian website designed for teenagers that contains information about puberty, sex, contraception, teenage pregnancy and periods.

The Mysterious Workings of the Adolescent Brain
www.brainneurofeedback.com/project/the-adolescent-brain-2
This is a film of a TED talk given by Professor Sarah-Jayne Blakemore of the Institute of Cognitive Neuroscience, University of London in 2012, in which she talks about how the brains of this age group function.

raising children network
www.raisingchildren.net.au
This site is described as the 'complete Australian resource for parenting newborns to teens'. The information for teens, which covers subjects such as behaviour, communicating, development, entertainment, school and education, as well as health and wellbeing, is reviewed by experts.

Sexual Health and Family Planning Australia (SH&FPA)
www.shfpa.org.au
SH&FPA is the national peak body for the family planning organisations that provide community education programs, and a range of sexual and reproductive health clinical services, including Pap tests and vaccinations, contraception and family planning services, and STI diagnosis and treatment. Each state has a family planning website with information regarding sexual and contraceptive health. Find the clinic nearest you on their national website at www.shfpa.org.au/find-clinic.

Somazone
www.somazone.com.au
An Australian youth service aimed at 14–18 year olds with information on youth mental health, depression, teenage pregnancy, sexuality, relationships, bullying, abuse, drugs and alcohol. On Somazone, young people can ask questions online, get free youth health advice, find youth services and share personal stories anonymously.

5 Food, physical activity and feeling good

Better Health Channel
www.betterhealth.vic.gov.au
The Better Health Channel provides health and medical information that is quality-assured, reliable, up-to-date, easy to understand, regularly reviewed and locally relevant. It does not have any advertising or sponsorship and is fully funded by the state government of Victoria. It has comprehensive sections on nutrition and physical activity:
www.betterhealth.vic.gov.au/bhcv2/bhcarticles.nsf/pages/hl_foodnutrition?open
www.betterhealth.vic.gov.au/bhcv2/bhcarticles.nsf/pages/hl_physicalactivity?open

Girls Health
www.girlshealth.gov
The shoutline of this website is 'Be healthy. Be happy. Be you. Beautiful'. It provides information for girls aged 10 to 16 and has sections on periods, bullying, body image, living with chronic illnesses, fitness and nutrition.

Kidshealth
www.kidshealth.org
This is an excellent website for both parents and kids with lots of advice on staying healthy and the right diet and fitness plans to follow. www.kidshealth.org/teen/food_fitness

6 Periods

Better Health Channel
www.betterhealth.vic.gov.au
The Better Health Channel provides health and medical information that is quality-assured, reliable, up-to-date, easy to understand, regularly reviewed and locally relevant. It does not have any advertising or sponsorship and is fully funded by the state government of Victoria. It has some useful and clear information on menstruation: www.betterhealth.vic.gov. au/bhcv2/bhcarticles.nsf/pages/Menstrual_cycle

Jean Hailes for Women's Health
www.jeanhailes.org.au
Jean Hailes for Women's Health is a national not-for-profit organisation providing a range of health services and information for women across Australia. Their website has a useful page on the menstrual cycle: www.healthforwomen.org.au/health-issues/92-understanding-your-menstrual-cycle

The Royal Women's Hospital
www.thewomens.org.au/health-information
The Royal Women's Hospital, Melbourne, was one of the first Australian hospitals to be given the World Health Organization designation of a Health Promoting Hospital and provides information on a wide range of women's health issues in English and other community languages. Women from anywhere in Australia can access this information online. The Women's also publishes downloadable fact sheets that are a useful reference tool. The health information covered includes periods.

7 Sexuality in adolescents

Kids Helpline
1800 55 1800 (free call)
www.kidshelp.com.au
This is a free, private and confidential telephone and online counselling service specifically for young people aged between 5 and 25.

likeitis
www.likeitis.org.au
This is an Australian website designed for teenagers that contains information about puberty, sex, contraception, teenage pregnancy and periods.

Love: the Good, the Bad and the Ugly
www.lovegoodbadugly.com
This site has lots of sound information for young people about all aspects of romantic relationships: meeting partners, breaking up, sex, abuse in relationships and advice on who you can talk to if you need help or support with a relationship.

Parentline
1300 30 1300
www.parentline.com.au
Parentline has offices in each state. It offers confidential telephone counselling to parents and carers of children aged from birth to eighteen years regarding issues that impact on parenting and relationships.

ReachOut
www.reachout.com
This website aimed at young people has useful information and advice about sexuality and personal identity, as well as about sex and relationships. It also has forums and emergency help and information phone and chat support.

Somazone
www.somazone.com.au
An Australian youth service aimed at 14–18 year olds with information on youth mental health, depression, teenage pregnancy, sexuality, relationships, bullying, abuse, drugs and alcohol. On Somazone, young people can ask questions online, get free youth health advice, find youth services, and share personal stories anonymously.

8 Genital irritations and infections

Let Them Know
www.letthemknow.org.au
This website was developed to help people who have been diagnosed with
an STI to (anonymously) inform their previous partners that they might
also be at risk.

Sexual Health and Family Planning Australia (SH&FPA)
www.shfpa.org.au
SH&FPA is the national peak body for the family planning organisations that provide community education programs, and a range of sexual
and reproductive health clinical services, including Pap tests and vaccinations, contraception and family planning services, and STI diagnosis
and treatment. Each state has a family planning website with information
regarding sexual and contraceptive health. Find the clinic nearest you on
their national website at www.shfpa.org.au/find-clinic.

The Royal Women's Hospital
www.thewomens.org.au/health-information
The Royal Women's Hospital, Melbourne, was one of the first Australian
hospitals to be given the World Health Organization designation of a
Health Promoting Hospital and provides information on a wide range
of women's health issues in English and other community languages.
Women from anywhere in Australia can access this information online.
The Women's also publishes downloadable fact sheets that are a useful
reference tool. The health information covered includes vulva and vagina
health.

Somazone
www.somazone.com.au
An Australian youth service aimed at 14–18 year olds with information
on youth mental health, depression, teenage pregnancy, sexuality, genital
health, relationships, bullying, abuse, drugs and alcohol. On Somazone,
young people can ask questions online, get free youth health advice, find
youth services, and share personal stories anonymously.

9 Plastic surgery in adolescence

Australasian Foundation for Plastic Surgery
www.plasticsurgeryfoundation.org.au
This is a not-for-profit organisation. Its website provides reliable and accurate information on cosmetic and reconstructive surgery, including comprehensive information on procedures and a range of other useful patient resources.
www.plasticsurgeryfoundation.org.au/patient-information/procedures/

Better Health Channel
www.betterhealth.vic.gov.au
The Better Health Channel provides health and medical information that is quality-assured, reliable, up-to-date, easy to understand, regularly reviewed and locally relevant. It does not have any advertising or sponsorship and is fully funded by the state government of Victoria. It devotes several pages to surgery of various kinds, including breast and cosmetic.

10 Mental health in adolescence

The Butterfly Foundation
www.thebutterflyfoundation.org.au
This is Australia's peak body for eating disorders. It provides support and education for people suffering from eating disorders and negative body image issues, and their families.

Headspace
www.headspace.org.au
This organisation is part of the Young Mental Health Initiative program. On their website you can locate a centre near you, or access online and telephone mental health counselling.

Kids Helpline
1800 55 1800 (free call)
www.kidshelp.com.au
This is a free, private and confidential telephone and online counselling service specifically for young people aged between 5 and 25.

ReachOut
www.reachout.com
This website aimed at young people has useful information and advice on lots of aspects of mental health. It also has forums and emergency help and information phone and chat support.

Youth beyondblue
www.youthbeyondblue.com
Youth beyondblue has a great deal of invaluable information for young people on depression and anxiety. Its adult website also has a useful page to visit:
www.beyondblue.org.au/resources/for-me/young-people

11 Drugs and alcohol

If you are in a crisis situation or need immediate medical assistance, call 000 or call DirectLine for 24/7 counselling and support on 1800 888 236 (free call).

Australian Drug Foundation (ADF)
1300 85 85 84
www.druginfo.adf.org.au
The ADF provides comprehensive information about alcohol and other drugs, and also about the prevention of harm related to drug use. Their resources include advice on talking to children about alcohol and other drugs, and information on the short- and long-term effects of particular drugs. National and state contacts for help and support are also available on the ADF website. For support (all states), visit:
www.druginfo.adf.org.au/contact-numbers/help-and-support

Australian Government National Drugs Campaign
www.health.gov.au/internet/drugs/publishing.nsf/content/youth
This government site has comprehensive information on drug use. It also has a free iPhone app (which is also available on iPod touch and iPads) that can provide information and support decisions not to use. It features GPS functionality to help find support services based on location.

Counselling Online
1800 888 236 (free call)
www.counsellingonline.org.au
This is a service on which you can communicate with a professional counsellor about an alcohol- or drug-related concern, online or on the phone. It is open 24 hours a day, seven days a week.

Family Drug Support
1300 368 186 (24-hour service)
www.fds.org.au
This is a volunteer organisation that assists and supports families dealing with drug and alcohol issues.

Girls Health
www.girlshealth.gov
The shoutline of this website is 'Be healthy. Be happy. Be you. Beautiful'. It has a section on drugs, alcohol and smoking:
www.girlshealth.gov/substance/index.html

Lifeline
13 11 14 (24-hour service)
www.lifeline.org.au
Lifeline provides crisis support and suicide prevention services, 24 hours a day, 7 days a week with confidential telephone counselling.

Quitnow
13 7848
www.quitnow.gov.au
This is an Australian government website that has information, links and resources to help you to quit smoking.

ReachOut
www.reachout.com
This website aimed at young people has useful information and support if you are concerned about your drinking, or need advice and support or facts about drug-taking.

The Royal Women's Hospital
www.thewomens.org.au/health-information
The Royal Women's Hospital, Melbourne, was one of the first Australian hospitals to be given the World Health Organization designation of a Health Promoting Hospital and provides information on a wide range of women's health issues in English and other community languages. Women from anywhere in Australia can access this information online. The Women's also publishes downloadable fact sheets that are a useful reference tool. The health information covered includes pregnancy, drugs and alcohol.

Somazone
www.somazone.com.au
An Australian youth service aimed at 14–18 year olds with information on youth mental health, depression, teenage pregnancy, sexuality, relationships, bullying, abuse, drugs and alcohol. On Somazone, young people can ask questions online, get free youth health advice, find youth services, and share personal stories anonymously.

12 Bullying

Australian Psychological Society
www.psychology.org.au/publications/tip_sheets/bullying
The society has tip sheets for parents including one on bullying.

Bullying. No Way!
www.bullyingnoway.com.au
This site was developed by the Safe and Supportive School Communities (SSSC) Project, which includes representatives from all Australian state, territory and federal education departments as well as national Catholic and independent schooling representatives. It provides information for parents, young children, students and teachers.

Bursting the Bubble
www.burstingthebubble.com
A website with information for young people experiencing family violence.

Cybersmart
www.cybersmart.gov.au
The site provides information and education to empower children to be safe online. It is part of the Australian government's commitment to cyber

safety, and is specifically designed for children, young people, parents, teachers and library staff.

Headspace
www.headspace.org.au
This website is part of the Young Mental Health Initiative program. On their website you can locate a centre near you, or access online and telephone mental health counselling.

Kids Helpline
1800 55 1800 (free call)
www.kidshelp.com.au
This is a free, private and confidential, telephone and online counselling service specifically for young people aged between 5 and 25.

Lifeline
13 11 14 (24-hour service)
www.lifeline.org.au
Lifeline provides crisis support and suicide prevention services as well as confidential telephone counselling.

Parentline
www.parentline.com.au
Parentline has offices in each state. It offers telephone confidential counselling to parents and carers of children aged from birth to eighteen years regarding issues that impact on parenting and relationships.

YOUNG WOMEN
13 Food and nutrition for young women

Diabetes Australia
www.diabetesaustralia.com.au
The national body for people affected by all types of diabetes and those at risk of it.

Dietitians Association of Australia (DAA)
www.daa.asn.au
The DAA site is a good place to look for nutrition tips or to find a dietician for advice.

Glycemic Index
www.glycemicindex.com
GI is a not-for-profit organisation supported by the University of Sydney and the Juvenile Diabetes Research Foundation, Australia. Their website has information, newsletters, resources and fact sheets on GI.

Heart Foundation
www.heartfoundation.org.au
For information on heart disease and healthy eating, including fats and cholesterol, food labels, BMI calculator and more, see their website.

14 Healthy weight management for young women

Australian Government Department of Health
www.health.gov.au
The National Physical Activity Guidelines for Australians outline the minimum level of physical activity required to gain a health benefit. They also provide ideas for incorporating incidental physical activity into everyday life. The guidelines can be found in the 'Education and Prevention' pages of the 'For Consumers' section under the 'Nutrition and Physical Activity' heading.

Heart Foundation
www.heartfoundation.org.au/Walking
The Heart Foundation runs walking groups. Find your nearest group on their website.

If Not Dieting Weight Management and Eating Behaviour Clinic
www.ifnotdieting.com.au/
A site to provide health and support for people who want to achieve and maintain a healthy weight without being deprived of food or quality of life. It has useful 'non-hungry' eating advice.

LocalFitness
www.localfitness.com.au
To find your local gym or swimming pool you can use this website. Also, check your local community health centre, library notice board and local paper for walking and exercise groups.

15 Periods – normal and not so normal

Jean Hailes for Women's Health
www.jeanhailes.org.au
Jean Hailes for Women's Health is a national not-for-profit organisation providing a range of health services and information for women across Australia. It has a separate website dedicated to endometriosis: www.endometriosis.org.au

The Royal Women's Hospital
www.thewomens.org.au/health-information
The Royal Women's Hospital, Melbourne, was one of the first Australian hospitals to be given the World Health Organization designation of a Health Promoting Hospital and provides information on a wide range of women's health issues in English and other community languages. Women from anywhere in Australia can access this information online. The Women's also publishes downloadable fact sheets that are a useful reference tool. The health information covers endometriosis, hysterectomies and period problems.

16 Contraception

Marie Stopes International Australia
1800 003 707 (free call)
www.mariestopes.org.au
Dr Marie provides help and advice on sexual and reproductive healthcare via their centres in the ACT, New South Wales, Queensland and Western Australia, as well as on their website (above), at www.contraceptioninfo. com.au and on their free, 24-hour phone line.

The Royal Women's Hospital
www.thewomens.org.au/health-information
The Royal Women's Hospital, Melbourne, was one of the first Australian hospitals to be given the World Health Organization designation of a Health Promoting Hospital and provides information on a wide range of women's health issues in English and other community languages. Women from anywhere in Australia can access this information online. The Women's also publishes downloadable fact sheets that are a useful reference tool, including ones on contraceptive choices.

Sexual Health and Family Planning Australia (SH&FPA)
www.shfpa.org.au
SH&FPA is the national peak body for the family planning organisations that provide community education programs, and a range of sexual and reproductive health clinical services, including Pap tests and vaccinations, contraception and family planning services, and STI diagnosis and treatment. Each state has a family planning website with information regarding sexual and contraceptive health. Find the clinic nearest you on their national website.

Their website also has a useful questionnaire, My Contraception Tool. The short version takes about 5 minutes to complete and the long version, which has some questions about your medical history, about 15 minutes. www.fpa.org.uk/helpandadvice/contraception

17 Pregnancy

health*insite*
www.healthinsite.gov.au
This is an internet gateway that links you to a wide range of up-to-date and reliable information on all areas of health and wellbeing for everyone in Australia. It has a page on dental health and pregnancy: www.healthinsite.gov.au/topics/Dental_Health_and_Pregnancy

Royal College of Obstetricians and Gynaecologists
www.ranzcog.edu.au
This website has some specially prepared patient information (under 'Women's Health' on the homepage) as well as guidelines for pregnancy care.

The Royal Women's Hospital
www.thewomens.org.au/health-information
The Royal Women's Hospital, Melbourne, was one of the first Australian hospitals to be given the World Health Organization designation of a Health Promoting Hospital and provides information on a wide range of women's health issues in English and other community languages. Women from anywhere in Australia can access this information online. The Women's also publishes downloadable fact sheets that are a useful reference tool. The health information available covers preparing for pregnancy and parenting, early pregnancy issues, and enjoying a healthy pregnancy.

18 Physical activity during and after pregnancy

Better Health Channel
www.betterhealth.vic.gov.au
The Better Health Channel provides health and medical information that is quality-assured, reliable, up-to-date, easy to understand, regularly reviewed and locally relevant. It does not have any advertising or sponsorship and is fully funded by the state government of Victoria. It has a page on exercising when pregnant:
www.betterhealth.vic.gov.au/bhcv2/bhcarticles.nsf/pages/Pregnancy_and_exercise

Bicycle Network
www.bicyclenetwork.com.au
This site provides useful advice about riding during pregnancy:
www.bicyclenetwork.com.au/general/bikes-and-riding/90457

Pelvic Floor First
www.pelvicfloorfirst.org.au
This website was developed by the Continence Foundation of Australia under the Australian Government's National Continence Program. It has lots of useful information and exercises on taking care of your pelvic floor muscles during and after pregnancy.

The Royal Women's Hospital
www.thewomens.org.au/health-information
The Royal Women's Hospital, Melbourne, was one of the first Australian hospitals to be given the World Health Organization designation of a Health Promoting Hospital and provides information on a wide range of women's health issues in English and other community languages. Women from anywhere in Australia can access this information online. The Women's also publishes downloadable fact sheets, including one on how to do pelvic floor exercises.

19 Having a baby

The Royal Women's Hospital
www.thewomens.org.au/health-information
The Royal Women's Hospital, Melbourne, was one of the first Australian hospitals to be given the World Health Organization designation of a Health Promoting Hospital and provides information on a wide range of women's health issues in English and other community languages. Women from anywhere in Australia can access this information online. The Women's publishes downloadable fact sheets, including ones on labour and birth.

20 Bleeding, miscarriage and stillbirth

The Royal Women's Hospital
www.thewomens.org.au/health-information
The Women's publishes downloadable fact sheets on pain and bleeding in early pregnancy, miscarriage and pregnancy loss.

Sands Australia
1300 0 Sands
www.sands.org.au
Sands Australia is a not-for-profit organisation that provides support and information for families following the death of a baby through miscarriage, stillbirth, newborn death or termination for medical purposes.

21 Motherhood and connecting with your baby

There are organisations throughout Australia – both in rural and metropolitan areas – that provide support and services for new parents and babies. Your GP or maternal and child health nurse will be able to offer you advice and if needed, refer you to specialist services.

Australian Association for Infant Mental Health
www.aaimhi.org
This organisation put out a paper in 2006 called 'Responding to babies' cues', which is available on their website:
www.aaimhi.org/inewsfiles/Position%20Paper%202.pdf

Raising Children Network
www.raisingchildren.net.au
This site is described as the 'complete Australian resource for parenting newborns to teens'. The site has information on mother–infant attachment and how attachment affects life-long social and emotional development.

22 Mental health and pregnancy

Beyondblue
www.beyondblue.org.au
Beyondblue has resources for the people who experience depression and anxiety, their partners, family and friends, and for health professionals who work in mental health. You can read them online, download them or order printed copies. They have an invaluable section on mental health and pregnancy:
www.beyondblue.org.au/the-facts/pregnancy-and-early-parenthood

Black Dog Institute
www.blackdoginstitute.org.au
The institute has information on the diagnosis, treatment and prevention of mood disorders such as depression and bipolar disorder, as well as general information on depression in and after pregnancy: www.blackdog institute.org.au/public/depression/inpregnancypostnatal/babyblues.cfm

Lifeline
13 11 14 (24-hour service)
www.lifeline.org.au
Lifeline provides crisis support and suicide prevention services. The organisation also has an advice line for confidential telephone counselling.

Post and Antenatal Depression Association (PANDA)
1300 726 306
www.panda.org.au
PANDA provides telephone support and information service for women with postnatal depression and their families.

23 Abortion and unplanned pregnancy

The Royal Women's Hospital
www.thewomens.org.au/health-information
The Royal Women's Hospital, Melbourne, was one of the first Australian hospitals to be given the World Health Organization designation of a Health Promoting Hospital and provides information on a wide range of women's health issues in English and other community languages. Women from anywhere in Australia can access this information online. The Women's also publishes downloadable fact sheets that are a useful reference tool. The health information includes an online decision-making guide for unplanned pregnancy as well as other information on unplanned pregnancies.

Sexual Health and Family Planning Australia (SH&FPA)
www.shfpa.org.au
SH&FPA is the national peak body for the family planning organisations that provide community education programs, and a range of sexual and reproductive health clinical services, including Pap tests and vaccinations, contraception and family planning services, and STI diagnosis and treatment. Each state has a family planning website with information regarding sexual and contraceptive health. Find the clinic nearest you on their national website at www.shfpa.org.au/find-clinic.

24 When pregnancy isn't happening

There are many private IVF clinics in Australia and New Zealand. Your GP can refer you to a reputable clinic in a convenient location for you.

Access Australia
www.access.org.au
A national, consumer-controlled organisation providing information, support and referrals for women and men who experience difficulties conceiving.

Dietitians Association of Australia
www.daa.asn.au
For an individualised assessment and advice about diet and lifestyle for PCOS, consult an accredited practising dietician through this website.

The Fertility Society of Australia
www.fertilitysociety.com.au
The Fertility Society Australia is the peak body representing health professionals, scientists and consumers in reproductive medicine in Australia and New Zealand. Its website has information to assist those requiring information relating to ART and ART services in both countries.

Jean Hailes for Women's Health
www.jeanhailes.org.au
Jean Hailes for Women's Health is a national not-for-profit organisation providing a range of health services and information for women across Australia. They have a separate website that deals with managing PCOS:
www.managingpcos.org.au/

PCOS Association of Australia
www.posaa.asn.au
This association is run by volunteers and enables you to become part of a network of women with PCOS offering support to one another. It also has information and advice on its website about the condition and how to find the right doctor for you.

Your Fertility
www.yourfertility.org.au
This resource has lots of information about the latest research findings on getting pregnant, fertility and infertility, fertility tips, as well as some useful videos and a blog.

25 Responding to pelvic pain

Jean Hailes for Women's Health
www.jeanhailes.org.au
Jean Hailes for Women's Health is a national not-for-profit organisation providing a range of health services and information for women across Australia. It has a separate website dedicated to endometriosis:
www.endometriosis.org.au/

Pelvic Pain
www.pelvicpain.org.uk
This site is run by a self-help group in the UK. Not surprisingly it is Euro-centric, but it is a good source of information and support, nevertheless, and provides links to other information sites.

The Royal Women's Hospital
www.thewomens.org.au/health-information
The Royal Women's Hospital, Melbourne, was one of the first Australian hospitals to be given the World Health Organization designation of a Health Promoting Hospital and provides information on a wide range of women's health issues in English and other community languages. Women from anywhere in Australia can access this information online. The Women's also publishes downloadable fact sheets, including one on chronic pelvic pain.

26 Genital irritations and infections

Better Health Channel
www.betterhealth.vic.gov.au
The Better Health Channel provides health and medical information that is quality-assured, reliable, up-to-date, easy to understand, regularly reviewed and locally relevant. It does not have any advertising or sponsor-ship and is fully funded by the state government of Victoria. It has a useful page with advice and information on STIs:
http://www.betterhealth.vic.gov.au/bhcv2/bhcarticles.nsf/pages/ct_sexuallytransmittedinfections?open

Let Them Know
www.letthemknow.org.au
This website was developed to help people who have been diagnosed with an STI to inform their previous partners that they might also be at risk.

Sexual Health and Family Planning Australia (SH&FPA)
www.shfpa.org.au
SH&FPA is the national peak body for the family planning organisations that provide community education programs, and a range of sexual and reproductive health clinical services, including pap smears and vaccina-tions, contraception and family planning services, and STI diagnosis and treatment. Each state has a family planning website with information

regarding sexual and contraceptive health. Find the clinic nearest you on their national website at www.shfpa.org.au/find-clinic.

27 Plastic surgery in young women

Australasian Foundation for Plastic Surgery
www.plasticsurgeryfoundation.org.au
This is a not-for-profit organisation. Its website provides reliable and accurate information on cosmetic and reconstructive surgery, including comprehensive information on procedures and a range of other useful patient resources.
www.plasticsurgeryfoundation.org.au/patient-information/procedures

Australian Society of Plastic Surgeons
www.plasticsurgery.org.au
This is the peak body for specialist plastic surgeons (both reconstructive and cosmetic). Their website includes a list of specialist plastic surgeons in each state.

Better Health Channel
www.betterhealth.vic.gov.au
The Better Health Channel provides health and medical information that is quality-assured, reliable, up-to-date, easy to understand, regularly reviewed and locally relevant. It does not have any advertising or sponsorship and is fully funded by the state government of Victoria. It devotes several pages to plastic surgery of various kinds, including breast and cosmetic.

Royal Australasian College of Surgeons
www.surgeons.org/find-a-surgeon
A website on which you can find a reputable plastic surgeon. You will need a referral from your GP.

28 Variations in sexual development

Congenital Adrenal Hyperplasia (CAH) Support Group
www.cah.org.au
This group provides support and education nationally for parents of newly diagnosed children with CAH, and adults living with CAH.

OII Australia
www.oii.org.au
OII Australia is the not-for-profit Australian affiliate of the International Organization for Intersex people. The site provides news, information and support for intersex people.

Turner Syndrome Association of Australia
www.turnersyndrome.org.au
This is a useful website for anyone looking for more information on Turner Syndrome.

29 Violence against women: sexual violence and sexual assault

Australian Centre for the Study of Sexual Assault
www.aifs.gov.au/acssa/crisis.html
The Australian Centre for the Study of Sexual Assault has a directory of crisis support services for sexual assault (women and men) for each state and also a specific support service for adult survivors of child sexual assault.

Australian Human Rights Commission
www.humanrights.gov.au/our-work/sex-discrimination
The 'Our Work' section of the Australian Human Rights Commission website has guides describing sex discrimination and sexual harassment and how to recognise and address them. There is also information on pregnancy discrimination, and articles on legislative and advocacy work being undertaken to ensure economic security for women and balance paid work and family responsibilities.

National Association of Services Against Sexual Violence (NASASV)
www.nasasv.org.au
Many victim/survivors find that healing and recovery from the trauma of past or recent sexual violence is assisted by talking with people who under-stand what they have experienced. Victim/survivors report that talking to counsellors or to other victim/survivors in facilitated support groups helps to gain perspective and insight, and to break through the silence and social isolation that surrounds sexual assault. NASASV is the peak body for organisations who work with victim/survivors of sexual violence and who work to prevent sexual violence. Their website has information about sexual assault services in each state:
www.nasasv.org.au/Sexual_Assault_Numbers.htm

The Royal Women's Hospital
www.thewomens.org.au/health-information
The Royal Women's Hospital, Melbourne, was one of the first Australian hospitals to be given the World Health Organization designation of a Health Promoting Hospital and provides information on a wide range of women's health issues in English and other community languages. Women from anywhere in Australia can access this information online. The Women's also publishes downloadable fact sheets that are useful reference tools. The health information covered includes violence against women.

30 Family violence

1800 RESPECT
1800 737 732 (24-hour service)
www.1800respect.org.au
RESPECT maintains a database of statewide and regional services, and services for Aboriginal and Torres Strait Islander women, and culturally and linguistically diverse women. Interpreters are provided.

Bursting the Bubble
www.burstingthebubble.com
A website with information for young people experiencing family violence.

Domestic Violence Resource Centre Victoria
www.dvrcv.org.au
The website has information, resources and stories about all aspects of family violence.

Kids Helpline
1800 55 1800 (free call)
www.kidshelp.com.au
A free, private and confidential telephone and online (web and email) counselling service specifically for young people aged between 5 and 25.

National Association of Community Legal Centres
www.naclc.org.au
Community legal services are available all around Australia, including specialist family violence services and services for Aboriginal women. This website provides information about the work of community legal services and a map to find your closest service.

Relationships Australia
1300 364 277
www.relationships.org.au
This organisation provides a range of services to assist those suffering
violence and/or abuse issues in their relationships.

MIDLIFE
31 Food and nutrition for midlife

Coeliac Australia
www.coeliac.org.au
The go-to website for people with coeliac disease.

Diabetes Australia
www.diabetesaustralia.com.au
The national body for people affected by all types of diabetes and those
at risk of it.

Dietitians Association of Australia (DAA)
www.daa.asn.au
The DAA site is a good place to look for nutrition tips or to find a dietician
for advice.

Glycemic Index
www.glycemicindex.com
This website has information about the glycaemic index, recipes, meal
plans.

The Gut Foundation
www.gutfoundation.com
The Foundation deals with the treatment and prevention of gastro-
intestinal diseases and conditions. It has a page dedicated to advice on the
best foods to eat for a healthy bowel:
www.gutfoundation.com/Dietary_Advice

A Healthy and Active Australia
www.healthyactive.gov.au
This Australian government website provides a range of information
and initiatives on healthy eating, regular physical activity and overweight
and obesity to assist all Australians to lead healthy and active lives.

Heart Foundation
www.heartfoundation.org.au
The Heart Foundation funds cardiovascular research, provides guide-lines for health professionals, informs the public and assists people with cardiovascular disease.

If Not Dieting Weight Management and Eating Behaviour Clinic
www.ifnotdieting.com.au
A site to provide health and support for people who want to achieve and maintain a healthy weight without being deprived of food or quality of life. It has useful, 'non-hungry' eating advice.

Jean Hailes for Women's Health
www.jeanhailes.org.au
Jean Hailes for Women's Health is a national not-for-profit organisa-tion providing a range of health services and information for women across Australia. They have a separate website about bone health: www.bonehealthforlife.org.au

Nutrition Australia
www.nutritionaustralia.org
This is a non-government, non-profit, community-based organisation that aims to promote the health and well-being of all Australians by encouraging food variety and physical activity. See their website for infor-mation on nutrition research and current food and health trends.

32 Common chronic medical conditions

Arthritis Australia
www.arthritisaustralia.com.au
The organisation provides support and information to people with arthritis, as well as to their families and friends. The website includes information on arthritis, its diagnosis and treatment, publications and links to resources.

Better Health Channel
www.betterhealth.vic.gov.au
The Better Health Channel provides health and medical information that is quality-assured, reliable, up-to-date, easy to understand, regu-larly reviewed and locally relevant. It does not have any advertising or

sponsorship and is fully funded by the state government of Victoria. It has a useful page on the thyroid:
www.betterhealth.vic.gov.au/bhcv2/bhcarticles.nsf/pages/ct_endocrine?
open&cat=Hormonal_system_(endocrine)_-_Thyroid_gland

Diabetes Australia
www.diabetesaustralia.com.au
Diabetes Australia helps all people affected by or at risk of diabetes. On their website you can access information on different types of diabetes, the diagnosis and treatment of diabetes, diabetes and pregnancy, diet and other relevant topics.

Heart Foundation
www.heartfoundation.org.au
A charity established to reduce premature death and suffering from heart, stroke and blood vessel disease. On their website you will find information including how to minimise the risk of cardiovascular disease, the warning signs of heart attack and how to get treatment.

National Asthma Council Australia
www.nationalasthma.org.au
A not-for-profit organisation working to improve health outcomes and quality of life for people with asthma. Their website includes information to help you understand asthma and best-practice asthma management.

Osteoporosis Australia
www.osteoporosis.org.au
The aim of the organisation is to communicate the positive and easy steps people can take to improve their bone health and prevent osteoporosis. It also provides information about the condition and has medical fact sheets on its website.

Stroke Foundation
www.strokefoundation.com.au
The foundation provides information to prevent strokes, support to help people who live with a stroke and resources to help staff work effectively in stroke health services.

Thyroid Australia
www.thyroid.org.au
Contains information and links to information on thyroid conditions; provides support to those with thyroid problems, and their families and friends. The full services of the site are only available to members.

33 Menopause

Australasian Menopause Society
www.menopause.org.au
The society has good resources, including information sheets, find-a-doctor, and links to clinical studies in recruitment.

Jean Hailes for Women's Health
www.jeanhailes.org.au
Jean Hailes for Women's Health is a national not-for-profit organisation providing a range of health services and information for women across Australia. It has separate pages on the menopause:
www.managingmenopause.org.au
www.earlymenopause.org.au

34 Complementary and natural therapies and medicines

There is a considerable amount of information on the internet on complementary and alternative medicine but not all of it is reliable. Below are some key resources to consider.

There are a number of peak organisations that represent health practitioners with expertise in complementary medicines who are regulated by the federal government's Australian Health Practitioner Regulation Agency (AHPRA, www.ahpra.gov.au). These health practitioners include doctors, nurses, midwives, dentists, physiotherapists, podiatrists, psychologists, osteopaths, chiropractors and Chinese medicine practitioners among others. See the AHPRA website for the full list of practitioners and links to the peak organisations.

Australasian College of Nutritional and Environmental Medicine
www.acnem.org
This College is the leading postgraduate training and membership body in nutritional and environmental medicine. This site can be used to find health professionals with specific interests.

Australasian Integrative Medicine Association (AIMA)
www.aima.net.au

The AIMA is constituted by a body of registered medical practitioners around Australia who integrate various forms of complementary medicine and holistic approaches into their medical practices. In recent decades there has been a steady and strong revival of interest in the general and medical communities for more holistic and natural forms of medicine. Many doctors seeking greater options to provide for their patients are safely and successfully integrating complementary medicine into their practices. AIMA was formed as a non-profit organisation in 1992 as a peer body and to make submissions to relevant government and medical authorities regarding the appropriate use of IM by medical practitioners. The AIMA website consists of a list of holistic GPs with an interest in integrative medicine.

Better Health Channel
www.betterhealth.vic.gov.au

The Better Health Channel provides health and medical information that is quality-assured, reliable, up-to-date, easy to understand, regularly reviewed and locally relevant. It does not have any advertising or sponsorship and is fully funded by the state government of Victoria. For more information on how to choose a complementary medicine practitioner, you can refer to the site's page, Complementary therapies – Choosing a Practitioner.

For more information to help you understand the safety and legal issues of using complementary medicines, you can refer to the site's page, Complementary Therapies – safety and legal issues.

Complementary and Alternative Medicine Guide, University of Maryland Medical Center
www.umm.edu/altmed

This University of Maryland Medical Center in the USA has a comprehensive complementary and alternative medicine guide that lists treatments for conditions, possible interactions between medicines and different herbs and supplements, and herb and supplement use, side effects and warnings.

35 Gynaecological cancers

BreaCan
www.breacan.org.au
An information and support service for people affected by breast, uterine, ovarian, cervical and other types of gynaecological cancer, their families and friends. Its resource centre is based in Melbourne, but its website has valuable information for sufferers or families of sufferers in any part of Australia.

Cancer Australia
www.canceraustralia.gov.au
This organisation's website provides information on different cancer types, including the different gynaecological cancers. It also provides an Australian-wide directory of gynaecological oncology services.

Cancer Council
13 11 20
www.cancer.org.au
This organisation's website provides information on different cancer types, including the different gynaecological cancers. The Council also runs a telephone helpline and online support group.

Ovarian Cancer Australia
www.ovariancancer.net.au
A website with information on the signs and symptoms, treatment and support available for those who have been diagnosed with this cancer.

36 Abnormal Pap tests – dysplasia

Better Health Channel
www.betterhealth.vic.gov.au
The Better Health Channel provides health and medical information that is quality-assured, reliable, up-to-date, easy to understand, regularly reviewed and locally relevant. It does not have any advertising or sponsorship and is fully funded by the state government of Victoria.

The National Cervical Screening Program
www.cancerscreening.gov.au/internet/screening/publishing.nsf/
Content/papsmear
An Australian government website on Pap tests and cervical cancer.

37 Breast health

Breast Cancer Network Australia
www.bcna.org.au
The network's website has information on breast cancer, including diagnosis and treatment. It also provides information for issues such as telling family members and colleagues and how to find support online and locally.

Cancer Australia
www.canceraustralia.gov.au
There is a page on which you can calculate your risk of breast cancer: www.canceraustralia.gov.au/affected-cancer/cancer-types/breast-cancer/your-risk/calculate

The Royal Women's Hospital
www.thewomens.org.au/health-information
The Royal Women's Hospital, Melbourne, was one of the first Australian hospitals to be given the World Health Organization designation of a Health Promoting Hospital and provides information on a wide range of women's health issues in English and other community languages. Women from anywhere in Australia can access this information online. The Women's also publishes downloadable fact sheets, including ones on breast health.

38 Plastic surgery in midlife

Australasian Foundation for Plastic Surgery
www.plasticsurgeryfoundation.org.au
This is a not-for-profit organisation. Its website provides reliable and accurate information on cosmetic and reconstructive surgery, including comprehensive information on procedures and a range of other useful patient resources.
www.plasticsurgeryfoundation.org.au/patient-information/procedures

Australian Society of Plastic Surgeons
www.plasticsurgery.org.au
This is the peak body for specialist plastic surgeons (both reconstructive and cosmetic). Their website includes a list of specialist plastic surgeons in each state.

Better Health Channel
www.betterhealth.vic.gov.au
The Better Health Channel provides health and medical information that is quality-assured, reliable, up-to-date, easy to understand, regularly reviewed and locally relevant. It does not have any advertising or sponsorship and is fully funded by the state government of Victoria. It devotes several pages to surgery of various kinds, including breast and cosmetic.

Royal Australasian College of Surgeons
www.surgeons.org/find-a-surgeon
A website on which you can find a reputable plastic surgeon. You will need a referral from your GP.

39 Prolapse and incontinence

Continence Foundation of Australia
www.continence.org.au
This is the peak body for continence promotion, management and advocacy. The website has information on preventing, managing, treating and curing incontinence, and where to get help.

Pelvic Floor First
www.pelvicfloorfirst.org.au
This website was developed by the Continence Foundation of Australia under the Australian Government's National Continence Program. It has lots of useful information and exercises on taking care of your pelvic floor muscles.

The Royal Women's Hospital, Melbourne
www.thewomens.org.au/health-information
The Royal Women's Hospital, Melbourne, was one of the first Australian hospitals to be given the World Health Organization designation of a Health Promoting Hospital and provides information on a wide range of women's health issues in English and other community languages. Women from anywhere in Australia can access this information online. The Women's also publishes downloadable fact sheets that are a useful reference tool. Health information covered includes prolapse, incontinence, surgery and how to do pelvic floor exercises.

40 Mental health in midlife

Beyondblue
www.beyondblue.org.au
This highly regarded organisation has resources for people who experience depression and anxiety, their partners, family and friends, and for health professionals who work in mental health. You can read their information online, download it or order printed copies.

Black Dog Institute
www.blackdoginstitute.org.au
Their website has information on the diagnosis, treatment and prevention of mood disorders such as depression and bipolar disorder.

The Royal Australian and New Zealand College of Psychiatrists (RANZCP)
www.ranzcp.org
RANZCP is responsible for training psychiatrists in Australia and New Zealand. Their website has information on finding a psychiatrist, how psychiatrists treat mental illness, resources on mental illness and treatments, what to do if someone is at risk of harming themselves and how to make a complaint.

SANE
1800 187 263 (free call)
www.sane.org
SANE provides information about mental health symptoms, treatments, medications, where to go for support and help for carers.

41 Being a carer

Better Start
1800 242 636
www.betterstart.net.au
If your child has a disability and you need to register them for the initiative, call your local Carers Association or visit the Better Start website.

Carers Association
1800 242 636
www.carersaustralia.com.au
Your local Carers Association is an excellent place to start if you want further information on being a carer. They can also tell you more about the Better Start for Children with Disability initiative. The association in your state or territory can provide you with information, support, counselling and referral to other services. Call during business hours to talk to someone who can help. Its resources include the Carers Advisory and Counselling Service and the National Carer Counselling Program.

You will also find lots of information on your local Carers Association website. From the main website choose *Resources* and then choose *State and territory Carers Associations*. From here, you can link to your local Carers Association website, which includes a wide range of information and fact sheets on all sorts of caring issues, with extra detail on many of the topics covered in this chapter.

You can ask for fact sheets in different community languages to be sent to you, or you can download them from the website.

Centrelink
132 717
131 202 (for languages other than English)
www.humanservices.gov.au
Contact Centrelink to see if you are eligible for payments to carers, pensions and concessions.

Commonwealth Respite and Carelink Centres
1800 052 222
www.health.gov.au/internet/main/publishing.nsf/Content/ageing-carers-respcent.htm
These centres are based throughout Australia and help you to find respite care. The centres can also help you to access local support services and aged care.

Dementia Care Australia (DCA)
www.dementiacareaustralia.com
DCA is an independent information and education organisation specialising in supporting both people with dementia and their carers, whether they are family members, professional carers, employers or friends.

Department of Veterans' Affairs (DVA)
133 254
www.dva.gov.au
The DVA provides some financial assistance to war veterans, war widows and widowers, their families and carers. You can call DVA to find out if you are eligible for DVA assistance. If you are unclear about what allowance you are eligible for, or have any problems completing application forms, your local Carers Association can provide you with assistance.

Emergency respite care
1800 059 059
This is the number to call if you need emergency respite care outside business hours.

My Aged Care
1800 200 422
www.myagedcare.gov.au
This Australian government website and national contact centre can help you access local support services and aged care and to organise an aged care assessment.

National Disability Insurance Scheme
1800 800 110
www.ndis.gov.au
The national disability insurance scheme is a new way of providing support for people with permanent and significant disability, their families and carers. Go online or call to find when the scheme will be available in your area and the type of help you can get.

Young People in Nursing Homes National Alliance
www.ypinh.org.au
The alliance works with young people with an acquired disability who are living in, or at risk of entry into, aged care facilities. The alliance ensures that these young people have a voice about where they live and how they want to be supported and also offers support for their families and carers.

LATER YEARS
42 Food and nutrition for older women

Aged Care Nutrition Services
www.agedcare-nutrition.com.au/resources/prevent-malnutrition-in-elderly
Information on how to detect and prevent malnutrition in older people.

Healthy Eating at Various Life Stages
www.health.gov.au/internet/healthyactive/publishing.nsf/Content/female-70
This Department of Health and Ageing site has suggestions about food quantities and physical activity guidelines.

Nutrition Screen
www.eatrightontario.ca/escreen/
This site has an interactive quiz that assesses your individual eating habits and gives recommendations based on your responses.

43 Sexuality in older women

National Institute on Aging
www.nia.nih.gov
The US National Institute on Aging has a publication on sexuality in later life available for download or viewing online at www.nia.nih.gov/health/publication/sexuality-later-life

44 Mental health in older women

Active Ageing Australia
www.activeageingaustralia.com.au
Active Ageing Australia promotes physical activity for health and well-being.

Aged Care Australia
www.agedcareaustralia.gov.au
The Aged Care Australia website is the Australian government's source of information about aged care and support services that are available locally and nationally.

Alzheimer's Australia
1800 100 500
www.fightdementia.org.au
Alzheimer's Australia is the peak body for advocacy, support and information about all forms of dementia. Each state also has its own local organisation providing information and services.

Council on the Ageing (COTA)
www.cota.org.au
COTA is a consumer organisation founded to protect and promote the wellbeing of older Australians. The organisation also has local offices in the states and territories.

Dementia Care Australia (DCA)
www.dementiacareaustralia.com
DCA is an independent information and education organisation specialising in supporting both people with dementia and their carers, whether they are family members, professional carers, employers or friends.

Contributors

Catarina Ang   MBBS, DSRH (RCOG), DUE, AFSA, Dip Epid, FRANZCOG, MBS
Dr Catarina Ang completed her MBBS at Monash University and obstetric and gynaecology training at Southern Health, Victoria. She trained extensively overseas, with posts at John Radcliffe Hospital and the University of Oxford in the United Kingdom in endometriosis and fertility, and advanced laparoscopic surgical training in France. She returned to a post at the Royal Women's Hospital and is head of Gynaecology Unit 1, which looks after abnormal menstrual bleeding. She is involved in the education of trainees and medical students at the Women's, the Royal Australian and New Zealand College of Obstetricians and Gynaecologists, the Australian Gynaecological Endoscopy Society and the Royal Australasian College of Surgeons.

Andrea Ball   BA (Professional Writing), Grad Cert Medical Writing
Andrea Ball is director of On the Ball Communications and has 20 years' experience specialising in health writing. With a strong focus on women's and family health, Andrea writes accurate and absorbing health information that promotes health literacy and empowers members of the community to be more actively involved in their own health and well-being. Andrea is author of Ovarian Cancer Australia's internationally acclaimed publication *Resilience*. Based on the success of this publication, Andrea was invited by the Prostate Cancer Foundation of Australia to develop a national resource for men with prostate cancer.

Shlomi Barak   MD, FRANZCOG
Dr Shlomi Barak is as obstetrician, gynaecologist and fertility specialist, supporting couples in all aspects of infertility, including IVF procedures, endoscopic surgery and testicular biopsies. He is also an andrologist, and manages many male reproductive health and infertility issues. A consultant specialist at the Women's, he runs designated IVF, male infertility and sexual dysfunction clinics. Shlomi is passionate about reproductive

medicine, pursuing his strong interest in finding better outcomes for patients through his research on preserving fertility in cancer patients and overcoming pregnancy complications. He also trains future fertility specialists, and is a senior lecturer in the Department of Obstetrics and Gynaecology at the University of Melbourne.

Chris Bayly   MD, BS, MPH, FRANZCOG, FRCOG

Dr Chris Bayly has practised as a gynaecologist mainly in the areas of infertility and fertility control, and has a particular interest in new and changing services offered to patients. She was involved in the establishment of IVF as a treatment option at the Women's and at Melbourne IVF; more recently she has worked on changing practice to accommodate new treatments such as nonsurgical methods of abortion, and to better meet the needs of diverse and changing health service users. As senior clinical adviser to the Women's Health Service at the Women's she contributes to policy work and to research into sexual and reproductive health.

Alison Bean-Hodges   M Women's Health (Hons), RN, RM

Alison Bean-Hodges was the first nurse practitioner specialising in women's health to be authorised in Australia and is a foundation fellow of the Australian College of Nurse Practitioners. Alison combines her clinical role at the Women's with leadership of a team of nurse practitioners providing outpatient gynaecological care. Alison is also manager of the Sexual Health Service at the Women's, supporting a team of specialist medical practitioners and nurse practitioners (a nurse with additional, advanced qualifications that allow them to prescribe medicines and perform some tasks usually performed by medical practitioners), and working collaboratively with community agencies in providing care for women and men who have experienced sexual assault. The principles of access, innovation and evidence-based care underpin Alison's healthcare philosophy.

Neelam Bhardwaj   FRANZCOG, FRCOG

Dr Neelam Bhardwaj has been involved in family planning since the 1970s. She has practised at the community clinic at Western Hospital, Footscray, and been in charge of the clinic at Sunshine Hospital. She ran the Choices Clinic at the Women's for more than 20 years. Neelam has seen the practice of this discipline evolve and consolidate over that time, with the introduction of many new methods. She is in full-time private practice in gynaecology.

Siobhan Bourke   MBBS, FAChSHM, RACP
Dr Siobhan Bourke is a Sexual Health Physician. Siobhan's strong interest in medical education led her to work in Medical and Humanitarian Aid in a number of countries including India as part of an HIV prevention program. She has particular expertise in the area of contraception. She has worked at the Victorian Cytology Service (VCS) since 2006 as a Liaison Physician helping in the provision of educational services to Pap screen providers across Victoria. She is a Medical Officer at Melbourne Sexual Health Centre and Family Planning Victoria, and Relieving Medical Officer at the Women's.

Shaun Brennecke   MBBS, BA, BMedSci(Hons), DPhil, FRANZCOG
Professor Brennecke is the Dunbar Hooper Professor of Obstetrics and Gynaecology at the Women's. He is director of the Hospital's Department of Perinatal Medicine, and a unit head within Maternity Services at the Hospital. His clinical and research interests include preterm labour, pre-eclampsia, fetal growth restriction, placental function, miscarriage, the endocrinology of human pregnancy and parturition, the assessment of fetal welfare, and factors influencing maternal and perinatal morbidity and mortality. He has published more than 200 research papers on these topics.

Christina Bryant   MA (Clin Psych), PhD
After training as a clinical psychologist, Dr Christina Bryant worked in a variety of clinical roles in public mental health, developing an interest in the wellbeing of older people. She completed a PhD in this area, and in 2007 was appointed to an academic position in the School of Psychological Sciences at the University of Melbourne, where she still contributes to the clinical psychology training program. In 2008, Christina joined the Women's as senior clinical psychologist based at the Centre for Women's Mental Health. In that role she has developed new services and research programs across a range of women's health issues, including healthy ageing.

Melissa Cameron   MBBS (Hons), MPH, FRANZCOG, MRMed
Dr Melissa Cameron trained in obstetrics and gynaecology at the Mercy Hospital for Women, Melbourne, obtaining her Fellowship of the Royal Australian and New Zealand College of Obstetricians and Gynaecologists in 2006. This included fellowships in paediatric and adolescent

gynaecology, and advanced laparoscopic gynaecological surgery. She has masters degrees in reproductive medicine and public health. With a focus on fertility issues affecting women with endometriosis, fibroids and uterine abnormalities, Melissa helps couples with some of the most challenging fertility problems. Melissa also has a special interest in helping same-sex couples and single women create a family through the Melbourne IVF donor program. Melissa holds public appointments at the Women's and the Mercy Hospital for Women, Melbourne.

Marcus Carey   MBBS, FRANZCOG

Dr Marcus Carey completed his undergraduate medical training at the University of Melbourne in 1982. He trained in obstetrics and gynaecology in Melbourne and the United Kingdom. Marcus completed urogynaecology subspeciality training in 1996. He is head of the Urogynaecology and Gynaecology 3 units at the Women's. His main research and clinical interests include minimal access (laparoscopic and robotic) prolapse and incontinence surgery and the conservative management of prolapse. Marcus has also worked at the Fistula Hospital in Ethiopia. He has published extensively in the field of urogynaecology.

Susan Carr   MB, CHB, DRCOG, MPhil, FFSRH

After a career as a consultant in sexual and reproductive health care in Scotland, looking after marginalised groups, and as a senior lecturer at Glasgow University, Dr Susan Carr moved to Melbourne in 2009. With a longstanding interest in the psychosocial and sexual care of patients she then took up a post as lead clinician for the Psychosexual Service at the Women's. She is a past president of the Sexuality section of the Royal Society of Medicine, London, and is currently president elect of the Australian Society for Psychosomatic Obstetrics and Gynaecology.

Jan Davies   BSc (Hons), PhD, MBA

After an early career of research and teaching in ethology, Dr Jan Davies trained and worked as a psychotherapist in the United Kingdom. Returning to Australia, she held senior positions in the public health system in New South Wales and Victoria, including Southern Health, Victoria. In 2000, Jan was invited to help establish the National Institute of Clinical Studies, a research translation agency, where she was executive officer and, after its merger with NHMRC, executive director. Jan is now an independent consultant in health care. She was an inaugural committee member of

CASSE, a non-profit organisation committed to creating safe, supportive environments for individuals, families and communities.

Jill Duncan   MA, BSc (Hons), Dip Teaching

Education and training have been core activities throughout Jill Duncan's professional life. Since 2003 she has coordinated CASA (Centre Against Sexual Assault) House's extensive community and professional training program. CASA House is based in Melbourne and is a department of the Women's. In 2006, Jill co-facilitated training in regional and remote Australia for medical, nursing and allied health practitioners about responding to adults who have experienced sexual assault. She is co-author of 'Addressing the ultimate insult: responding to women experiencing intimate partner sexual violence', commissioned in 2011 by the Australian Domestic and Family Violence Clearinghouse.

Geraldine Edgley   MBBS, MAppSci (Sexual Health)

Dr Geraldine Edgley has worked in women's sexual and reproductive health for more than 20 years. She has consulted in this area at the Women's for 15 years. She has extensive knowledge and experience in the area of contraception. She is also a general practitioner at Jean Hailes for Women's Health.

Dale Fisher   RN, BA (Business), MBA

Dale Fisher was the creative force behind *The Women's Health Book*. As chief executive of the Women's from 2004 to 2013, Dale delivered the $250 million Women's Hospital redevelopment project, modernised clinical models of care, re-engaged the community in the Women's work, secured the organisation as an employer of choice, developed a population health framework, and established six clinical research centres. Dale is a board member of Women's Hospitals Australia and of the Victorian Comprehensive Cancer Centre. She is an associate fellow of the Australian College of Health Service Executives, and was inducted into the Victorian Honour Roll of Women in 2011. Dale was named as one of Australia's Top 100 Women of Influence for 2013 in the category of public policy for her work in women's health.

Suzanne M. Garland   MBBS, MD, FRCPA, FRANZCOG ad eundem, FAChSHM

Professor Garland is an internationally recognised clinical microbiologist and sexual health practitioner, with particular expertise in infectious diseases in relation to reproductive health and newborns. With her team, Professor Garland has published more than 400 peer-reviewed papers on the clinical epidemiology of sexually transmitted infections. A key research interest is cervical cancer and the role of human papillomaviruses (HPV). She is a regular adviser to the World Health Organization and is the inaugural and past president of the Asian Oceania Research Organization on Genital Infection and Neoplasia. Her research was recognised when one of her projects was named in the NHMRC 10 Best Research Projects 2010 list. Professor Garland is the clinical director of Microbiology and Infectious Diseases and director of Microbiology Research at the Women's, and senior consultant in Microbiology at the Royal Children's Hospital Melbourne.

Elisabeth Gasparini   BSc, GradDip, APD, GradDip BA
Elisabeth Gasparini has spent most of her working life as a dietician and has devoted the last 20 years to working in women's health. Elisabeth is the manager of Nutrition and Dietetics at the Women's, where she leads a team of highly skilled dieticians. She oversees the extensive clinical services of the department, and is also involved in research, teaching and the development of consumer health information.

Martin Healey   MBBS, MD, FRANZCOG, MRCOG
Following the completion of his obstetrics and gynaecology training, Dr Martin Healey undertook an 18-month advanced laparoscopy fellowship at the Mercy Hospital for Women, Melbourne. Moving to the Women's as a consultant gynaecologist in 1998, Martin helped expand the role of operative laparoscopy, and completed an MD thesis on pain, nerve function and endometriosis. Martin became head of the Gynaecology 2 Unit, and specialises in endometriosis and pelvic pain. He continues to pursue research in the areas of endometriosis, adenomyosis and pelvic pain, while also being actively involved in training medicine graduates.

Martha Hickey   BA (Hons) Psychology, MSc (Clin Psych), MB, ChB, MRCOG, FRANZCOG, MD
Professor Martha Hickey is Professor of Obstetrics and Gynaecology at the University of Melbourne and the Women's. She runs the Menopause and Menopausal Symptoms after Cancer Service at the Women's and has research and clinical interests in surgical menopause and menopause after cancer.

Alice Huang   MBBS (Hons), FRANZCOG, MRepMed
Dr Alice Huang is a consultant gynaecologist specialising in fertility, reproductive endocrinology and fertility preservation at the Women's Reproductive Service Unit, Melbourne IVF and in private practice. Her interests are in polycystic ovarian syndrome (PCOS), management of fibroids, laparoscopic surgery, microsurgery to reverse tubal ligation and vasectomy, fertility preservation and infertility issues. She graduated from Monash University's medicine program with honours and the final-year Robert Power Scholarship in Surgery in 2002. She then completed her obstetrics and gynaecology training, as well as a Masters in Reproductive Medicine at the University of New South Wales, Sydney.

Yasmin Jayasinghe   MBBS, FRANZCOG, PhD
Yasmin Jayasinghe is a gynaecologist at the Royal Children's Hospital Melbourne, the Women's, and the Victorian Aboriginal Health Service. She is a senior lecturer in the Department of Obstetrics and Gynaecology – Royal Women's Hospital, University of Melbourne. She obtained her FRANZCOG in Queensland in 2002, during which she was a member of the Far North Regional Obstetric and Gynaecological Service, providing gynaecological outreach services to remote communities. Since then, she has focused largely on young women's health. She completed a fellowship in paediatric and adolescent gynaecology at the Royal Children's Hospital Melbourne in 2004, and underwent research training at the Department of Pediatric Gynecology, Mayo Clinic, Rochester, Minnesota, in 2005–06. She completed a PhD on cervical cancer and pre-cancer in young women in 2012. She is current president of the Australian and New Zealand Society of Paediatric and Adolescent Gynaecology.

Maureen Johnson   Dip Prof Writing and Editing, MPH
Maureen Johnson has 15 years' experience and expertise in women's health, health information and consumer engagement. Currently manager of Women's Consumer Health Information at the Women's, Maureen has expertise in professional writing and editing. She co-authored a chapter in a book on improving communication with women in a hospital setting. In 2011, Maureen was a recipient of the Victorian Quality Council travelling fellowship and travelled to North America and Europe to investigate health literacy. She has led several projects to improve women's access to health information, using a range of media and other strategies to improve health communication in sexual and reproductive health, family

violence and reproductive loss, particularly for women with disabilities, refugee and immigrant women, young women and lesbians.

Fiona Judd   MBBS, DPM, MD, FRANZCP

Professor Fiona Judd is a professorial fellow in the Department of Psychiatry at the University of Melbourne and director of the Women's Centre for Women's Mental Health. She has worked at the interface of physical health/illness and mental health throughout her career as a psychiatrist. Since joining the Women's in 2007, her clinical and research interests have focused on perinatal and infant mental health, the health of women in midlife and healthy ageing, and the mental health care of women with breast and gynaecological cancers.

Jane Karpavicius   BSc (Food Sc & Nut), B Nut & Diet

Jane Karpavicius is an accredited practising dietician with a background in women's and children's nutrition. In 2007 she joined the Women's, where she developed a special interest in diabetes and weight management during pregnancy. She has trained health professionals both locally and overseas in the management of diabetes and is also now the dietician team leader at Diabetes Australia – Victoria.

Rachael Knight   MBBS, BMedSci, MD, FRANZCOG

Dr Rachael Knight studied medicine at the University of Tasmania before training in obstetrics and gynaecology at the Women's and Mercy Hospital for Women, Melbourne. She also undertook further study for a doctorate of medicine at Melbourne University and three years of specialty training in reproductive endocrinology and infertility. She furthered her expertise in infertility with two years working in the United Kingdom. Back in Melbourne, she works in private practice at Melbourne IVF and as a consultant gynaecologist and infertility specialist at the Women's Reproductive Services, where she is head of the Polycystic Ovarian Syndrome Clinic. She is actively involved in research.

Vicki Kotsirilos   MBBS, FRACGP (honorary), FACNEM

Dr Vicki Kotsirilos is a respected general practitioner with more than 20 years' clinical experience specialising in women's health. Vicki combines general practice with evidence-based complementary medicine such as acupuncture and nutritional medicine. She is founder of the Australasian Integrative Medicine Association and has the honour of working closely with the Royal Australian College of General Practitioners as chair of the Integrative Medicine working group. Vicki has published numerous articles in a wide range of publications, lectures widely, and is often quoted in the media on issues relating to general healthcare matters and complementary medicine. She is co-author of the textbook *A Guide to Evidence-based Integrative and Complementary Medicine.*

Gillian Lang   MPH, MEd
Gillian Lang has more than 20 years' experience in the design and implementation of training for primary healthcare programs and has held several overseas positions in maternal and child health programs. She has also worked in community health, in health promotion and community participation roles. Gillian currently works at Dental Health Services Victoria as a health promotion project officer.

Amelia Lee   BSc (Hons), MND, APD
Amelia Lee began her dietetics career in community health in 2001, developing an interest in working with young women and women's health. In 2005, she became the team leader for a chronic conditions program and provided nutrition consultation for people who were homeless or at risk of homelessness. She has been with the Women's since 2007, providing nutrition consultation to a number of maternity clinics specialising in young women, alcohol and drugs, and multiple pregnancies. Her continuing interest in women's health has led her to commence a PhD in pregnancy nutrition.

John McBain   AO, MB, ChB, MRCOG, FRANZCOG
Associate Professor John McBain has worked in the IVF field longer than any other specialist in the world. Born in Glasgow, John graduated in medicine from Glasgow University, then trained in obstetrics and gynaecology in Scotland. He joined the Women's in 1976, developing ovarian stimulation for the early IVF program. He was a founder of Melbourne IVF and its chairman from 1998 to 2005 and was elected president of the Fertility Society of Australia in 1991. He campaigned in the 1990s for de facto couples in Victoria to be allowed to use IVF, and brought landmark action against the Victorian state government allowing access to infertility treatment, including IVF, for single women and women in lesbian relationships. John is head of reproductive services at the Women's and a member of the Low Cost IVF Foundation, which

establishes affordable IVF in developing countries. He is an officer in the Order of Australia.

Ian McCahon   MBBS, Dip Ed, FRANZCOG, FRCOG

Dr Ian McCahon is clinical head of the Women's Alcohol and Drug Service. He is an honorary senior lecturer at the University of Melbourne, a fellow of the Royal Australian and New Zealand College of Obstetricians and Gynaecologists, fellow of the Royal College of Obstetricians and Gynaecologists, and member of the American College of Obstetricians and Gynecologists. Ian's interests include group dynamics, cooperation with the Chapter of Addiction Medicine of the Royal Australasian College of Physicians. He seeks to improve links with community and Indigenous services and providers.

Orla McNally   MB, BAO, BCh, FRCSI, MRCOG, FRANZCOG, CGO

Miss Orla McNally embarked on a career in general surgery after completing her medical training in Ireland. During that time she was exposed to the serious outcomes for women with gynaecological cancer, in particular ovarian cancer, and decided to pursue a career as a gynaecological oncologist. Orla completed a fellowship in Melbourne in 1998, after which she returned to the United Kingdom to complete her training. As a consultant in the NHS for five years, Orla set up a gynaecological cancer centre in Somerset before returning to Melbourne, where she is now director of Oncology and Dysplasia at the Women's.

Sarah McQuillan   MD, FRCPSC O&G

Dr Sarah McQuillan completed her obstetrics and gynaecology training in Canada then travelled across the globe to complete a fellowship in paediatric gynaecology at the Women's. On completion of the fellowship she will return to Canada to work at the Alberta Children's Hospital and South Health Campus – Calgary as a clinical assistant professor of obstetrics and gynaecology. Sarah has helped coordinate paediatric gynaecology updates for physicians throughout Australia.

Helena Maher   BA (Hons), M Public Policy & Management

After graduating Helena Maher began her career in health working in policy and planning for the Commonwealth and Northern Territory health departments and Aboriginal community-controlled health services. In 2002 she was appointed senior project officer and policy coordinator at

Health Issues Centre, Melbourne. Helena joined the Women's in 2005 as coordinator of consumer participation. Now in Strategy and Planning, she is focused on service innovations, the Population Health Strategic Framework, violence against women as a health issue and advocacy for women's health.

Bruce Mann   MBBS, PhD, FRACS
After graduating from medical school at the University of Melbourne and surgery training at the Royal Melbourne Hospital, Professor Bruce Mann completed a PhD in cancer genetics at the Ludwig Institute for Cancer Research and a fellowship in surgical oncology at the Memorial Sloan Kettering Cancer Center in New York. Throughout this time he developed his interest and skills in various aspects of the surgical management of cancer, but in particular specialised in breast disease and breast cancer. After some time at Royal Melbourne Hospital, he was appointed director of the combined Women's/Royal Melbourne Breast Service in 2007. He has many outside appointments, including chair of the Surgical Oncology Group of the Royal Australasian College of Surgeons, and is a past president of the Clinical Oncology Society of Australia.

Alexandra Marceglia   MBBS, Dip Ven, GradDip EpiBiostat, FRACGP, FAChSHM
Dr Alex Marceglia is a sexual health practitioner and unit head of the Sexual Health Service at the Women's. She also undertakes clinical roles in other specialist services at the Women's, including the family planning and unplanned pregnancy service, in addition to her role as a colposcopist within the Dysplasia Service. Alex plays a key role in the provision of undergraduate and postgraduate medical training, in particular in the field of sexual health. She has a long professional association with collaborating agencies including Family Planning Victoria and the Melbourne Sexual Health Centre, and has a special interest in caring for women with HIV infection.

Jennifer Marino   BA, BSN, MPH, PhD
After an early career in basic science research and nursing, Dr Jen Marino studied reproductive epidemiology at the University of California, Berkeley, and the University of Washington. In 2008, she came to Australia to pursue postdoctoral research with the Lifecourse and Intergenerational Health Research Group at the University of Adelaide. She moved to

Melbourne in 2011 to join the Women's Gynaecology Research Centre and the University of Melbourne, where she works closely with Professor Martha Hickey.

Tram Nguyen   MBBS, FRANZCP
Since completing her training in psychiatry, Dr Tram Nguyen has specialised in the field of perinatal mental health. She joined the Centre for Women's Mental Health at the Women's in 2009 and is the consultant psychiatrist for the Women's Alcohol and Drug Service. She has an interest in improving outcomes for women with psychiatric disorders and their babies, and in the parent–infant attachment relationship. She has been on the expert panel for *Therapeutic Guidelines – Psychotropics* (7th edition) and numerous panels for the Department of Human Services' Perinatal Mental Health Initiative. Tram is also an honorary clinical lecturer in the University of Melbourne's Department of Psychiatry.

Ross Pagano   MBBS, FRCOG, FRANZCOG
Dr Ross Pagano is a practising specialist obstetrician and gynaecologist with a special interest in benign vulvar disorders. He is the gynaecologist in charge of the Vulvar Disorders Clinic and the DES Follow-up Clinic at the Women's. Ross established the Australian and New Zealand Vulvovaginal Society, is a past president of that society and is the current treasurer. He is a fellow of the International Society for the Study of Vulvovaginal Disease as well as the past vice president of the Australian Society for Colposcopy and Cervical Pathology. He works predominantly in the private sector, with a clinical attachment to the Women's.

Jo Payne   BSc (Hons), BHSc
Jo Payne has more than nine years' government and private sector experience in health promotion. Her background includes health promotion roles in South Australia at the Centre for Health Promotion – Children, Youth and Women's Health Service, Hepatitis South Australia and the Centre for Culture, Ethnicity and Health in Melbourne. She joined Dental Health Services Victoria as a health promotion project officer in 2011.

Anne Florence Plante BA BSc PT
Anne Florence Plante trained in France as a physiotherapist and specialised in women's health in 1992. She moved to Australia in 2008, and began working in physiotherapy at the Women's. She is an APA-titled member

in Australia, a member of the Continence Foundation of Australia, and a Committee member of CFA Victoria Physiotherapy Group. Anne Florence was involved in setting up the Chronic Pelvic Pain Clinic. Her postgraduate qualifications in victimology and criminology have helped her to develop a strong multidisciplinary commitment. She lectures widely internationally, and is a current peer reviewer for the *Journal of Sexual Medicine*. She has published six articles (in French and English) since 2008.

Alessandra Radovini   MBBS, DPM, FRANZCP, Cert Child Psych

Dr Alessandra Radovini is a child and adolescent psychiatrist who has worked in public mental health for more than 25 years. She has a particular interest in children, young people and their families with multiple and complex needs. She is currently director of Mindful – Centre for Training and Research in Developmental Health, a joint venture of the University of Melbourne and Monash University and a state-wide unit delivering postgraduate courses and professional development programs in child and adolescent mental health. Dr Radovini is also the clinical director of headspace – Australia's National Youth Mental Health Foundation, an innovative program encouraging young people aged between 12 and 25 to seek early help by providing services face to face, online and in schools.

Leslie Reti   MBBS, SM, FRCOG, FRANZCOG

Associate Professor Leslie Reti has been a practising gynaecologist with an interest in the macro issues of Women's Health for more than 30 years. He is clinical director of Gynaecology, Cancer Services and Clinical Governance at the Women's. Committed to improving quality and safety systems, he was an executive member and deputy chair of the Victorian Quality Council as well as some other peak bodies. Formerly senior lecturer in obstetrics and gynaecology at the University of Leicester and the University of Melbourne, he is now adjunct associate professor of public health at La Trobe University. Les was the founding chair of the committee of management of the Centre Against Sexual Assault (CASA).

Allison Ridge   BAppSc (EnvHlth), MPH

After starting her career in regulatory public health, Allison Ridge became involved in municipal public health planning and has since worked in health promotion. Her background includes local government health planning and project management in the Primary Care Partnership program before joining Dental Health Services Victoria in late 2010.

She is currently health promotion program manager for Healthy Families, Healthy Smiles, an oral health promotion initiative.

Ines Rio   MBBS (Hons), MPH, FRACGP, GAICD, DRACOG, GradDip Ven
After becoming a general practitioner, Dr Ines Rio worked as a medical educator and then obtained a masters in public health while working in public health advisory and development roles. She joined the Women's in 2001 and is currently one of their senior medical staff and head of their general practice liaison unit. Ines is inaugural chair of the local primary healthcare organisation, medical officer for the City of Melbourne and sits on a number of government committees. She has provided care to women and their families in both the community and hospital settings across a very broad range of health issues over many years and is committed to the development of person-centred, quality, equitable and integrated healthcare services, and the central role in this of general practice and primary care.

Penelope Sheehan   MBBS, GDEB, FRANZCOG
Dr Penny Sheehan is the obstetric head of one of four maternity units at the Women's. She also runs a specialist clinic dedicated to women at high risk of preterm labour. Penny is a clinical research fellow with the Pregnancy Research Centre and lecturer in the Department of Obstetrics and Gynaecology, University of Melbourne. She is actively interested in pregnancy research related to the role of hormones in childbirth. She has worked in a number of collaborative models of maternity care and been involved in the development of guidelines for antenatal care.

Margaret Sherburn   BAppSc (Physio), M Women's Health, PhD, FACP
Dr Margaret Sherburn is head of the Physiotherapy Department at the Women's and an academic in physiotherapy at the University of Melbourne. In these roles she has research, teaching, clinical and managerial responsibilities. Her main areas of research are the conservative management of pelvic floor dysfunction in women with prolapse or incontinence, and the role of exercise for pre- and postnatal women. Marg has been the recipient of two NHMRC grants for large multicentre studies. She is a member of the Physiotherapy Committee of the International Continence Society, and is on the editorial board of *The Australian and New Zealand Continence Journal*.

Kate Stern   MBBS, FRANZCOG, MMed, CREI

Associate Professor Kate Stern graduated in medicine from the University in Melbourne and trained in obstetrics and gynaecology at the Women's and the Mercy Hospital for Women, Melbourne. After two years' work in this field in the United Kingdom, she spent three years specialising in infertility and reproductive endocrinology. Kate is head of the Endocrine and Metabolic Service and the Fertility Preservation Services at the Women's and head of clinical research and a senior specialist at Melbourne IVF. She is clinical associate professor of obstetrics and gynaecology at the University of Melbourne. Kate's research interests include fertility preservation for people with cancer and other serious diseases who are undergoing treatment that can damage fertility.

Jenny Taylor   BSc, BND, APD

Ms Jenny Taylor, an accredited practising dietician, began her professional life as a science graduate working in a lab with lizards. Deciding she needed to broaden her horizons, Jenny completed a postgraduate qualification in nutrition and dietetics and now has 22 years' experience in women's health nutrition. Her role includes helping women achieve eating patterns that optimise their health or help them cope with illnesses.

Frances Thomson-Salo   LlB, MCPP, PhD

Associate Professor Frances Thomson-Salo joined the Women's as the consultant infant mental health clinician in the Centre for Women's Mental Health after working for 15 years in the clinical infant mental health group of the Consultation/Liaison service of the Royal Children's Hospital, Melbourne. At the Women's, Frances works with women and their partners before and after the birth of their baby to help them feel more connected to their baby and consolidate their baby's happiness and social–emotional wellbeing.

Dean Trotter   MBBS, FRACS

Mr Trotter is a specialist plastic and reconstructive surgeon with a particular interest in breast surgery. He completed his MBBS at the University of Melbourne in 1999 and was awarded Fellowship of the Royal Australasian College of Surgeons (FRACS) in 2009. In 2010, Dean completed a 12-month microsurgical fellowship at St Andrews Centre for Plastic Surgery and Burns, Chelmsford, United Kingdom. During this fellowship, Dean focused on microsurgery, particularly breast reconstruction, working with world-renowned expert Mr Venkat Ramakrishnan. Dean has also received fellowship training in the United Kingdom and Argentina in aesthetic plastic surgery, skin cancer surgery and cosmetic breast surgery, including correction of congenital breast asymmetry. Dean has public hospital appointments at the Women's, Royal Melbourne and Northern hospitals.

Sarah L. White   BSc (Hons), PhD
After completing a PhD in genetics, Dr Sarah White worked as a breast cancer researcher for several years before becoming director of communications for an international cancer research institute. She joined the Women's in 2010 as the director of Communications and Foundation. Sarah oversees external and internal communications, fundraising, and the production of consumer health information for the Women's, and is also the executive sponsor of the hospital's research program and its community participation efforts.

C. David H. Wrede   MA, MB, BChir, FRCS, MRCOG, FRANZCOG
Mr David Wrede studied medicine at Cambridge and St Thomas' Hospital, London. He pursued postgraduate training in surgery and obstetrics and gynaecology in London, Oxford and the West Midlands, including a period of laboratory-based research on HPV and cervical cancer. After holding consultant appointments in Scotland and England, David moved to Australia in 2009 as a gynaecologist and lead for dysplasia at the Women's. His main focus is now women's cancer prevention, laparoscopic surgery and the surgical management of placental adhesive disorders. David is an investigator on a number of therapeutic and preventative cancer research projects.

Index

For extra information
and updated resources about
the topics covered in
The Women's Health Book, visit:

thewomenshealthbook.com

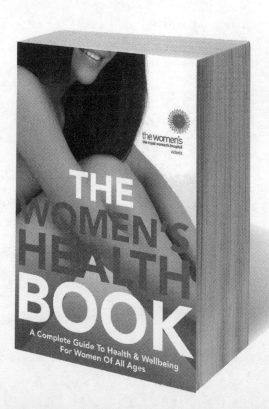